ATLAS OF
CLINICAL NEUROLOGY

THIRD EDITION

G. David Perkin, BA, MB, FRCP
Consultant Neurologist
Charing Cross and HIllingdon Hospitals
London, UK

Douglas C. Miller, MD, PhD, FCAP
Clinical Professor of Pathology and Anatomical Sciences
University of Missouri School of Medicine
Columbia, MO
USA

Russell J.M. Lane, BSc, MD, FRCP
Consultant Neurologist
Charing Cross Hospital
London, UK

Maneesh C. Patel, BSc(Hons), MBBS, MRCP, FRCR
Consultant Neuroradiologist
Imperial College NHS Trust
London

Fred H. Hochberg, MD
Attending Neurologist
Massachusetts General Hospital
Associate Professor of Neurology
Harvard Medical School
Cambridge, MA
USA

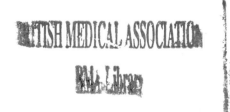

ELSEVIER
SAUNDERS

SAUNDERS
ELSEVIER

1600 John F. Kennedy Blvd.
Ste 1800
Philadelphia, PA 19103-2899

Notice

Knowledge and best practice in this field are constantly changing. As new research and experience broaden our
understanding, changes in research methods, professional practices, or medical treatment may become necessary.

Practitioners and researchers must always rely on their own experience and knowledge in evaluating
and using any information, methods, compounds, or experiments described herein. In using such information
or methods they should be mindful of their own safety and the safety of others, including parties for whom they
have a professional responsibility.

With respect to any drug or pharmaceutical products identified, readers are advised to check the most
current information provided (i) on procedures featured or (ii) by the manufacturer of each product to be
administered, to verify the recommended dose or formula, the method and duration of administration, and con-
traindications. It is the responsibility of practitioners, relying on their own experience and knowledge of their
patients, to make diagnoses, to determine dosages and the best treatment for each individual patient, and to take
all appropriate safety precautions.

To the fullest extent of the law, neither the Publisher nor the authors, contributors, or editors, assume
any liability for any injury and/or damage to persons or property as a matter of products liability, negligence
or otherwise, or from any use or operation of any methods, products, instructions, or ideas contained
in the material herein.

Library of Congress Cataloging-in-Publication Data or Control Number

Atlas of clinical neurology / G. David Perkin ... [et al.]. -- 3rd ed.
    p. ; cm.
    Rev. ed. of: Atlas of clinical neurology / G. David Perkin, Fred H. Hochberg, Douglas C. Miller. 2nd ed. 1993.
    Includes index.
    ISBN 978-0-323-03275-9
    1. Nervous system--Diseases--Atlases. I. Perkin, G. D. (George David) II. Perkin, G. D.
(George David). Atlas of clinical neurology.
    [DNLM: 1. Nervous System Diseases--Atlases. WL 17 A8815 2010]
    RC348.A78 2010
    616.80022'2--dc22

                                                                        2010002722

Acquisitions Editor: Adrianne Brigido
Developmental Editor: Taylor Ball
Project Manager: Janaki Srinivasan Kumar
Design Manager: Lou Forgione
Illustration Manager: Kari Wszolek
Marketing Manager: Courtney Ingram

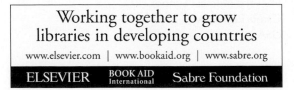

To Harry, George, Jo, Tom, Ted, Elsie and Ella.

G. David Perkin

To my wife and love, Sherry, for her constant support and immense patience.

Douglas C. Miller

To Neeta, Anoushka, Kelan and Rahul for their understanding.

Maneesh C. Patel

CONTENTS

PREFACE

Some 17 years have elapsed since the second edition of *Atlas of Clinical Neurology*. Major advances have occurred in neurology during this period, particularly in the field of imaging. With such advances, the need to add a neuroradiologist to the authorial team was evident. I am delighted that Maneesh Patel from Imperial College NHS Trust accepted the offer. He has provided a wealth of information regarding "state of the art" imaging, along with a critical revision of relevant text.

In addition, this third edition has benefited from the contribution of another Charing Cross colleague, Russell Lane. Russell has completely revised the "Myopathies and Myasthenia" chapter and substantially modified the "Motor Neurone and Peripheral Nerve Diseases" chapter, incorporating anterior horn cell disease. Finally, he rewrote the chapter on "Pain Syndromes and Trauma," producing an outstanding review in the process.

It remains a pleasure to record the ongoing contribution of Douglas Miller. He provided the majority of the pathology slides in the second edition, and he has, for this edition, revised and enlarged the pathology material.

A significant number of slides have been derived from other sources for this edition and acknowledgement is made with our great thanks.

In addition, I would like to thank the staff of the Medical Illustration unit of Charing Cross Hospital, and particularly Sam Bristol, for the invaluable help I have received in the preparation of the illustrations, and to Ann McGarry for her help in the preparation of the manuscript.

Finally, it is a great pleasure to record our dcbt to the staff of Elsevier. This edition has undergone a long gestation, and I am grateful for Susan Pioli for her encouragement and support, as well as the subsequent support provided by Adrianne Brigido and Taylor Ball.

George D. Perkin

NEUROLOGIC INVESTIGATION

THE CEREBROSPINAL FLUID

The cerebrospinal fluid (CSF) is formed partly from the choroid plexuses of the ventricular system and partly by diffusion through the ependymal lining of the ventricles. The total CSF volume is around 120 mL, with a production rate of around 0.3 to 0.4 mL/min. The fluid leaves the fourth ventricle through the median and lateral recesses and then circulates over the surface of the spinal cord and cerebral hemispheres before it is resorbed through the arachnoid villi of the superior sagittal sinus and to a lesser extent through arachnoid villi in the spinal canal. The ionic composition of the fluid indicates that it is not simply an ultrafiltrate of blood but is formed by an active secretion process through the epithelium of the choroid plexuses. The Na/K pump is the main mechanism underlying CSF secretion. Na/K-ATPase has been detected in the surface of the choroid plexus epithelium.

CSF is normally obtained from the lumbar or cervical subarachnoid space, the cisterna magna, or the lateral ventricle. In adults, the spinal cord terminates at the lower border of the first lumbar vertebra, but the subarachnoid space continues to the level of the second or third sacral vertebra. Insertion of an 18- to 21-gauge needle, usually between the third and fourth, or fourth and fifth, lumbar vertebrae, allows CSF to be assessed without injury to the spinal cord (Fig. 1-1).

After infiltration of local anesthetic, the beveled hollow needle with stylet is introduced through the skin, subcutaneous tissues, and finally the dura. The CSF pressure, maximally about 180 mm of fluid in normal, nonobese subjects, is measured with a manometer (Fig. 1-2). The CSF pressure of perhaps as much as 5% of the normal population exceed 200 mm, and this is usually attributable to obesity.

For many patients, measurement of pressure along with protein and glucose concentrations and cell count suffices as a screening procedure. The upper limit of normal for CSF protein concentration is 0.45 g/L, although the value varies between laboratories. The protein concentration tends to rise with age and is higher in lumbar than ventricular CSF. The cell count should not exceed five lymphocytes per cubic millimeter. Other measurements frequently performed include syphilis serology, IgG concentrations, and electrophoresis (Fig. 1-3). A variety of other measurements are used to identify the presence of unusual proteins, enzymes, infectious agents, and tumor cells (Table 1-1).

PLAIN RADIOGRAPHY

Skull Radiography
Skull radiography is not used in the routine investigation of the common neurologic disorders. Plain radiographs have a role in the investigation of nonaccidental injury or penetrating injury and in the assessment of ventriculoperitoneal-shunt tubing connections.

Spinal Radiography
Spinal radiography is still performed widely as part of the primary survey for patients with acute spinal trauma, and less often for those suspected of having cervical or lumbar nerve root compression, although it is incapable of providing evidence, at least directly, of any cord or root entrapment. Lateral and anteroposterior views of the lumbar spine allow identification of the components of the neural

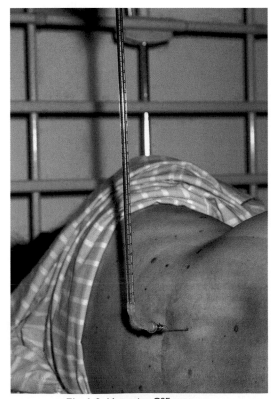

Fig. 1-2. Measuring CSF pressure.

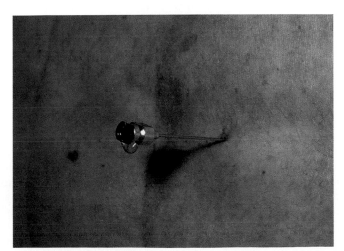

Fig. 1-1. Lumbar puncture needle in situ.

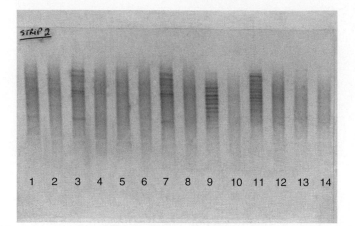

Fig. 1-3. CSF electrophoresis. Oligoclonal bands are present in samples 7, 9, and 11.

TABLE I-I.	CEREBROSPINAL FLUID ANALYSES IN COMMON USE	
TECHNIQUE	**TARGET CELL OR DISEASE**
Markers of Reactive/Tumor Cells (Immunocytochemistry)	
CLA	Marks leukocytes
T2000	Marks "reactive" T lymphocytes
B1, B2	Mark B lymphocytes
Anti-kappa, anti-lambda	Clonal B lymphocytes (lymphoma)
HMB 45	Melanoma
Cytokeratin	Epithelial cells (carcinoma)
CA-125	Ovarian cancer
Tumor Protein Markers	
HCG/α-fetoprotein/placental alkaline phosphatase	Pineal tumors
β_2-microglobulin	Carcinoma
Markers of Infection	
ELISA or Western blot	Lyme disease or other antigen assays
	HIV-1 infection
	Toxoplasmosis
	Cysticercosis
	Herpes simplex
	JC virus
	Cryptococcus
	Syphilis
Viral antigens or antibodies	Herpes zoster
	Epstein-Barr virus
	Arbovirus, enterovirus

CLA, Cationic leukocyte antigen; ELISA, enzyme-linked immunosorbent assay; HCG, human chorionic gonadotropin.

arch, together with the shape and size of the intervertebral foramina (Fig. 1-4). Although many views of the cervical spine have been described, anteroposterior, lateral, and oblique views suffice other than for traumatic cases (Figs. 1-5 and 1-6). Views of the cervical or lumbar spine in flexion and extension (Fig. 1-7) are performed if there is a suggestion of instability of the spine—for example, after injury. However, most spinal imaging is now performed with computed tomography (CT) or magnetic resonance imaging (MRI).

ULTRASOUND: NONINVASIVE SCANNING

Duplex scanning combines an ultrasound image with a pulsed Doppler flow detector. The neck vessels are first imaged with the ultrasound system and then scanned with the pulsed Doppler system to identify any significant stenosis and the direction of the flow. The common, internal, and external carotid arteries are assessed, and then the subclavian and vertebral arteries (Fig. 1-8). The technique provides a safe and accurate analysis of the state of the extracranial vessels, and it can be used serially to assess the progression of atherosclerotic disease or its modification by surgery.

Transcranial Doppler sonography has been used to evaluate intracranial arterial disease, the existence of vasospasm, and the absence of flow in patients who are brain dead. It allows the detection of asymptomatic cerebral emboli (Fig. 1-9). Vessels that can be scanned include the distal carotid siphon, and proximal segments of the anterior, middle, and posterior cerebral arteries.

COMPUTED TOMOGRAPHIC SCANNING

Computed tomographic scanning was originally called computerized axial tomographic (CAT) scanning, but the term *axial* was dropped because, although the images are acquired axially, they are now routinely visualized in any plane. Once the mainstay of neurologic imaging, it is still the first choice in the acute setting. It is of primary use in trauma cases, for excluding intracranial hemorrhage, for assessing bones, and in many cases when assessment of vessels (arteries, veins, and dural sinuses) is necessary. It is used to obtain myelographic images and in the assessment of acute stroke to obtain cerebral blood flow and volume maps. Most CT scans are now obtained using helical (spiral) scanning and using multidetector arrays (multislice scanners). If used in a spiral mode, with table movement, they enable coverage of a large volume of patient in a short time and allow arterial and venous phase imaging with one bolus of IV contrast (e.g., CT angiography and venography). If the table is not moved, the same volume (e.g., the brain) can be scanned repetitively during the passage of a bolus of contrast, enabling CT perfusion maps to be obtained. At present, 256-slice scanners are available (Fig. 1-10).

CT Myelography
CT myelography is now seldom performed, but it may be necessary if MRI is contraindicated—for example, in a patient with a pacemaker. The contrast can be inserted into either the lumbar or the cervical region (Fig. 1-11). Although the latter is a more hazardous procedure, it may be necessary if there is a spinal block between the lumbar and cervical regions (Fig. 1-12).

CT Angiography
Computed tomography–angiography (CTA) can be performed on all multislice scanners with spiral capability and can be performed immediately after standard CT imaging. Intravenous nonionic contrast medium is injected using a pump injector. The technique is particularly applicable for the assessment of carotid and vertebral artery stenosis (particularly the origins of the vertebral arteries) (Fig. 1-13), and for assessment of intracranial aneurysm morphology (Fig. 1-14).

CT Perfusion
The injection of a bolus of contrast with continuous scanning enables the alteration of contrast with time to be plotted. Various parameters can be measured (time to peak, mean transit time, change in contrast), which enables other parameters to be calculated (cerebral blood flow, cerebral blood volume) using certain assumptions. These parameters can be overlaid on a structural slice of brain for ease of interpretation and have been validated with gold standard cerebral blood flow measurements (using positron emission tomography [PET]) (Fig. 1-15).

MAGNETIC RESONANCE IMAGING

The ability of MRI to allow visualization of bodily structures depends on the presence in those structures of charged hydrogen atoms (protons), whose alignment can be influenced by the application of an external magnetic field. If the magnetic field is parallel to the body's axis, the protons align so that the majority point to the north end of the magnet, producing a bulk magnetization vector whose amplitude is determined partly by proton density and partly by the strength of

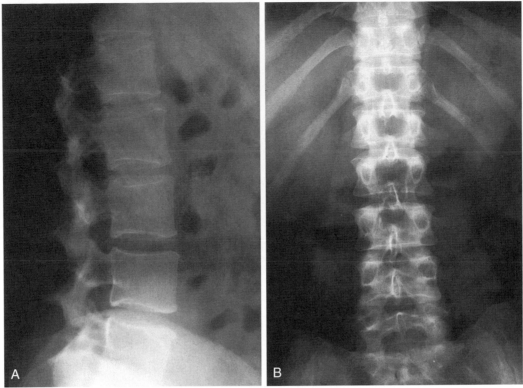

Fig. 1-4. Normal lumbar spine radiographs. **A,** Lateral. **B,** Anteroposterior.

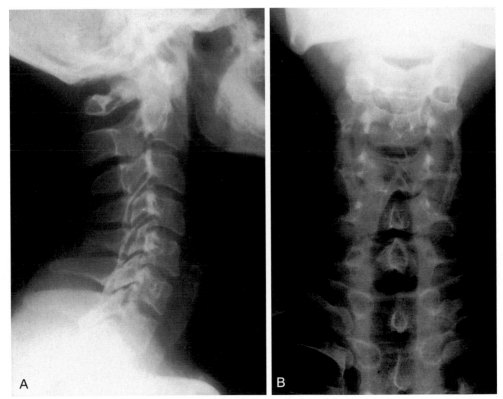

Fig. 1-5. Normal cervical spine radiographs. **A,** Lateral. **B,** Anteroposterior.

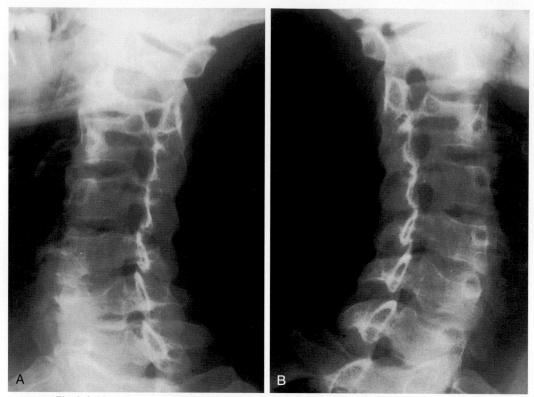

Fig. 1-6. Normal cervical spine radiographs. **A,** Left posterior oblique. **B,** Right posterior oblique.

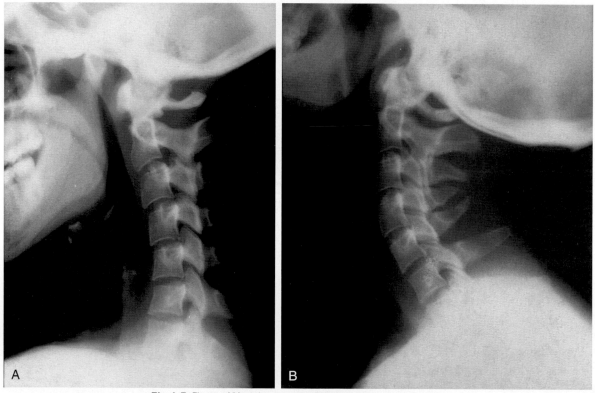

Fig. 1-7. Flexion **(A)** and extension **(B)** views of the cervical spine.

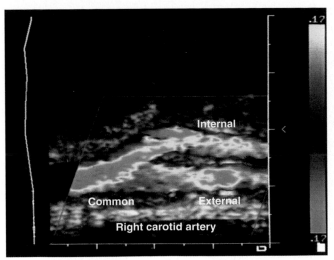

Fig. 1-8. Duplex scan of the carotid bifurcation.

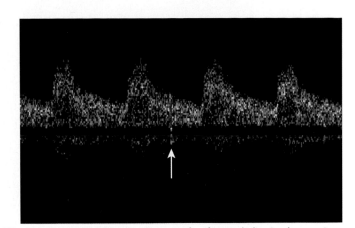

Fig. 1-9. Transcranial Doppler. An example of an embolic signal appearing as a short-duration, high-intensity signal in the Doppler spectrum.

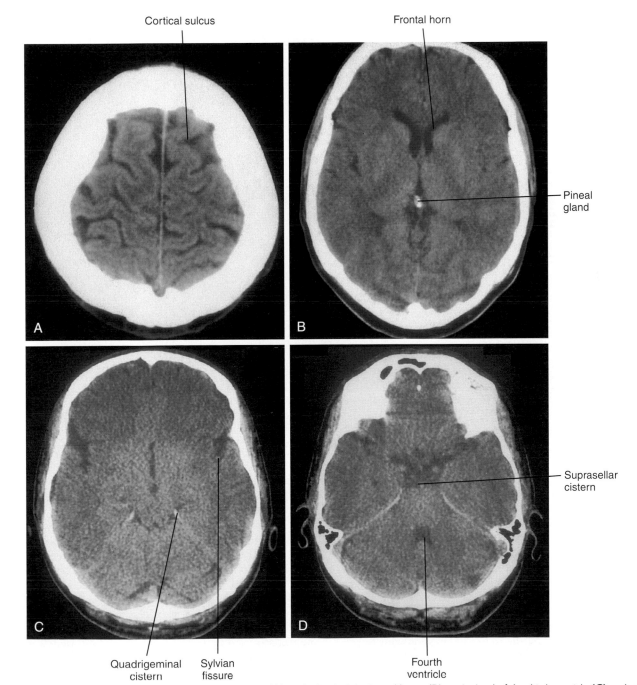

Fig. 1-10. Normal noncontrasted CT scan at four levels: at the vertex **(A)**, at the level of the frontal horns **(B)**, at the level of the third ventricle **(C)**, and at the level of the pons **(D)**.

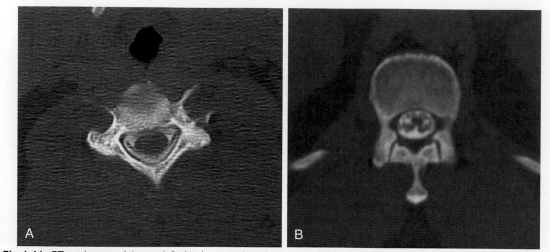

Fig. 1-11. CT myelogram of the cord. **A,** Axial source data showing normal cervical cord and dorsal roots. **B,** Conus and filum.

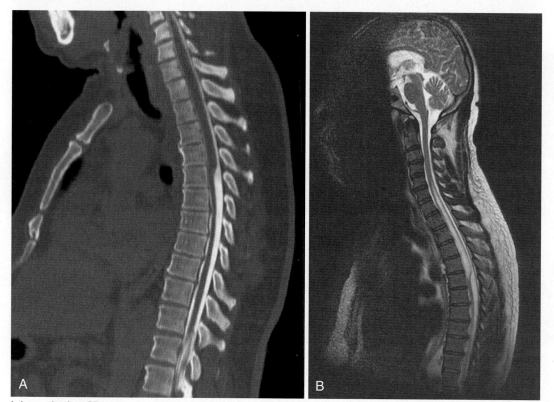

Fig. 1-12. Reformatted thoracolumbar CT myelogram **(A)** and MRI **(B)** showing intramedullary signal change and anterior cord displacement with MRI, but with no posterior mass seen with MRI and myelography.

the applied magnetic field. Magnetic field strength ranges between 0.25 and 3.0 tesla (T), compared with Earth's magnetic field of 0.3 to 0.6 Gauss (1T = 10,000 G).

After equilibration, an electric current is passed through coils mounted inside the magnet core so that a magnetic field is produced at a chosen angle (often 90 or 180 degrees) to the main magnet's field. In practice, many and varying currents are used, and it is the movement of these coils during switching of the powerful currents that causes MRI scanning to be noisy. The alignment of the charged protons can be changed by any angle up to 360 degrees. When the electric current is switched off, the protons gradually return to their previous alignment, emitting energy as they do so. Capturing this emitted energy and positioning the source of emission with receiver coils is the fundamental process that enables images to be obtained.

Two time measures of this decay are determined: T1 and T2. T1 measures time taken to recover the bulk magnetization vector in the north–south plane of the main magnet. T2 measures the time taken

for the individual charged particles to fall out of the coherent resonance induced by the radio frequency signal. T1-weighted images produce pictures in which CSF is dark; in T2-weighted images, the CSF appears lighter, and the contrast between gray and white matter is particularly prominent. Fluid-attenuated inversion recovery (FLAIR) images are similar to T2 images but with suppressed CSF. These are the three common sequences used in neurologic imaging (Fig. 1-16). One of the advantages of MR over CT (in addition to the improved soft tissue contrast resolution) is that images can be acquired in the sagittal, axial, or coronal (or indeed any) plane. At higher field strengths, spatial resolution is improved for a given acquisition time (Fig. 1-17). Three-dimensional (3D) data sets can be reconstructed in a 3D format. A midline sagittal image displays midline structures, including the third and fourth ventricles (Fig. 1-18). Axial images display horizontal brain slices at any level from the vertex to the foramen magnum and can be targeted to show particular features of interest (Fig. 1-19).

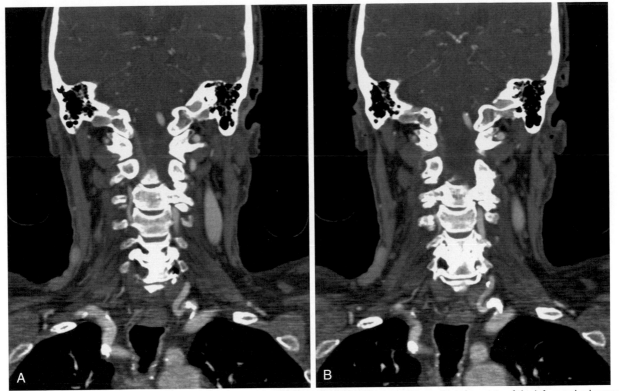

Fig. 1-13. A, B: CT angiography showing origins of vertebral arteries, with calcified plaque and stenosis at the origin of the left vertebral artery.

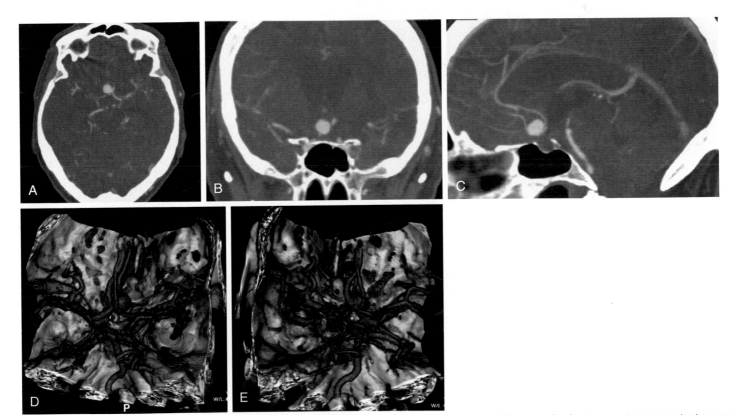

Fig. 1-14. Axial **(A)**, coronal **(B)**, and sagittal **(C)** maximum-intensity projection reconstructions of an intracranial CT angiography showing anterior communicating artery aneurysm morphology, with 3D superior oblique volume reconstructions **(D** and **E)**.

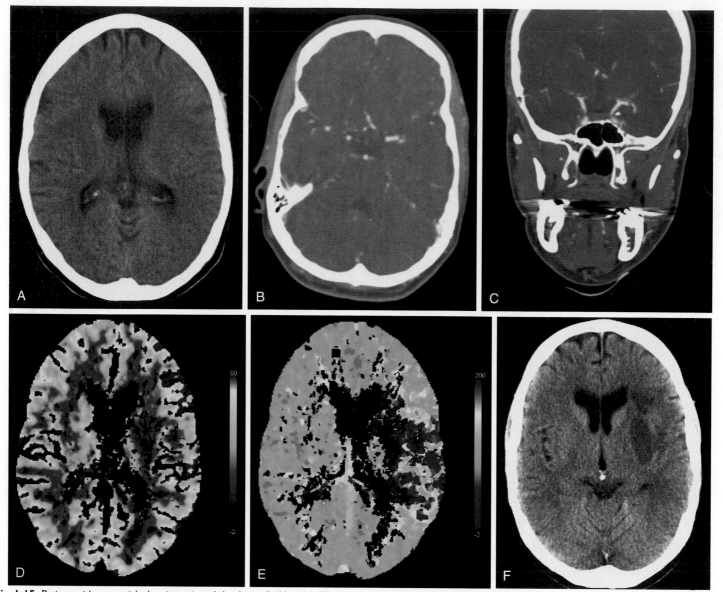

Fig. 1-15. Patient with acute right hemiparesis and dysphasia. **A,** Normal CT (at ictus +2 hrs). **B** and **C,** CT angiography showing left middle cerebral artery occlusion. Cerebral blood volume (CBV) **(D)** and time-to-peak (TTP) **(E)** maps show irreversible ischemia in deep white matter and gray matter, and critical ischemia in cortex. (TTP and cerebral blood flow maps show ischemic and infarcted tissue; CBV shows infarcted tissue.) **F,** Follow-up CT at 48 hours shows preserved cortex with infarct corresponding to CBV map.

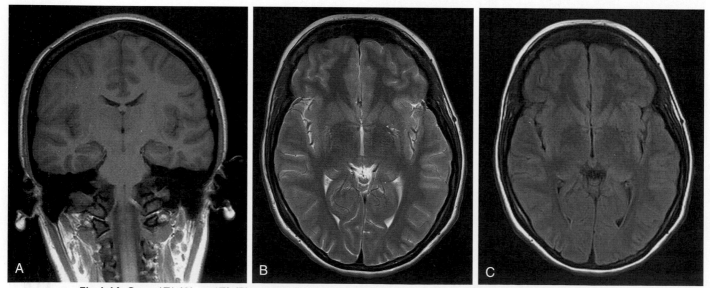

Fig. 1-16. Coronal T1 **(A),** axial T2 **(B),** and axial fluid-attenuated inversion recovery (FLAIR) **(C)** images through normal brain.

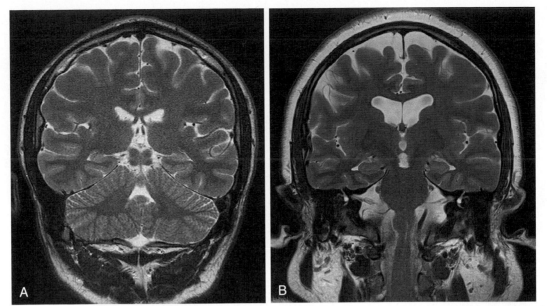

Fig. 1-17. Coronal 3-mm T2-weighted slices through the hippocampi at 1.5T **(A)** and 3T **(B)**. Note the improved resolution at 3T, with improved detail of hippocampal substructures.

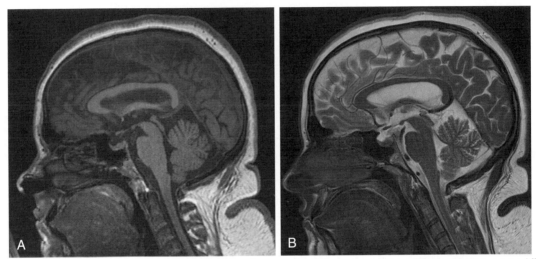

Fig. 1-18. Midline sagittal T1-weighted **(A)** and T2-weighted **(B)** images demonstrating different appearances of the same structures on different sequences.

Conventional MRI techniques (e.g., spin echo) require a considerable time (up to 15 minutes). Accordingly, faster imaging techniques have been developed—for example, fast spin echo and gradient echo imaging. Although many thousands of sequences are now available, the standard sequences suffice in most clinical settings. The IV contrast media used for MRI scanning are all gadolinium based. Shortening the T1 relaxation times of lesions enhances the imaging discrepancy between the lesion and its surrounding tissue.

MRI is also used to visualize the spinal cord and its surrounding structures. A midline sagittal image is supplemented by axial images at the relevant levels. Structures demonstrated on the sagittal images of the cervicothoracic region include the spinal cord, the vertebral bodies, and the intervertebral discs (Fig. 1-20). Axial views, according to the level, demonstrate the vertebral body, the facet joints, the spinal cord and nerve roots, and the epidural space (Fig. 1-21). Images of the lumbar spine demonstrate the vertebral body and neural arches, the discs, and the contents of the spinal canal (Fig. 1-22).

MR Angiography or Venography
Signal from vessels can be obtained using many types of sequences with MR. Most commonly, 3D time of flight (3D TOF) (Fig. 1-23) or 2D TOF is used (neither needs IV contrast), but contrast-enhanced MR angiography (MRA) and black blood MRA are also available if needed. MR venography (MRV) is often produced using phase contrast techniques. Carotid MRA does have a tendency to overestimate tight stenoses.

Contrast-enhanced MRA requires a 3D gradient echo sequence with a short repetition time of 3 to 7 msec and a short echo time of 1 to 3 msec. With correctly timed gadolinium infusion, high-signal vascular imaging is obtained because of the T1 shortening of blood caused by the gadolinium. By using the coronal plane, both carotid and vertebral arteries can be assessed throughout their cervical and intracranial portions. Carotid stenoses exceeding 30% are detected on contrast-enhanced MRA with high sensitivity and specificity. Contrast-enhanced MRA is a more sensitive technique than time-of-flight MRA. The technique is less successful for detecting stenoses of the vertebral artery origins.

Diffusion-Weighted MRI
Diffusion-weighted imaging (DWI) is of particular value in detecting signal changes in early cerebral infarction, but it is also useful for differentiating abscesses from metastases (Fig. 1-24). DWI obtains images sensitized to the distance diffused by water molecules in a set time. Cytotoxic edema (e.g., caused by ischemia) entails cell swelling, a reduction in intercellular space, and a reduction in the distance a water molecule can diffuse. This causes restricted diffusion. DWI images are usually obtained in three orthogonal planes (right-left, anteroposterior, superoinferior). These are summed to produce an

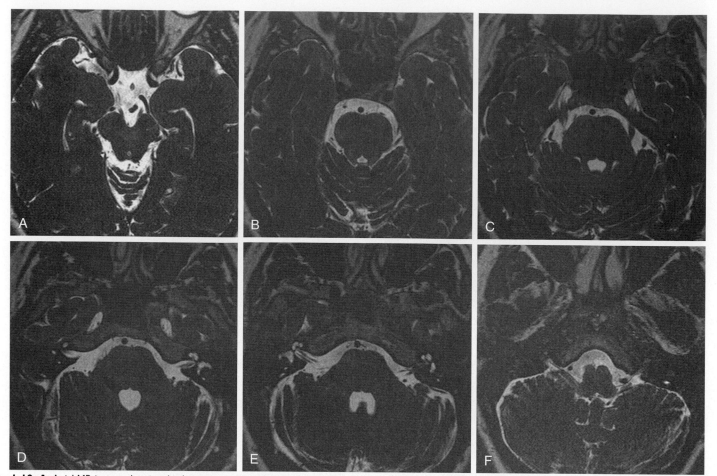

Fig. 1-19. A, Axial MR images showing third nerves in interpeduncular cistern. **B,** Left fourth nerve crossing prepontine cistern. **C,** Left fifth nerve exiting pons, and right entering Meckel's cave. **D,** Both sixth nerves entering Dorello's canal in the clivus. **E,** Seventh and eighth nerves in the internal auditory meat; **F,** Twelfth nerve and fifth nerve leaving lateral medulla and traversing hypoglossal canals.

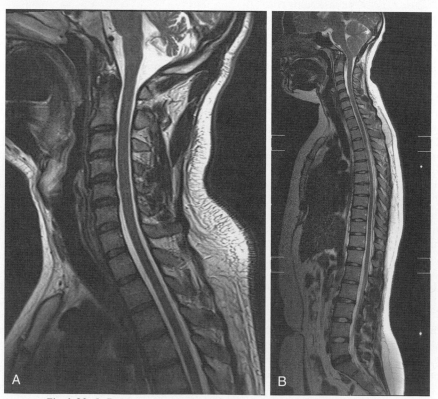

Fig. 1-20. A, B: T2-weighted sagittal MRI of cervical and upper thoracic spine.

apparent diffusion coefficient (ADC) map that allows for the differences in diffusion distances in normal tissue, which depend on whether the underlying tissue has myelinated tracts running parallel or perpendicular to the direction of measurement (one DWI sequence measures distance traveled in one direction only), and that compensates for any T2 "shine through" (T2 signal that can shine through on DWI sequences and give spurious results). Using DWI sequences, it is also possible to obtain maps of fractional anisotropy, which is related to diffusion direction and magnitude, particularly in white matter. This may have clinical uses in white matter diseases, including multiple sclerosis, diffuse axonal injury, and dementia or mild cognitive impairment.

MRI Tractography

In vitro, water diffuses freely in any plane—that is, it is a vector, having both direction and distance. Using diffusion-weighted sequences in multiple directions, it is possible to measure both the extent of diffusion and its direction, which, in vivo, is not free in any plane but is altered by the presence of myelinated white matter tracts, which severely restricts diffusion in directions tangential to the direction of the myelinated fibers. In MRI tractography, these vectors are overlaid on a structural image and displayed as color maps with brightness equivalent to increased magnitude (i.e., greater distance of diffusion), and color can be used to encode direction (Fig. 1-25). White matter tracts can be displayed using mathematical formulas that use various assumptions to link neighboring voxels (Fig. 1-26).

MR Perfusion

The principles of MR perfusion are similar to those of CT perfusion coupled with an IV bolus injection of contrast agent to calculate time-to-peak (TTP), relative cerebral blood volume (rCBV), and relative cerebral blood flow (rCBF) maps ("relative" because in MR techniques the measured values are relative, as opposed to the absolute values obtained with CT perfusion). This is useful in the assessment of acute stroke and in imaging gliomas. Glioblastoma multiforme typically demonstrates higher CBV than low-grade gliomas (Fig. 1-27). It is possible that a progressive elevation of CBV in tumors is one of the earliest markers of transformation of a low-grade glioma to a high-grade glioma. It is possible to obtain MR perfusion data without IV contrast using arterial spin labeling techniques, but this is not widely used.

Functional MR

Blood oxygen level–dependent (BOLD) functional MRI (fMRI) is the most commonly used method. It measures changes in blood flow by detecting changes in intravascular oxyhemoglobin concentration. This occurs because in activated cortex there is an increase in blood flow, mediated by vasodilation, that exceeds the local metabolic requirement, and this results in an increase in the intravascular oxyhemoglobin concentration (Figs. 1-28 and 1-29). This increase can be measured, usually using gradient echo sequences. The BOLD effect is greater at 3T than at 1.5T, so the former (if available) is preferred.

MR Spectroscopy

The speed of precession (or spinning) of hydrogen atoms is governed by the strength of the external magnetic field. However, when H is incorporated into chemicals, other atoms vary slightly in local field strength. This slight variation in local magnetic field strength (measured in parts per million) can tell us what chemical the hydrogen atom is part of, and modern scanners allow us to

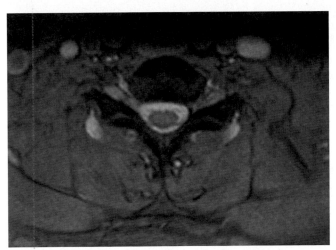

Fig. 1-21. T2-weighted MRI at the midcervical level.

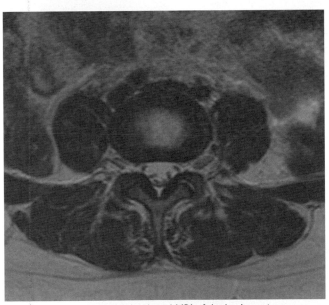

Fig. 1-22. T2-weighted axial MRI of the lumbar spine.

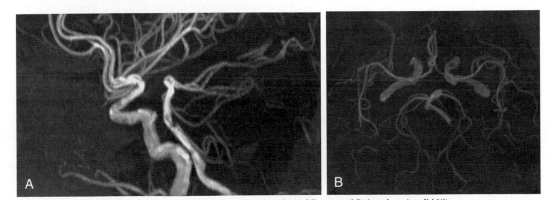

Fig. 1-23. A and **B,** Reconstructed data from 3D time of flight of circle of Willis.

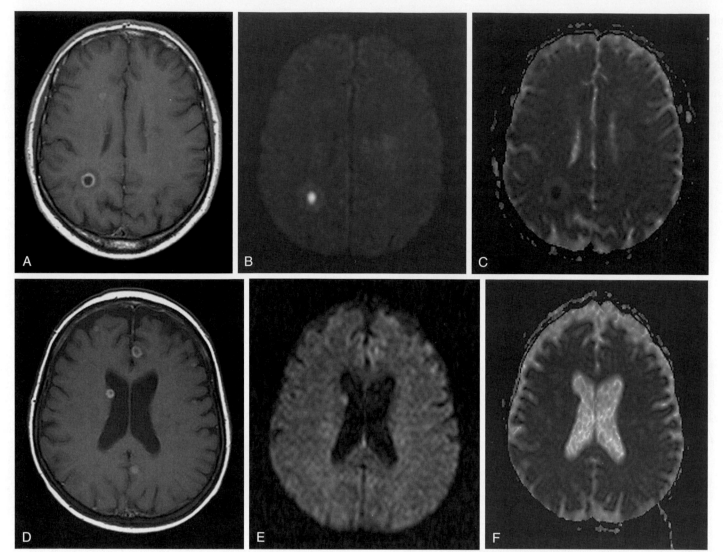

Fig. 1-24. Axial postcontrast T1-weighted **(A, D)**, diffusion-weighted **(B, E)**, and apparent diffusion coefficient **(C, F)** images of abscesses **(A, B, C)** and metastases **(D, E, F)**, showing similar ring enhancement on postcontrast T1 but with characteristically restricted diffusion in bacterial abscesses.

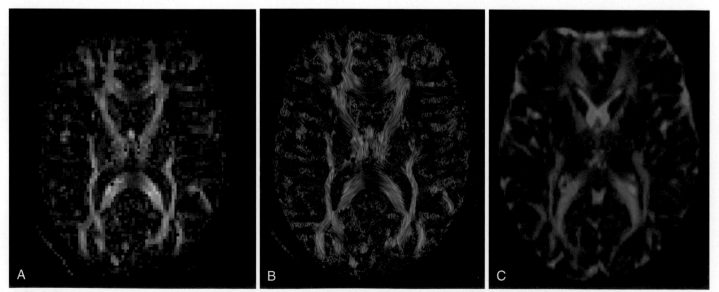

Fig. 1-25. Diffusion tensor imaging showing color (superoinferior, *blue;* anteroposterior, *green;* right-left, *red-orange*) encoding of tracts **(A)**, with "texture" **(B)**, and with anatomic overlay **(C)**.

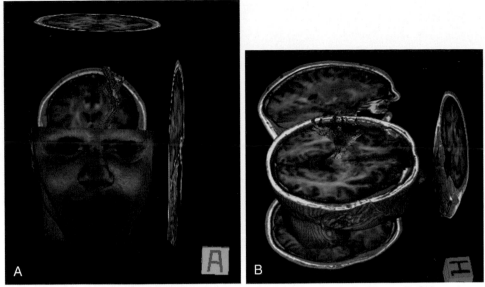

Fig. 1-26. Fiber tracking of motor fibers from cortex into cerebral peduncle. **A,** AP view. **B,** Oblique view.

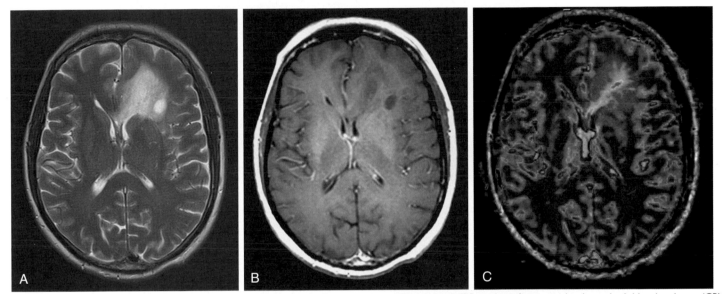

Fig. 1-27. Biopsy-proven glioblastoma multiforme. Axial T2-weighted **(A)**, postcontrast T1-weighted **(B)**, and perfusion-weighted cerebral blood volume (CBV) **(C)** MR images showing "bland," nonenhancing mass with markedly raised CBV.

localize the position. Commonly, MR spectroscopy of the brain is used to assess choline, creatine, *N*-acetylaspartate, inositol, lactate, and mobile lipid resonances. The varying proportions can help in grading of primary tumors and assessing dementia (Figs. 1-30 and 1-31).

DIGITAL SUBTRACTION ANGIOGRAPHY

Catheter angiography allows visualization of the carotid and vertebral arteries via injection of contrast medium through a catheter inserted via the femoral artery into the aortic arch. For visualization of intracranial vessels, the catheter is then manipulated into the relevant neck artery before injection of contrast medium. Digital subtraction angiography employs a computerized technique to eliminate background detail and summate successive images (Figs. 1-32 through 1-35). Visualization of spinal cord arteries is achieved by catheterizing the relevant vessels from the thoracic and abdominal aorta (Fig. 1-36). The need for intracranial angiography is declining as CT angiography and MR angiography have improved.

INTERVENTIONAL TECHNIQUES

Using the arterial (or sometimes venous) tree as an access pathway, it is now possible to position a microcatheter almost anywhere in the central nervous system (CNS). Endovascular techniques are now the first-line treatment for intracranial aneurysms and for most dural fistula. Arteriovenous malformations are now often treated endovascularly to obliteration or to reduce their size prior to surgery or stereotactic radiosurgery (gamma knife treatment).

It is possible to place stents in the middle and anterior cerebral arteries, as well as in the internal carotid artery and the carotid bifurcation, although randomized trial data for benefit are lacking, and these techniques are often used only in medically refractory cases.

Intraarterial clot lysis and aspiration catheters are available and may be of benefit in the anterior intracranial circulation, but benefit has not yet been shown in large randomized trials. In the posterior circulation (particularly with basilar artery occlusion), the outcome is so poor that intervention is often tried. Major dural venous sinus occlusion can also be treated this way if there is no improvement with IV heparin.

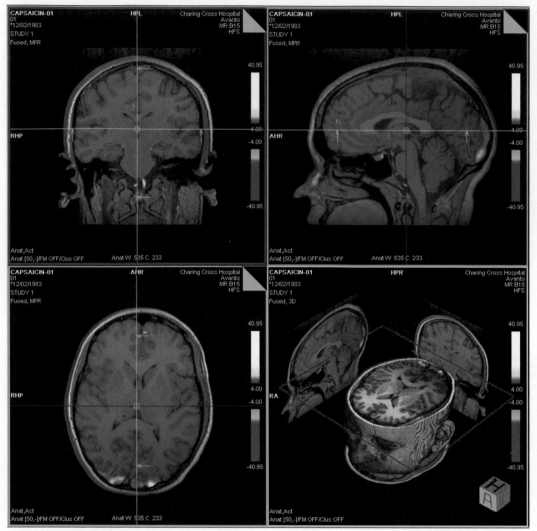

Fig. 1-28. Functional MRI after visual stimulation showing increased activity in visual cortex.

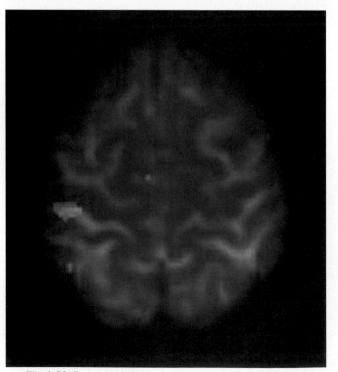

Fig. 1-29. Functional MRI after voluntary movement of left hand.

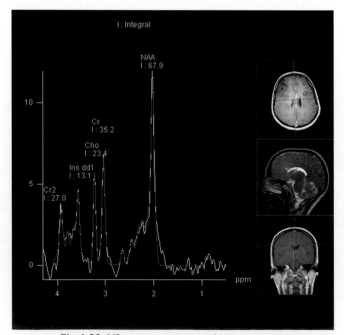

Fig. 1-30. MR spectroscopy, normal brain spectrum.

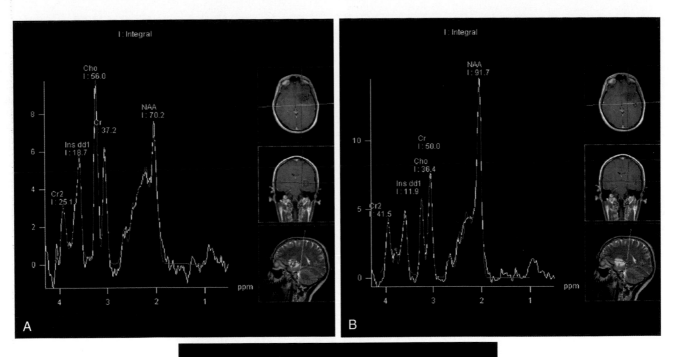

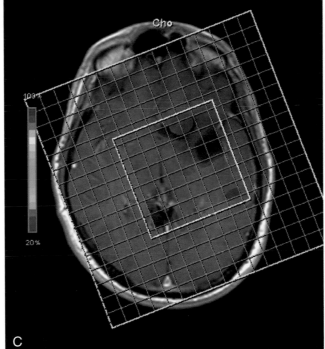

Fig. 1-31. MR spectroscopy spectrum in **(A)** and out of tumor **(B)**, showing increased choline in low-grade tumor. **C,** Metabolite map of choline.

RADIOISOTOPE IMAGING

Single-Photon Emission CT

Single-photon emission computed tomography (SPECT) can be carried out with either multidetector or rotating gamma camera systems. Using a radioactively labeled isotope, usually technetium-99m labeled hexamethylpropylene amine oxide, the system allows quantitative assessment of regional cerebral blood flow. In normal individuals, symmetrical activity is greatest in a strip corresponding to cortical gray matter at the periphery of the frontal, temporal, parietal, and occipital lobes. In addition, high flow is found in the region of the thalami and basal ganglia (Fig. 1-37).

Positron Emission Tomography

Positively charged electrons (positrons) are emitted during the decay of certain unstable nuclei. When a positron collides with an electron, the two particles destroy each other and in doing so release energy in the form of paired photons, which then travel in opposite directions. Using detectors placed around the head, the origin of the signal can be localized to a particular tomographic slice of the brain. Accurate measurement of activity requires a tissue volume of the order of 1 cm^3. The isotopes commonly used are of oxygen, carbon, and nitrogen, with a fluorine isotope substituted for hydrogen.

Cerebral perfusion and blood volume are measured, the former with H_2O labeled with radioactive oxygen ($H_2^{15}O$), and the latter with labeled CO_2. Assessment of metabolic activity is achieved either by calculating an oxygen extraction fraction using $^{15}O_2$, or by the use of a labeled glucose analogue (Fig. 1-38).

Transmitter systems in the brain can be studied in conditions such as Parkinson's disease. PET with radioactively labeled dopa ([^{18}F] dopa PET) is used to visualize the nigrostriatal dopaminergic system. [^{18}F]Dopa PET reflects presynaptic dopa uptake, decarboxylation to dopamine, and storage, with [^{18}F]dopa uptake rate constants correlating with the number of functional dopaminergic neurons.

Similarly, PET techniques can be used to assess dopaminergic receptor systems. PET studies with selective D_2 receptor ligands such as ^{11}C-raclopride show a mild increase in D_2 site availability in the putamen of de novo Parkinson's patients (Fig. 1-39). PET studies have been applied to the study of other neurotransmitter systems, such as those involving serotonin.

ELECTROPHYSIOLOGY

Electroencephalography

For an electroencephalography (EEG) recording, 16 to 20 scalp electrodes record, amplify, and convert the basic brain rhythms into a trace drawn on paper moving at 3 cm/sec. Bipolar recording measures the potential difference between two electrodes. Unipolar recording measures the difference between a single electrode and, most commonly, an average reference electrode summating potentials from the other recorders.

The electrodes are attached to the scalp with an adhesive material as the patient sits or lies on a couch (Fig. 1-40). The recording is performed with the patient's eyes closed and also with eyes open. In addition to the resting trace, recording is carried out during overbreathing and while the patient is exposed to a light flashing at frequencies from 1 to 20 Hz.

During maturation, the basic EEG rhythms accelerate, so that the initially predominant theta and delta activities are replaced in the adult by a dominant alpha rhythm, at 8 to 13 Hz, most conspicuous in the post-central areas (Fig. 1-41). The alpha rhythm disappears when the eyes are opened. Intermingled with the alpha rhythm is beta activity, defined as rhythmic activity faster than 13 Hz. During overbreathing, particularly in children, slower activity in the form of theta and even delta activities can appear.

In an attempt to identify epileptic foci, additional techniques have been devised, either using alternative electrode placements or exposing the patient to a stimulus theoretically capable of activating an otherwise silent focus. Both nasopharyngeal and sphenoidal electrodes are sometimes used in the investigation of patients with suspected epilepsy, and the former are generally more successful. Activation procedures such as sleep deprivation or injection of Metrazol are now seldom undertaken, but an EEG recording, with the patient asleep or ambulatory with portable equipment, can be of value in the search for epileptic activity. Increasingly, recording of activity is performed from the cortex or with depth electrodes at the time of craniotomy.

Computer-assisted EEG interpretation has been used to permit a topographic representation of normal and abnormal activity. For example, the distribution of alpha rhythm can be presented in the form of a brain map (Fig. 1-42).

Magnetoencephalography

Magnetoencephalography (MEG) is used to localize focal epileptic discharges by measuring the changes in extracranial magnetic fields that those discharges generate (Fig. 1-43). There is, in general, a good correlation between the sites of foci localized by MEG and those discovered by the use of depth electrodes.

Evoked Potentials

Evoked potentials measure conduction along visual, auditory, somatosensory, and motor pathways, either from the periphery to the central nervous system (the first three) or vice versa (the last). Averaging techniques allow the evoked response to be distinguished from random background activity. Latency measurements are more reliable than those of amplitude, because the latter are more susceptible to technical error.

Visual Evoked Potentials. Stimulation of the retina by an alternating pattern of light and dark squares produces a well-defined positive potential over the occipital cortex. Typically, 100 to 200 visual presentations are required to obtain a satisfactory averaged response. A pattern-reversal stimulus (Fig. 1-44) is the most effective, the response being recorded by a string of electrodes above and below the inion together with a horizontal row along a line 5 cm above the inion. Monopolar recordings are made with the reference electrode placed anteriorly. Full-field stimulation produces a triphasic potential

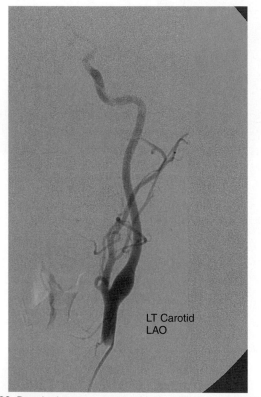

Fig. 1-32. Digital subtraction angiography. Normal left carotid bifurcation.

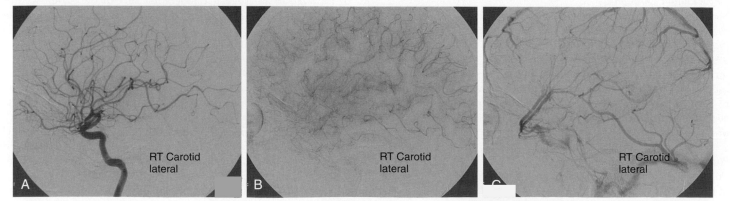

Fig. 1-33. Digital subtraction angiography. Normal lateral internal carotid artery arteriogram. Arterial (**A**), late arterial/capillary (**B**), and venous (**C**) phases.

with a large positive component, preceded and followed by smaller negative potentials (Fig. 1-45). Topographic mapping confirms the occipital localization of the evoked response (Fig. 1-46).

Abnormal responses, particularly with respect to latency, have been identified, most commonly in patients with multiple sclerosis (MS). Many other neurologic disorders (e.g., Friedreich's ataxia and Parkinson's disease) can affect latency, although to a lesser degree than in MS.

Alteration of both waveform and latency can occur with compression of the visual pathway at any site.

Auditory Evoked Responses. Auditory evoked responses are obtained by applying a click stimulus via earphones. The clicks, applied unilaterally, are repeated at a frequency of 10 Hz. A masking noise is used contralaterally. Click intensity is set at about 70 dB above the hearing threshold. The response to 1000 to 2000 clicks is summated using electrodes over the earlobe and vertex (Fig. 1-47). The brainstem components are separated into waves I to VII (Fig. 1-48). Measurements are made of the interwave latencies and the amplitude ratio of waves I to V.

Wave I represents the eighth nerve activation potential, and waves II and III are derived from the cochlear nucleus and superior olivary complex, respectively. The origin of waves IV and V is less certain, although the latter may represent arrival of the signal at the inferior colliculus. Waves VI and VII are variable and seldom used in clinical studies.

Measurement of auditory evoked responses has been used in the investigation of vestibular neurinomas, MS, and intrinsic brainstem tumors, although this role is now largely historical.

Somatosensory Evoked Potentials. After limb stimulation, an evoked potential can be recorded not only from the relevant peripheral nerve but also from over the spine or the cortex (Fig. 1-49). If the median nerve is stimulated at the wrist, with recording electrodes over the neck, four distinct negative potentials can be recorded: N9, N11, N13, and N14 (Figs. 1-50 and 1-51). A later negative wave with a latency of about 20 msec can be recorded over the contralateral sensory cortex (N20). Late (vertex) potentials can be evoked by visual, auditory, or somatosensory stimulation. Their latencies extend up to about 300 msec.

Measurement of somatosensory evoked potentials (SSEPs) has found less clinical application than either visual or auditory evoked potentials. Abnormalities have been found, particularly in patients with MS, but also in those with cervical spondylosis, spinal trauma, or brachial plexus lesions. Monitoring of SSEPs has been used during the course of spinal cord surgery.

Central Motor Conduction

The corticospinal tract can be stimulated through the scalp either electrically or by an electromagnetic system. The latter method is preferable as it causes less discomfort. After transcranial activation of the motor system, a response can be recorded, principally contralaterally, from the muscles of the limbs or trunk. The type of response and its latency depend on the stimulus mode (Fig. 1-52).

Subclinical abnormalities of central motor conduction have been found in patients with MS. The technique has also been used to study conduction time in patients with motor neuron disease or cervical myelopathy, and during surgery of the spinal cord.

Nerve Conduction Studies and Electromyography

Nerve conduction studies are of great value in the assessment of peripheral nerve function. A short-duration stimulus is used, usually 0.2 msec, with a repetition rate of 1 Hz. The stimulating electrode is either positioned at sites where the nerve is close to the skin surface, or around the digits in the form of a ring (Fig. 1-53). The resulting

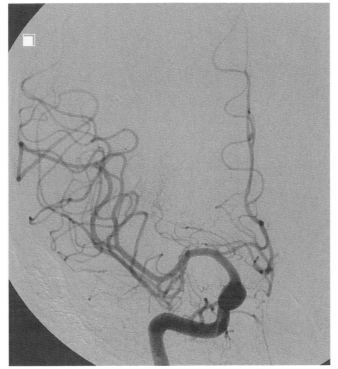

Fig. 1-34. Digital subtraction angiography. Normal frontal (Towne's projection) internal carotid artery view.

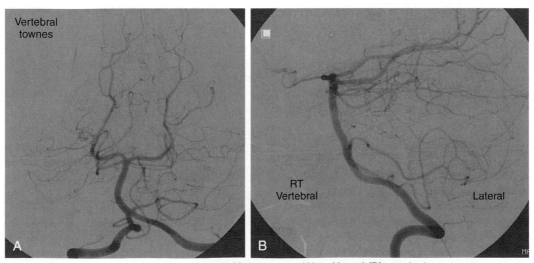

Fig. 1-35. Digital subtraction angiography. Normal frontal **(A)** and lateral **(B)** vertebral arteriograms.

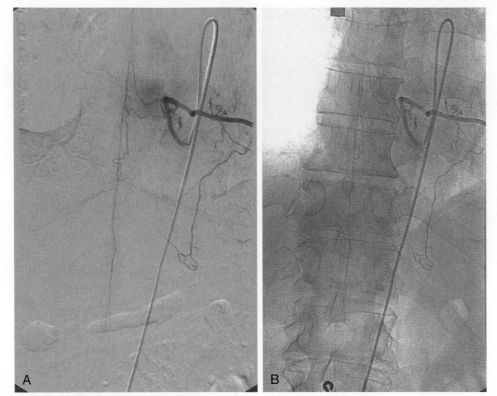

Fig. 1-36. A and **B,** Digital subtraction angiography, two views. Radicular injection demonstrating filling of anterior spinal artery from artery of Adamkiewicz.

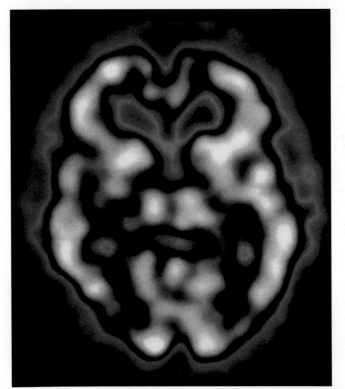

Fig. 1-37. Single-photon emission computed tomography (SPECT). Normal study. Low-flow areas (e.g., the skull) appear *blue,* high-flow areas are *yellow.*

sensory action potential is satisfactorily recorded by a surface electrode (Fig. 1-54). Conventionally, about 30 repetitive stimulations are used, with the responses being averaged.

Conduction velocity in the fast conducting fibers in the nerve can be expressed as a distal latency or as an actual velocity. Conduction velocity declines with age and slows with a fall in limb temperature. Cooling increases compound muscle action potential amplitude.

Nerve conduction, particularly as measured by H reflexes and F responses, is also influenced by height. Commonly studied nerves for sensory conduction include the median, ulnar, and radial nerves in the upper limbs, and the sural, medial, and lateral plantar nerves in the lower limbs.

Motor conduction velocities are measured by stimulating the peripheral nerve at two or more separate sites while recording the response from the relevant muscle using surface or needle electrodes (Fig. 1-55). A velocity is obtained by dividing the distance between any two stimulating sites by the latency difference of the two responses (Fig. 1-56). The figure obtained applies to the most rapidly conducting fibers in the nerve.

The H Reflex.   The H reflex is a monosynaptic reflex response that can be obtained from the soleus muscle after stimulation of the tibial nerve. Stimulation of afferent fibers in the tibial nerve triggers a reflex response in the motor nerves to the soleus via the spinal cord (Fig. 1-57).

The F Wave.   The F wave requires a more potent stimulus than the H reflex. With such a stimulus, a depolarizing wave is transmitted both centrally and distally, with the former then activating anterior horn cells. The resulting action potential propagates down the motor nerve, producing a potential several milliseconds after the direct response. Variation in latency and amplitude of successive F wave responses occurs because the anterior horn cells activated vary from stimulation to stimulation (Fig. 1-58). The latency of the F response is a measure of conduction time in the proximal segment of the relevant nerve. It is particularly valuable in the evaluation of those demyelinating neuropathies in which proximal involvement is likely—for example, in chronic inflammatory demyelinating polyneuropathy.

Repetitive Stimulation.   Nerve stimulation over a range of frequencies is used in the evaluation of the neuromuscular junction. In normal individuals, a small decrement can occur in the size of the muscle evoked potential when the nerve is stimulated at 10 Hz or less. At faster rates of stimulation (10 to 50 per second), a small increment is sometimes seen initially, and the compound action potential subsequently remains stable.

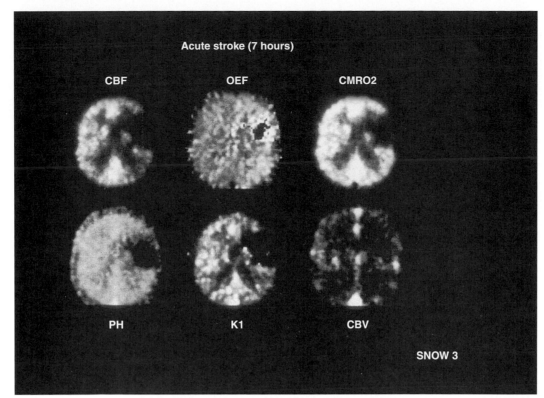

Fig. 1-38. Cerebral blood flow (CBF), cerebral oxygen metabolism (CMRO₂), oxygen extraction fraction (OEF), cerebral blood volume (CBV), and pH in patient 7 hours after an acute stroke. The OEF image displays a central zone of reduced oxygen extraction, with enhanced extraction at its periphery.

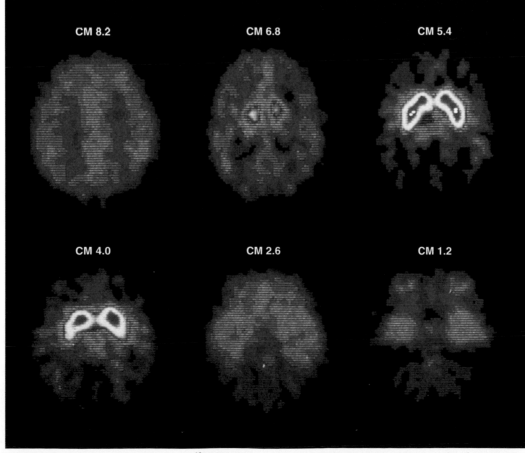

Fig. 1-39. PET images of a normal subject injected with ^{18}F-labeled N-methylspiperone, demonstrating intense uptake of tracer in the basal ganglia.

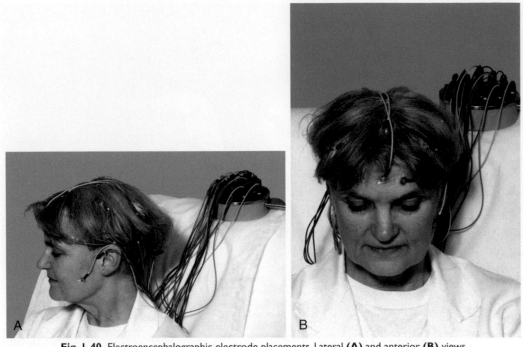

Fig. 1-40. Electroencephalographic electrode placements. Lateral **(A)** and anterior **(B)** views.

NORMAL 16 CHANNEL ELECTROENCEPHALOGRAM

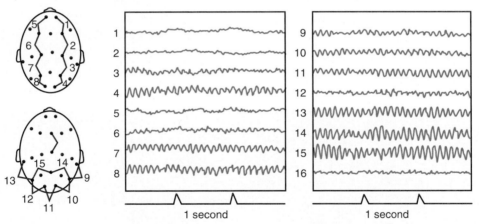

Fig. 1-41. Normal 16-channel EEG. The electrode placements are shown on the *left* (position 6).

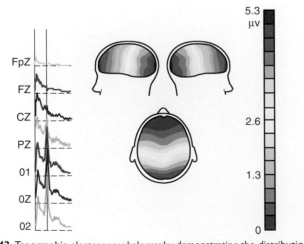

Fig. 1-42. Topographic electroencephalography demonstrating the distribution of alpha rhythm in a normal subject. A frequency analysis for alpha rhythm is shown on the *left*. It reaches its maximal amplitude *(red)* over the occipital electrodes (O$_2$ and Oz).

ELECTROMYOGRAPHY

Most sampling of muscle for analysis of motor unit activity is done with a concentric needle electrode (Fig. 1-59). In the relaxed state, no spontaneous activity can be recorded from healthy muscle except in the region of the motor endplate. As the needle is inserted, a brief burst of electrical activity occurs (insertional activity), and it becomes prolonged in a variety of neuropathic and myopathic disorders.

Abnormal spontaneous activity includes fibrillation potentials, positive sharp waves, and fasciculation potentials. Fibrillation potentials are biphasic or triphasic and arise from single, or a small number of, muscle fibers. They are particularly associated with denervation of muscle (Fig. 1-60, *A*). Positive sharp waves have a similar connotation (see Fig. 1-60, *B*).

Fasciculation potentials are larger and readily visible to the naked eye. They are believed to represent the spontaneous contraction of fibers belonging to a single motor unit. They can be found in normal muscle but are particularly associated with motor neuron disease (see Fig. 1-60, *C*).

MAGNETOENCEPHALOGRAM

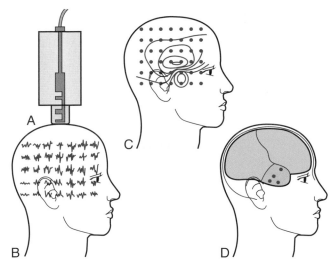

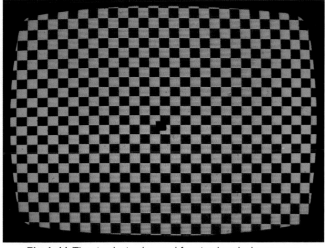

Fig. 1-44. The visual stimulus used for visual evoked responses.

Fig. 1-43. Magnetoencephalogram (MEG). **A,** Schematic of a squid (superconductive quantum interference device) magnetometer, which is connected to a detection coil and immersed in liquid helium. The magnetometer is positioned close to the patient's head. The output is in voltage proportional to the magnetic field detected. **B,** Magnetic spikes were measured at more than 20 sensor positions located 2 cm apart. In this patient, one similar, unaveraged magnetic spike, out of a total of four spike types, was displayed over the right temporal region. **C,** *Dots* represent the locations where the magnetic measurements were made. From the distribution of the amplitude of the same magnetic spike, sampling the signal at the spike peak, an isofield contour map was made and the equivalent current source was calculated for this particular field pattern. **D,** Each of four dots in the temporal tip represents a different spike type. Electrocorticography (ECoG) showed epileptiform activity in the *shaded area* of the right temporal lobe, which was surgically removed. In this case, the MEG results matched well with the ECoG findings.

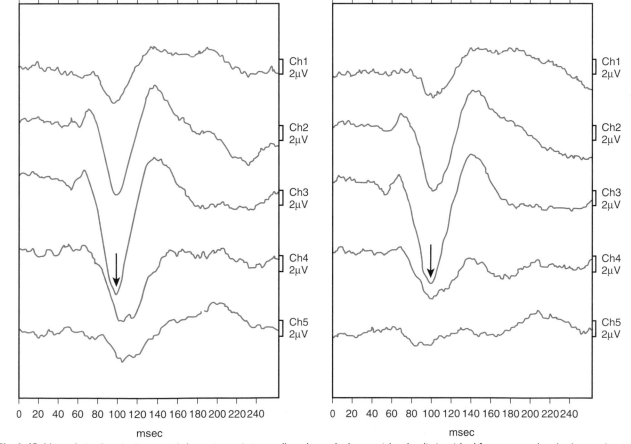

Fig. 1-45. Normal visual evoked potential. Averaging techniques allow the evoked potential to be distinguished from any random background activity.

During muscle contraction, the nature of the motor unit potentials can be assessed. As the force of contraction increases, the motor unit potentials coalesce to form an interference pattern that eventually completely obscures the baseline (see Fig. 1-60, *D*). In neuropathic disorders, the motor units lessen in number and tend to be prolonged and polyphasic. In primary muscle disease, amplitude and duration of the potentials lessen, often, again, with polyphasia.

Single-Fiber Studies

Recording action potentials from individual muscle fibers shows that for two fibers belonging to the same motor unit, a slight difference in timing occurs, which varies slightly between consecutive discharges because of variability in delay of conduction at their respective neuromuscular junctions (known as jitter) (Fig. 1-61). This phenomenon is accentuated in myasthenia gravis.

BIOPSY

Muscle Biopsy

Muscle biopsy can be performed by needle or as an open procedure. The former is less invasive and allows multiple samples to be obtained; the latter allows better assessment of tissue architecture and is more sensitive for the detection of focal processes such as inflammation. In normal muscle, the fibers lie in close relationship to one another, with one or more peripheral nuclei. Some variability of fiber size occurs in normal subjects (Fig. 1-62).

Staining techniques allow separation of muscle into different fiber types. Myofibrillar adenosine triphosphatase (ATPase) at pH 9.4 produces a dark-staining reaction in type II (fast-reacting) fibers and a light reaction in type I fibers (Fig. 1-63). With nicotinamide dinucleotide tetrazolium reductase (NADH-tr), the reverse staining reaction is found, with some differential staining among type II fibers.

The distribution of fiber type varies from muscle to muscle. An increased proportion of one fiber type, or a selective atrophy, is a recognized consequence of certain muscle disorders.

Nerve Biopsy

Nerve biopsy is sometimes of value when attempting to clarify the diagnosis or classification of certain peripheral nerve disorders. The sural nerve is usually chosen, largely because it is very commonly affected by the peripheral neuropathies, and also because its sacrifice is of little consequence to most patients. It is of sufficient size to allow a number of fascicles, each around 3 to 4 cm in length, to be dissected free from the main trunk (Fig. 1-64). Part of the material is used for the preparation of teased fibers and part for the preparation of transverse and longitudinal sections.

The teased fiber preparation demonstrates the nodes of Ranvier and the Schwann cells (Fig. 1-65). The internodal length and its variability can be calculated, along with the thickness of the myelin sheath. In transverse section, the nerve fibers appear as circles, the size of which is determined by the thickness of the myelin sheath. Groups of fibers are bound together by an encircling connective tissue (the perineurium) (Fig. 1-66), forming a fasciculus. In turn, the fasciculi are bound together in a further layer of connective tissue, the epineurium. Blood vessels run within the epineurium and then divide to supply capillary branches to the individual fibers and their surrounding endoneurium (Fig. 1-67).

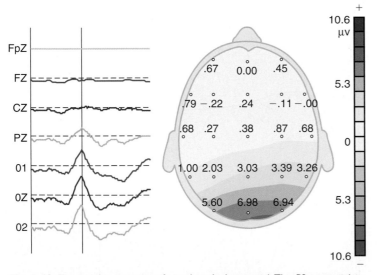

Fig. 1-46. Topographic mapping of visual evoked potential. The P2 potential is shown pointing upward on the *left side* of the figure and has a maximal amplitude (*red* on the *right-hand side*) at the O₂ and Oz channels.

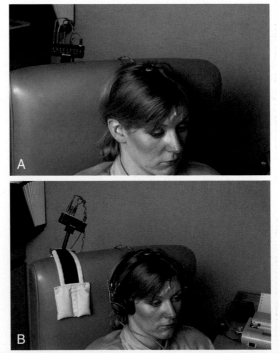

Fig. 1-47. Electrode placement **(A)** and headphones in position **(B)** for measurement of auditory evoked responses.

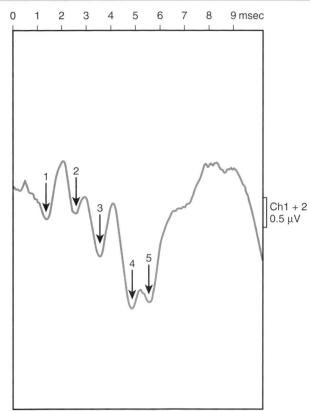

Fig. 1-48. Normal brainstem evoked potentials using a 70-dB stimulus. Waves VI and VII are often ill defined and have not been demonstrated here.

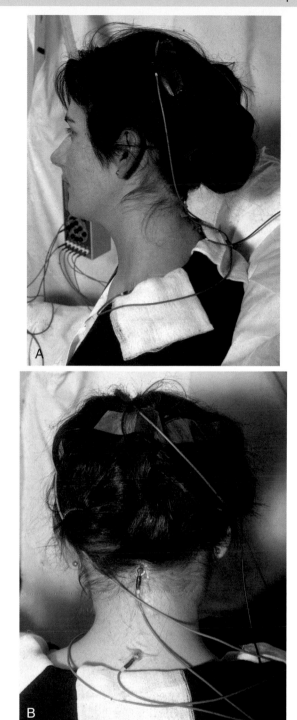

Fig. 1-49. Electrode placement for somatosensory evoked potentials. Lateral **(A)** and posterior **(B)** views.

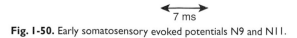

Fig. 1-50. Early somatosensory evoked potentials N9 and N11.

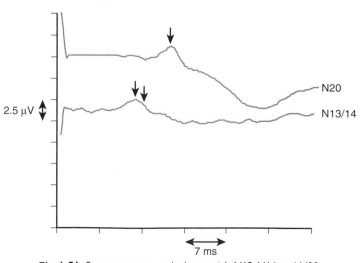

Fig. 1-51. Somatosensory evoked potentials N13, N14, and N20.

ELECTROMAGNETIC STIMULATION

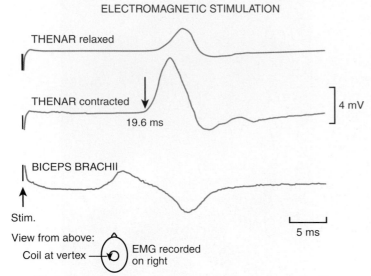

THENAR relaxed

THENAR contracted

19.6 ms

4 mV

BICEPS BRACHII

Stim.

View from above:

Coil at vertex ——— EMG recorded on right

5 ms

Fig. 1-52. Central motor conduction. Response from a normal subject.

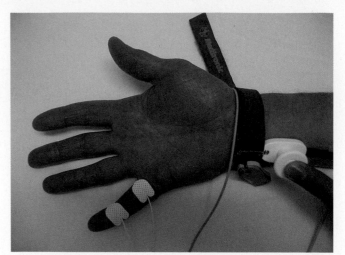

Fig. 1-53. Electrodes attached to the little finger with the recording electrode over the ulnar nerve at the wrist.

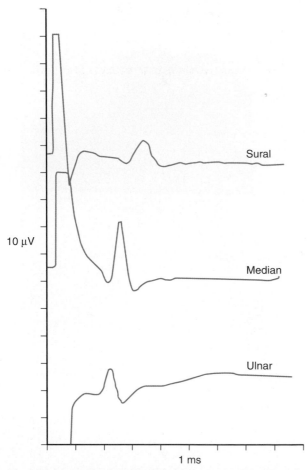

Sural

Median

10 µV

Ulnar

1 ms

Fig. 1-54. Normal sural, median, and ulnar sensory action potentials.

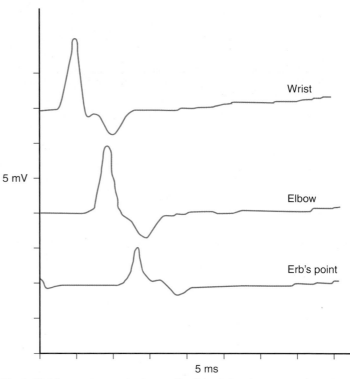

Wrist

5 mV

Elbow

Erb's point

5 ms

Fig. 1-55. Ulnar motor conduction studies. Stimulating the nerve at the wrist, at the elbow, and at Erb's point.

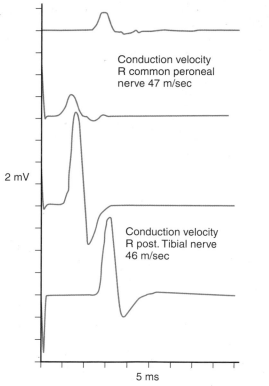

2 mV

Conduction velocity
R common peroneal
nerve 47 m/sec

Conduction velocity
R post. Tibial nerve
46 m/sec

5 ms

Fig. 1-56. Measurement of motor conduction velocity in the right common peroneal and right posterior tibial nerves.

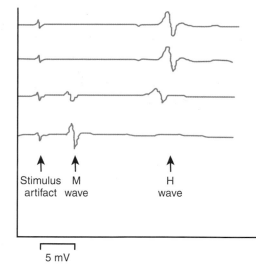

Stimulus   M   H
artifact   wave   wave

5 mV

Fig. 1-57. As the stimulus strength increases (from higher to lower), the H reflex diminishes and the M response appears.

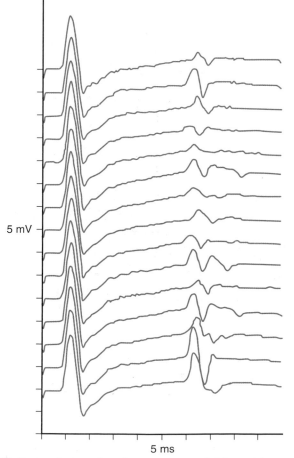

5 mV

5 ms

Fig. 1-58. F wave. A succession of responses recorded from abductor pollicis brevis after stimulation of the median nerve at the wrist.

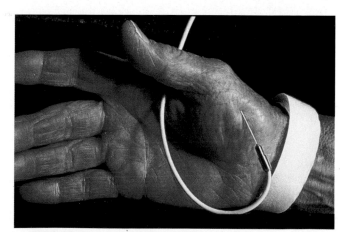

Fig. 1-59. Concentric needle electrode in abductor pollicis brevis.

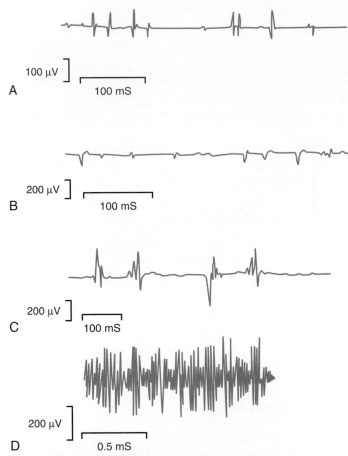

A   100 µV

100 mS

B   200 µV

100 mS

C   200 µV

100 mS

D   200 µV

0.5 mS

Fig. 1-60. Electromyographic findings. **A,** Fibrillation potentials. **B,** Positive sharp waves. **C,** Fasciculation potentials. **D,** Normal interference pattern.

JITTER

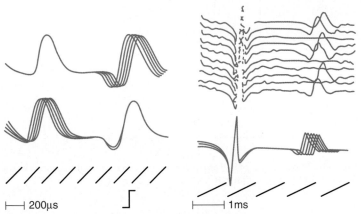

200µs   1ms

Fig. 1-61. In normal subjects, the slight variability of delay in conduction at the neuromuscular junctions of two fibers belonging to the same motor unit can be recorded.

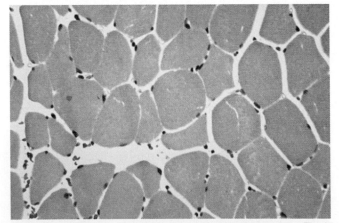

Fig. 1-62. Normal muscle cells are approximately hexagonal in shape. The blue-staining nuclei are visible beneath the cell membrane (H&E ×600).

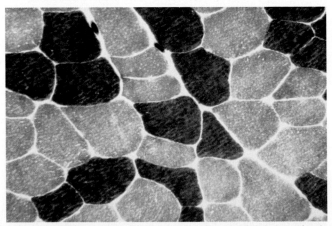

Fig. 1-63. Normal muscle. Type I (slow-reactive) fibers are lightly stained and type II (fast-reactive) fibers are darkly stained (ATPase [at pH 9.4]; ×600).

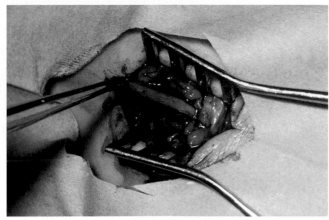

Fig. 1-64. Sural nerve biopsy.

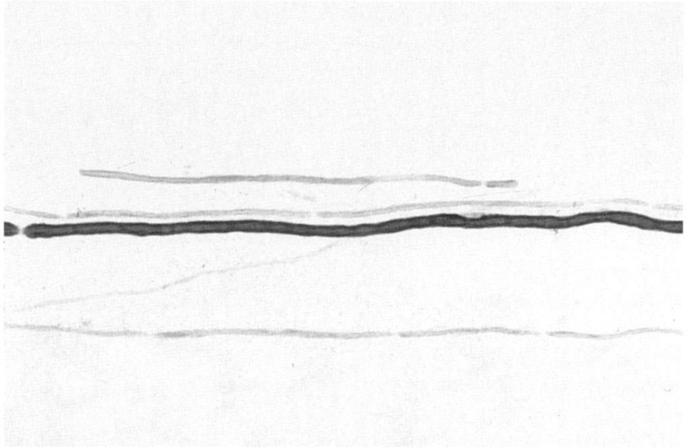

Fig. 1-65. Teased-fiber preparation of normal peripheral nerve. A node of Ranvier is seen toward the left end of the fiber, with a Schwann cell toward the right.

Blood vessel

Endoneurium

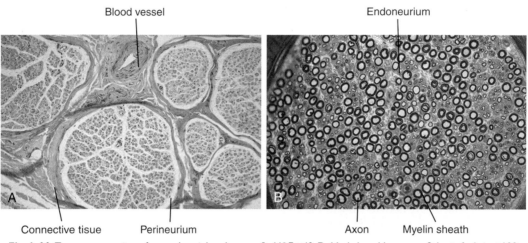

Connective tisue   Perineurium

Axon   Myelin sheath

Fig. 1-66. Transverse section of normal peripheral nerve. **A,** H&E ×40. **B,** Methylene blue, azure 2, basic fuchsin; ×100.

Longitudinally
arrayed fibers

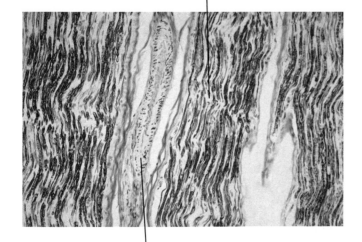

Blood vessel

Fig. 1-67. Longitudinal section of normal peripheral nerve (Luxol fast blue/Nissl; ×40).

MOTOR NEURON AND PERIPHERAL NERVE DISEASES

Motor neuron diseases (MND) comprise a number of conditions, generally sporadic but occasionally inherited, characterized by lower motor neuron degeneration (anterior horn cell disease), usually in combination with signs of degeneration in other neuronal systems. Amyotrophic lateral sclerosis (ALS), the classic form of motor neuron disease first described by Charcot, is the most common, with an annual incidence of 2 per 100,000 per year and a prevalence of 4 to 7 per 100,000. This form of MND has signs of both anterior horn cell disease and upper motor neuron dysfunction. Cells and tracts in other systems are also involved in the pathology, however. This may not be evident clinically, although in some cases there may be features of frontotemporal dementia (FTD) and, rarely, progressive supranuclear gaze paresis and extrapyramidal features.

The common idiopathic sporadic form of motor neuron disease includes the clinically defined variants sporadic ALS (SALS), progressive bulbar palsy, progressive muscular atrophy (PMA), and primary lateral sclerosis. This disease is probably caused by interactions between certain genes, some of which have been identified, and environmental factors. There are also acquired sporadic motor neuron diseases, secondary to systemic disease, drugs, or toxins. These exclusively lower motor neuron syndromes include postpolio muscular atrophy, the rare Hopkins' postasthmatic amyotrophy, and paraneoplastic amyotrophy (Box 2-1).

Genetic motor neuron diseases include the spinal muscular atrophies and familial motor neuron diseases (referred to collectively as familial amyotrophic lateral sclerosis [FALS]). A number of genes causing FALS have been identified. Some mutations produce a condition indistinguishable from SALS (indeed, rare cases of apparently sporadic disease harbor mutations in these genes), whereas other forms largely entail lower motor neuron disease and additional atypical features. Also, a number of other rare nonfamilial conditions are definitely or probably genetically determined, in which the clinical signs of lower motor neuron disease are associated with prominent bulbar symptoms and signs. These include Kennedy's disease, the Madras form of motor neuron disease, Brown–Vialetto–Van Laere syndrome, and Fazio-Londe disease.

PATHOGENESIS OF MOTOR NEURON DISEASE

The common form of MND is caused by degeneration of upper and lower motor neurons in the spinal cord and brainstem, resulting in degeneration of corticobulbar and corticospinal tracts (Fig. 2-1) and thinning of the anterior nerve roots (Fig. 2-2). Interneurons are also affected, and there may be pathologic involvement of other neuronal systems and pathways in atypical forms. Vague sensory symptoms may occur, but there is no objective clinical evidence of sensory impairment. Cramps are a common complaint, and patients are often aware of fasciculation, especially in the early stages.

The destruction of anterior horn cells begins with accumulation of skeins of ubiquitinated proteins in the cytoplasm of affected motor neurons (Fig. 2-3) and the formation of characteristic cytoplasmic masses—Bunina bodies and Hirano bodies—together with axonal spheroids derived from neurofilaments in the proximal parts of axons (Fig. 2-4). It has recently been established that the principal ubiquitinated protein in the neurons in SALS is *TDP-43* (TAR DNA binding protein, 43 kD). Mutations in the *TARDBP* gene also cause a form of FALS, and this ubiquitinated protein accumulates in the neurons in the commonest form of FTD.

Loss of neurons is followed by gliosis and shrinkage of the anterior horn. The motor neurons of the lateral aspect of the ventral horns of the sacral cord—Onuf's nucleus—are typically spared, so sphincteric function is preserved. The motor neurons supplying the extraocular muscles are usually involved only late in the course of the disease.

CLINICAL VARIANTS OF CLASSIC MOTOR NEURON DISEASE

The four clinical variants of the common form of MND reflect differences in the extent of upper and lower motor neuron involvement and the site of onset of the disease, but the underlying pathology is the same in all forms.

Amyotrophic lateral sclerosis is characterized by signs of both lower motor neuron involvement (muscular atrophy and fasciculation) and upper motor neuron signs (such as spasticity, hyperreflexia, and Babinski responses). As a rule, lower motor neuron symptoms and signs are asymmetrical at the outset, and the next area of involvement is contiguous. For example, wasting of the small muscles of one hand, indicating cervical cord disease, is usually followed by involvement of other parts of the same arm, and then the other hand and arm, before lower motor neuron signs appear in the legs (Fig. 2-5).

In progressive bulbar palsy, disease begins in the lower brainstem, causing dysphagia, dysarthria, and dysphonia. Bilateral wasting and fasciculation of the tongue are virtually pathognomonic of the condition (Fig. 2-6). The symptoms and signs of the disease may remain localized to this area for some time, and it can be difficult to confirm the diagnosis electrophysiologically in the limb muscles. Aspiration, with the risk of pneumonia, is a common complication at an early stage. Pseudobulbar palsy, characterized by tongue spasticity, spastic dysarthria, and emotional lability, with inappropriate laughing and crying, results from degeneration of the corticobulbar tracts.

Progressive muscular atrophy is a predominantly lower motor neuron syndrome, in which slowly progressive muscular atrophy of the limbs occurs with few or no upper motor signs. Fasciculation may not be prominent. The reflexes are usually preserved despite the atrophy, at least in the early stages. The condition tends to be more benign than classic ALS.

Recent work has shown that homozygous deletions of exon 7 of *SMN2,* the centromeric homologue of the telomeric survival motor neuron gene *(SMN1)* implicated in the common form of spinal muscular atrophy (see later), predispose to an adult-onset lower motor neuron disease. However, it is not yet clear that this condition is a form of typical MND, and the role of copy number variations in *SMN1* and *SMN2* in the pathogenesis of MND is currently unclear.

The obverse of PMA is primary lateral sclerosis, a rare disorder that appears with progressive spastic tetraparesis, often with early bulbar dysfunction (progressive bulbospinal spasticity). Evidence of lower motor neuron involvement may be difficult to demonstrate, even by electromyography (EMG). Atrophy of the prefrontal gyrus may be seen on magnetic resonance imaging (MRI) brain scan. The natural history of this form, like that of PMA, tends to be more benign and protracted than ALS.

BOX 2-1   SPORADIC MOTOR NEURON DISEASE

Motor Neuron Disease (MND)
- Amyotrophic lateral sclerosis (ALS)
- Progressive bulbar palsy (PBP)
- Progressive muscular atrophy (PMA)
- Primary lateral sclerosis (PLS)
- Atypical ALS
  - With frontotemporal dementia
  - With ophthalmoplegia and extrapyramidal features
  - Western Pacific ALS

Monomelic Amyotrophy
- Upper extremity (Hirayama)
- Lower extremity

Acquired Sporadic Motor Neuron Diseases
- Postpolio syndrome
- Hopkins syndrome
- Paraneoplastic amyotrophy

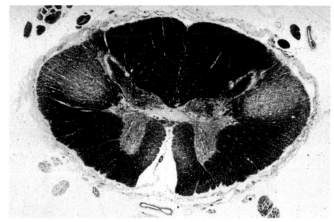

Fig. 2-1. Myelin preparation of thoracic cord in motor neuron disease, showing marked pallor of lateral and anterior corticospinal tracts.

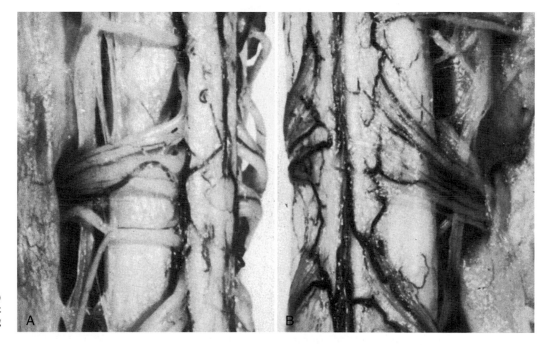

Fig. 2-2. Posterior **(A)** and anterior **(B)** nerve roots from the cervical cord of a patient with motor neuron disease. Note the thinning of the anterior roots.

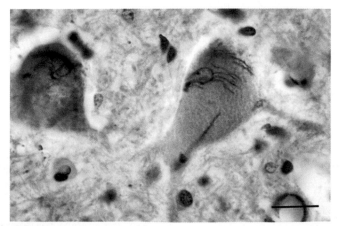

Fig. 2-3. Motor neuron disease. Ubiquitinated protein skeins in the cytoplasm of the cell body of a motor neuron. (Marker = 20 μm; ×100.)

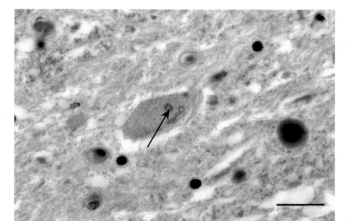

Fig. 2-4. Motor neuron disease. Bunina body in an anterior horn cell neuron. (Marker = 20 μm; ×100.)

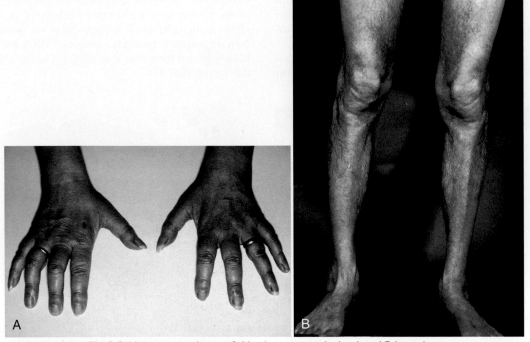

Fig. 2-5. Motor neuron disease. **A** Muscle wasting in the hands and **B** lower legs.

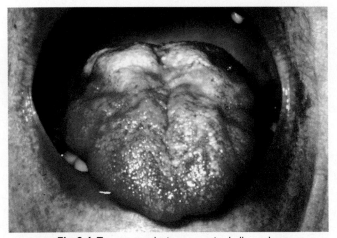

Fig. 2-6. Tongue atrophy in progressive bulbar palsy.

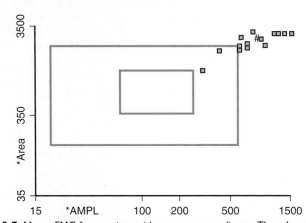

MACRO EMG

Fig. 2-7. Macro-EMG from patient with motor neuron disease. The values for the median amplitude and area of the motor unit potentials should lie within the small rectangle, and those for the 20 individual motor units within the large rectangle (shaded squares). Only two individual motor units have normal values for macro amplitude and area in this patient. The median is also well above the upper normal limits for amplitude and area. This pattern is typical of chronic denervation and reinnervation.

Diagnosis can usually be made on clinical grounds but needs to be supported by electromyography. A combination of fibrillation and fasciculation potentials at rest in muscles of several limbs, together with other features of denervation and reinnervation, is characteristic, and particularly clearly shown by macro-EMG (Fig. 2-7). There may be slight slowing of motor conduction in peripheral nerves as a result of dropout of large axons, and slowing of conduction in central motor pathways may be demonstrated by transcranial magnetic stimulation. Occasionally, degeneration of the corticospinal tracts can be seen as symmetrical high-signal abnormalities on MRI of the brainstem and spinal cord.

The serum creatine kinase level is modestly increased in half of all cases, largely relative to the degree of limb involvement. A level of more than 1000 U/L would be unusual.

Muscle biopsy is rarely required but may be helpful in difficult cases. The changes are typical of chronic denervation, with target cells, small denervated atrophic fibers, grouped-fiber atrophy, and fiber-type grouping. Recent studies also suggest that expression of neuronal nitric oxide synthetase (nNOS) at the sarcolemma is lost in denervation, and this can be a useful marker of a primary denervating process such as MND when the clinical picture is atypical (Fig. 2-8).

The diagnosis of motor neuron disease is defined by the El Escorial criteria, which can be summarized as follows:

Definite ALS: evidence of disease (upper and lower motor neuron signs, plus compatible neurophysiologic or pathologic abnormalities) in three regions of the body
Probable ALS: two regions affected
Possible ALS: one region affected

ATYPICAL AMYOTROPHIC LATERAL SCLEROSIS

Rarely, additional clinical and pathologic features can complicate ALS. The commonest of these is frontotemporal dementia, characterized by dementia, dysphasia, and personality and behavioral abnormalities, particularly loss of judgment and insight, which may either precede or follow the development of ALS. Another rare form is associated with vertical supranuclear gaze paresis, in isolation or with involuntary movements, including tremor, rigidity, and ballism.

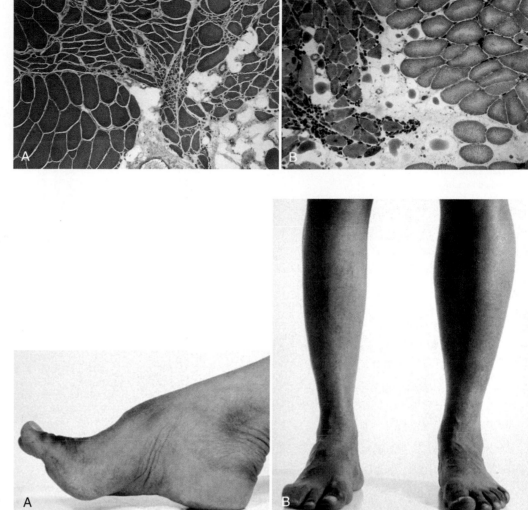

Fig. 2-8. Muscle biopsy from patient with motor neuron disease. **A,** Grouped-fiber atrophy (H&E). **B,** NADH-tr stain shows that the atrophic denervated fibers are of both main types (type 1, dark; type 2, paler), whereas the larger reinnervated fibers are type 2.

Fig. 2-9. Polio. **A,** Pes cavus deformity. **B,** Wasting of the right leg.

Western Pacific ALS, sometimes referred to as Guamanian ALS–parkinsonism–dementia complex, occurs in clusters in the Mariana Islands, Guam, and the Kii peninsula of Japan. It may result from ingested neurotoxins in a genetically susceptible population. However, Guamanian-type ALS can occasionally be seen elsewhere.

MONOMELIC AMYOTROPHY

Occasionally, a single limb develops slowly progressive atrophy. If upper motor neuron features are also present, careful EMG studies usually demonstrate subclinical involvement in other areas, and most such patients prove to have ALS. However, progressive weakness and wasting of one arm with features of a purely lower motor neuron syndrome may occur (Hirayama disease). This has been attributed to cervical cord compression by an inelastic dura. Most of these patients are male, and the condition may be familial. A rare lower limb amyotrophy syndrome, affecting particularly the posterior compartment muscles below the knee, has also been described.

ACQUIRED SPORADIC MOTOR NEURON DISEASES

Several lower motor neuron syndromes are believed to result from disease of anterior horn cells unrelated to the processes described thus far. These need to be distinguished from motor neuropathies and neuronopathies.

Postpolio muscular atrophy is defined as the development of new weakness and wasting in muscles previously affected by polio, or in additional muscle groups remote from the original involvement, after more than 15 years of stability. EMG shows active denervation in these newly affected areas. There are no upper motor neuron signs

(Fig. 2-9). If this is associated with chronic fatigue, myalgia, and other nonspecific symptoms, the diagnosis is postpolio syndrome. However, most cases of "postpolio syndrome" result from secondary musculoskeletal disorders and are not associated with postpolio muscular atrophy. There is some evidence that postpolio muscular atrophy may result from a chronic inflammatory process associated with raised levels of cytokines in the CSF, and this may respond to intravenous immunoglobulin.

Hopkins' syndrome (postasthmatic amyotrophy) is a very rare condition in adolescents, in which rapidly progressive weakness and wasting of a limb develops some 2 weeks after an acute asthmatic attack. Again, this may be immunologically mediated, with meningism, CSF pleocytosis, and signal abnormality in the spinal cord.

Rarely, a paraneoplastic lower motor neuron syndrome accompanies or precedes the development of a neoplasm, particularly non-Hodgkin's lymphoma, other lymphomas, and myeloproliferative disorders.

GENETIC MOTOR NEURON DISEASES

Conditions comprising the main groups of hereditary and familial motor neuron diseases are shown in Box 2-2.

SPINAL MUSCULAR ATROPHIES

Spinal muscular atrophies result from degeneration of motor neurons in the anterior horns. They are exclusively lower motor neuron syndromes. The common form of spinal muscular atrophy (SMA1) is an autosomal recessive disease, caused in greater than 95% of cases by

BOX 2-2   SOME HEREDITARY AND FAMILIAL MOTOR NEURON DISEASES

Spinal Muscular Atrophies (SMAs)
- Recessive 5q11-13 *SMN* (survival motor neuron gene)
  - Werdnig-Hoffmann disease
  - Intermediate form
  - Kugelberg-Welander disease
  - Adult onset
- Other forms: dominant, recessive, X-linked, including the following:
  - Scapuloperoneal SMA
  - Distal SMA

Bulbar Syndromes
- X-linked recessive
  - Xq12-13 Kennedy's disease *Androgen receptor*
- Recessive
  - Fazio-Londe disease
  - Brown–Vialetto–van Laere syndrome
  - Madras motor neuron disease

Familial (Hereditary) Amyotrophic Lateral Sclerosis (FALS)
- Dominant
  - FALS-1 21q22.1 superoxide dismutase (SOD1)
  - Other dominant forms, including the following:
    - With frontotemporal dementia 9q21-22
    - Others, such as 9q34 *sentaxin* and neurofilament heavy-chain subunit
- Recessive
  - FALS-2 2q33 *alsin*
- X-linked

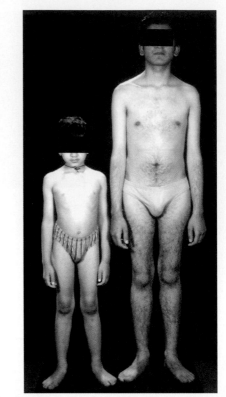

Fig. 2-11. Kugelberg-Welander disease. The older brother presented with suspected polymyositis with a high creatine kinase level and a "myopathic" biopsy. His younger brother had very mild weakness but biopsy changes of chronic denervation and reinnervation. Both patients had deletions of exons 7 and 8 of the telomeric *SMN* gene.

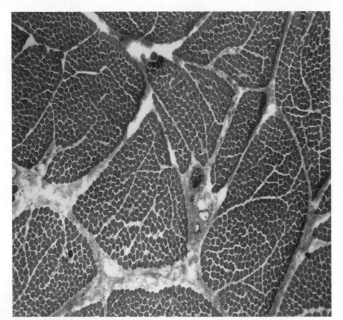

Fig. 2-10. Werdnig-Hoffmann disease. Muscle biopsy shows swathes of atrophic, denervated fibers.

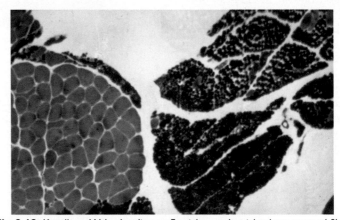

Fig. 2-12. Kugelberg-Welander disease. Fascicles on the right show grouped fiber atrophy, reflecting denervation of both main fiber types. The fascicle on the left shows fiber-type grouping, the result of reinnervation of large numbers of fibers by surviving motor neurons—in this case, type 2.

mutations in the telomeric survival motor neuron *(SMN1)* gene on 5q11-13. SMA1 is the commonest human autosomal recessive disease after cystic fibrosis. A rare form not linked to this locus (SMA2) has also been described.

The expression of the centromeric homologue of the survival motor neuron gene *(SMN2)* influences the severity of the disease: Milder forms are associated with larger numbers of *SMN2* copies. The most severe form, type 1 SMA or Werdnig-Hoffmann disease, usually results from *SMN1* deletions together with a low *SMN2* gene copy number of less than 2. The affected infant is grossly hypotonic and areflexic, with breathing and suckling difficulties. Tongue fasciculations are diagnostic. There may be arthrogryposis. Death occurs within 6 months. Muscle biopsy shows generalized muscle fiber denervation without evidence of reinnervation (Fig. 2-10).

SMN2 copy numbers of 3 or more are associated with the intermediate infantile form (type II) and the milder Kugelberg-Welander disease (type III or adolescent SMA) (Fig. 2-11). Ambulation may be achieved with walking aids, and survival to adult life is possible. Neurophysiologic studies typically demonstrate chronic denervation changes with large-amplitude, long-duration potentials. Muscle biopsy shows grouped fiber atrophy and fiber type grouping in varying degrees (Fig. 2-12). However, the diagnosis can now be made by genetic testing, which usually demonstrates deletions of both copies of the *SMN1* gene (typically exons 7 and 8), although some cases have missense point mutations.

Patients with type IV SMA present in adult life with proximal weakness, suggesting a proximal myopathy but with reduced or absent reflexes (Fig. 2-13).

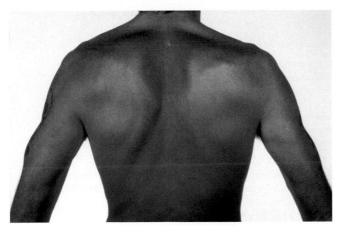

Fig. 2-13. Adult proximal spinal muscular atrophy.

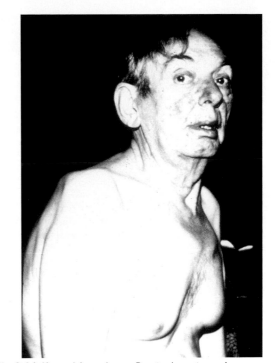

Fig. 2-14. Kennedy's syndrome. Proximal wasting and gynecomastia.

OTHER FORMS OF SPINAL MUSCULAR ATROPHY

A number of rare forms of SMA are caused by other genetic mutations, involving dominant, recessive, and X-linked inheritance, and with predilection for either proximal or distal muscles. The distal forms of SMA are difficult to distinguish from the hereditary motor neuropathies. SMA is also one cause of the scapuloperoneal syndrome (see Chapter 3).

BULBAR SYNDROMES

Several lower motor neuron syndromes affect particularly the bulbar musculature. Kennedy's disease (X-linked bulbospinal muscular atrophy) is the commonest adult-onset SMA. It affects only males. The causative mutation at Xq13 is a CAG triplet repeat expansion in the androgen receptor gene, which produces polyglutamine aggregates in the nuclei of motor neurons. It is thought that these interfere with nuclear function. Gynecomastia (Fig. 2-14) and testicular atrophy result from the associated androgen receptor deficiency.

The condition is characterized by slowly progressive dysphagia and dysarthria, difficulty with chewing, and bilateral facial and limb weakness, usually distal. Cramps and fasciculations are a common early feature, and mild tremor is also typical, affecting the fingers and sometimes the jaw. There are no upper motor signs, and the reflexes are depressed to absent. There may be subtle distal sensory impairments, and sensory nerve action potentials may show reduced amplitude. The diagnosis can be confirmed by genetic testing.

There is also a rare autosomal dominant condition with very similar features.

Fazio-Londe disease, or progressive bulbar palsy of childhood, is characterized by ptosis, bilateral facial and jaw weakness, and bulbar dysfunction, which may include respiratory stridor.

Brown-Vialetto-van *Laere* syndrome has similar features, but ptosis is not typical and there is severe sensorimotor deafness.

The *Madras* form of motor neuron disease, found mainly among peoples of southern India, shares some of these features, but there are often clinical features of ALS and sometimes other evidence of more widespread pathology, such as optic atrophy and cerebellar ataxia.

FAMILIAL MOTOR NEURON DISEASE

Some 5% to 10% of cases of MND are hereditary or familial. The discovery that mutations in the cytoplasmic superoxide dismutase gene on 21q22.1 (SOD1) account for only about 10% to 20% of such cases prompted a search for other loci, and nine additional genes have been identified, often in only one or two large families. Some of these are catalogued in Box 2-2. Six of these genotypes cause typical ALS, and in some the culpable gene and protein have been identified. Most are dominantly inherited.

ALS1, caused by SOD1 mutations, is the commonest. SOD1 mutations have also been reported in occasional cases of SALS. The disease appears to result from a toxic "gain of function" of SOD1 rather than loss of the antioxidative function of the enzyme.

Subtle cognitive abnormalities resulting from frontal lobe dysfunction can often be demonstrated in patients with sporadic ALS, and mutations in TARDP, resulting in TDP-43 accumulation in neurons in a form of FTD, also cause a form of FALS, although FALS-FTD can also be caused by mutations in genes on chromosome 9 (*ALS with FTD*, 9q21-22, 9p21-13).

PERIPHERAL NERVE DISEASES

The peripheral nervous system contains sensory, motor, and autonomic components. They are combined in the peripheral nerves, which communicate with the spinal cord through 21 paired nerve roots, each consisting of a dorsal (sensory) and ventral (motor) component. According to the distribution of the pathologic process, a number of peripheral nervous system disorders can be defined on anatomic grounds from clinical examination.

Peripheral neuropathy, or *polyneuropathy:* A disorder affecting the peripheral nerves diffusely, although sometimes predominantly affecting sensory, motor, or autonomic components
Radiculopathy (polyradiculopathy): A disorder affecting one or multiple nerve roots
Mononeuropathy: A disorder of a single peripheral nerve
Mononeuritis multiplex: A disorder of several anatomically disparate peripheral nerves, usually characterized by rapidly evolving pain and sensory abnormality followed by weakness and wasting in the innervated muscles. More insidious but clinically similar forms are sometimes referred to as *multiple mononeuropathy*.
Plexopathy: A disorder of the brachial or lumbosacral plexus.

PERIPHERAL NEUROPATHY

In polyneuropathy, there is a generalized involvement of peripheral nerve function, usually symmetrically and with a distal predominance. Typically, there is distal sensory loss with muscle weakness and hypoflexia or areflexia. In some cases, the major site of nerve

---

BOX 2-3 ETIOLOGIC CLASSIFICATION OF PERIPHERAL NEUROPATHIES

- Genetic
- Metabolic and endocrine disorders
- Nutritional and deficiency disorders
- Infectious
- Immune mediated
  - Postinfectious (Guillain-Barré syndrome, Miller Fisher syndrome)
  - Chronic inflammatory demyelinating polyradiculoneuropathy, multifocal motor neuropathy with conduction block
  - Paraproteinemic
  - Paraneoplastic
  - Vasculitic
  - Polyarteritis nodosa
  - Antineutrophil cytoplasmic antibody associated (Churg-Strauss, Wegener's)
  - Connective tissue disease (rheumatoid, Sjögren's, systemic lupus erythematosus)
  - Hypersensitivity vasculitis (drugs, malignancy)
  - Isolated peripheral nerve vasculitis
- Drugs, toxins
- Drug-induced
- Unknown cause
  - ?Age-related degeneration

BOX 2-4 CLASSIFICATION OF THE GENETIC NEUROPATHIES

Neuropathies with Neuropathy as the Sole or Predominant Part of the Disease
- Hereditary motor and sensory neuropathies (HMSN; Charcot-Marie-Tooth disease)
- Hereditary sensory and autonomic neuropathy (HSAN)
- Hereditary neuralgic amyotrophy
- Hereditary neuropathy with liability to pressure palsies (HNPP)
- Distal hereditary motor neuropathies (distal HMN)

Neuropathies with Neuropathy as Part of a More Widespread Genetic Neurologic or Multisystem Disorder
- Porphyria
- Disorders of lipid metabolism
- Familial amyloid polyneuropathies (FAP)
- Disorders with defective DNA
- Neuropathies associated with mitochondrial disease
- Neuropathy in hereditary ataxias

---

damage is proximal, although this more often applies to the motor than the sensory component.

The predominant locus of damage can be either the axon or the myelin sheath. This selectivity can be used as a pathologic classification of peripheral neuropathy; thus, neuropathies can be described as axonal or demyelinating. However, secondary axonal and demyelinating changes are commonly superimposed on the primary process, which can cause confusion.

Neuropathies can be further classified with regard to the relative degree of motor, sensory, or autonomic fiber involvement (e.g., axonal sensory polyneuropathy, predominantly motor demyelinating polyneuropathy).

Classification can also be based on the etiology of the disease process underlying the nerve damage (Box 2-3).

GENETICALLY DETERMINED NEUROPATHIES

The most common forms of genetic neuropathy are caused by mutations in genes that determine factors such as compaction and maintenance of myelin, neuronal cytoskeletal function, axonal transport, and mitochondrial metabolism. In other forms, there are abnormalities in specific metabolic pathways that may involve nerves exclusively, although in most the neuropathy is part of a multisystem disorder (Box 2-4). Only the most commonly encountered conditions will be considered here.

CHARCOT-MARIE-TOOTH DISEASE

Hereditary sensory and motor neuropathy (HSMN) is the commonest hereditary neuromuscular disorder, with an estimated prevalence of 1 in 2500. The Charcot-Marie-Tooth (CMT) phenotype is characterized by slowly progressive distal weakness and wasting, resulting in a characteristic appearance of the feet and lower legs, variable wasting of the intrinsic hand muscles, depressed or absent reflexes, and impaired distal sensation. When clinical and neurophysiologic studies show only motor involvement, the condition is referred to as distal hereditary motor neuropathy (dHMN) but this is very rare.

HSMN is reasonably homogeneous clinically but is highly heterogeneous genetically. At least 25 genes causing the disease have now been defined, and a precise genetic diagnosis can be provided in about 70% of cases. Many subtypes of CMT are now recognized,

therefore, but the classification is complex, not least because some phenotypes can be caused by mutations in several different genes.

Mild forms of CMT may be asymptomatic, but the condition usually comes to attention in the first 2 decades of life because of symptoms such as progressive foot deformity, tendency to trip or twist the ankles, numbness, cramps, gait disturbance, cold feet, and loss of dexterity. The symptoms and signs show a distal-to-proximal evolution. Motor symptoms start in the feet, with intrinsic muscle atrophy resulting in pes cavus and hammer toes (Fig. 2-15, *A*). The atrophy spreads proximally, involving particularly the lower third of the peronei (hence the older term peroneal muscular atrophy); and anterior tibial muscles, which may result in the classic "champagne bottle" appearance of the legs. Axonal forms may demonstrate more diffuse distal atrophy (see Fig. 2-15, *B*). Motor involvement of the hands and arms follows (Fig. 2-16), again from distal to proximal. Sensory loss follows a similar anatomic pattern and can involve all modalities, although the extent and characteristics of impairment vary in different subtypes. Finger and hand tremors, leg and foot cramps, acrocyanosis, and pain are common. CMT is also a very rare cause of floppy baby syndrome and delayed motor development.

Some CMT subtypes can be associated with white matter lesions in the brain (e.g., CMT1X, CMT2A) and pyramidal tract signs (CMT2A, CMT5). Very rare forms can have vocal cord paresis, facial nerve involvement, sensorineural deafness (CMT2A, CMT4), diaphragmatic weakness (CMT4), and optic atrophy with severe visual impairment (CMT2A, CMT6).

The family history is usually helpful. Most forms of CMT are inherited as autosomal dominants, but some affected family members may be largely asymptomatic. It is often helpful to examine other family members clinically and neurophysiologically to define the mode of inheritance more clearly. X-linked dominant inheritance, characterized by no male-to-male transmission and more severe manifestations in hemizygous males than heterozygous females, is also common (CMTX1). Autosomal recessive disease is rare, except in consanguineous families, and tends to be more severe, often appearing in childhood or infancy.

Before molecular genetic diagnosis became widely available (Table 2-1), diagnosis and classification were based on nerve conduction and sural nerve biopsy criteria:

Type 1. Demyelinating forms. Upper limb motor conduction less than 38 m/sec. Sural nerve biopsy shows clear evidence of demyelination and remyelination, with "onion bulb" formation (Fig. 2-17).

Type 2. Axonal forms. Mild upper limb motor slowing, but greater than 38 m/sec, with chronic denervation changes on EMG. Sural nerve biopsy shows typical axonal degeneration.

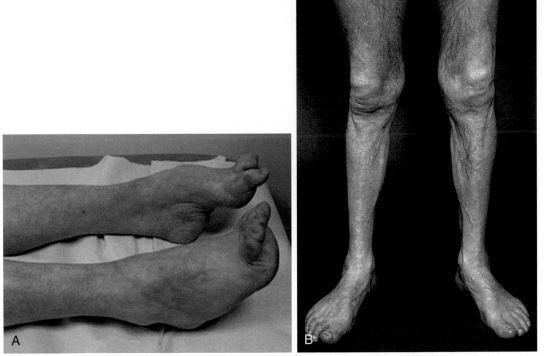

Fig. 2-15. Charcot-Marie-Tooth disease, type IA. **A,** Pes cavus and hammer toes. **B,** Diffuse distal lower limb wasting in CMT2.

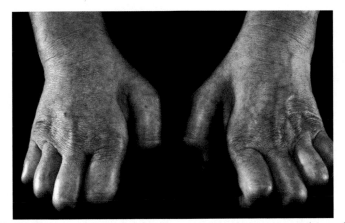

Fig. 2-16. Wasting of the hands in hereditary sensory and motor neuropathy type I.

the peripheral myelin protein PMP22 gene at 17p11.2, but some cases are the result of point mutations. However, deletions of this locus produce hereditary neuropathy with liability to pressure palsies (see later). CMT1B is a more severe disease that results from mutations in the myelin protein P_0 gene on 1q22. Other CMT1 genotypes are very rare.

X-linked dominant CMT (CMTX1) closely resembles CMT1A. The disease is caused by point mutations in the connexin 32 gene at Xq13 (Fig. 2-18). X-linked recessive CMT is severe, very rare, and largely confined to infants and children. Autosomal recessive demyelinating CMT (CMT4) is also very rare and has been linked to eight loci to date. Most patients present in infancy or childhood.

CMT1 may also be associated with sensory ataxia and tremor of the fingers, referred to as Roussy-Levy syndrome, and these features are also a feature of the rare CMT1F.

Dejerine-Sottas disease (CMT3) is a severe phenotype that appears in childhood and leads to marked disability. There is striking reduction of conduction velocities associated with segmental demyelination, endoneural fibrosis, and Schwann cell proliferation (Fig. 2-19) with palpable nerve hypertrophy. The condition most often results from point mutations and homozygous mutations in the genes that determine the CMT1 phenotype, but both dominant and recessive forms are described.

However, secondary demyelination and axonal degeneration are common, and, in practice, many *intermediate* cases are seen. In addition, certain forms of CMT have intrinsic intermediate characteristics. In practice, therefore, it is now usual to consider the results of the neurophysiologic data in conjunction with the phenotype and pedigree data, and to screen for the more common genetic mutations in the first instance, rather than proceeding immediately to biopsy.

Demyelinating Charcot-Marie-Tooth

The vast majority of patients with CMT1 present before the age of 20 years. Distal weakness and wasting of the lower limbs are prominent, with a predilection for the peroneal and anterior tibial muscles. Pes cavus is characteristic and may suggest the diagnosis if a family history is lacking. Some sensory loss is present in the majority. Depression or absence of the deep tendon reflexes, at least at the ankles, is almost invariable. Distal wasting and weakness of the upper limbs usually follow. Enlargement of peripheral nerves is detectable in some patients with CMT1, reflecting the segmental demyelination and remyelination, with onion-bulb formation seen on biopsy.

Autosomal dominant demyelinating CMT (CMT1) is subdivided into types A, B, C, D, and F, according to the genetic basis. CMT1A is the commonest, accounting for about half of all cases of CMT. It is usually caused by a 1.5-Mb duplication of

Axonal Charcot-Marie-Tooth

Axonal CMT (CMT2) is genetically very heterogeneous and can be autosomal dominant or recessive (Fig. 2-20). Recessive disease is more severe. CMT2A, caused by mutations in the mitofusin gene, is the most prevalent subtype, accounting for 20% of axonal CMT. The phenotype can be complicated by white matter abnormalities in the brain, with pyramidal signs, optic atrophy, and sensorineural deafness. Mutations in MPZ account for a further 5% of cases (CMT2I/J), often with later onset of symptoms. Pupillary abnormalities, dysphagia, and pain can be features. Pes cavus, present in about two thirds of patients with CMT1, is less conspicuous in CMT2, and diffuse wasting is typical (see Figs. 2-15 and 2-20) and nerve enlargement is absent (see Fig. 2-18). Histology shows axonal degeneration with little segmental demyelination (Fig. 2-21).

TABLE 2-1.   GENETICS OF SOME COMMON FORMS OF CHARCOT-MARIE-TOOTH (CMT) DISEASE

TYPE AND PROPORTION OF CMT CASES	INHERITANCE	GENE	PROTEIN	FUNCTION
Demyelinating CMT				
CMT1A (40%–50%)	AD	*PMP22* 17p11.2 Duplication Point mutation (1%)	Peripheral myelin protein, 22 kD	Myelin compaction and maintenance
CMT1B (3%–5%)	AD	*MPZ* 1q22	Myelin protein zero (P₀)	
CMT3 (Dejerine-Sottas) <1%	Variable	*PMP 22, MPZ*, other genes	—	
CMTX1 (10%)	XD	*GJB1* Xq13.1	Connexin 32	Gap junction protein in myelin
CMT4 <1%	AR	*GDAP1* 8q13-q21.1 most commonly, but at least nine genes identified	Ganglioside-induced differentiation-associated protein 1, and others	Maintenance of mitochondrial network
Axonal CMT				
CMT2A (20% of CMT2)	AD	*MFN2*, 1p36.2	Mitofusin	Mitochondrial membrane functions

AD, autosomal dominant; AR, autosomal recessive; XD, X-linked dominant.

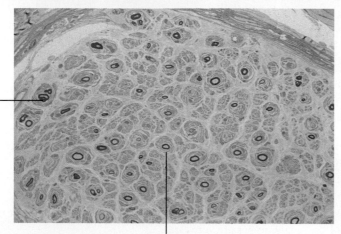

Onion bulb formation —

Increase in endonenrinm

Fig. 2-17. Nerve biopsy in hereditary sensory and motor neuropathy type 1. There is a major loss of large myelinated fibers. Surviving fibers show proliferation of Schwann cell processes resulting in "onion bulbs" (Thionine and acridine orange; ×100).

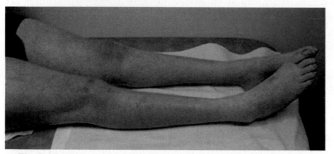

Fig. 2-18. Charcot-Marie-Tooth disease, type 1X in a female patient.

HEREDITARY NEUROPATHY WITH LIABILITY TO PRESSURE PALSIES

Hereditary neuropathy with liability to pressure palsies is associated with a deletion of the same 1.5-Mb portion of chromosome 17 that, when duplicated, causes CMT1A. Typically, patients develop a low-grade demyelinating neuropathy, superimposed on which are episodes of pressure palsies of individual nerves. The nerves particularly susceptible, therefore, are the median nerve at the wrist, causing carpal tunnel syndrome; the lateral popliteal nerve at the knee, resulting in footdrop; the radial nerve in the spiral groove, causing wrist drop; and the ulnar nerve at the elbow, causing tardy ulnar nerve palsy. Generally, the pressure palsies recover but permanent deficits can result (Fig. 2-22). Nerve conduction studies demonstrate a background neuropathy with, in addition, conduction block or severe slowing of motor conduction if relevant entrapment has occurred. Nerve biopsy reveals globular thickenings of the myelin sheath called tomacula, from the Greek word for sausage (Fig. 2-23).

HEREDITARY SENSORY AND AUTONOMIC NEUROPATHY

Hereditary sensory and autonomic neuropathy (HSAN) is classified into five subtypes, with three causative genes identified to date. Type 1 usually appears in the second decade. It is inherited as a dominant. Presenting features include sensory loss over the feet, pes cavus, and foot ulceration. Later, some muscle weakness with distal wasting may appear. Lancinating pains in the feet are characteristic. If foot care is unsatisfactory, progressive mutilation of the feet occurs, accompanied by bony changes as the result of recurrent osteomyelitis (acrodystrophic neuropathy) (Fig. 2-24). The sensory loss is initially dissociated, with loss of pain and temperature but preserved light touch, although this discrimination fades as the condition progresses. Sweating is lost or decreased over the areas of sensory change, but there is no involvement of sphincter function.

There is little or no change in motor conduction velocities, but sensory action potentials are absent. Peripheral nerves show a marked reduction of unmyelinated fibers, with relative preservation of large myelinated fibers. Examination of the dorsal roots shows a fallout of fibers, with secondary degeneration of the posterior columns (Fig. 2-25).

The other forms of HSAN are rare. Type III is also known as Riley-Day syndrome or familial dysautonomia. Type IV is associated with congenital insensitivity to pain (pain asymbolia) and anhidrosis. Self-mutilating behavior and mental retardation are associated features.

HEREDITARY NEURALGIC AMYOTROPHY

Hereditary neuralgic amyotrophy, also referred to as hereditary brachial plexus neuritis, is inherited as a dominant and usually appears between the ages of 10 and 30 years. It has been mapped

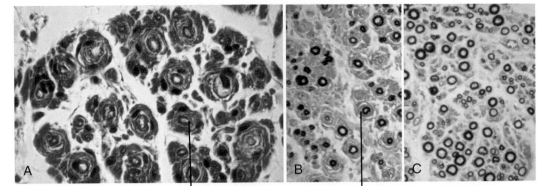

Fig. 2-19. Nerve biopsy from patient with Dejerine-Sottas disease. Collagen proliferation can be seen around the myelin sheaths (staining blue-green in **A**), with a reduction in the number of myelinated fibers in **B**. **C** control section. **A,** Masson's trichrome stain, ×350. **B** and **C,** Osmic acid stain, ×375.

Collagen thickening

Thickening around myelin sheath

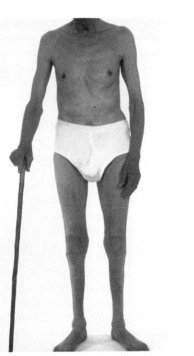

Fig. 2-20. Distal wasting in hereditary sensory and motor neuropathy type II.

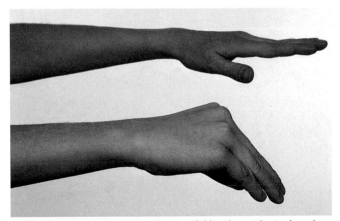

Fig. 2-22. Posterior interosseous palsy in a child with an inherited tendency to pressure palsies. There is a R wrist drop.

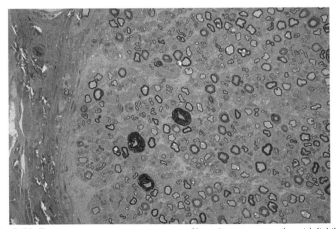

Fig. 2-23. Transverse nerve section in a case of hereditary neuropathy with liability to pressure palsies, showing tomaculous bodies (methylene blue, azure 2, basic fuchsin; ×100).

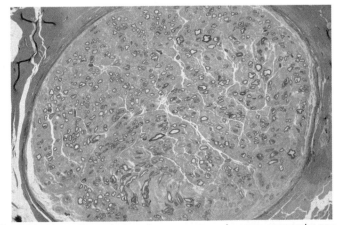

Fig. 2-21. Nerve biopsy in hereditary sensory and motor neuropathy type II. Note the absence of large fibers (methylene blue, azure 2, basic fuchsin; ×40).

to chromosome 17q24-q25. Affected individuals are often of short stature, with hypotelorism, small palpebral fissures, and syndactyly. Typically, there are recurrent episodes of pain with weakness predominantly affecting the proximal flexors of the arm and forearm supplied by the upper trunk of the plexus. Cranial nerves can be involved, and Horner's syndrome can occur. Sensory change is less conspicuous. With recurring episodes, residual deficit is likely

NEUROPATHIES AS PART OF GENETIC SYSTEMIC NEUROLOGIC DISEASES

PORPHYRIA

Acute neurovisceral attacks occur in acute intermittent porphyria, hereditary coproporphyria, variegate porphyria, and Doss porphyria (δ-aminolevulinic acid dehydratase deficiency). All but the last are

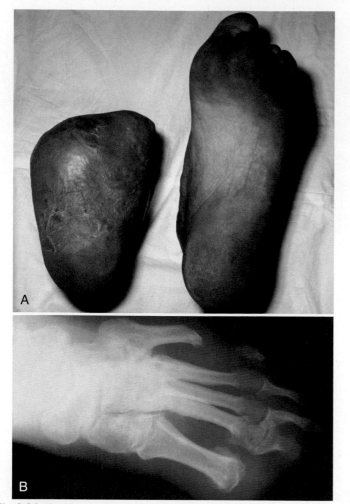

Fig. 2-24. Hereditary sensory and autonomic neuropathy type I. **A,** Foot mutilation in acrodystrophic neuropathy. **B,** Radiograph of the foot, showing bone destruction.

inherited as an autosomal dominant. Characteristic features of the attack include abdominal pain, usually with constipation rather than diarrhea, limb pain followed by substantial weakness, and various psychiatric phenomena including restlessness, delusions, and hallucinations. Sympathetic hyperactivity leads to hypertension, sweating, and tachycardia. Tonic–clonic seizures occur in about 10% of cases.

The neurologic presentation is identical to that of Guillain-Barré syndrome but with sensory sparing and evidence of axonal rather than demyelinating pathology. Typically, the patient's urine becomes discolored on standing because of the formation of oxidation products of porphobilinogen.

DISORDERS OF LIPID METABOLISM

Abetalipoproteinemia
Abetalipoproteinemia (Bassen-Kornzweig disease) is inherited as an autosomal recessive. Serum levels of cholesterol and triglyceride are severely reduced as a result of the absence of apolipoprotein B. Concentrations of fat-soluble vitamins, including vitamin E, are reduced. Clinical features include atypical retinitis pigmentosa (see Refsum's Disease, later), ataxia, peripheral neuropathy, and fat malabsorption. Hypobetalipoproteinemia is inherited as an autosomal dominant and is less severe (Fig. 2-26).

Tangier Disease
Tangier disease is inherited as a recessive. There is deficiency of high-density lipoproteins with reduced serum cholesterol concentrations. The condition appears in childhood with an axonal neuropathy and

enlarged, orange-colored tonsils. Occasionally, ptosis and ophthalmoplegia are seen (Fig. 2-27).

Refsum's Disease
The cardinal features of Refsum's disease (heredopathia atactica polyneuritiformis) include demyelinating polyneuropathy, pigmentary retinal degeneration, and sensorineural deafness. The retinal degeneration, a form of atypical retinitis pigmentosa, involves relatively fine granules (salt-and-pepper as opposed to the bone spicule pattern of typical retinitis pigmentosa) located forward of the periphery of the retina (Fig. 2-28) and leads to tunnel vision.

The neuropathy is symmetrical and results in distal weakness and wasting (Fig. 2-29). Other findings may include anosmia, cardiomyopathy, ichthyosis (Fig. 2-30), and a variety of skeletal abnormalities, particularly shortening of the fourth metatarsal bones (Fig. 2-31). All forms are autosomal recessive.

The commonest form usually appears in childhood or within the first 3 decades of life, and is caused by a deficiency of phytanoyl CoA hydroxylase, a peroxisomal enzyme coded at 10pter-p11.2. The enzyme deficiency results in defective chlorophyll metabolism and accumulation of phytanic acid. Distal sensory loss is common, and there may be palpable enlargement of peripheral nerves. Histology reveals reduction in the number of myelinated nerve fibers, with collagen thickening and Schwann cell proliferation. This syndrome may also result from peroxisomal dysfunction resulting from other genetic enzyme defects, with presentations in infancy to adult life.

FAMILIAL AMYLOID POLYNEUROPATHIES

Familial amyloid polyneuropathies (FAPs) are caused by extracellular deposition of amyloid derived from a mutated protein in the circulation. The most frequently involved protein is transthyretin (TTR), but the same clinical presentation may be caused by different variant proteins and different mutations, and individuals with the same mutation may have different clinical manifestations.

TTR-related familial amyloid polyneuropathy is inherited as an autosomal dominant. It appears in early adult life with sensory loss: pain and temperature sense are conspicuously affected. Lancinating pains are common. Later, other sensory modalities are affected and there is distal wasting and weakness (Fig. 2-32). Autonomic involvement is prominent, leading to impotence, constipation (sometimes alternating with diarrhea), incontinence, and loss of sweating. Postural hypotension is common, along with cardiac conduction defects. Pupillary abnormalities are characteristic, with an irregular indentation of the pupillary margins secondary to involvement of the ciliary body (Fig. 2-33). Nerve histology reveals, in addition to amyloid deposition, a substantial loss of unmyelinated fibers (Fig. 2-34). Focal deposits of amyloid can lead to compression of adjacent nerve tissue. Deposition in the flexor retinaculum, for example, is associated with the development of carpal tunnel syndrome. Deposits are also found in other organs, including the kidney and the brain.

Liver transplantation halts the progression of FAP.

METACHROMATIC LEUKODYSTROPHY

Most forms of metachromatic leukodystrophy are the consequence of arylsulfatase A deficiency. As a result, there is degeneration of myelin in the peripheral and central nervous systems. Different forms are described according to the age of onset, with the late infantile form (onset at 5 to 18 months) being the most common. Development of walking difficulty is associated with increasing lower limb weakness and flaccidity. Later, pyramidal signs can obscure the neuropathic features, although the reflexes are depressed; this condition is one cause of areflexia with upgoing plantar responses.

Peripheral nerve histology reveals segmental demyelination and remyelination, with an accumulation of metachromatic granules in Schwann cells and macrophages (Fig. 2-35). Electron microscopy demonstrates a number of different types of inclusions (Fig. 2-36).

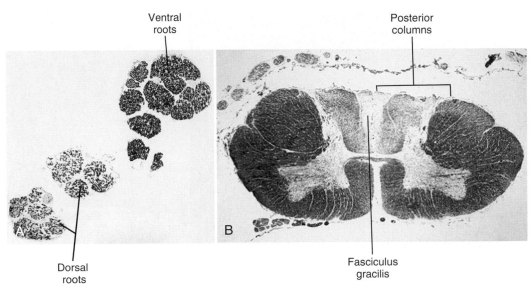

Fig. 2-25. Hereditary sensory and autonomic neuropathy type I. **A,** Root and spinal cord histology shows fiber fallout in dorsal roots (×25). **B,** Note degeneration of posterior columns at the cervical level, maximal in fasciculus gracilis (×6).

Ventral roots

Posterior columns

Dorsal roots

Fasciculus gracilis

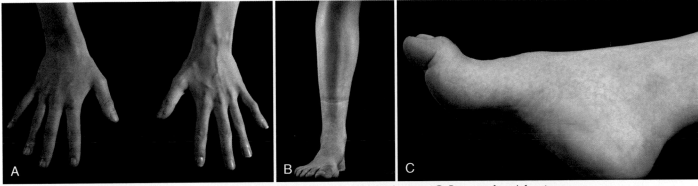

Fig. 2-26. Hypobetalipoproteinemia. **A** and **B,** Mild distal wasting. **C,** Pes cavus foot deformity.

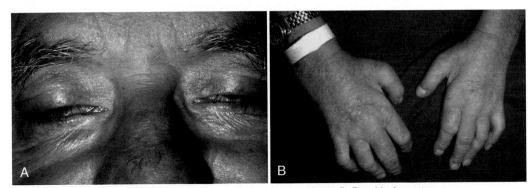

Fig. 2-27. Tangier disease. **A,** Bilateral facial weakness. **B,** Distal limb wasting.

POLYNEUROPATHIES IN ACQUIRED SYSTEMIC DISEASES

Many other metabolic disorders are associated with peripheral neuropathy, including renal and hepatic failure and endocrine disease. In hypothyroidism, for example, there is an increased incidence of mononeuropathy, particularly of the median nerve in the carpal tunnel (carpal tunnel syndrome [see later]) as well as a predominantly sensory polyneuropathy.

DIABETIC NEUROPATHY

Diabetes is now the most common cause of generalized neuropathy in the world. Its prevalence, in patients with a history exceeding 20 years, may be as high as 50%. The main clinical types are the following:

Symmetrical, mainly sensory polyneuropathy, which is often painful
Proximal, asymmetrical, and predominantly motor neuropathy (diabetic amyotrophy)

Isolated or multiple mononeuropathies
Autonomic neuropathy

Sometimes, more than one of these forms is evident in a particular patient. Subclinical autonomic dysfunction is particularly common. The pathogenesis of diabetic polyneuropathy involves both metabolic and vascular factors. Increased activity of aldose reductase leads to the accumulation of sorbitol and fructose and a decrease in free nerve myoinositol. This and other metabolic derangements lead to oxidative stress and impaired mitochondrial function. Ischemic injury involving endoneural capillaries also leads to nerve fiber damage, and a mixed axonal and demyelinating neuropathy is commonly found on nerve conduction studies.

Diabetic sensory polyneuropathy is the commonest form. An insidious onset is usual, and the condition may remain asymptomatic for some time. Early signs include loss of the ankle jerks and depression of vibration sense in the feet. The clinical features reflect, to some extent,

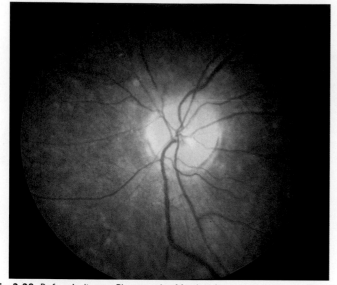

Fig. 2-28. Refsum's disease. Photograph of fundus shows pigmentary retinopathy.

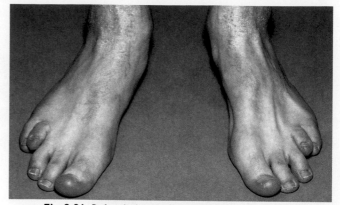

Fig. 2-31. Refsum's disease. Shortening of the fourth toes.

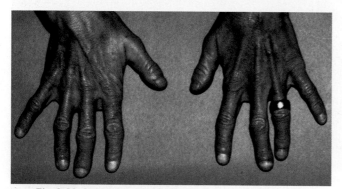

Fig. 2-29. Refsum's disease. Wasting of the small hand muscles.

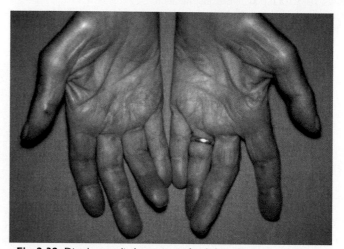

Fig. 2-32. Distal upper limb wasting in familial amyloid polyneuropathy.

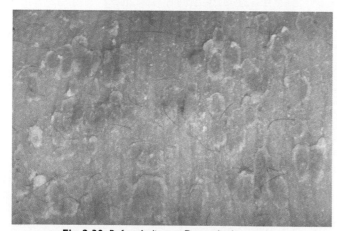

Fig. 2-30. Refsum's disease. Dry scaly skin patches.

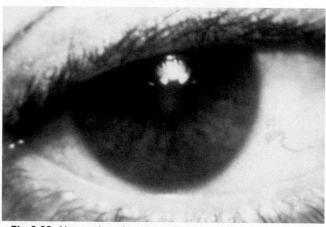

Fig. 2-33. Abnormal pupil in a case of familial amyloid polyneuropathy.

the fiber type affected. Where small myelinated and unmyelinated nerve fibers bear the brunt of the damage, distal pain and paresthesias are prominent symptoms. Pain and temperature loss can lead to persistent foot ulceration, and occasionally neuropathic (Charcot) joints, inadvertent foot injury, and painless fractures (Fig. 2-37). Intensive treatment of type 1 diabetes reduces the subsequent appearance of neuropathy, and pancreatic transplantation halts its progression.

Diabetic amyotrophy tends to occur in older individuals with type 2 diabetes. Typically, a painful, asymmetrical proximal lower limb weakness appears, and it evolves and progresses over weeks or even months. Wasting is often prominent (Fig. 2-38). Recovery is slow and may be incomplete, although the prognosis is generally reasonably good. The underlying mechanism is thought to be a microvasculopathy involving the vasa nervorum of the lumbosacral roots, plexus, and peripheral nerves in various combinations.

Diabetic mononeuropathies can affect both the limbs and cranial nerves, typically the third (painless or occasionally painful, and usually pupil-sparing) and the sixth. A thoracic radiculopathy results in truncal pain with segmental sensory loss. *Acute femoral neuropathy* is also a typical manifestation and can be confused with diabetic amyotrophy.

Autonomic dysfunction can be profound in diabetic patients. Consequences include impotence, bladder atony with recurrent infection and incontinence, diarrhea, and postural hypotension. Loss of the normal cardiac response to the Valsalva maneuver may be detectable in the clinic.

The pathologic changes in diabetic neuropathy are mixed. In addition to axonal loss affecting both myelinated and unmyelinated fibers, there is evidence of segmental demyelination. In long-standing cases, evidence of axonal degeneration is reflected in the appearance of regenerative clusters (Fig. 2-39). Where there has been repeated demyelination, onion bulb formation is seen.

NUTRITIONAL AND DEFICIENCY DISORDERS

Deficiency of the B group vitamins is particularly associated with the development of a peripheral neuropathy. Vitamin B deficiency is rare in developed countries except in association with alcoholism. It is

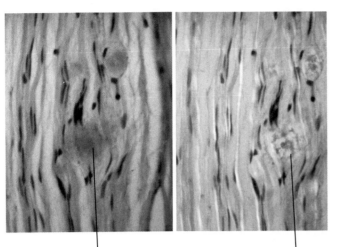

Amyloid deposit

Birefringence

Fig. 2-34. Amyloid neuropathy. **A,** Longitudinal section of peripheral nerve showing amyloid deposit. **B,** Characteristic green birefringence on polarization microscopy (Congo red; ×100).

deficiency of this vitamin that is the predominant cause of alcoholic neuropathy, a condition with many similarities to dry beriberi. A mixed neuropathy occurs, affecting principally or solely the lower limbs, with a combination of weakness, paresthesias, and pain. The patients often complain bitterly of intense burning paresthesias in the soles of their feet. Proximal weakness in these patients may be either neuropathic or myopathic (see alcoholic myopathy, Chapter 3). Autonomic fiber loss leads to segmental anhidrosis and disordered vagal function.

Pellagra is the consequence of a mixed deficiency, in which vitamin B_6 (pyridoxine) deficiency is paramount. The neuropathy induced by isoniazid is secondary to pyridoxine deficiency.

In addition to its effect on the spinal cord, vitamin B_{12} deficiency secondary to pernicious anemia, malabsorption, or gastrectomy can lead to peripheral nerve degeneration, which is commonly present in subacute combined degeneration.

The basic pathologic process in these conditions is an axonal degeneration. Consequently, there is a relatively mild reduction of motor and sensory conduction velocities, with severely depressed sensory action potentials. When small-diameter neurons are particularly affected, routine nerve conduction studies may show no abnormality, and measurement of sensory thresholds to pain and temperature may be required to confirm the diagnosis.

PARAPROTEINEMIC NEUROPATHIES

Myeloma is associated with clinical evidence of a sensorimotor or motor neuropathy in about 10% of cases. In the osteosclerotic form of the disease, the incidence is considerably higher. The neuropathy is usually mixed, it predominates in the lower limbs, and it occasionally involves the cranial nerves. Pain is often prominent. The peripheral nerves and roots show abnormalities of both myelin and axon cylinders, with lymphocytic infiltration. Amyloid deposition is not a feature.

Monoclonal gammopathy is found in 1% of the population older than 50 years and in 3% of those older than 70 years. When the

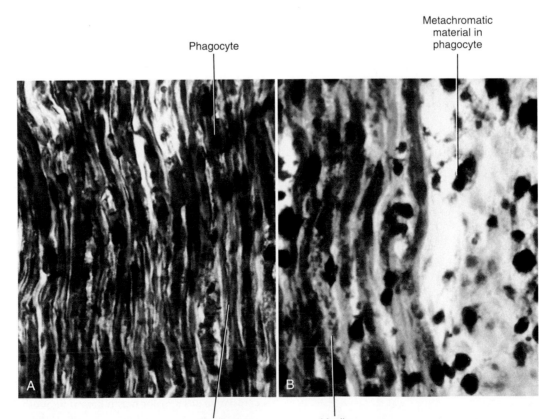

Metachromatic material in phagocyte

Phagocyte

Myelin fragmentation

Myelin fragmentation

Fig. 2-35. Metachromatic leukodystrophy. Peripheral nerve showing myelin fragmentation with phagocytic infiltration **(A)** and myelin fragmentation with phagocytes containing metachromatic material **(B)** (**A,** Sharlach R hematoxylin, ×540; **B,** toluidine blue, ×540).

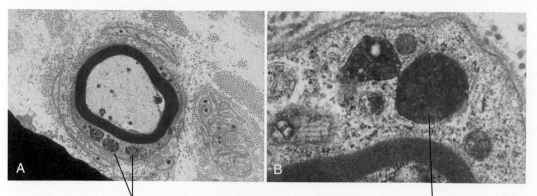

Tuffstone
bodies

Tuffstone
body

Fig. 2-36. Metachromatic leukodystrophy. Electron microscopy showing Tuffstone bodies in the Schwann cell cytoplasm. **A,** ×25,000. **B,** ×100,000.

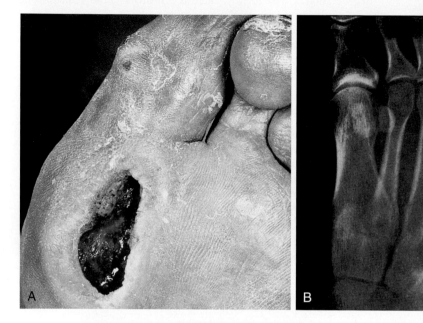

Fig. 2-37. Diabetes. **A,** Perforating foot ulcer. **B,** Metatarsal fracture.

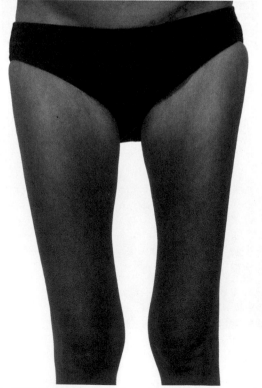

Fig. 2-38. Proximal lower limb wasting in diabetic amyotrophy.

monoclonal gammopathy is of unknown significance, between 8% and 37% of patients develop a symptomatic neuropathy. The gammopathy may be of subtype IgA, IgG, or IgM. The IgM subtype has been best characterized in terms of its neurologic associations, producing a chronic sensorimotor neuropathy accompanied by tremor and ataxia (Fig. 2-40). In about 50% of patients with neuropathy and IgM monoclonal gammopathy, the M-protein reacts with myelin-associated glycoprotein (MAG) and cross-reacting nerve glycoconjugates. Histology studies reveal a demyelinating neuropathy with axonal loss (Fig. 2-41, *A*). Electron microscopy demonstrates separation of the myelin lamellae by deposits of IgM (see Fig. 2-41, *B*), which can also be identified in peripheral nerve sections (Fig. 2-42).

In other patients, anti-sulfatide IgM antibodies have been demonstrated. The associated neuropathy is usually predominantly sensory or may target small fibers. The relationship between neuropathy and IgG or IgA gammopathy is less well defined.

Neuropathy can also be a feature of macroglobulinemia and cryoglobulinemia. Involvement of the vasa nervorum is important in the genesis of the neuropathy associated with the latter, which often produces a mononeuritis multiplex.

INFECTIOUS AND POSTINFECTIOUS CAUSES

Leprosy remains a major health hazard in South America and the Far East and is found among émigrés from those countries. The disease is classified into three major forms: tuberculoid, lepromatous, and borderline (indeterminate). The manifestations of the disease depend more on the host reaction than on the innate properties of the bacillus.

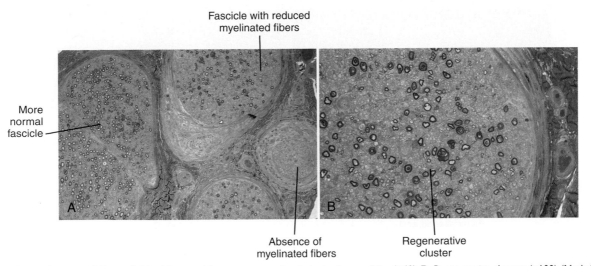

Fascicle with reduced
myelinated fibers

More
normal
fascicle

A

B

Absence of
myelinated fibers

Regenerative
cluster

Fig. 2-39. Peripheral nerve biopsy in diabetes. **A,** Fascicle containing a spectrum of pathologic abnormalities (×40). **B,** Regenerative clusters (×100) (Methylene blue, azure 2, basic fuchsin).

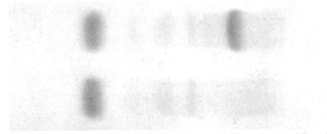

Fig. 2-40. IgM paraprotein band *(right, upper strip).* Normal control *(lower).*

In lepromatous leprosy, there is a defect of host cell–mediated immunity, leading to uncontrolled proliferation of the bacilli and their hematogenous dissemination. In tuberculoid leprosy, the dissemination of the bacilli is much more limited and the number of skin lesions correspondingly fewer. The neuropathic features also differ in the two forms. In tuberculoid leprosy, there are few areas of cutaneous loss that coincide with the skin lesions (Fig. 2-43). In lepromatous leprosy, both the skin lesions and the areas of sensory loss are more extensive, although usually predominantly in the exposed areas. Intermediate forms can have features of both types. Thickened peripheral nerves are found in both the tuberculoid and lepromatous forms of the disease (Fig. 2-44). Tuberculoid leprosy is associated with granuloma formation in the nerves adjacent to the skin lesion (Fig. 2-45, *A*). In lepromatous leprosy, the greatly enlarged nerve trunks are infiltrated by histiocytes and bacilli (see Fig. 2-45, *B*).

Sarcoid Neuropathy
In sarcoidosis, granulomatous infiltration of the nerve roots or peripheral nerves can lead to an asymmetrical radiculopathy or polyneuropathy. Sural nerve biopsy is diagnostic.

Guillain-Barré Syndrome
Guillain-Barré syndrome (GBS) is an immunologically driven polyneuropathy that occurs in all age groups. About two thirds of patients give a history of an antecedent illness, typically a sore throat, flulike symptoms, or gastrointestinal disturbance, some 2 weeks or so before the onset of the neuropathic symptoms. GBS can also be precipitated by vaccinations. The clinical spectrum of the disease embraces the following:

A classic form, consisting of an acute inflammatory demyelinating
  polyneuropathy
Axonal variants
  With both sensory and motor features
  Without sensory involvement (acute motor axonal neuropathy)

The Miller Fisher syndrome
A rare, almost exclusively pure autonomic form, which can appear
  with gastrointestinal paresis

Campylobacter jejuni infection is the commonest specific precipitating infective agent, particularly in China and the Far East. In a European cohort, it accounts for about a quarter of cases. Patients with this trigger are more likely to develop axonal involvement and have a pure motor syndrome than when other agents are the trigger. Some of the serotypes of this organism possess capsular lipopolysaccharide epitopes that are shared with peripheral nerve myelin glycoproteins. A vast array of antibodies to different glycolipids have been identified in GBS, including GM1, asialo-GM1, GM1b, GD1b, and GQ1b. Anti-GD1b antibodies appear to correlate with the common demyelinating neuropathy with the sensory-involvement form of GBS, and GQ1b with the Miller Fisher variant.

The clinical picture evolves gradually, usually over several days, although fulminant onset is recognized. The motor deficit predominates over any sensory loss and can be profound. Facial weakness is common (Fig. 2-46). Autonomic fiber involvement is associated with sinus tachycardia, postural hypotension, and loss of sweating.

The EMG findings reflect the underlying pathology. Wasting is sometimes prominent and may reflect axonal damage. Electrophysiologic evidence of denervation implies a worse prognosis. Some 5% to 10% of patients are left with substantial disability (Fig. 2-47).

The Miller Fisher syndrome is characterized by external ophthalmoplegia, ataxia, and areflexia (Fig. 2-48). Circulatory antibodies to GQ1b are found in the majority of cases.

CHRONIC INFLAMMATORY DEMYELINATING POLYRADICULONEUROPATHY

Although the clinical features of chronic inflammatory demyelinating polyradiculoneuropathy (CIDP) are similar to those of GBS, CIDP is characterized by a subacute onset and chronic course, sometimes interrupted by relapses and remissions. As a general rule, neurologic deficit in GBS is maximal within a month of onset, whereas CIDP evolves over a longer period.

In addition to a typical mixed motor and sensory picture, variants are described, including pure motor involvement, ataxic sensory forms, and cases where the condition is limited to the lower limbs, or even to one limb. The reflexes may be preserved. Root pain is sometimes conspicuous, and scans or surgery may (but rarely) demonstrate striking hypertrophy of cervical or lumbosacral nerve roots (Fig. 2-49). The CSF protein level is typically increased. Sural nerve biopsy may be helpful in diagnosis, in terms of establishing the presence of macrophages expressing inflammation-associated antigens,

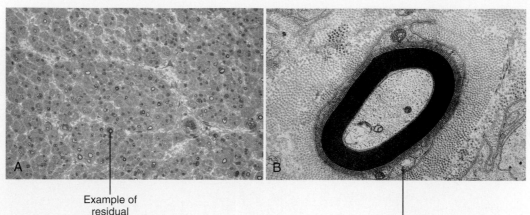

Example of
residual
thin-walled fiber

IgM deposit

Fig. 2-41. Nerve biopsy in IgM paraproteinemia. **A,** Light microscopy demonstrating a reduced population of fibers with thin sheaths (methylene blue, azure 2, basic fuchsin; ×100). **B,** Electron microscopy demonstrates outer separated lamellae of myelin containing deposits of IgM (×25,000).

IgM

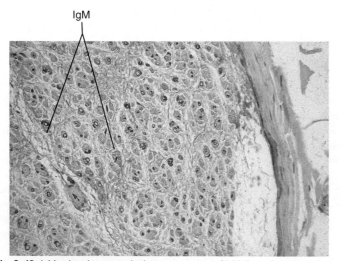

Fig. 2-42. IgM-related neuropathy. Immunostaining of IgM *(brown)* over myelinated fibers (avidin-biotin immunoperoxidase method for IgM).

not seen with other noninflammatory or hereditary neuropathies. An equivalent chronic inflammatory axonal polyneuropathy is also described but is rare.

CONNECTIVE TISSUE DISORDERS

The large-vessel vasculitides (e.g., giant cell arteritis) are seldom associated with a peripheral neuropathy. Among the medium-size-vessel vasculitides, neuropathy occurs only in patients with polyarteritis nodosa. Conditions considered to involve small vessels include rheumatoid disease, Wegener's granulomatosis, and the Churg-Strauss syndrome, in which mononeuritis multiplex may be the presenting feature.

Rheumatoid Neuropathy
Necrotizing arteritis with consequent ischemic neuropathy is not uncommon in rheumatoid arthritis. A digital neuropathy is associated, with vasculitic lesions affecting individual digital nerves (Fig. 2-50). Less than 1% of patients with rheumatoid arthritis have an arteritis of small and medium-size arteries indistinguishable from that occurring in polyarteritis nodosa. Pathologic changes include perivascular cellular infiltration, fibrinoid necrosis, vessel occlusion, and intimal proliferation (Fig. 2-51).

Polyarteritis Nodosa and Churg-Strauss Syndrome
A neuropathy occurs in about 50% of patients with polyarteritis nodosa and is typically a mononeuritis multiplex, particularly affecting the radial, median, and sciatic nerves, although it often evolves

into a symmetrical polyneuropathy. Other neurologic manifestations include cranial neuropathy and a picture suggesting Guillain-Barré syndrome. Sural nerve biopsy shows a necrotizing vasculitis in about 50% of the patients with Churg-Strauss syndrome. Rarely, vasculitis can be confined to the peripheral nerves, and nerve biopsy is then the essential investigation (Fig. 2-52).

Critical Illness Polyneuropathy
Critical illness neuropathy (and its counterpart, critical illness myopathy) occurs relatively commonly in the setting of an intensive care unit. It is suggested that some 70% to 80% of patients with severe sepsis and multiple organ failure develop critical illness neuropathy. An acute axonal neuropathy develops, which then resolves as the underlying triggers are reversed. Typically, there is marked wasting with weakness of all four limbs (Fig. 2-53). Tendon reflexes are typically decreased or absent, but they are reported as preserved in up to one third of patients. EMG confirms an axonal neuropathy with active widespread denervation. Conduction velocities are relatively preserved. Sensory axons are relatively spared. The prognosis is usually good. Chronic weakness and wasting in this clinical context are usually the result of critical illness myopathy (see Chapter 3).

TOXIC NEUROPATHIES

Toxic neuropathies include neuropathies caused by industrial toxins (e.g., the organophosphates, acrylamide, and *n*-hexane) and drug-induced forms. Sometimes the adverse reaction to a particular drug is determined by the metabolic status of the individual. For example, isoniazid-induced neuropathy is more common in those individuals who are slow acetylators of the drug.

Drug-induced neuropathies are usually axonal, appearing some weeks or months after initial response to the drug. Demyelinating neuropathies are unusual but are encountered with perhexiline and amiodarone.

PARANEOPLASTIC NEUROPATHIES

Any form of polyneuropathy can occur in the context of malignancy, but a painful sensorimotor polyneuropathy is the most frequent manifestation. It may be difficult to distinguish neuropathy secondary to the malignancy from toxic neuropathy, as many anticancer drugs can cause neuropathy. A purely sensory, painful small-fiber neuropathy is particularly common in association with small cell lung cancer. This and subacute sensory neuropathy are frequently associated with anti-Hu antibodies, although a variety of other antibodies have been described with the former. In many patients with anti-Hu antibodies, autonomic involvement is also prominent.

A variety of pure motor syndromes have also been described as a feature of paraneoplastic encephalomyelitis, including subacute

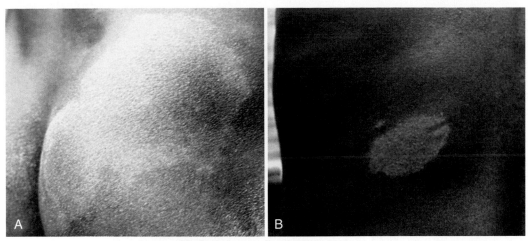

Fig. 2-43. Leprosy. Skin depigmentation.

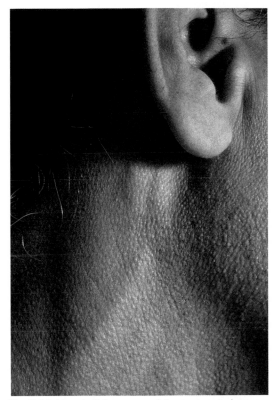

Fig. 2-44. Leprosy. Enlargement of the great auricular nerve.

motor neuropathy and typical motor neuron disease (see earlier). Anti-Yo antibodies have been found in some of these cases.

NEUROPATHY OF UNKNOWN CAUSE

The cause of peripheral neuropathy remains undiscovered in at least 25% of cases, especially when the patient is older and presents with an insidious axonal neuropathy, particularly affecting small fiber modalities. Distal numbness is typical and pain may be a feature. Usually only symptomatic treatment for the discomfort can be offered, often with a rather disappointing effect.

THE MONONEUROPATHIES

An external force can affect a peripheral nerve in a number of ways. External compression damages particularly those nerves that pursue, at least for a short distance, a superficial course (e.g., the common peroneal nerve at the head of the fibula), and entrapment can occur where a nerve passes through a confined space. The damage in such cases is often cumulative over time.

All forms of nerve damage up to complete transection are possible with penetrating injuries. After complete transection, spontaneous regeneration can occur only if the divided ends of the nerve are reasonably contiguous. Otherwise, surgical anastomosis or nerve grafting is required. Neuromas can develop at the ends of divided nerves (Figs. 2-54 and 2-55). Percussion over an injured nerve trunk typically produces transient paresthesias in the distal distribution of the nerve (Tinel's sign).

Median Nerve Lesions
Carpal Tunnel Syndrome.   Carpal tunnel syndrome is the commonest entrapment neuropathy, and it predominantly affects women. It can be a transient feature during pregnancy. Those who develop the condition have anatomically smaller canals than normal individuals, and various diseases, such as acromegaly, hypothyroidism, and rheumatoid arthritis, are associated with median nerve compression at this site by virtue of their effects on the adjacent soft tissues. Nocturnal pain, numbness, and paresthesias are highly characteristic, although the symptoms are often diffusely distributed in the fingers and even, in the case of the pain, referred to the forearm or upper arm. A complaint of being awakened in the night by symptoms and shaking the hands or running them under cold water to gain relief are characteristic.

Examination may reveal surprisingly little. Rather than dramatic sensory loss over the palmar aspect of the three and a half fingers innervated by the nerve, it is more common to find a subtle difference in the appreciation of touch between the radial and ulnar aspects of the ring finger. Weakness of the median innervated muscles of the thenar eminence is likely in more advanced cases (Fig. 2-56, A). Involvement of the opponens pollicis is detected either as a reduction of the pressure that can be exerted between the tips of the thumb and fifth finger or by the failure of the thumb to rotate as it moves to the base of the fifth finger (see Fig. 2-56, B). Tinel's sign, with tingling sensations in the fingers elicited by percussion of the nerve at the wrist, can be elicited in perhaps a quarter of the patients. Rather more frequently, symptoms can be duplicated by sustained wrist flexion (Phalen's sign). In many cases, the involvement is bilateral, although symptoms may be unilateral (Fig. 2-57). In some cases, compression of the nerve follows deformity of the wrist caused by a malunited wrist fracture (Fig. 2-58).

Electrophysiologic investigation is of major value in diagnosis. Typically, the median sensory action potential is depressed and delayed, with prolonged distal motor latency to the abductor pollicis brevis (Fig. 2-59). Sensory and mixed nerve conduction studies appear more sensitive than motor studies.

If conservative treatment fails, decompression of the nerve in the carpal tunnel is required. Focal constriction of the nerve confirms the site of compression (Fig. 2-60). The success rate exceeds 95%, with a complication rate of less than 3%. Endoscopic techniques have been introduced as an alternative to a traditional open procedure.

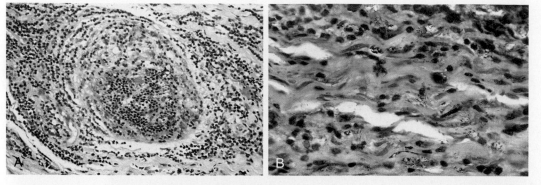

Fig. 2-45. Leprosy. Nerve section. **A,** Tuberculoid form with noncaseating granuloma formation (H&E). **B,** Lepromatous form. Hypertrophic nerve infiltrated with histiocytes. Profuse bacillary infiltration is seen (Wade-Fite).

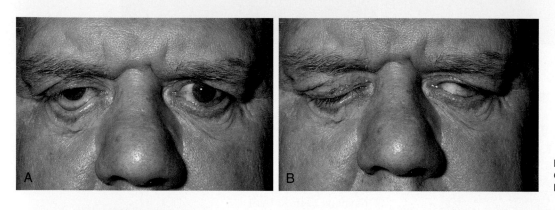

Fig. 2-46. Bilateral facial weakness in Guillain-Barré syndrome. **A,** Eyes open. **B,** Attempting eye closure.

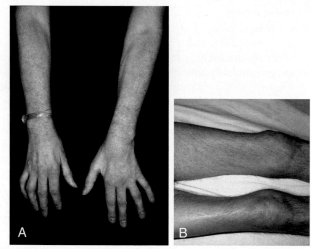

Fig. 2-47. **A** Hand and thigh **B** muscle wasting in Guillain-Barré syndrome.

Proximal Median Nerve Lesions. Proximal median nerve lesions are rare. Entrapment of the anterior interosseous branch of the nerve by the origin of the deep head of pronator teres (pronator syndrome) appears with pain in the forearm flexors and is worsened by pronation against resistance. The muscles affected are pronator quadratus, flexor pollicis longus, and flexor digitorum profundus to the second and third digits, leading to weakness of pinch grip (Fig. 2-61). Sensation is unaffected. Decompression of the nerve may be required.

Ulnar Nerve Lesions. Although the ulnar nerve can be damaged at both the wrist and the shoulder, the vast majority of ulnar nerve palsies arise at the level of the elbow. Some cases follow deformity caused by previous fracture, but most result from trauma to the nerve as it lies in the epicondylar groove and from compression by the aponeurosis of flexor carpi ulnaris (cubital tunnel syndrome) (Fig. 2-62). Pain may be felt, radiating from the elbow to the ulnar border of the hand.

Muscles affected in the hand include the interossei, adductor pollicis, and the muscles of the hypothenar eminence (Fig. 2-63). Involvement of the lumbricals to the fourth and fifth digits produces a characteristic deformity in which hyperextension of the metacarpophalangeal joints of the fourth and fifth fingers is accompanied by

flexion at the proximal interphalangeal joints (Fig. 2-64). The fifth finger is liable to take up an abducted position, and writing is affected by the impairment of thumb adduction. When the patient attempts to grip a piece of paper between the thumb and the radial side of the index finger, flexion of the terminal phalanx of the thumb appears to compensate for weakness of the adductor pollicis (Froment's sign) (Fig. 2-65). Testing of the long flexors supplied by the ulnar nerve is of value, because, if one or more of them is weak, the lesion is at the level of the elbow or above (Fig. 2-66).

Sensory change in an ulnar lesion is confined to the ulnar one-and-a-half digits and the ulnar border of the hand ending at the wrist, on both the palmar and dorsal aspects. The loss may be confined to an alteration of the two-point threshold.

Electrophysiologic testing may demonstrate an absent ulnar sensory action potential if axonal damage has occurred, but the most sensitive techniques involve demonstrating either selective slowing of motor conduction across the elbow or a prolonged latency to the flexor carpi ulnaris after stimulation of the nerve above the medial epicondyle (Fig. 2-67).

Decompression of the nerve in the cubital tunnel or its transposition from the ulnar groove may serve to prevent further damage (Fig. 2-68).

Radial Nerve Lesions. The radial nerve is susceptible to damage, as it winds around the spiral groove of the humerus. Triggering factors including blunt trauma and fractures of the humerus, but the commonest cause is so-called Saturday night palsy, typically a result of alcohol excess. The nerve is damaged during sleep, with the arm draped over the back of a chair. The triceps is usually spared but weakness is conspicuous in the wrist and finger extensors, brachioradialis, and the supinator muscle (Fig. 2-69). Sensory loss is often slight.

Posterior Interosseous Palsy. The posterior interosseous nerve is susceptible to entrapment as it passes through the supinator muscle immediately below the tip of the lateral epicondyle. Following pain in the elbow and forearm, weakness appears in the extensors of the wrist, fingers, and thumb. As there is relative sparing of the radial extensors, radial deviation occurs during attempted wrist extension (Fig. 2-70). There is no sensory loss. If spontaneous recovery does

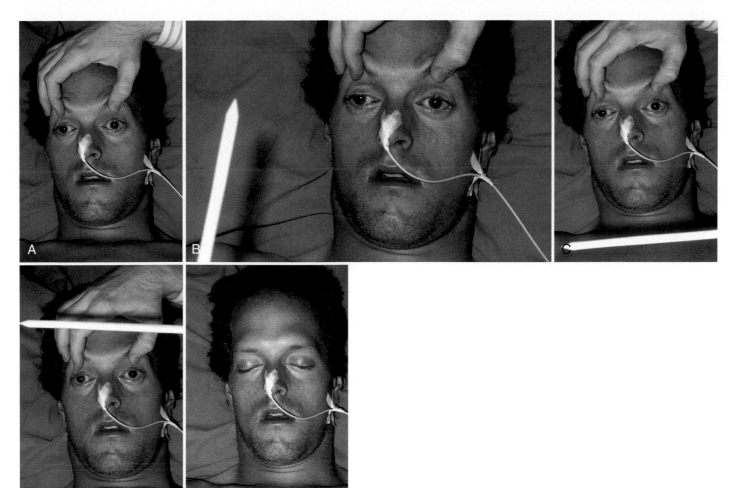

Fig. 2-48. Miller Fisher syndrome. Failure of gaze to left **(A)**, right **(B)**, down **(C)**, and up **(D)**. There is also bilateral facial weakness **(E)**.

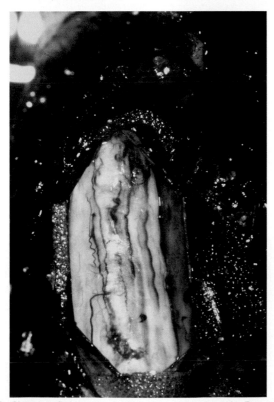

Fig. 2-49. Chronic inflammatory demyelinating polyneuropathy. Exposed lumbar canal at surgery showing grossly thickened nerve roots.

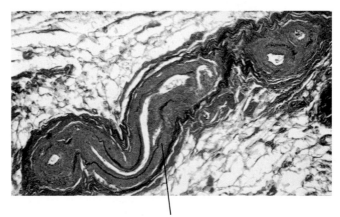

Intimal thickening

Fig. 2-50. Rheumatoid arthritis. A digital nerve showing intimal thickening of the vasa nervorum (elastic–van Gieson; ×180).

not occur over a 2-month period, exploration of the nerve may be indicated (Fig. 2-71).

Musculocutaneous Nerve Palsy. Musculocutaneous nerve palsy is rare. The affected muscles are the biceps and brachialis (Fig. 2-72). Sensory loss, if present, occurs on the radial aspect of the forearm.

Thoracic Outlet Syndrome. Thoracic outlet syndrome results from compression of the lower trunk of the brachial plexus, sometimes by a cervical rib but more commonly by a fibrous band passing from the transverse process of the seventh cervical vertebra to the first rib. Pain, usually referred to the ulnar aspect of the hand and forearm, is prominent and may sometimes be the only symptom, but usually

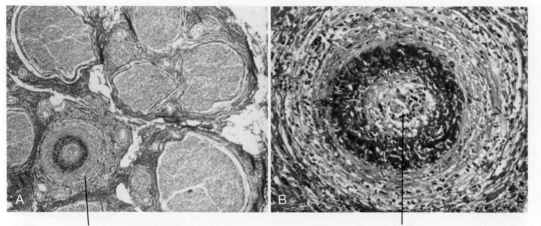

Arteriole

Arteriole

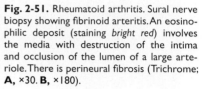

Fig. 2-51. Rheumatoid arthritis. Sural nerve biopsy showing fibrinoid arteritis. An eosinophilic deposit (staining *bright red*) involves the media with destruction of the intima and occlusion of the lumen of a large arteriole. There is perineural fibrosis (Trichrome; **A,** ×30. **B,** ×180).

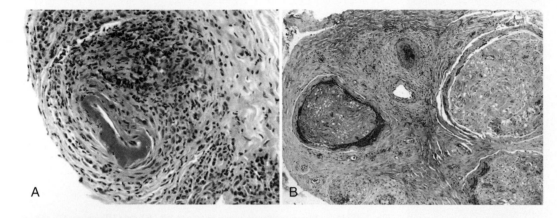

Fig. 2-52. Vasculitic neuropathy. **A,** Epineural artery with fibrinoid necrosis. **B,** Late stage: epineural and perineural fibrosis with mild inflammation (H&E).

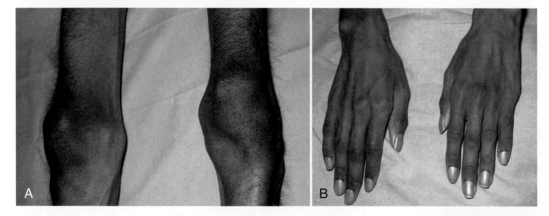

Fig. 2-53. Critical illness neuropathy. Severe wasting of the lower limbs **(A)** and the hands **(B).**

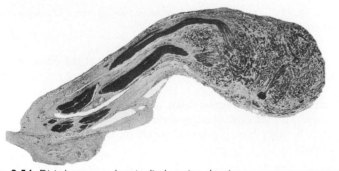

Fig. 2-54. Digital neuroma. Longitudinal section showing a neuroma composed of interwoven, thin, myelinated nerve fibers, connective tissue, and Schwann cells (×85).

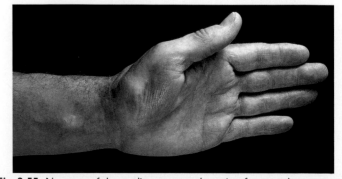

Fig. 2-55. Neuroma of the median nerve at the wrist after complete severance of the nerve.

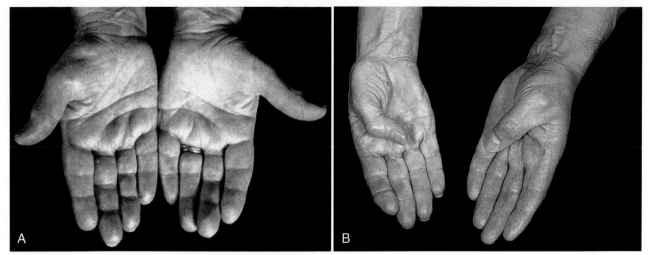

Fig. 2-56. Carpal tunnel syndrome. **A,** Wasting of the thenar eminence. **B,** Failure of right opposition.

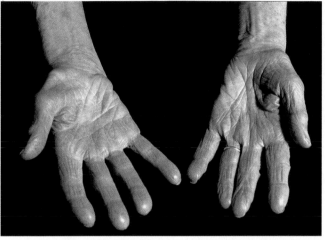

Fig. 2-57. Bilateral carpal tunnel syndrome.

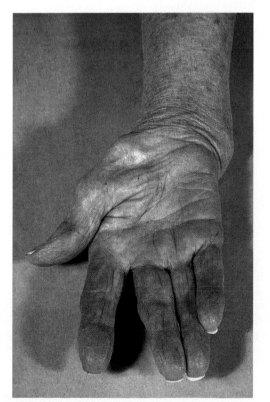

Fig. 2-58. Carpal tunnel syndrome. Wasting of the thenar eminence. The patient's wrist was previously fractured.

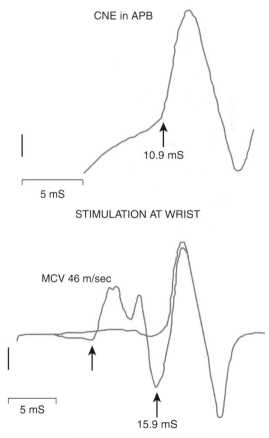

CNE in APB

10.9 mS

5 mS

STIMULATION AT WRIST

MCV 46 m/sec

5 mS

15.9 mS

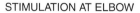

STIMULATION AT ELBOW

Fig. 2-59. Carpal tunnel syndrome. EMG shows marked prolongation of distal latency to the abductor pollicis brevis (10.9 msec). The earlier response with proximal stimulation was a spurious ulnar response.

weakness and wasting appear eventually. In the hand, the thenar eminence muscles are more often affected than the ulnar innervated muscles, and weakness is accompanied by muscular wasting on the medial aspect of the forearm (Fig. 2-73). Sensory change occurs over the medial aspect of the forearm, extending into the fourth and fifth digits of the hand. The patient's symptoms can sometimes be reproduced by downward traction on the arm as it is held against the back, and by pressure over the thoracic inlet.

Radiologic findings on the affected side are more likely to show beaking of the C7 transverse process than a formed cervical rib. Measurement of somatosensory evoked responses is a sensitive technique for providing evidence of the syndrome. Typically, there is reduced amplitude and increased latency of N9 and N13 (Fig. 2-74). In some

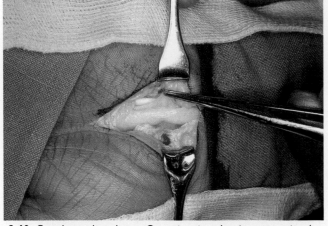

Fig. 2-60. Carpal tunnel syndrome. Operative view showing a constricted nerve in the carpal tunnel.

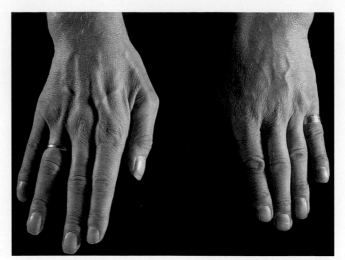

Fig. 2-63. Right ulnar nerve palsy with wasting.

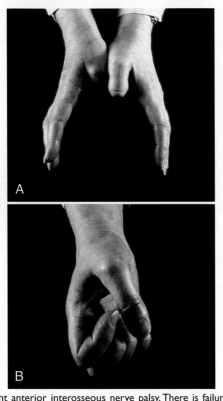

Fig. 2-61. Right anterior interosseous nerve palsy. There is failure of flexion of the thumb **(A)** and an inability to make a circle with thumb and index finger **(B)**.

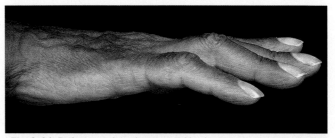

Fig. 2-64. Deformity of the fourth and fifth fingers in a right ulnar palsy.

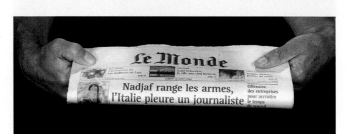

Fig. 2-65. Froment's sign. There is flexion of the thumb on the right because of weakness of the adductor pollicis.

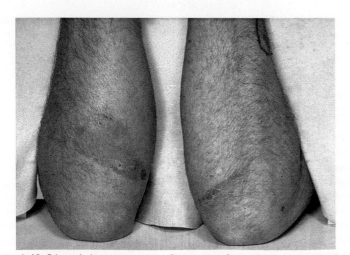

Fig. 2-62. Bilateral ulnar nerve palsies. Pressure marks on the skin were acquired during a period of drug-induced coma.

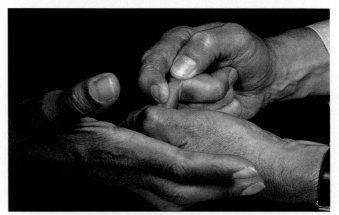

Fig. 2-66. Testing flexor digitorum profundus to the fifth finger.

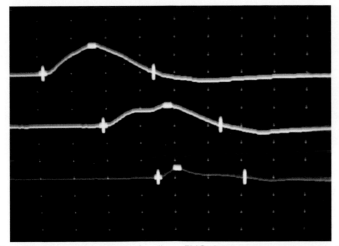

Fig. 2-67. Ulnar nerve palsy at the elbow. EMG showing motor action potential amplitudes from abductor digiti minimi after stimulation at the wrist *(top)*, below the elbow *(middle)*, and above the elbow *(bottom)*.

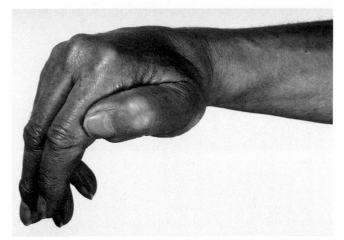

Fig. 2-70. Posterior interosseous palsy. Radial deviation of the right hand during attempted wrist extension.

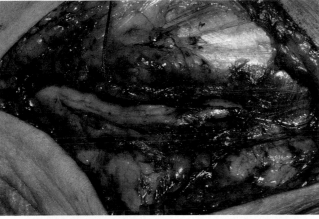

Fig. 2-68. Ulnar nerve decompression. Operative photograph.

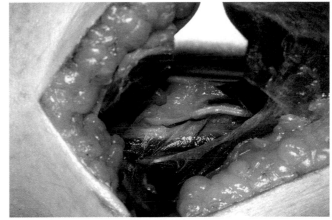

Fig. 2-71. Exploration of the posterior interosseous nerve in a patient with a posterior interosseous palsy.

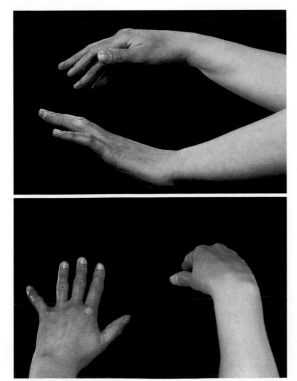

Fig. 2-69. Radial palsy. Failure of right wrist and finger extension.

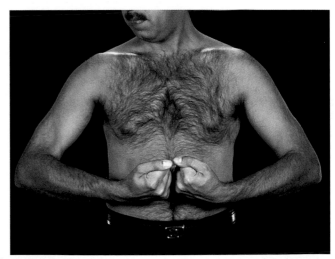

Fig. 2-72. Musculocutaneous nerve palsy. There is wasting of the biceps muscle on the right.

cases, it is possible to demonstrate deviation of the plexus by the compressing structure by MRI imaging, using special radiofrequency coils.

Median sternotomy–related brachial plexopathy is another form of lower trunk brachial plexopathy, but here the picture tends to overlap with an ulnar neuropathy, and the predominant neurogenic involvement is of C8-innervated structures. Measurement of the sensory action potential of the medial cutaneous nerve of the forearm appears to distinguish these entities, and this is potentially

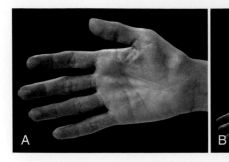

Fig. 2-73. Thoracic outlet syndrome. **A,** The hand. **B,** The forearm.

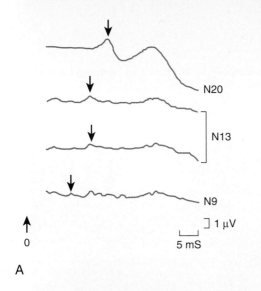

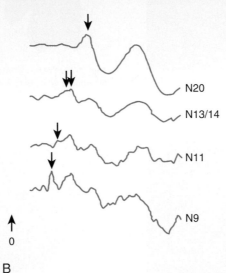

Fig. 2-74. Thoracic outlet syndrome. The N9 and N13 potentials from the right hand **(A)** are depressed compared with those from the left **(B)**.

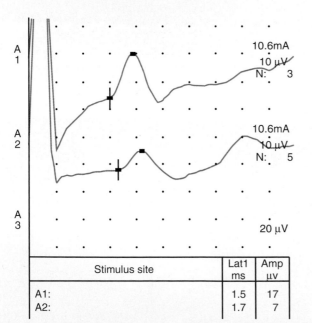

Fig. 2-75. Depressed medial cutaneous nerve of forearm sensory action potential in thoracic outlet syndrome. Normal *(upper)* and depressed *(lower)* potential.

Stimulus site	Lat1 ms	Amp μv
A1:	1.5	17
A2:	1.7	7

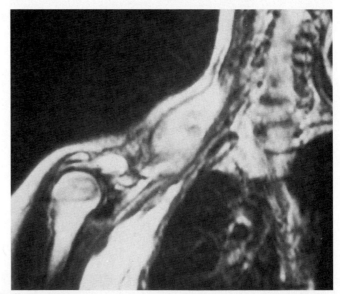

Fig. 2-76. MRI demonstrating sarcoma of the brachial plexus secondary to previous irradiation.

sensitive for the diagnosis of neurogenic thoracic outlet syndrome (Fig. 2-75).

Other Brachial Plexus Lesions. Brachial plexus damage can result from trauma, irradiation, or tumor infiltration (Fig. 2-76). The first two commonly produce pain in the distribution of the upper plexus. When the damage is extensive, there is global weakness of the arm, with wasting, flaccidity, and areflexia (Fig. 2-77, *A*). Involvement of sympathetic fibers results in an ipsilateral Horner's syndrome (see Fig. 2-77, *B*), classically in Pancoast's syndrome.

Neuralgic Amyotrophy. Neuralgic amyotrophy (brachial plexus neuritis) may occur spontaneously but is sometimes triggered by intercurrent infection, trauma, or a surgical procedure. Typically, onset is heralded by severe pain in one shoulder. This usually resolves over a day or two but is then quickly followed by weakness and wasting of various muscles. There may be sensory impairment, most often in the distribution of the axillary nerve. The wasting is often confined to the deltoid and spinati muscles (Fig. 2-78) or, as a consequence of involvement of the long thoracic nerve, to the serratus anterior, with winging of the scapula (Fig. 2-79). The weakness can rarely follow

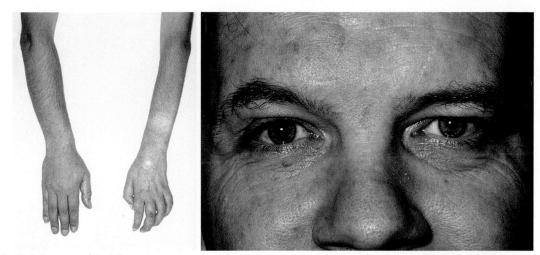

Fig. 2-77. A, Global wasting of the left arm in a posttraumatic brachial plexopathy. **B,** Horner's syndrome associated with a left brachial plexopathy.

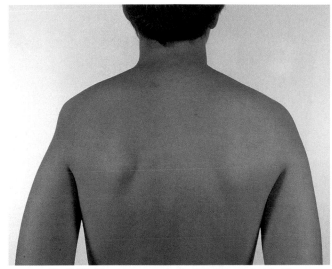

Fig. 2-78. Neuralgic amyotrophy. Wasting of left deltoid.

the distribution of a single peripheral nerve or nerve root, or even appear to reflect anterior horn cell involvement. The condition can also occasionally be bilateral, painless (aneuralgic amyotrophy), and recurrent. The appropriate reflexes are usually preserved unless wasting is profound, a point of distinction from nerve root lesions.

Sciatic Nerve Lesions
The sciatic nerve can be damaged by pelvic trauma or injury to the buttock as a result of a fall, iatrogenically by injection into the nerve, or by prolonged recumbency (e.g., after a protracted period of unconsciousness caused by a drug overdose). Rarely, hemorrhage into the buttock in a patient on anticoagulant therapy damages the nerve.

Weakness affects the hamstring muscles and all the muscles supplied by the medial and lateral popliteal branches of the nerves, although often the latter, supplying the dorsiflexors of the foot and toes, are affected to a greater degree (Fig. 2-80). Sensation is affected over the lateral aspect of the foot and over the inferior aspect of the calf. The ankle jerk is depressed or absent. Wasting, reflecting axonal interruption, worsens the prognosis for recovery (Fig. 2-81).

Femoral Neuropathy. The femoral nerve can be compressed during passage through the psoas muscle by retroperitoneal tumor, localized infection, or hematoma. With nerve damage at this level, there is weakness of hip flexion in addition to the changes produced by more distal damage to the nerve (e.g., after a surgical procedure), in which there is weakness of the quadriceps, accompanied by depression of the knee jerk, and sensory loss over the anterior thigh and the medial aspect of the lower leg as a result of involvement of the saphenous branch of the nerve

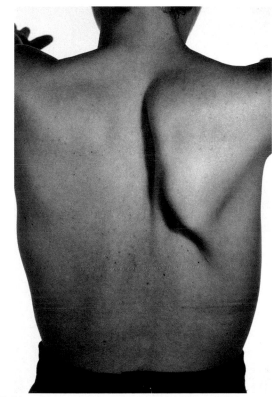

Fig. 2-79. Neuralgic amyotrophy. Winging of the right scapula as a result of weakness of serratus anterior.

(Fig. 2-82). The main distinguishing feature from a root lesion at the L3 level is the involvement of the adductors of the thigh with the latter. Femoral and saphenous nerve conduction studies can be helpful, comparing the affected and unaffected sides, but can be technically difficult.

Meralgia Paresthetica. The lateral cutaneous nerve of the thigh is commonly entrapped at the level of the groin, where it pierces the lateral aspect of the inguinal ligament. Meralgia paresthetica is not confined to the obese. There results a combination of pain, typically burning in quality, and paresthesia over a circumscribed area of the anterolateral aspect of the thigh. Sensory change on examination is often restricted to a smaller area than the theoretical total distribution of the nerve. Nerve conduction studies may be helpful but (again) can be technically challenging.

Peroneal (Lateral Popliteal) Nerve Lesions. The common peroneal nerve is susceptible to compression as it winds around the neck of the fibula. The damage may result from external trauma (Fig.

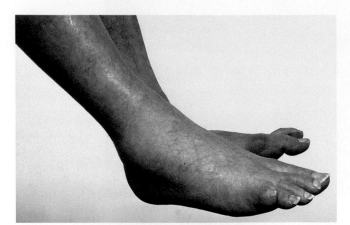

Fig. 2-80. Sciatic palsy secondary to a buttock hematoma. Right foot - and toe drop.

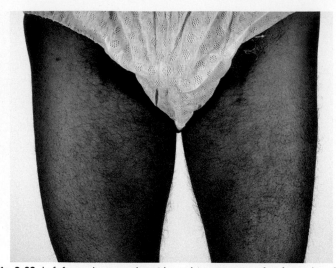

Fig. 2-82. Left femoral nerve palsy with quadriceps wasting after femoral profundoplasty.

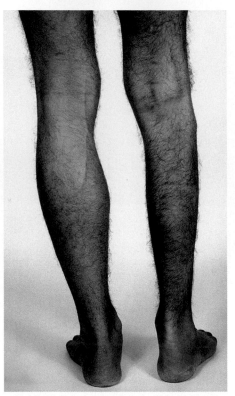

Fig. 2-81. Sciatic palsy. Wasting of the right calf.

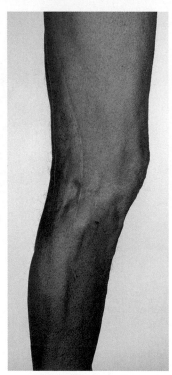

Fig. 2-83. Common peroneal palsy. Traumatic damage to the nerve at the level of the knee.

2-83), including crouching (e.g., while gardening), pressure resulting from poor positioning of the patient during surgical procedures, or simply from a period of bed rest in a relatively immobile subject. Weakness appears in the evertors of the foot and the dorsiflexors of the foot and toes. Typically, the extensor hallucis longus is most affected. Sensory change occurs over the lateral aspect of the calf and the dorsum of the foot, but it is confined to a small area between the first and second toes if only the deep branch of the nerve is affected. There is no reflex change (Fig. 2-84). In some cases, the peronei are spared.

Tarsal Tunnel Syndrome. The posterior tibial nerve passes through a tunnel analogous to the carpal tunnel in the wrist. Compression in the tunnel leads to pain, numbness, and paresthesias in the sole of the foot. Either the medial or lateral plantar branch of the nerve can be individually affected, with sensory symptoms then referred to the medial or lateral aspects of the foot, respectively. Percussion over the nerve behind the medial malleolus may trigger pain and tingling in the foot. Weakness of the intrinsic foot muscles is difficult to elicit

but may occur. The medial plantar sensory action potential, obtained by stimulating the great toe and recording behind the medial malleolus, is absent in the majority of patients.

Morton's Metatarsalgia. Compression of the interdigital nerves between adjacent metatarsals leads to pain and paresthesias in the foot or toes, classically affecting the web space between the third and fourth toes. Typically, the nerve develops a painful swelling, excision of which relieves the symptoms. Histology of the swelling (Morton's neuroma) demonstrates nerve fiber loss coupled with fibrosis and Schwann cell proliferation and encircling fibrosis, so this is an entrapment neuropathy rather than a true neuroma (Fig. 2-85).

Mononeuritis Multiplex

Mononeuritis multiplex is a clinical syndrome characterized by sequential palsies of individual nerves in an asymmetrical fashion over a relatively short period, resulting in weakness usually accompanied by significant pain and sensory impairment. As noted earlier, this picture often evolves into a more typical symmetrical polyneuropathy.

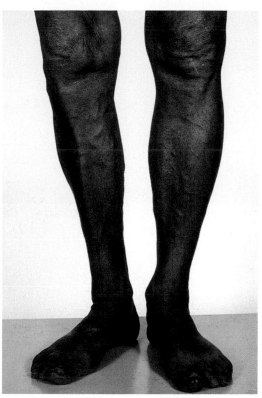

Fig. 2-84. Severe wasting of the right anterior tibial compartment resulted from a traumatic common peroneal palsy.

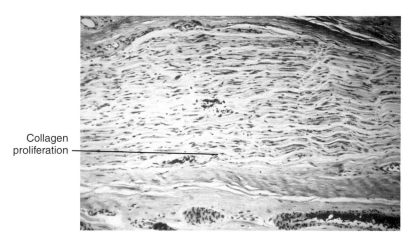

Collagen
proliferation —

Fig. 2-85. Morton's neuroma. Nerve fiber atrophy with collagen proliferation.

In most cases, the pathology is centered in the axon rather than the myelin sheath, and it usually results from a microinfarction after thrombosis of the vasa nervorum. Causes include vasculitides, collagen vascular diseases, diabetes, and dysproteinemias. Cranial nerves can also be affected (Fig. 2-86).

More insidious evolutions of this type, referred to as multiple mononeuropathy, are seen in leprosy, sarcoidosis, and neoplastic infiltration.

Multifocal Motor Neuropathy with Conduction Block
In multifocal motor neuropathy with conduction block, slowly progressive and mainly distal weakness evolves over a period of years. The arms are more affected than the legs. The affected muscles atrophy. Fasciculation is often prominent, and, as there are no sensory signs or symptoms, the condition is commonly misdiagnosed as motor neuron disease before investigation. Although the EMG findings vary, multifocal conduction block is usually found in peripheral motor nerves (Fig. 2-87).

There is increasing consensus that multifocal motor neuropathy is part of the CIDP spectrum, but, unlike that disorder, it does not respond to steroids. However, there is often a good response to immunosuppressive therapy, notably intravenous immunoglobulins, at least at the outset.

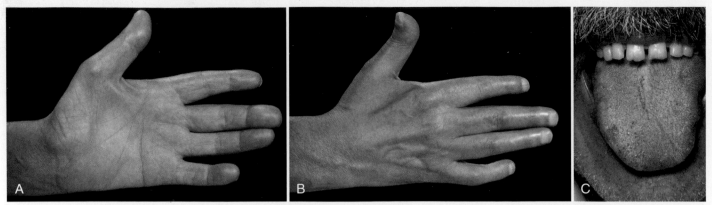

Fig. 2-86. Mononeuritis multiplex. Involvement of left median and ulnar **(A)**, right ulnar **(B)**, and left hypoglossal **(C)** nerves.

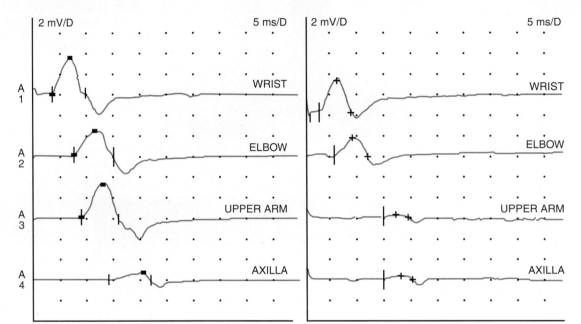

Fig. 2-87. Multifocal motor neuropathy. EMG. Partial conduction block in the right median nerve in the region of the axilla *(left)* and left median nerve in the upper arm *(right)*.

MYOPATHIES AND MYASTHENIA

Myopathies may be genetic or acquired and can be classified in several ways. In general, myopathies resulting from inflammatory, toxic, and metabolic processes cause nonselective, symmetrical, and largely proximal weakness, whereas genetic myopathies tend to result in selective weakness and wasting in particular patterns. Diagnosis is influenced by the age of onset, rate of progression, and family history of the disorder; the pattern of weakness and wasting; the presence of muscle enlargement and signs such as myotonia; evidence of cardiac and respiratory involvement; and skeletal abnormalities such as contractures and kyphoscoliosis.

Measurement of creatine kinase (CK) levels, neurophysiological studies, and muscle imaging can help establish the nature and extent of the process. Other investigations may determine if the myopathy is primary, or secondary to systemic disease. However, muscle biopsy with immunohistochemical, genomic, and proteomic analysis, and sometimes biochemical analysis of muscle tissue is usually essential for accurate diagnosis.

Box 3-1 provides a clinically based classification of the myopathies. Only the most common of these many diseases are discussed here. The interested reader can visit http://neuromuscular.wustl.edu/ for further details.

GENETIC MYOPATHIES

MUSCULAR DYSTROPHIES AND RELATED DISORDERS

Muscular dystrophies are genetically determined, progressive muscle diseases, characterized histologically by muscle fiber necrosis and degeneration, with replacement of muscle by fat and fibrous connective tissue. In some conditions, these dystrophic changes are less pronounced and the more general term myopathy is preferred. Three main clinical patterns of weakness can be discerned (Box 3-2).

Axial and limb-girdle pattern. This pattern includes Duchenne's muscular dystrophy (DMD), Becker's muscular dystrophy (BMD), and the limb-girdle muscular dystrophies (LGMDs). It is also evident in the congenital muscular dystrophies (CMDs and in) Bethlem myopathy and Emery-Dreifuss muscular dystrophy (EDMD) but these conditions have prominent muscle contractures developing at

an early stage as an additional feature. Some of these diseases also have cardiac involvement.

Non–limb girdle weakness pattern with prominent involvement of cranial musculature. This pattern includes facioscapulohumeral muscular dystrophy (FSHD) and oculopharyngeal muscular dystrophy (OPMD). Note that myotonic dystrophy falls into this group but is generally classified with the myotonic disorders (see p. 65).

Distal pattern. Selective distal weakness is unusual in muscle disease, but distal myopathies need to be considered in the differential diagnosis of this pattern of weakness, which is more commonly associated with neurogenic processes.

Pathogenesis of Axial and Limb-Girdle Pattern Dystrophies and Myopathies

This pattern of disease is usually caused by protein defects in the following:

Muscle cytoskeleton, including proteins of the sarcolemma and the extracellular matrix.

Sarcomeric structures (the contractile apparatus). Such conditions are now referred to as myofibrillar myopathies.

Cytosolic enzymes, which appear to play a part in maintenance of the cytoskeleton.

These structures are shown diagrammatically in Figure 3-1. In addition, defects of certain nuclear membrane proteins can cause this clinical phenotype, although here the pathogenic mechanism is less clear.

Cytoskeletal Protein Defects. The muscle cytoskeleton comprises the structural proteins of the sarcolemma and the extracellular matrix, which includes the basal lamina and a diffuse collagen network embedded in amorphous ground substance. To date,

---

BOX 3-1   CLINICAL CLASSIFICATION OF MYOPATHIES

Genetic Myopathies
- Muscular dystrophies and related disorders
- Myotonic dystrophies
- Muscle channelopathies (non-dystrophic myotonias and periodic paralyses)
- Congenital myopathies
- Myofibrillar myopathies and hereditary inclusion body myopathies
- Mitochondrial myopathies
- Metabolic myopathies

Acquired Myopathies
- Inflammatory myopathies
- Myopathies in systemic diseases
- Toxic and drug-induced myopathies

BOX 3-2   CLINICAL PATTERNS OF MUSCULAR DYSTROPHIES AND GENETIC MYOPATHIES

Axial and Limb-Girdle Pattern Dystrophies and Myopathies
- Duchenne's dystrophy (DMD)*
- Becker's dystrophy (BMD)*
- Limb-girdle muscular dystrophies (LGMD)
- Congenital muscular dystrophies (CMD)*†
- Bethlem myopathy
- Emery-Dreifuss muscular dystrophy (EDMD)*†

Non–Limb-Girdle Pattern with Cranial Musculature Involvement
- Facioscapulohumeral muscular dystrophy (FSHD)
- Oculopharyngeal muscular dystrophy (OPMD)
- (Myotonic dystrophy)*

Distal Myopathies
- Welander disease
- Myoshi myopathy
- Tibial muscular dystrophy
- Nonaka myopathy
- Laing-type myopathy

*Conditions with cardiac involvement.
†Conditions with prominent early contractures.

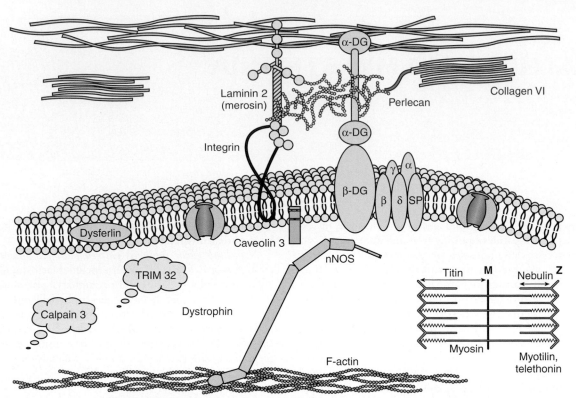

Fig. 3-1. Muscle fiber cytoskeleton, extracellular matrix, and sarcomeric proteins.

muscle diseases caused by deficiencies of dystrophin, the sarcogly-cans and dystroglycans, caveolin 3, and dysferlin have been defined. The sarcoglycans and dystroglycans are together referred to as dystrophin-associated glycoproteins (DAGs). Alpha-dystroglycan is sometimes referred to as adhalin.

The basal lamina proteins include merosin (now more commonly referred to as lamininα-2), the integrins, and collagen 6. Defects in basal lamina proteins result chiefly in forms of CMD.

Dystrophinopathies: Duchenne's and Becker's Dystrophies. Dystrophin is the lynch pin of the muscle cytoskeleton. Defects in this molecule can produce a wide range of phenotypes, of which Duchenne's and Becker's dystrophies are the most common and most severe.

Duchenne's muscular dystrophy is the archetypal muscular dystrophy and the first condition of this type to be recognized. It the most common X-linked recessive disease in man, with an incidence of about 1 per 3500 male live births. About one third of cases are born to mothers who are carriers of dystrophin mutations, but this huge gene has an extremely high mutation rate and other 'new mutation' cases result from gonadal mosaicism in mothers, grandmothers and grandfathers: a further proportion result from gonadal mosaicism in mothers, grandmothers and grandfathers and the remainder from somatic mutations in affected boys. Although the disease can be diagnosed at birth and even prenatally, diagnosis is often delayed until age 3 to 6 years, by which time a carrier mother may already have conceived another affected child.

Muscular enlargement, particularly of the calves, is a notable feature (Fig. 3-2). The first classifications of dystrophies were based partly on the presence or absence of this feature (pseudohypertrophic muscular dystrophy). The enlargement results chiefly from replacement of muscle fibers by fat and fibrous tissue, giving an unusually firm rubbery feel to the muscle. Other muscles may also be affected, including the tongue.

The condition causes delay in motor milestones, and most affected boys fail to walk by 18 months of age. Muscle involvement is typically selective, affecting the girdles, axial muscles, and proximal limbs, particularly the legs. This results in problems rising from the floor. The affected boy compensates for the loss of axial strength and stability

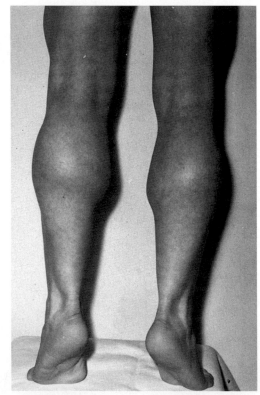

Fig. 3-2. Calf enlargement in Duchenne's dystrophy.

by "climbing up his legs," using his arms when attempting to stand (Gowers' maneuver) (Fig. 3-3). This is typical of DMD but can be a feature of all myopathies with this clinical pattern. Another major problem is the development of excessive lumbar lordosis, kyphoscoliosis, and disabling contractures (Figs. 3-4 and 3-5), although dramatic abnormalities of this type are now less common with modern orthotics and spinal surgery. The ability to walk is lost by about 12 years of age, and death from respiratory or cardiac failure usually occurs in the 20s or early 30s. Some degree of mental retardation occurs in about one third of patients.

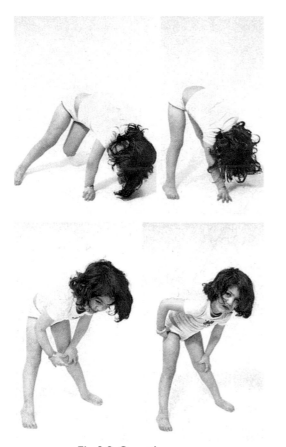

Fig. 3-3. Gowers' maneuver.

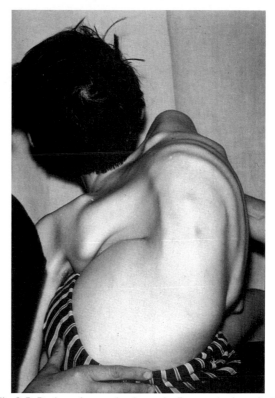

Fig. 3-5. Duchenne's muscular dystrophy. Extreme kyphoscoliosis.

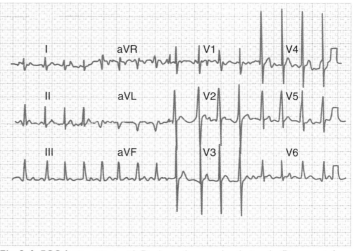

Fig. 3-6. ECG from patient with Duchenne's muscular dystrophy. Deep noninfarction Q waves and large-amplitude RS complexes are seen in chest leads.

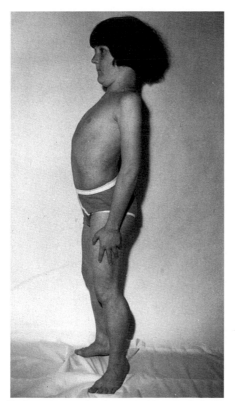

Fig. 3-4. Duchenne's muscular dystrophy. Hyperlordosis ("swayback").

Cardiac involvement, with selective atrophy and scarring of the posterobasal and lateral wall of the left ventricle and interventricular septum, causes a progressive hypertrophic and dilated cardiomyopathy and dysrhythmias. This is inevitable by age 18, although only about half of the patients become symptomatic. A characteristic electrocardiographic (ECG) appearance develops, with deep,

noninfarction Q waves and large-amplitude RS waves in the chest leads (Fig. 3-6).

Becker's muscular dystrophy has a much more variable clinical picture and can appear from childhood to early adult life. Lifespan may be normal. The pattern of muscle involvement is similar to that of DMD, but weakness is less severe and patients often remain ambulant into their 30s or later. Exertional myalgia is a common presenting symptom and may be the only manifestation. Calf muscle enlargement is typical and often striking (Fig. 3-7), but some patients have little evidence of disease in the early stages (Fig. 3-8).

The serum CK in dystrophinopathies is usually very high (at least 10-fold greater than normal and often 100 times greater), at least in the early stages of disease. Most patients require muscle biopsy (Figs. 3-9 and 3-10), and the diagnosis and nature and position of the mutation can generally be confirmed by standard lymphocyte DNA analysis, which detects the common dystrophin gene deletions in 70% of patients. Duplications may also be found, but detection of point mutations requires complete sequencing of the gene.

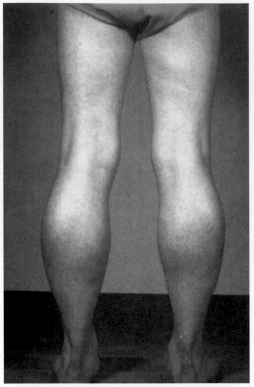

Fig. 3-7. Becker's dystrophy. Calf enlargement.

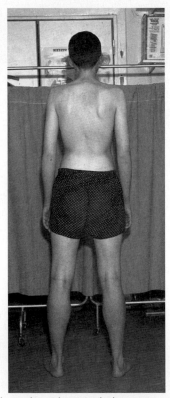

Fig. 3-8. Becker's dystrophy with minimal phenotypic expression. The patient presented with exertional myalgia. Equivocal calf enlargement and mild scapular winging.

Dystrophin. Dystrophin, one of the largest proteins in the body (427 kD), is encoded by a gene at Xp21.2 of over 2.5 million base pairs, including 79 exons. The molecule links F-actin to the sarcolemma (see Fig. 3-1), and the dystrophin molecules are arranged in a costameric (rib-like) fashion that provides mechanical bracing for the sarcolemma (Fig. 3-11). Deficiency results in loss of structural integrity of the muscle surface membrane, allowing ingress of calcium and

other noxious agents into the muscle fibers through splits called delta lesions (Fig. 3-12). The calcium excess causes focal fiber hypercontraction (hyaline fibers) and fiber necrosis (Fig. 3-9).

Mutations of the dystrophin gene may be out of frame, resulting in complete absence of dystrophin causing DMD, or in frame, producing partial dystrophin deficiency characteristic of BMD and other dystrophinopathy phenotypes such as idiopathic hyperCK-emia, X-linked cardiomyopathy (young males present with congestive cardiac failure and carrier females with "atypical" chest pain), isolated quadriceps weakness, exertional myalgia, and episodic myoglobinuria. Deficiency can usually be demonstrated immunohistochemically using specific anti-dystrophin antibodies (Fig. 3-13), although false-positive staining can occur using standard antibodies, when small mutations affect certain rod domains. Western blotting can demonstrate dystrophin deficiency quantitatively in equivocal cases (Fig. 3-14).

Manifesting Carriers
Some 10–20% of carrier females have symptoms of the recessive mutation. This results from skewed X-inactivation, resulting in a high proportion of mutated dystrophin genes. The resulting myopathy usually has a limb-girdle phenotype, although the chance intimate relationship of nuclear domains lacking dystrophin genes in individual muscles may result in only particular muscles being affected, such as one calf (Fig. 3-15, A). Biopsies from female carriers may show a mosaic pattern of dystrophin-positive and dystrophin-negative fibers (see Fig. 3-15, B and C).

Limb-Girdle Muscular Dystrophies
The limb-girdle pattern of muscular weakness affects perhaps 1 in 100,000 of the population. Since 90% of LGMDs are autosomal recessive disorders, a sporadic presentation is typical. The same clinical picture can also result from other pathologies, including spinal muscular atrophy, dystrophin deficiency, and inflammatory and mitochondrial myopathies, so full investigation is mandatory. Two forms of LGMD, dysferlinopathy and titin deficiency, also cause forms of distal myopathy (see p.60). Indeed, the same mutation in these genes can cause either clinical pattern in different members of the same family but the reason for this intrafamilial phenotypic heterogeneity is unknown.

Currently, there are six classified autosomal dominant LGMDs (LGMD1A to 1F) and ten autosomal recessive diseases (LGMD2A to 2J). Some conditions, such as LGMD2A (calpain deficiency) and LGMD2I (fukutin related protein deficiency), are common, whereas others have been reported in only a few families worldwide. More than a quarter of cases of LGMD result from as yet undefined protein defects.

In general terms, LGMDs result from defects of sarcolemmal proteins (sarcoglycans, dysferlin, and caveolin), cytosolic enzyme deficiencies (e.g., calpain 3, TRIM 32), and defects of sarcomeric (myofibrillar) proteins (e.g., titin, telethonin).

Adult-onset LGMDs usually appear in the second to third decade with progressive difficulty in walking followed by proximal arm weakness. Ambulation is often lost after 20 to 30 years, but age of onset and progression vary considerably even within families. Cranial and bulbar musculature is unaffected. The neck muscles become weak and the muscles of the shoulder and pelvic girdles and the proximal arm and leg muscles become weak and wasted, although the quadriceps are sometimes spared (Fig. 3-16). Hip abduction is often strong compared with adduction and may result in a Charlie Chaplin type of gait. Distal involvement and calf hypertrophy is variable. In some forms, muscular hypertrophy can be marked, with appearances suggestive of Becker's dystrophy (Fig. 3-17). Bilateral scapular winging is a typical and often an early feature (Fig. 3-18), and there is eventually marked muscular wasting, particularly of proximal muscles (Fig. 3-19).

Childhood-onset LGMDs produce a DMD-like phenotype referred to as severe childhood autosomal recessive muscular dystrophy. However, being autosomal, the condition affects girls as well as boys.

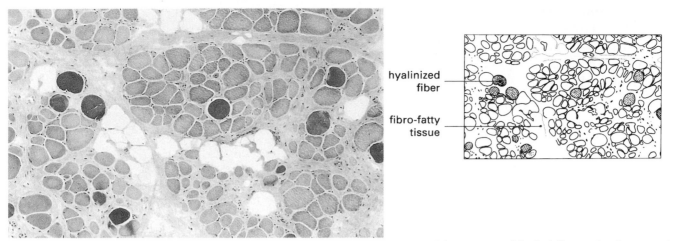

Fig. 3-9. Duchenne's muscular dystrophy. Section from muscle biopsy shows marked fiber size variation, with hypercontracted (hyaline) fibers and replacement of muscle by fat and fibrous tissue (dystrophic change) (H&E).

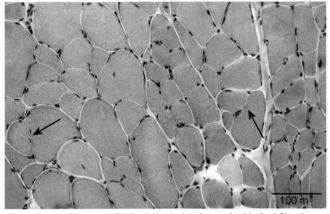

Fig. 3-10. Biopsy findings in Becker's muscular dystrophy. Marked fiber hypertrophy sometimes with fiber splitting *(arrows),* and regenerative activity characterized by basophilic fibers.

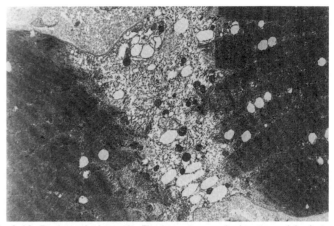

Fig. 3-12. Duchenne's dystrophy. Electron micrograph showing a delta lesion, a split in the sarcolemma caused by loss of cytoskeletal integrity caused by lack of dystrophin. The split has resulted in homogenization of sarcomeres representing early fiber necrosis.

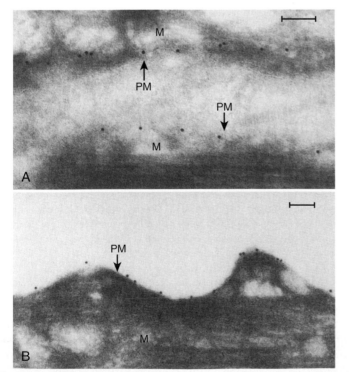

Fig. 3-11. Immunogold labeling with antibody to 43-kD dystrophin-associated glycoprotein showing normal costameric disposition of dystrophin on the sarcolemma. M, myofibrils; PM, plasma membrane. (Reproduced from Russell J. M. Lane, editor: *Handbook of Muscle Disease,* 1996, by permission of Marcel Dekker, Inc.)

CK levels are increased in patients with LGMDs but vary considerably with the specific conditions. A very high CK suggests LGMD2B (dysferlinopathy). Muscle biopsy changes tend to be rather nonspecific, but lobulated and moth-eaten fibers seen with histochemical staining are suggestive (Fig. 3-20). Specific diagnoses require immunohistochemical and multiplex immunoblotting techniques (Fig. 3-21).

Congenital Muscular Dystrophies. Congenital muscular dystrophies are generally severe diseases that appear at birth or within the first few months of life, with marked hypotonia, limb contractures, and breathing and feeding problems. The prognosis is usually poor. However, the increasing availability of molecular markers has shown that the mutations causing these diseases are more common than previously thought, and milder phenotypic variants can appear in later childhood and even very rarely in adult life, as forms of LGMD. Some CMDs comprise muscle disease alone, and others have significant central nervous system involvement.

The locations of the defective proteins are shown in Figure 3-1. They include defects in structural proteins of the extracellular matrix, including proteins of the basal lamina (merosin) or laminin α 2 (6q2) and integrin α 7 (12q) and, defects in enzymes involved with the glycosylation of dystroglycan and of selenoprotein N1 (SEPN1), an endoplasmic reticulum protein (1p3). Defects in collagen 6 (COL6, 21q22.3, 2q37) in the extracellular matrix cause the Ullrich form of CMD but also cause Bethlem myopathy, a relatively benign autosomal dominant myopathy in adults, with an axial limb-girdle pattern characterized by rigid spine and striking limb

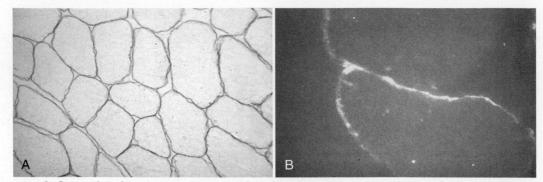

Fig. 3-13. Dystrophin staining. **A,** Crisp outline of the protein on the inner surface of the sarcolemma in a normal biopsy. In Duchenne's muscular dystrophy, staining would be absent. **B,** Patchy staining in Becker's muscular dystrophy (immunofluorescent stain) caused by the presence of truncated dystrophin.

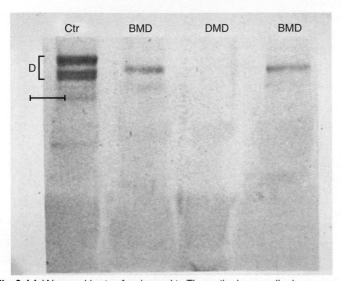

Fig. 3-14. Western blotting for dystrophin. The antibody normally demonstrates a doublet comprising full-length dystrophin and a smaller dystrophin isoform band (D). Dystrophin is absent in the case of Duchenne's muscular dystrophy, whereas in Becker's muscular dystrophy, the dystrophin isoforms are smaller (more mobile on the gel) and reduced in quantity.

contractures, notably of the long-finger flexors, causing the "prayer sign" (Fig. 3-22).

Deficiency of another matrix protein, perlecan (see Fig. 3-1), causes Schwartz-Jampel syndrome. This disease can be considered a CMD, but its cardinal neuromuscular feature, continuous myotonia, is so atypical that it is usually considered with the group of myotonic dystrophies.

To date, 10 genes underlying CMDs have been defined, but these do not account for all cases, and other loci remain to be identified.

Other Axial and Limb-Girdle Pattern Dystrophies

Nuclear Membrane Protein Defects: Emery-Dreifuss Muscular Dystrophy. Patients with Emery-Dreifuss muscular dystrophy (EDMD) present in childhood with progressive weakness and wasting of the scapulohumeral, anterior tibial, and peroneal muscle groups. It accounts for some instances of scapuloperoneal syndrome p7, Box 3-3. Muscle contractures develop at an early stage, leading to a pathognomonic posture, with elbow flexion, equinovarus ankle deformities, fixed neck flexion, scoliosis, and rigid spine (Fig. 3-23). Unlike DMD, the muscles tend to be slim, and hypertrophy is unusual. Cardiac involvement is prominent, leading to serious conduction disorders and sometimes sudden death. Prophylactic pacemaker insertion can be life saving.

This phenotype results from mutations in genes that code for structural proteins of the inner nuclear membrane. In X-linked forms, muscle immunohistochemistry demonstrates deficiency of the nuclear membrane protein emerin (Fig. 3-24). The autosomal

dominant form of EDMD is caused by deficiency of lamin A/C and can also be identified immunohistochemically.

Non–Limb-Girdle Weakness Pattern Dystrophies with Prominent Involvement of Cranial Musculature

Facioscapulohumeral Muscular Dystrophy. Facioscapulohumeral muscular dystrophy (FSHD) is a common autosomal dominant disease with a prevalence of about 3 in 100,000. A family history may not be evident because the disease can be mild and even remain undiagnosed. New mutations also account for some 10% of cases. Phenocopies due to spinal muscular atrophy, mitochondrial myopathy, and inclusion body myositis have been reported, but lymphocyte DNA analysis has greatly reduced diagnostic uncertainty in recent years.

The disease is defined by the demonstration of abnormally small (<35 kb) 4q35-derived DNA fragments after digestion with restriction site enzymes. Disease severity tends to correlate inversely with the size of the fragments, and milder phenotypes, including cases of scapuloperoneal syndrome caused by this mutation usually have larger fragments, between 35 and 40 kb.

Weakness typically begins in the face, although the face is unaffected in some individuals. The deltoids are usually strong compared with the biceps and triceps muscles, which become progressively wasted. There is anterior rotation of the shoulders, and the clavicles become horizontally displaced (Fig. 3-25). The extraocular, pharyngeal, and lingual muscles are spared. Inability to whistle is characteristic but not invariable. In later stages, dramatic scapular winging usually develops. Weakness of the scapular fixators allows overriding of the scapulae above the shoulders, like a pair of wings (Fig. 3-26). Lower limb weakness may not be conspicuous, but footdrop caused by weakness of the tibialis anterior and peronei, and later proximal weakness, is common.

Creatine kinase levels may be normal or only mildly increased, and electromyography (EMG) and muscle biopsy often show only minimal abnormalities. However, dramatic changes are occasionally found (Fig. 3-27).

Oculopharyngeal Muscular Dystrophy. Oculopharyngeal muscular dystrophy presents with ptosis and weakness of the extraocular muscles and the muscles of the pharynx and larynx, causing progressive dysphagia and dysphonia (Fig. 3-28). This may be followed by weakness of facial, limb-girdle, and even distal muscles. It is an autosomal dominant disorder, but gene penetrance varies considerably. Cases may be mild to severe, and patients can present at almost any age, though typically in the sixth decade and beyond.

Creatine kinase levels may be normal or only minimally increased. Biopsy can show a range of changes that may include rimmed vacuoles, "ragged red" fibers, and cytochrome c oxidase–negative fibers typical of a mitochondrial myopathy (Fig. 3-29, A). Ultrastructural studies may reveal pathognomonic accumulations of 8.5-nm filaments in a small proportion of myonuclei (Fig. 3-29, B).

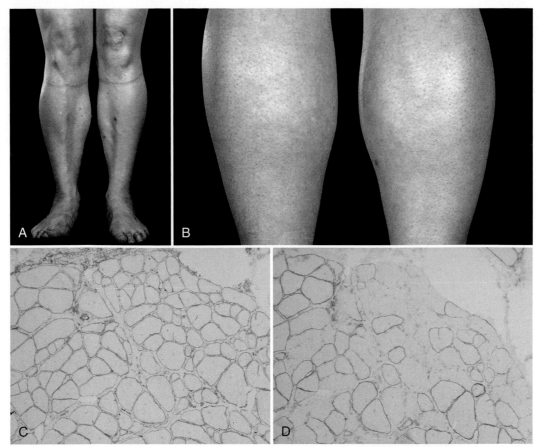

Fig. 3-15. Dystrophinopathy. Manifesting Carrier **A** and **B**, Presenting complaint was of right calf hypertrophy. No family history of muscle disease. **C,** β-Spectrin immunohistochemistry demonstrated structural integrity of the sarcolemma. **D,** Dystrophin staining showed a mosaic of positive and negative fibers.

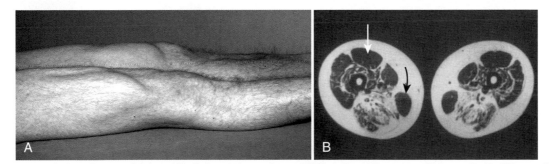

Fig. 3-16. Quadriceps sparing in limb-girdle muscular dystrophy. **A,** Prominent quadriceps. Weak and wasted posterior thigh muscles. **B,** CT scan of thighs confirms selective involvement of the posterior leg compartment (high signal) with sparing of the quadriceps *(arrows).* The abductors were also strong compared with the adductors.

The disease is caused by a GCG triplet expansion at the poly-A binding protein 2 (PABP2) gene coded at 14q11, and can be diagnosed by lymphocyte DNA analysis. The expansion causes mutated PABP2 monomers to aggregate in nuclei, resulting in the filament accumulations.

Scapuloperoneal Syndrome. Weakness and wasting in a distribution similar to that seen with FSHD but sparing the face is referred to as scapuloperoneal syndrome. There are several neurogenic and myopathic causes, and the pathogenesis can be determined only by detailed investigation (Box 3-3). Mutations in the FSHD gene are the most common cause.

Distal Myopathies
Progressive symmetrical distal weakness is usually a result of neurogenic disease but can be a feature of a number of rare myopathies. The five well-defined forms of distal myopathy are classified by inheritance pattern, age at onset, and muscle groups initially involved (Table 3-1). Some affect mainly the anterior compartment of the lower limbs, causing footdrop, others the posterior compartment,

BOX 3-3	CAUSES OF SCAPULOPERONEAL SYNDROME

Neurogenic
Scapuloperoneal neuronopathies
Davidenkow's syndrome

Myopathic
Facioscapulohumeral dystrophy
Polymyositis
Scapuloperoneal muscular dystrophy
Calpainopathy (LGMD 2A)
Emery-Dreifuss dystrophy
Centronuclear myopathy
Mitochondrial myopathy
Acid maltase deficiency

causing difficulty standing on the toes. Involvement of the hands, forearms, and occasionally proximal muscles may develop later, and upper limb involvement is the presenting feature in Welander's disease. Rimmed vacuoles in muscle fibers are a feature of several of these conditions (see also Inclusion Body Myositis, below).

TABLE 3-1.   DISTAL MYOPATHIES

	SITE OF ONSET	AGE OF ONSET	CK LEVEL	RV	PROTEIN	LOCUS
Autosomal Dominant						
Welander disease	Hands, forearms	Adult	N↑	+	?	2p13
Tibial muscular dystrophy	Anterior compartment	Adult	↑↑	+	Titin	2q31
Laing myopathy	Anterior compartment	Infancy	↑↑	−	Myosin	14q11
Autosomal Recessive						
Miyoshi myopathy	Posterior compartment	Adult	↑↑↑	−	Dysferlin	2p12-14
Nonaka myopathy	Posterior compartment	Adult	↑	+	GNE	9p21-q12

CK, creatine kinase; GNE, UDP-*N*-acetylglucosamine 2-epimerase/*N*-acetylmannosamine kinase; RV, rimmed vacuoles in muscle fibers.

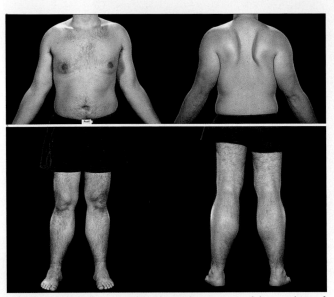

Fig. 3-17. Limb-girdle muscular dystrophy in an adult, resulting from α-sarcoglycanopathy. The patient presented with a Becker-type clinical picture, but dystrophin analysis was normal.

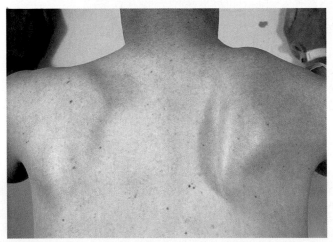

Fig. 3-18. Limb-girdle muscular dystrophy. Scapular winging is typical and often asymmetrical.

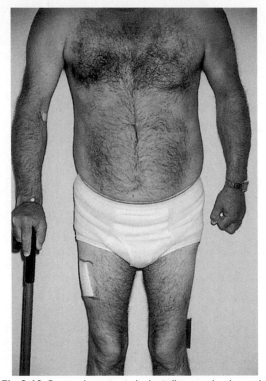

Fig. 3-19. Proximal wasting in limb-girdle muscular dystrophy.

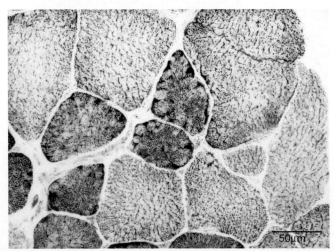

Fig. 3-20. Limb-girdle muscular dystrophy. Fiber hypertrophy and typical lobulated muscle fibers on NADH-TR staining.

Miyoshi myopathy is the most common of the distal myopathies. As noted earlier, this autosomal recessive disease is an alternative phenotypic manifestation of dysferlinopathy, the cause of LGMD2B. Both phenotypes can occur in the same family. Patients present with slowly progressive weakness of the posterior compartment muscles of the lower legs (although very rarely the anterior compartment is affected first), causing difficulty standing on the toes, followed by more general lower leg weakness and wasting (Fig. 3-30). The CK level is typically very high (often > 10,000 U/L). Later, weakness may affect the distal arms and then more proximal muscles, as in the LGMD form. Muscle biopsy shows nonspecific myopathic abnormalities. Rimmed

vacuoles are not present. The diagnosis can be confirmed by immunohistochemistry and immunoblotting for dysferlin (see Fig. 3-21). The location of the defective proteins causing distal myopathies is shown in Figure 3-1.

Laing-type distal myopathy is usually severe and starts in infancy with footdrop, wrist drop, and finger drop. Udd's tibial muscular dystrophy is an autosomal dominant disease occurring in the Finnish population. It is characterized by weakness and wasting of the tibial muscles and results from the same titin mutations that cause LGMD2J. Nonaka myopathy (Fig. 3-31) is clinically similar but is inherited as an autosomal recessive. It is allelic with a form of

hereditary inclusion body myopathy (see p. 71) caused by mutations in the GNE gene (UDP-*N*-acetylglucosamine 2-epimerase/*N*-acetylmannosamine kinase, 9p21-q12). Both conditions are rimmed vacuolar myopathies.

MYOTONIC DYSTROPHIES AND NON-DYSTROPHIC MYOTONIAS

The finding of clinical or electromyographic myotonia (inability to relax muscles after contraction) in a patient with neuromuscular symptoms opens a new range of diagnostic possibilities. Myotonias can be classified as dystrophic (the myotonic dystrophies) or non-dystrophic. Non-dystrophic myotonias are part of the group of conditions now also referred to as muscle channelopathies, as they are caused by mutations in muscle ion channel genes. The muscle channelopathies also include the periodic paralyses and some forms of malignant hyperthermia.

Myotonic Dystrophies

There are two forms of myotonic dystrophy: DM1 (Steinert's disease) and DM2, which most often presents as proximal myotonic myopathy. However, there are also rare cases of myotonic dystrophy not linked to the genes for these diseases. A condition previously designated DM3 is caused by a mutation in the valosin gene and is considered to be one of the hereditary inclusion body myopathies.

DM1 is the most common inherited neuromuscular disease. The prevalence is about 5 in 100,000. Although neuromuscular dysfunction is the most prominent clinical feature, it is a multisystemic disease with many other manifestations (Box 3-4). It is caused by a trinucleotide expansion $(CTG)_n$ at 19q13.3, in which *n* is increased from 5 to 37 repeats in normal individuals to anything from 50 repeats in mild DM (manifest perhaps by cataracts alone) to more than 1000 repeats in congenital DM. In general, the larger the repeat size, the more severe the disease is. Individuals in successive generations usually inherit larger expansions and thus have more severe disease and an earlier onset (genetic anticipation) (Fig. 3-32).

The mutation involves the 3′ untranslated region of the dystrophia myotonica phosphorylase kinase (DMPK) gene. Current evidence indicates that the long CUG RNA transcripts of the trinucleotide intronic repeats accumulate in nuclei and sequester pre-mRNA alternate splicing regulatory proteins, such as Muscleblind1, disrupting transcription of a number of genes in many tissues. This accounts for the multisystemic features characteristic of myotonic dystrophies. There are prominent far

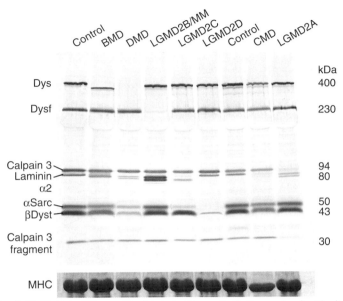

Fig. 3-21. Multiplex Western blot labeled with a cocktail of monoclonal antibodies to proteins associated with some of the axial limb-girdle pattern muscular dystrophies. The lanes (from left to right) show:

Lane 1: Normal control muscle sample (Dys, dystrophin, 400 kD; Dysf, dysferlin, 230 kD; calpain 3, 94 kD and 30 kD; laminin α2, 80 kD; α-sarcoglycan, 50 kD; and β-sarcoglycan, 43 kD)

Lane 2: Shortened (more mobile) dystrophin fragment caused by in-frame mutation in BMD

Lane 3: Total absence of dystrophin caused by out-of-frame mutation in Duchenne's muscular dystrophy, plus secondary reduction in labeling of other bands

Lane 4: Total absence of dysferlin in LGMD2B/MM (Miyoshi myopathy)

Lanes 5 and 6: Deficiency of sarcoglycans and dystroglycan in cases of severe childhood autosomal recessive muscular dystrophy (LGMD2C and LGMD2D, respectively). (Courtesy of the late Dr. Louise Anderson, Newcastle University, Newcastle upon Tyne, UK.)

Lane 7: Normal control

Lane 8: Deficiency of laminin α2 chain in congenital muscular dystrophy

Lane 9: Absence of calpain 3 in LGMD2A

MHC: Myosin heavy chain band stained with Coomassie blue shows amount of muscle protein loaded in each lane.

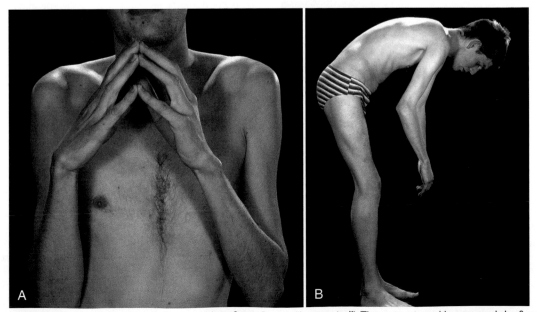

Fig. 3-22. Bethlem myopathy. **A,** Flexion contractures of elbows and long-finger flexors ("prayer sign"). The patient is unable to extend the fingers. **B,** Rigid spine sign. The patient is unable to flex the spine any further.

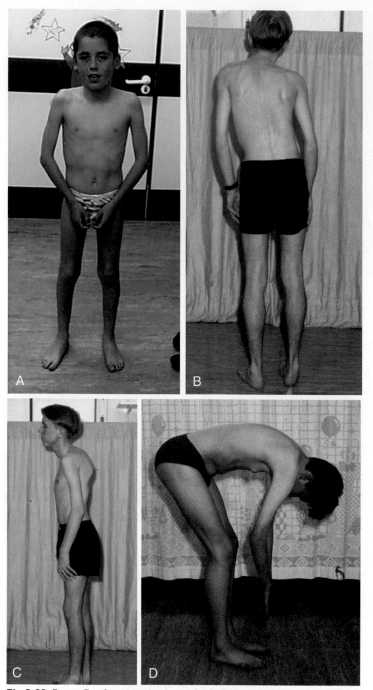

Fig. 3-23. Emery-Dreifuss muscular dystrophy. **A,** Early elbow contractures. **B** and **C,** Scoliosis and scapular winging. **D,** Rigid spine.

<table>
<tr><td>

BOX 3-4 CLINICAL FEATURES OF MYOTONIC DYSTROPHY DM1

Neuromuscular
• Grip and percussion myotonia
• Progressive muscular weakness and wasting, starting distally
• Bilateral ptosis
• Facial muscle weakness
• Sternomastoid wasting
• Bulbar and respiratory muscle weakness

Eye
• Cataracts, ptosis, ophthalmoparesis, retinopathy

Endocrinopathy
• Diabetes, testicular atrophy, pituitary dysfunction

Cardiovascular
• Conduction defects, hypotension

Gastrointestinal
• Dysphagia, pseudo-obstruction

Respiratory
• Aspiration pneumonia, sleep apnea

Skin
• Frontal balding, pilomatricoma

Central Nervous System
• Mental retardation, apathy

</td></tr>
</table>

field effects on SIX5, the DM-associated homeodomain gene that lies close to DMPK, which is involved in the regulation of eye formation This may explain the prominence of cataract in the phenotype. There are also changes in Cl⁻ channel function, resulting in the myotonia.

The availability of a specific genetic test for DM1 has largely superseded the need for nonspecific investigations such as muscle biopsy and slit lamp examination of the eyes for early signs of cataract. The condition is sometimes first ascertained in an undiagnosed patient when myotonia is found during a routine EMG examination.

Gene expression can vary from asymptomatic cases, with no clinical signs, to severe congenital disease. In the classic form, the lugubrious facies is characteristic, with bilateral ptosis and facial weakness (Fig. 3-33). The sternomastoids are selectively wasted. Limb weakness is the most disabling symptom. It begins distally, notably in the hands, and spreads proximally, involving the deltoids, a distinction from FSHD (Fig. 3-34).

Myotonia may be a prominent clinical sign but it is rarely disabling. Myotonia of grip is usually easy to demonstrate (Fig. 3-35).

Percussion myotonia is elicited at the thenar eminence by striking this region with a tendon hammer, which causes sustained abduction and opposition of the thumb. Myotonia can also be demonstrated in the tongue in some cases (Fig. 3-36).

The most common non-neuromuscular manifestations are cataracts, cardiac disease, and diabetes. Cataracts are usually asymptomatic until later stages of the disease but can be a presenting feature (Fig. 3-37). Glucose intolerance due to insulin resistance, caused by changes in insulin receptor function, is common, but clinical diabetes is relatively infrequent. Cardiac symptoms resulting from conduction defects may be life-threatening, requiring a pacemaker (Fig. 3-38).

Pilomatricomas (calcifying epithelioma of Malherbe) are found more commonly in DM1 than expected. Often multiple, these skin lesions may require excision. Muscle biopsy, now rarely required for diagnosis, may be normal but often demonstrates "trucking" of centrally placed myonuclei (Fig. 3-39).

Congenital myotonic dystrophy usually appears as floppy baby syndrome in an infant with breathing and suckling difficulties. Myotonia is not demonstrable at this age, and the diagnosis is often made by recognizing the condition in the mother; the mother rather than the father is the carrier in nearly all cases. There is a significant degree of mental and physical handicap.

Proximal myotonic myopathy (or DM2) is a rare disorder caused by an expansion in the number of CCTG repeats in the gene encoding zinc finger protein 9 (ZNF9, 3q21). Like DM1, it is a multisystemic disorder, but there are a number of distinctive features. In particular, weakness is usually confined mainly to proximal muscles. Muscle pain is also more prominent, although the myotonia is generally less severe than in DM1. Muscle hypertrophy, particularly of the calves, rather than atrophy, is common, and facial and sternomastoid weakness is only mild. Cognitive changes are less prominent, and although there is some intergenerational instability in the number of CCTG repeats, genetic anticipation is less evident.

Like DM1, DM2 appears to be a "spliceopathy" in which the aggregation of mRNA transcripts of the expanded CCTG repeats interferes with normal mRNA splicing, although the reason that DM2 is generally milder than DM1 is unclear.

It should be stressed that this disease may present as a rather featureless, nonselective, symmetrical proximal myopathy with little increase in serum CK level. Myotonia may be minimal and easily overlooked, so patients may undergo muscle biopsy before the

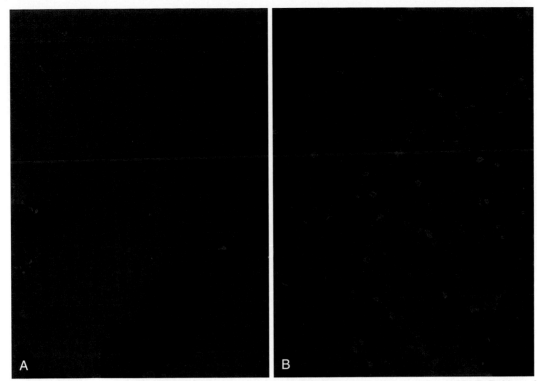

Fig. 3-24. Emery-Dreifuss muscular dystrophy (EDMD), emerin staining. **A,** Absent nuclear staining in X-linked EDMD. **B,** Normal control.

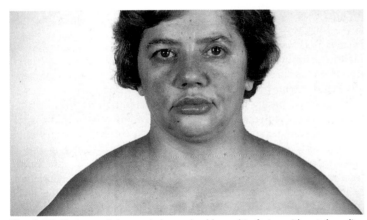

Fig. 3-25. Facioscapulohumeral dystrophy. Myopathic facies with patulous lips, anterior shoulder rotation, and horizontally displaced clavicles.

TABLE 3-2.   MUSCLE CHANNELOPATHIES

CHANNEL	DISEASE	INHERITANCE	GENE	LOCUS
Sodium	Hyperkalemic periodic paralysis Paramyotonia congenita Potassium-aggravated myotonia	AD	SCN4A1	17q23
Chloride	Myotonia Congenita (Thomsen's and Becker's disease)	AD AR	CLCN1	7q35
Calcium	Hypokale-mic periodic paralysis	AD	CACNA1S	1q31-32
	Malignant hyperthermia	AD AD?	CACNA1S RYR	1q31-32 19q12-13.2
Potassium	Andersen's disease	AD	KCNJ2	17q23

CACNA1S, dihydropyridine receptor; *RYR,* ryanodine receptor.

diagnosis is considered. Muscle biopsy, however, can suggest the correct diagnosis, because there are usually rather characteristic pyknotic nuclear clumps, consisting of very atrophic type 2 muscle fibers with prominent nuclear aggregates (Fig. 3-40).

Schwartz-Jampel syndrome (chondrodystrophic myotonia), as noted previously, is fundamentally a rare CMD and is unique in that it presents in infancy with continuous severe myotonia, particularly of the face. Affected children have a characteristic fixed expression, with microstomia, pursed lips, puckered chin, and blepharospasm (Fig. 3-41). The continuous myotonia leads to muscular hypertrophy, notably of the thighs. Associated skeletal malformations include micrognathism, kyphoscoliosis, and contractures. Patients have short stature and adopt a crouched posture, with a waddling gait.

The condition results from loss of perlecan, a heparan sulphate proteoglycan component of the extracellular matrix, caused by in-frame mutations in the perlecan gene at 1p34-36 (see Fig. 3-1). This protein interacts with integrins to anchor the basal lamina to the sarcolemma and is involved with the regulation of bone growth. It also has a major role in clustering of acetylcholinesterase to the neuromuscular junction. Lack of acetylcholinesterase results in persistent muscle depolarization and the continuous myotonia. This differs, however, from endplate acetylcholinesterase deficiency, one of the congenital myasthenias (see p. 85).

Non-dystrophic Myotonias

Non-dystrophic myotonias and other muscle channelopathies are caused by mutations in skeletal muscle sodium, chloride, calcium, and potassium ion channel genes (Fig. 3-42). In the non-dystrophic myotonias, the main feature is myotonia, whereas periodic paralyses are characterized by attacks of muscular weakness, although mild myotonia can also be a feature in some forms. Muscle channelopathies also underlie most instances of susceptibility to malignant hyperthermia (MH).

Ion channel dysfunction results in electrical instability of the muscle fiber surface membranes. Some mutations result in partial depolarization, causing membrane hyperexcitability (myotonia), and others cause loss of excitability (weakness, paralysis). Table 3-2 shows the main associations between genes and syndromes.

Periodic paralyses are usually associated with changes in serum K^+ during attacks (hyperkalemic and hypokalemic periodic paralyses); normokalemic periodic paralysis is a variant of the hyperkalemic form. A periodic paralysis very similar to the genetic hypokalemic form can also be caused by chronic hypokalemia due to a variety of

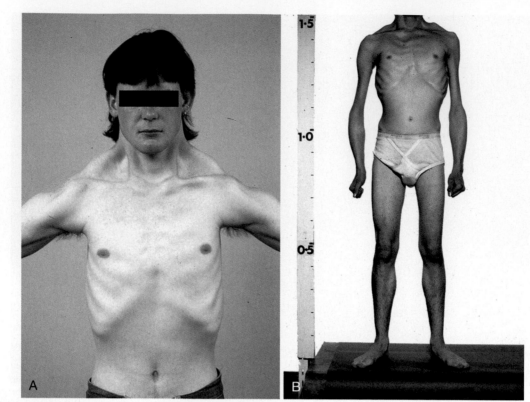

Fig. 3-26. Facioscapulohumeral dystrophy. Overriding of the scapulae *(left)*. Note the preserved bulk of the deltoids compared with the wasted biceps and triceps muscles *(right)*.

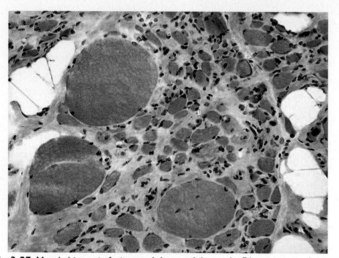

Fig. 3-27. Muscle biopsy in facioscapulohumeral dystrophy. Fiber necrosis, dramatic variation in fiber sizes, increased endomysial connective tissues, and numerous small immature regenerating fibers. In some cases, however, changes are minimal.

systemic disorders (secondary periodic paralysis) and may also be a manifestation of thyrotoxicosis (thyrotoxic periodic paralysis).

Myotonia congenita is caused by mutations in the muscle chloride channel gene. Myotonia rather than weakness is the major feature. Myotonia is also a feature of muscle sodium channelopathies that cause hyperkalemic periodic paralysis but is not found in hypokalemic periodic paralysis, which is a muscle calcium channelopathy.

Sodium Channelopathies. Different mutations in the SCN4A1 gene cause a variety of syndromes. Some mutations result in increased membrane excitability, causing myotonia. Others cause episodic membrane depolarization and weakness. These conditions include hyperkalemic periodic paralysis, paramyotonia congenita (Eulenburg's disease), and potassium-aggravated myotonia (PAM).

Hyperkalemic periodic paralysis (HyPP) is an autosomal dominant disease that usually begins in infancy or childhood. Attacks of flaccid, areflexic paralysis lasting between 15 minutes and an hour may be triggered by rest after exercise and by ingestion of foods and drink high in potassium. The serum K$^+$ is usually increased, up to 7 mM, during an attack. Some patients have myotonia between attacks, usually demonstrable by EMG and sometimes clinically.

Myotonia typically lessens with exercise (the warm-up phenomenon) but in paramyotonia congenita, myotonia worsens rather than improves with exercise (paradoxical myotonia). It is also strikingly worsened by cold. The myotonia affects particularly the facial muscles, neck, and forearms. Eyelid myotonia is characteristic. Some families have mutations that also cause attacks of paralysis independently of the paramyotonia.

Potassium-aggravated myotonia is also characterized by myotonia rather than by paralysis, and is typically precipitated by rest after exercise, and worsened by cold and by potassium loading.

Chloride Channelopathies. Muscle chloride channelopathies cause myotonia congenita. Unlike myotonic dystrophies, where weakness and wasting are the predominant neuromuscular symptoms, myotonia is the chief manifestation and the resulting generalized muscular hypertrophy is the striking clinical characteristic (Fig. 3-43). The Becker form is the most common. This is an autosomal recessive disorder that causes generalized myotonia of moderate severity, and sometimes weakness. Thomsen's disease, an autosomal dominant condition, tends to be milder. It usually appears in the first decade but tends to stabilize in adolescence.

Calcium Channelopathies. *Hypokalemic periodic paralysis* (HoPP), the most common form of periodic paralysis, is an autosomal dominant condition of variable penetrance. The attacks tend to be less frequent than in the hyperkalemic form, but they last longer, hours to days. Attacks are precipitated by stress and high carbohydrate intake. Oliguria is typical during attacks because of sequestration of water in muscle. The serum K$^+$ may fall to 1 to 2 mM, sufficient to cause cardiac dysrhythmia. Recurrent attacks can eventually lead to a progressive proximal myopathy with vacuolar change on biopsy (Fig. 3-44).

This disease results from mutations in the CACNA1S gene. This gene codes for the dihydropyridine receptors, voltage-dependent Ca^{2+} channels located on the transverse tubules, which interact with

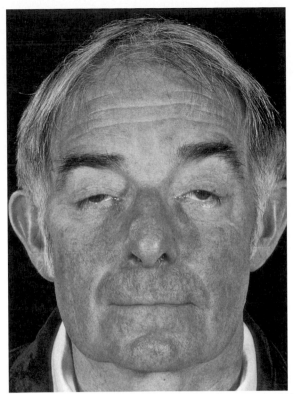

Fig. 3-28. Oculopharyngeal muscular dystrophy. Bilateral ptosis and mild bilateral facial weakness.

the ryanodine receptors of the sarcoplasmic reticulum to initiate excitation–contraction coupling (Fig. 3-45).

Malignant hyperthermia is a syndrome characterized by the rapid onset of muscular rigor, usually in the context of general anesthesia, caused by sudden release of Ca^{2+} from the sarcoplasmic reticulum into the myoplasm. Mutations in the ryanodine and dihydropyridine receptor genes account for many cases of MH, suggesting that defects in proteins regulating muscle Ca^{2+} homeostasis may be the common mechanism. MH is genetically heterogeneous, and some forms are inherited as an autosomal dominant trait.

Patients with a variety of genetic myopathies are susceptible to MH. Patients with central core disease (CCD) (see end of this page), a form of congenital myopathy resulting from mutations of the ryanodine receptor gene (RYR1, 19q12-13.2), are especially vulnerable. Mutations of this gene have also been found in MH families without evident myopathy. Some patients with otherwise unexplained hyper-CKemia also carry MH susceptibility mutations.

Potassium Channelopathies. *Andersen's syndrome* is a rare autosomal dominant condition in which potassium-sensitive periodic paralysis is associated with electrocardiographic abnormalities, notably a long QT interval (unrelated to the serum K^+), and often dysmorphic features, including hypertelorism, low-set ears, broad nose, hypognathism, and skeletal abnormalities such as clinodactyly and syndactyly.

Secondary periodic paralysis. Persistent intracellular hypokalemia can cause periodic weakness as well as a progressive myopathy (see p. 80) and can be difficult to distinguish from HoPP. Onset of symptoms after age 30 and the demonstration of significant hypokalemia with a potentially causative underlying condition, such as a renal, endocrine, or gastrointestinal disorder, or excessive use of kaliuretics (e.g., diuretics and licorice) would be suggestive. Thyrotoxic periodic paralysis is particularly associated with individuals of Chinese extraction (Fig. 3-46).

CONGENITAL MYOPATHIES

Congenital myopathies are defined by histopathologic and ultra-structural changes on muscle biopsy. Some features, such as nemaline rods and central and multiple cores, have been shown to result from

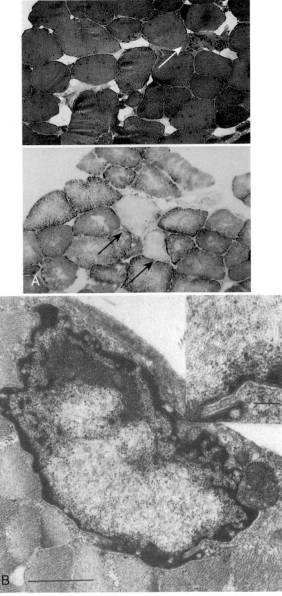

Fig. 3-29. Muscle biopsy in oculopharyngeal muscular dystrophy. **A,** Cytoplasmic protein accumulations *(white arrow) (above)*. Pale cytochrome c oxidase–negative fibers *(black arrows) (below)*. **B,** Electron micrograph of myonucleus showing 8.5-nm filaments *(inset)*.

specific genetic mutations, but these structures can sometimes be epiphenomena. Rarely, a mixture of such structures can be found in a single patient, illustrating the complexity of the pathogenesis. The term 'congenital myopathy' is also something of a misnomer, because although many patients infants do present as "floppy infants" and the signature pathologic changes are probably present from birth, diagnosis may not be made until adult life, because these conditions often show little progression, and disability may be modest.

Typical clinical features include a characteristic long face, high arched palate (Fig. 3-47), and generally slim musculature. Sometimes, a limb-girdle phenotype is evident (Fig. 3-48), perhaps complicated by eye closure weakness. CK is often normal or only slightly increased. The heart, respiratory, and extraocular muscles may be involved in some forms.

Central Core Disease
Central core disease, which is caused by ryanodine receptor (RYR1) gene mutations, has already been mentioned in connection with malignant hyperthermia. However, although many different RYR mutations have been identified in MH families, relatively few cause CCD.

This is a dominantly inherited condition and usually appears in infancy or childhood with hypotonia and delayed motor milestones.

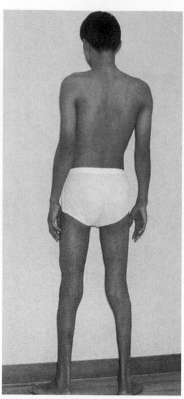

Fig. 3-30. Miyoshi myopathy. Marked wasting of distal leg muscles, especially the calves. The patient had difficulty standing on his toes.

Congenital dislocation of the hips is a common manifestation. Biopsy findings are diagnostic (Fig. 3-49).

Multicore-minicore disease is a rare autosomal recessive congenital myopathy resulting from mutations in the selenoprotein N1 gene (1p36) (see p. 61). The histologic features are similar to those of CCD, which can cause diagnostic difficulties. However, the individual cores run for only a few sarcomeres along the fibers.

Nemaline Myopathies

Nemaline myopathies are caused by defects in a number of contractile proteins, including slow α-tropomyosin, nebulin, α-actin, β-tropomyosin, and slow troponin T. Nemaline rods are generally composed of Z-line–derived proteins (Fig. 3-50) and are readily identified in biopsies stained by the Gomori trichrome or toluidine blue method.

Centronuclear and Myotubular Myopathies

Centronuclear and myotubular myopathies are so called because of the accumulation of myonuclei along the long axis of fibers rather than at the periphery as is normal. The appearance is thus reminiscent of myotubes formed during fiber maturation. The severe X-linked form results from mutations of the myotubularin gene (MTMX, Xq28). Affected males almost always die in infancy but survival to adult life has been reported. Milder dominant and recessive forms also occur, but the genes for these have not yet been defined. The clinical and pathologic features can be easily confused with those of congenital myotonic dystrophy (see p. 65).

Congenital Fiber-Type Disproportion

It has been suggested that centronuclear and myotubular myopathies might represent abnormalities of muscle fiber maturation. The same can be said of congenital fiber type disproportion, in which there is an increase in the proportion of type 1 fibers, which are also hypotrophic, together with hypertrophy of type 2 fibers. The pathologic appearances are reminiscent of some cases of spinal muscular atrophy, but the process is not neurogenic.

This condition is genetically heterogeneous and currently ill defined. Patients can present with floppy infant syndrome, but there is a wide range of severity.

Myofibrillar Myopathies and Hereditary Inclusion Body Myopathies

A number of myopathies are characterized histologically by muscle fiber inclusions, such as cytoplasmic bodies, spheroid bodies, and granulofilamentous material, in which there is accumulation of intermediate-filament proteins. Generally considered to be rare, such processes are increasingly recognized to underlie many otherwise undiagnosed degenerative muscle diseases. These conditions are usually, but not invariably, autosomal dominant, and mutations in a number of genes including desmin, alpha-B-crystallin, myotilin, BAG3, and ZASP have been defined. These diseases can present with a variety of phenotypes and diagnosis rests on laboratory identification of the molecular defect.

Desminopathies are the most common of this group of "surplus protein myopathies." Desmin is one of a group of structural proteins that link myofibrils to the sarcolemma and other organelles to provide stability during muscle contraction. Patients can present with scapuloperoneal, limb-girdle, or distal muscle weakness. Respiratory muscle involvement can occur, and cardiomyopathy is common and can be prominent. Desmin accumulation can be demonstrated immunohistochemically (Fig. 3-51).

Mutations in desmin also cause one form of hereditary inclusion body myopathy (hIBM), which can resemble inclusion body myositis clinically (see p. 76). The most common hIBM, however, results from mutations in GNE, mentioned earlier in connection with a form of distal myopathy. As mentioned above, another form, previously classified as DM3 (see p. 65), is caused by mutations in the valosin gene, in which the muscle disease is associated with Paget's disease and frontotemporal dementia. These complex clinical and pathologic overlaps illustrate the need to define and classify genetic muscle diseases by genotype.

MITOCHONDRIAL MYOPATHIES

The demonstration that a large number of diseases of hitherto unknown cause were the result of mitochondrial dysfunction was a major advance. Many of these diseases are multisystemic, with particular predilection for the nervous system, but skeletal muscle is usually involved. Indeed, a diagnosis can often be made by muscle biopsy even in the absence of clinical myopathy.

The presence of ragged red fibers, in a Gomori trichrome preparation, caused by accumulations of structurally abnormal mitochondria beneath the sarcolemma, is the histologic hallmark of a mitochondrial myopathy (Fig. 3-52). On electron microscopy, these mitochondria may have bizarre appearances, such as whorled and "parking lot" paracrystalline structures (Fig. 3-53). Mitochondrial dysfunction can, however, be present in the absence of structural mitochondrial abnormalities, and diagnosis may then rest on biochemical and genetic studies.

Most mitochondrial myopathies result from mutations in mitochondrial DNA (mtDNA) and are therefore maternally transmitted, but sporadic cases are common, as mtDNA has a high spontaneous mutation rate. The mutations are either major deletions or duplications of mtDNA, or point mutations or insertions in mitochondrial transfer RNA genes, which result directly or indirectly in impaired oxidative phosphorylation. Somatic gene mutations can also cause mitochondrial disease, so autosomal dominant and recessive inheritance can also be seen.

Defective oxidative phosphorylation can be demonstrated using cytochrome c oxidase staining (Fig. 3-54). Impaired aerobic metabolism results in increased anaerobic glycolysis and an increase in plasma lactate, so useful screening tests include measurement of fasting plasma and cerebrospinal fluid lactate, and measurement of lactate responses to exercise. By contrast, the CK level may well be normal, and there may be little abnormality on EMG.

Direct mtDNA mutational analysis is increasingly available. Mutations may not be detectable in lymphocyte DNA but are usually detectable in muscle, so muscle biopsy is usually necessary. Polarographic studies of oxygen consumption and respiratory chain enzyme activity in isolated mitochondrial preparations may be required in some instances.

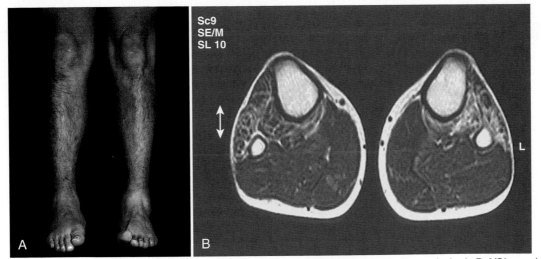

Fig. 3-31. Nonaka myopathy. **A,** Wasting and weakness of the anterior compartment muscles causes difficulty standing on the heels. **B,** MRI scan shows high-signal abnormality confined to the tibialis anterior muscles and the peronei.

Classification of Mitochondrial Disorders

The classification of mitochondrial disorders is difficult because identical phenotypes can result from many different mutations of both mitochondrial and somatic DNA, and yet specific mutations may cause different phenotypes. Moreover, in any tissue, only a proportion of mitochondria may be defective (heteroplasmy), and the manifestations of the disease in that tissue are to a degree determined by the proportion of abnormal mitochondria.

"Pure" Mitochondrial Myopathy

Some mitochondrial disorders affect skeletal muscle almost exclusively. Intuitively, one might anticipate that mitochondrial myopathy would be characterized by exertional myalgia and fatigue, but although such symptoms may indeed be induced or exacerbated by exercise in some cases, this is actually a less common manifestation than a progressive myopathic picture.

Lactic acidosis is usually demonstrable at rest or after mild exercise. Some patients also experience migrainous headaches, nausea, and vomiting after exertion. In extreme cases, myoglobinuria may occur.

Chronic progressive external ophthalmoplegia (CPEO) is the most common form of mitochondrial myopathy. This comprises slowly progressive external ophthalmoplegia and ptosis, which is usually bilateral but sometimes unilateral (Fig. 3-55). Chronic ocular myasthenia is an important differential. In the CPEO-plus form, these features are associated with limb weakness and a variety of other symptoms and signs, which may include atypical (pepper-and-salt type rather than the bone spicule type) retinitis pigmentosa, cerebellar ataxia, sensorineural deafness, short stature, endocrine and maturational defects, and cardiac conduction defects. CPEO and CPEO-plus are a continuum of Kearns-Sayre syndrome, which is defined by ptosis, external ophthalmoplegia, and pigmentary retinopathy, together with one of the following: heart block, cerebellar ataxia, or cerebrospinal fluid protein greater than 1 g/L, with onset under age 20. These syndromes most often result from major mtDNA deletions.

Other Mitochondrial Cytopathies

Neuromuscular dysfunction is a common feature of a variety of other mitochondrial disorders affecting the central and peripheral nervous systems, and often other systems. Some of these are summarized in Table 3-3. MELAS (mitochondrial encephalomyopathy with lactic acidosis and strokelike episodes), in particular, has several distinguishing features with regard to muscle involvement. This syndrome is characterized by short stature, recurrent secondary migraine headache with nausea and vomiting, blackouts and seizures, mental impairment, and recurrent lactic acidosis. Strokelike

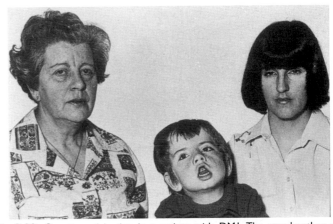

Fig. 3-32. Genetic anticipation in a patient with DM1. The grandmother was asymptomatic but had cataracts. Her daughter has the classical phenotype, and her daughter's child has congenital myotonic dystrophy. (Courtesy of Professor Keith Johnson, University of Glasgow)

TABLE 3-3. OTHER MITOCHONDRIAL CYTOPATHIES WITH PROMINENT NEUROMUSCULAR ABNORMALITIES

ACRONYM	CYTOPATHY	SIGNS AND SYMPTOMS
MELAS	Mitochondrial encephalopathy with lactic acidosis and strokelike episodes	Migraine headaches, strokelike episodes, intermittent metabolic acidosis
MERRF	Myoclonic epilepsy with ragged red fibers	Myoclonic epilepsy, ataxia, deafness, sometimes neuropathy, optic atrophy
NARP	Neurogenic weakness, ataxia, and retinitis pigmentosa	Retinitis pigmentosa, ataxia, seizures, dementia, proximal weakness, sensory neuropathy
MNGIE	Myoneurogastrointestinal encephalopathy	Ophthalmoplegia, gastric and intestinal dysfunction, peripheral and autonomic neuropathy

events often cause cortical blindness and hemiplegia, but the cortical damage does not follow anatomic vascular territories. The disease results essentially from a mitochondrial capillary angiopathy (Fig. 3-56).

Finally, there is some evidence that a small proportion of patients with chronic fatigue syndrome (CFS), a common problem in clinical practice, may have defective mitochondrial function secondary to viral induced damage.

TABLE 3-4.   GLYCOGEN STORAGE DISEASES OF MUSCLE

TYPE*	ENZYME	TISSUE INVOLVEMENT	CLINICAL PRESENTATION	GENE LOCUS
II (Pompe's)	Acid maltase (α-glucosidase)	Generalized	Floppy baby Cardiomyopathy Respiratory failure Limb weakness	17q23
III (Cori-Forbes)	Debrancher (amylo-1,6-glucosidase)	Heart Liver Muscle	Hepatosplenomegaly Distal weakness	1p21
IV (Andersen's)	Brancher (1,4-α-glucan branching enzyme)	Liver Spleen Muscle	Hepatosplenomegaly Cirrhosis	3p12
V (McArdle's)	Myophosphorylase	Muscle	Exertional myalgia Cramps Myoglobinuria	11q13
VIa	Phosphorylase b kinase	Liver Muscle	Hepatomegaly Growth retardation	Xq12-13
VII (Tarui's)	Phosphofructokinase	Muscle Red blood cells	Exertional myalgia "Cramps" Myoglobinuria	1 cen-q32
IX	Phosphoglycerokinase	Red blood cells Central nervous system	Hemolytic anemia Seizures Limb weakness	Xq13
X	Phosphoglyceromutase	Muscle	Exertional myalgia Myoglobinuria	7p12-p13
XI	Lactate dehydrogenase	Muscle	Exertional myalgia Myoglobinuria	11p14.1-15.1

*Types II to VI are glycogenolytic, and types VII to XI are glycolytic.

METABOLIC MYOPATHIES

A number of genetically determined enzyme defects affect intermediary metabolism of glucose and fatty acids, resulting in impaired ATP synthesis in muscle. Most patients present with exertional myalgia and sometimes myoglobinuria, although, as with mitochondrial myopathies, progressive weakness may also occur. They are all rare, and only the most common are described here.

Glycogen Storage Diseases of Muscle

The commonly used term glycogen storage disease is something of a misnomer, because several of these diseases do not in fact cause conspicuous glycogen accumulation in muscle. Some glycogen storage diseases also affect liver and cardiac muscle, and these features may dominate the clinical picture, particularly in infancy. Muscle biopsy with immunohistochemical analysis is the key to diagnosis, but assay and characterization of glycogen and measurements of specific enzyme activities in a biopsy sample are sometimes required.

Enzyme defects that inhibit glycogen metabolism (glycogenolytic diseases) generally produce a progressive myopathy, although exertional myalgia can also be a feature, whereas glycolytic disorders, caused by deficiency of enzymes involved in glucose catabolism, typically cause exertional myalgia and myoglobinuria. Table 3-4 shows the main clinical features of the different diseases.

Glycogenolytic Diseases.   Glycogenolytic diseases include acid maltase deficiency (referred to as Pompe's disease, although strictly speaking the eponym relates to presentation in infancy) and McArdle's disease.

Acid Maltase Deficiency, Pompe's Disease.   Acid maltase is a lysosomal enzyme, and deficiency results in glycogen accumulation in lysosomes. Pompe's disease in infancy is characterized by gross accumulation of glycogen in muscle, liver, and heart causing cardiorespiratory failure and hepatomegaly. In later childhood, it causes a myopathy with raised CK, which may at first suggest a dystrophy. In adults, a common presentation is with type 2 respiratory failure, although again a dystrophy may be suspected from the clinical features (Fig. 3-57). Hepatomegaly and cardiac involvement are very rare in older patients, and acid maltase deficiency may also cause macroglossia (Fig. 3-58). Rarely, exertional myalgia is the only manifestation.

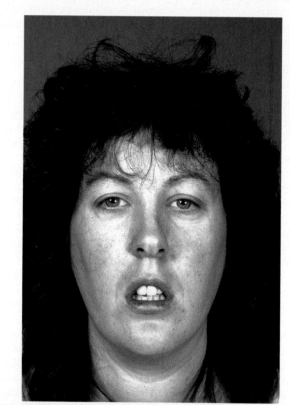

Fig. 3-33. Facies in myotonic dystrophy. Bilateral facial weakness, "carp mouth," and sternomastoid wasting.

Muscle biopsy in infancy shows a vacuolar myopathy. The glycogen content of the vacuoles is periodic acid–Schiff positive, and the amount stored tends to lessen in patients presenting at older ages (Fig. 3-59). Electron microscopy of muscle is useful to identify the engorged lysosomes (Fig. 3-60), but the biopsy may in fact be normal in adults. Blood film analysis may allow identification of glycogen accumulation in white cells (Fig. 3-61), but the only reliable diagnostic test is direct measurement of acid maltase activity in blood. **This should be performed in *any* case of otherwise undiagnosed progressive myopathy,** because enzyme replacement therapy can significantly improve the condition.

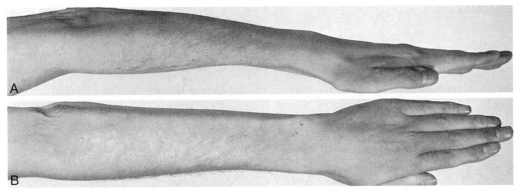

Fig. 3-34. Distal wasting in the upper limbs in a patient with DM1 muscular dystrophy.

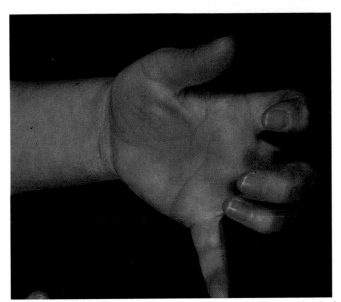

Fig. 3-35. Grip myotonia. The patient is attempting to open her hand after gripping.

McArdle's Disease. Patients with McArdle's disease, the first metabolic myopathy to be described, present with exertional myalgia and "cramps," with weakness and stiffness in the exercising muscles. The cramps are in fact contractures—localized rigor—which, unlike true cramps, are electrically silent.

The symptoms begin early in the course of exercise, when glucose is the most important fuel source. Muscle fiber damage occurs and, if severe or widespread, can result in rhabdomyolysis and myoglobinuria with the risk of renal failure. Curiously, attacks are unpredictable. Exercise of similar severity on some occasions may produce few or no symptoms. This presumably relates to the variable use of alternative fuel substrates. Most patients experience the second-wind phenomenon, whereby if they exercise at a low rate at the outset, they can work through the symptoms and endurance is increased.

Most patients have a raised CK, but the EMG may show little abnormality outside attacks. Although an ischemic forearm exercise test is often advocated as part of the workup, the diagnosis is made most easily by biopsy, which typically demonstrates subsarcolemmal glycogen blebs on histology, and absence of myophosphorylase staining (Fig. 3-62). The ischemic forearm exercise test may then be helpful if the biopsy fails to demonstrate myophosphorylase deficiency. A flat or defective lactate response might indicate one of the rarer glycolytic diseases.

Glycolytic Diseases. Glycolytic diseases are even less common than the glycogenolytic diseases. They typically cause exertional myalgia and rhabdomyolysis. A mild hemolytic anemia may be found, reflecting the importance of glycolysis to red cell metabolism. The most common, Tarui's disease, results from phosphofructokinase deficiency, which can be demonstrated immunohistochemically.

Lipid Storage Diseases of Muscle
Fatty acids derived from lipid digestion are transported into mitochondria either directly (short and medium chain) or via carnitine palmitoyltransferases (CPT) (long chain) on the inner mitochondrial membranes, to undergo β-oxidation. Defects in the complex system of lipid-catabolizing enzymes in mitochondria can result in hepatic, cardiac, and skeletal muscle disease. Presentation in neonates and infants may include hepatic encephalopathy, cardiomyopathy, and hypotonia, often recurrent and sometimes following otherwise mild viral infection or anorexia. In adults, muscle symptoms tend to predominate, with exertional myalgia with rhabdomyolysis in CPT deficiency and a progressive proximal lipid-storage myopathy and intermittent hepatic encephalopathy in carnitine or acyl-CoA dehydrogenase deficiency.

Diagnostic clues to lipid storage myopathies include the following:

• A history of episodic rhabdomyolysis or myoglobinuria precipitated by fasting or *prolonged* exercise (as opposed to glycolytic diseases)
• Demonstration of hypoglycemia and hypoketosis with raised levels of free fatty acids in plasma with prolonged fasting
• Hyperammonemia and raised transaminases

Screening for urinary organic acids during or shortly after attacks may yield a pattern of dicarboxylic acids specific for a particular dehydrogenase deficiency. A provocative fast for at least 18 hours (which should be undertaken only in the hospital) may precipitate a number of these symptoms and biochemical abnormalities between episodes. However, ultimately the diagnosis rests on in vitro tests such as measurement of CPT activity and fatty acid flux studies in cultured fibroblasts from a skin biopsy.

Carnitine Deficiency and Acyl Dehydrogenase Deficiencies. Primary carnitine deficiency is rare. The systemic form is caused by the absence of the carnitine transporter (5q31) in gut and kidney, and patients present with myopathy and hepatic encephalopathy. Secondary deficiency is common with β-oxidation enzyme defects and mitochondrial disorders. Acyl-CoA dehydrogenase deficiencies have a similar spectrum of presentations, in combination with lipid storage myopathy, which can be demonstrated histochemically with Sudan black or oil red O staining (Fig. 3-63, A). Electron microscopy demonstrates accumulations of lipid droplets between the myofibers (see Fig. 3-63, B)

Carnitine Palmitoyltransferase Deficiency. Carnitine palmitoyltransferase deficiency is the most common lipid storage myopathy, although lipid accumulation may be rather inconspicuous on biopsy. Patients tend to present with exertional myalgia and myoglobinuria after prolonged or severe exercise, especially when fasting. Mild weakness may be evident between attacks.

ACQUIRED MYOPATHIES

INFLAMMATORY IMMUNE-MEDIATED MYOPATHIES

Inflammation is a histological feature of many muscle diseases and does not necessarily indicate that the primary pathologic process is immune driven . The term myositis refers to muscle inflammation caused by either infection or by autoimmune and autoinflammatory processes. Box 3-5 shows the main forms of idiopathic myositis and immune-mediated myopathies.

The myopathic features of polymyositis and dermatomyositis are similar: symmetrical, nonselective proximal weakness occasionally associated with myalgia and tenderness, usually with well-preserved reflexes. The presence of skin rash is the defining clinical feature of dermatomyositis, but this can sometimes be subtle. The features of inclusion body myositis are quite different, and it is not yet clear how this disorder relates to other diseases in this group.

Polymyositis

Patients with polymyositis typically present with symmetrical proximal weakness, sometimes associated with myalgia and muscle tenderness. It is rare in children. Patients may also present with selective distal or neck and upper limb weakness, or with dropped head syndrome but these presentations are uncommon. In chronic cases, patients may eventually develop clinical features suggestive of a limb-girdle or scapuloperoneal syndrome, referred to as chronic polymyositis (Fig. 3-64). Indeed, terms such as menopausal muscular dystrophy were once used erroneously to describe forms of indolent chronic myositis.

Symptoms may rarely be confined to skeletal muscle (organ-specific polymyositis), but more often the myositis is a complication of an underlying connective tissue disease, particularly Sjögren's syndrome, rheumatoid disease, systemic sclerosis, and mixed connective tissue disease (overlap myositis, Fig. 3-65). Serum CK is nearly always increased, and the EMG typically shows a mixed picture of increased insertional and spontaneous activity, together with myopathic changes.

Muscle biopsy (Fig. 3-66) typically shows endomysial and perimysial lymphocytic infiltration, with fiber necrosis, degeneration, and regeneration, but the process is patchy and inflammation may be inconspicuous. Demonstration of diffuse major histocompatibility complex (MHC) class I antigen expression on muscle fibers is helpful for diagnosis (Fig. 3-67). Occasionally, it is possible to see nonnecrotic fibers invaded by lymphocytes, which is evidence of the CD8+ T-cell–mediated cytotoxicity that is the basis of the inflammatory

attack (see Fig. 3-67, inset). Indeed, the pathologic diagnosis of polymyositis now depends on the demonstration of the MHC class I-CD8+ 'lesion'.

Dermatomyositis

Dermatomyositis in its classical form, is clinically and pathogenetically distinct from polymyositis. It is a humorally mediated microangiopathy affecting principally skin and muscle, although childhood dermatomyositis can also include gut involvement, resulting in gastrointestinal hemorrhage.

The skin features are diagnostic: erythematous and violaceous lesions often affecting light-exposed areas (heliotrope cyanosis) such as the supraorbital ridges, eyelids, malar areas, chest, knuckles, knees, and elbows (Fig. 3-68). The skin lesions may sometimes occur without muscle weakness (amyopathic dermatomyositis), but careful investigation usually confirms muscle involvement. Extensive skin calcification may occur in childhood dermatomyositis. This is uncommon in adults, although it is a feature of CREST (calcinosis, Raynaud's, esophageal dysmobility, sclerodactyly, telangiectasia) syndrome, which may include an inflammatory myopathy.

BOX 3-5 CLASSIFICATION OF INFLAMMATORY AND IMMUNE-MEDIATED MYOPATHIES

Polymyositis
- Organ specific (variants include distal polymyositis, brachiocervical inflammatory myopathy, neck extensor myopathy)
- Overlap myositis

Dermatomyositis
- Juvenile
- Adult

Inclusion body myositis

Necrotizing Myopathy
- Cancer associated
- Anti-SRP associated

Granulomatous Myopathies
- Sarcoidosis

Focal and Localized Myositis
- Focal myositis
- Localized nodular myositis
- Orbital myositis

SRP, signal recognition protein.

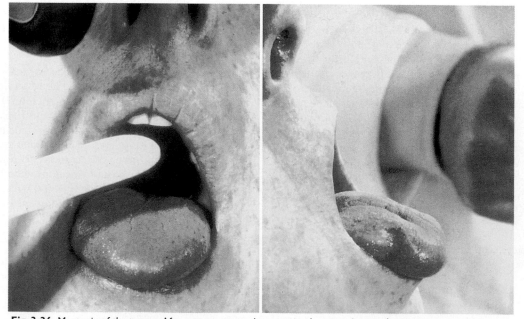

Fig. 3-36. Myotonia of the tongue. After tongue percussion, sustained contraction produces a groove at the margin.

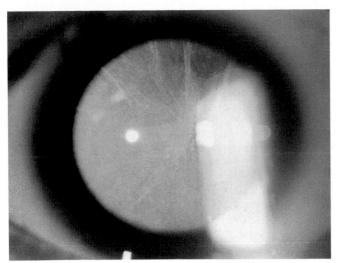

Fig. 3-37. Cataract in a patient with muscular dystrophy. Posterior lens opacities with characteristic radiating-spokes pattern.

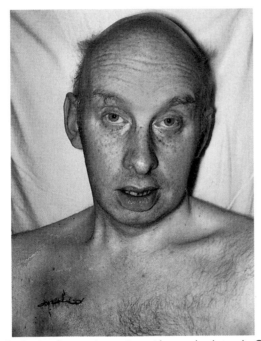

Fig. 3-38. Cardiac involvement in a patient with muscular dystrophy. Cardiac conduction defects are a cause of sudden death in DM1. This patient, who has the typical facies and sternomastoid wasting, has had a pacemaker inserted.

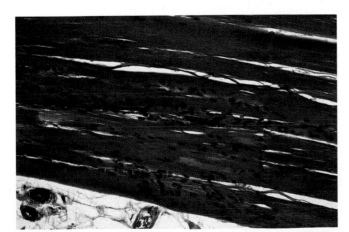

Fig. 3-39. Muscle biopsy in DM1 muscular dystrophy. Longitudinal section showing "trucking" of central nuclei.

Muscle biopsy from patients with dermatomyositis typically shows perivascular and perifascicular inflammation (Fig. 3-69), but in dermatomyositis this comprises mainly CD4+ T lymphocytes and B cells, in keeping with a significant humoral component to the immunopathogenesis (Fig. 3-70). Immunoglobulin and complement deposition can be demonstrated on the vascular endothelium of endomysial vessels. The endothelial injury results in a paucity of muscle capillaries, which is thought to lead to relative ischemia at the edges of muscle fascicles, causing perifascicular muscular atrophy, a pathognomonic feature of the muscle biopsy in dermatomyositis (Fig. 3-71). Electron microscopy may reveal tubuloreticular inclusions in the capillary endothelial cells, indicative of local interferon synthesis (Fig. 3-72).

In addition to joint and skin involvement, polymyositis and dermatomyositis may also be complicated by interstitial lung disease and inflammatory cardiomyopathy, causing conduction defects and dysrhythmias. Autoantibodies associated with specific collagen vascular diseases may be demonstrated in overlap syndromes, but in addition there may be a number of myositis-specific antibodies directed against cytoplasmic enzymes and proteins. However, these antibodies relate more to involvement of tissues other than muscle; anti-Jo1 (anti-histidyl-tRNA synthetase), in particular, is associated with pulmonary fibrosis disease.

Myositis and Cancer

There is good epidemiologic evidence that inflammatory myopathy, and particularly dermatomyositis, may be a manifestation of underlying malignancy. This association is strongest for men older than 50,

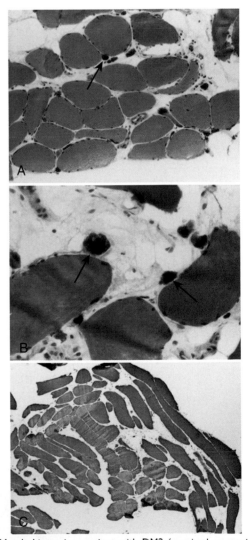

Fig. 3-40. Muscle biopsy in a patient with DM2 (proximal myotonic myopathy). **A** and **B,** Pyknotic nuclear clumps (arrows), consisting of severely atrophic type 2 fibers with prominent accumulations of nuclei. **C,** Slow myosin antibody stain shows nearly all fibers are type 1.

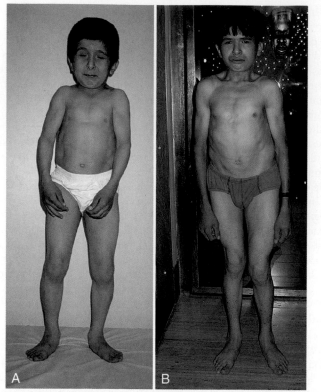

Fig. 3-41. Schwartz-Jampel syndrome. Eleven-year-old patient *(left)*. At age 15 *(right)*.

and any form of cancer may be involved, including lymphomas and hematologic malignancies. It is common practice to screen for cancer in patients with polymyositis or dermatomyositis, but the yield is generally low. Whole-body PET may be useful. Malignancies can also cause necrotizing myopathy.

Necrotizing Myopathy

Occasionally, a biopsy from a patient presenting with possible myositis may show inflammation composed mainly of macrophages, associated with prominent fiber necrosis. Like dermatomyositis, necrotizing myopathy may also indicate an underlying malignancy, but some cases are associated with pathogenenic antibodies to signal recognition protein (anti-SRP) (Fig. 3-73). The myopathy is therefore probably humorally mediated.

Other Inflammatory Myopathies

Muscle is often involved in sarcoidosis. This may be asymptomatic, and muscle is a useful tissue for diagnostic biopsy for systemic disease (Fig. 3-74). However, on occasions, a secondary inflammatory response is generated, referred to as sarcoid myositis. Granulomatous change in muscle may also occur in other immune-mediated disorders, such as forms of vasculitis and systemic granulomatous diseases.

Occasionally, inflammation is restricted to a single muscle, a group of muscles, or a limb. Such focal myositis may persist for years and induce localized wasting. In localized nodular myositis, inflammatory muscle masses develop in several sites. The features may superficially resemble thrombophlebitis, but the multifocal process usually evolves into a more typical polymyositis picture.

Orbital myositis, or orbital pseudotumor, is a particular form of focal myositis, in which the extraocular muscles are involved, causing

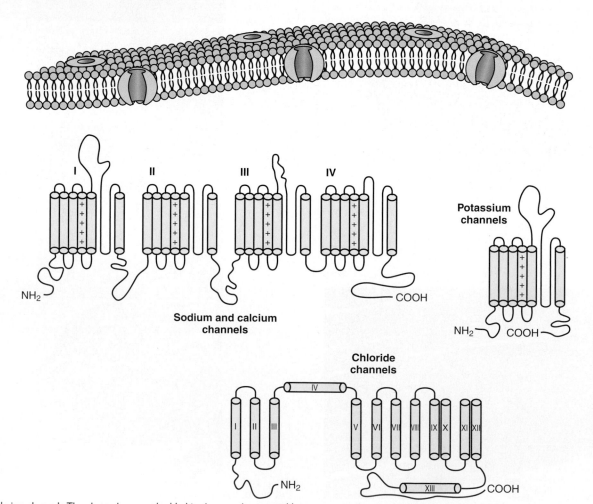

Fig. 3-42. Muscle ion channels. The channels are embedded in the sarcolemma and have transmembrane, extracellular, and intracellular domains. Mutations affecting proteins that make up these channels result in forms of non-dystrophic myotonia, periodic paralysis, and malignant hyperthermia.

proptosis and diplopia (Fig. 3-75). The main differential diagnosis is ophthalmic Graves' disease (see p. 78).

Sporadic Inclusion Body Myositis (sIBM)

Inclusion body myositis is sometimes indistinguishable from organ-specific polymyositis at the outset although it more often develops insidiously. The characteristics of the inflammation in muscle are the same as polymyositis, but notable clinical and pathologic differences emerge as the condition progresses, and the typical phenotype is then very different.

Although it can occur at any age, onset is after age 50 in the great majority of cases. It is more common in men than women, unlike other forms of inflammatory myopathy, most cases are refractory to steroids and immunosuppressants. Weakness is associated with progressive wasting, which, unlike in typical inflammatory myopathies, tends to be selective, with a distinctive pattern, different from that of other myopathies.

In the upper limbs, the forearm flexors are prominently involved, leading to a characteristic scalloped appearance, whereas in the legs the quadriceps are affected at an early stage, resulting in the knees giving way on descending stairs (Fig. 3-76). Early involvement of the muscles of the hands and feet is typical. There may be mild facial weakness, and dysphagia is a common complaint. The reflexes may be diminished or absent.

About 20% of patients have diabetes and 10% have other autoimmune diseases. The CK level may be normal and is rarely high, and EMG often gives a mixed myopathic and neurogenic picture.

Diagnosis rests ultimately on muscle biopsy (Fig. 3-77). The pathological hallmarks of sIBM are: inflammation; rimmed vacuoles in at least a proportion of fibres; ubiquitinated sarcoplasmic protein aggregates in some fibres and a significant proportion of fibers negative for cytochrome c oxidase, indicating mitochondrial dysfunction. As noted, the inflammation characteristics are typical of polymyositis (see Fig. 3-66). The vacuoles are not membrane lined but contain membrane fragments and other debris, which results in basophilic staining of the vacuole walls. None of these features is unique to the condition, however, and further immunohistochemical and ultrastructural examination is essential (Fig. 3-78). The protein aggregates include amyloid (Fig. 3-78, A), β-amyloid precursor protein, phosphorylated tau and apo-E (Fig. 3-78, B). With electron microscopy, in addition to structural mitochondrial abnormalities and accumulations of membranous structures on the walls of vacuoles (Fig. 3-79, A), characteristic filaments may be identified in the cytoplasm and nuclei (Fig. 3-79, B) and cytoplasm (Fig. 3-79, C). Some of these are paired helical filaments, and in a number of ways, some of the pathological characteristics of sIBM are reminiscent of the brain pathology of Alzheimer's disease, raising the possibility that some forms of inclusion body myositis are primary degenerative disorders, any inflammation being a secondary response.

A number of genetic myopathies, including the hereditary inclusion body myopathies and some distal myopathies, share some of these pathologic features, but inflammation is absent or less conspicuous.

MYOPATHIES IN SYSTEMIC DISEASES

Muscle constitutes some 40% of body mass and is affected to some extent in most systemic illnesses, although the clinical features of the primary disorder usually predominate. Muscle disease can be a feature of many infections, connective tissue diseases, vasculitic disorders, and occasionally a paraneoplastic phenomenon. Myopathy may also be a presenting feature of most forms of endocrinopathy.

Diabetes

Muscular weakness and wasting in patients with diabetes is usually neurogenic. Infarction of muscle can occur rarely in poorly controlled diabetics, causing myalgia and sometimes a painful muscle mass.

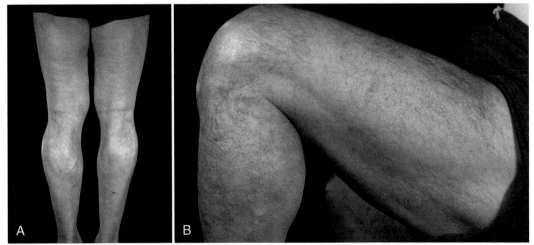

Fig. 3-43. Myotonia congenita. Muscular hypertrophy of the calves and thighs. Percussion myotonia was readily elicited from all limb muscles.

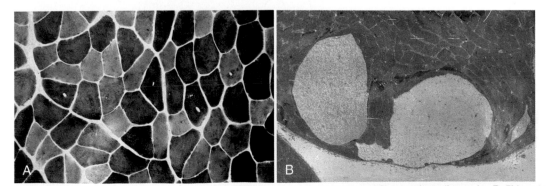

Fig. 3-44. Muscle biopsy in hypokalemic periodic paralysis. **A,** Myophosphorylase preparation shows several fibers with small vacuoles. **B,** EM study showing non-rimmed vacuoles.

Dysthyroid Myopathies

The triad of proximal weakness, delayed relaxation of the tendon reflexes, and raised CK level is typical of hypothyroid myopathy. In severe cases, patients may present with Hoffman's syndrome, comprising weakness, stiffness, myalgia, and muscle hypertrophy. Thyrotoxicosis causes detectable weakness in the majority of cases, but this is clinically significant in only a minority. Thyrotoxic myopathy sometimes has features reminiscent of amyotrophic lateral sclerosis, with marked muscle wasting, cramps, fasciculations, and brisk reflexes, but scapular winging is usually prominent (Fig. 3-80). As noted earlier, thyrotoxicosis may be associated with periodic paralysis, especially in patients of Chinese extraction. There is also an increased incidence of myasthenia gravis in patients with thyroid disease, and comorbidity can produce a confusing clinical picture (Fig. 3-46).

Patients with exophthalmic Graves' disease present with diplopia, external ophthalmoparesis, and painful proptosis with lid retraction, which is typically bilateral. Patients are usually, but not invariably, biochemically hyperthyroid. The proptosis is caused by edema and inflammation of the orbital contents and extraocular muscles, which may be sufficient to compress the optic nerves (Fig. 3-81). The differential diagnosis includes orbital pseudotumor (Fig. 3-75) and Tolosa-Hunt syndrome (see Chapter 15).

Cushing's syndrome, caused by excess glucocorticoids resulting from adrenal hyperplasia, adrenal tumor, or ectopic secretion of adrenocorticotropic hormone, usually causes a slowly progressive, painless proximal myopathy (Fig. 3-82). The serum CK level is normal, and the biopsy typically shows selective type 2 fiber atrophy (see also steroid myopathy, p 80).

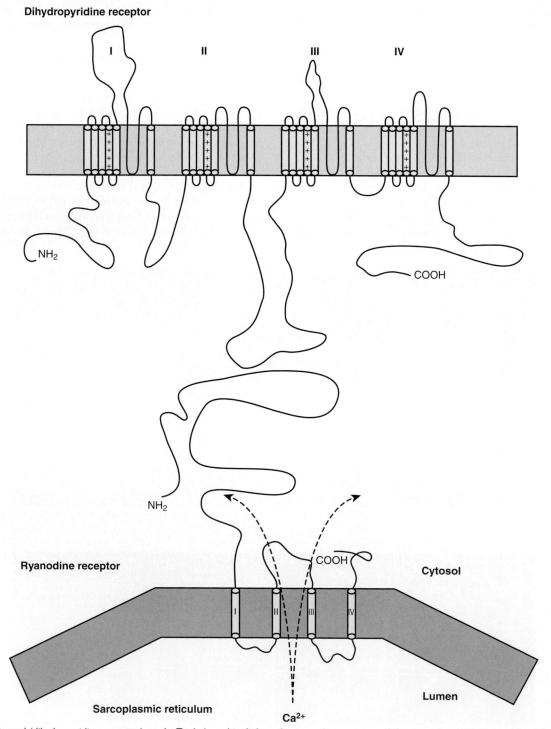

Fig. 3-45. Calcium channel (dihydropyridine receptor) on the T-tubule and its link to the ryanodine receptor of the sarcoplasmic reticulum. This linkage serves excitation contraction coupling.

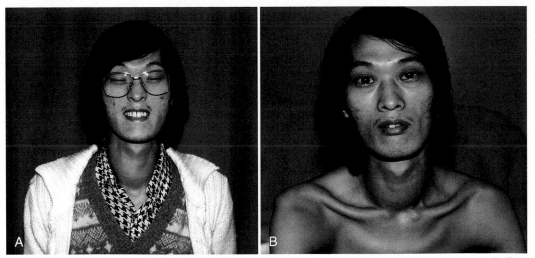

Fig. 3-46. A patient with thyrotoxic periodic paralysis and ocular myasthenia gravis. **A,** Bilateral ptosis, myopathic facies and thyromegally. **B,** Resolution of ptosis after intravenous edrophonium. Note proximal muscle wasting due to the thyrotoxicosis.

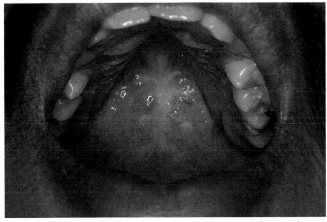

Fig. 3-47. "Cathedral" palate in patient with congenital myopathy.

Muscle Involvement in Infectious Diseases

Many viruses, bacteria, fungi, and parasites can infect muscle. Viral myositis can result in symptoms ranging from mild generalized myalgia to rhabdomyolysis. Influenza, parainfluenza, and adenoviruses are common causes. Enteroviruses are particularly myotoxic and may be a common cause of postviral fatigue syndrome.

Human immunodeficiency virus infection causes a range of myopathies, including an inflammatory myopathy and a progressive muscle wasting syndrome. Bacterial pyomyositis, resulting in skeletal muscle abscesses, is largely confined to the tropics (tropical myositis). It is most often caused by Staphylococcus aureus. Clostridial infection causes myonecrosis (gas gangrene).

One of the most common of all muscle infections is cysticercosis, resulting from infestation by Taenia solium, the pork tapeworm. This may be asymptomatic, but it can result in muscle hypertrophy and sometimes weakness. The cysticerci often calcify and plain radiography of the leg muscles can be helpful in the general diagnosis of this disease (Figs. 3-83 to 3-85).

The three organs commonly affected by hydatid disease are the liver, lung, and muscle. The paravertebral and proximal lower limb muscles are particularly affected. The usual finding is a painless mass that may later calcify. Weakness is not a feature.

TOXIN- AND DRUG-INDUCED MYOPATHIES

Many drugs and other toxins, including alcohol, can damage muscle. The resulting clinical picture can range from asymptomatic hyperCK-emia to acute rhabdomyolysis. The most common presentations are acute or subacute, painful, proximal myopathy and chronic painless

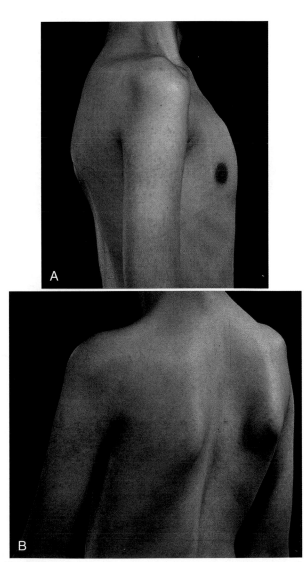

Fig. 3-48. Limb-girdle phenotype in a patient with nemaline myopathy.

proximal myopathy. Some drugs and toxins can cause either, and a number of pathogenetic mechanisms have been identified (Table 3-5).

Acute and Subacute Painful Proximal Myopathy

Alcohol can cause an acute painful necrotizing myopathy through direct myotoxicity, as can opiates, but statins are now the most common cause of this problem in routine clinical practice (Fig. 3-86).

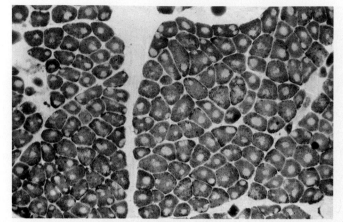

Fig. 3-49. Central core disease (NADH-TR staining). The fibers are all type I and exhibit typical loss of myofibrillar structure in the center of each fiber. These "cores" extend along the whole length of the fibers, usually in the center. Occasionally, they appear multiple *(arrows)*, causing diagnostic difficulties with multicore-minicore disease.

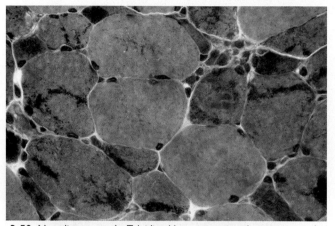

Fig. 3-50. Nemaline myopathy. Toluidine blue preparation showing accumulations in Z-line–derived proteins in many fibers.

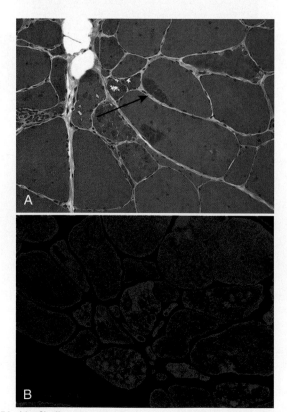

Fig. 3-51. Myofibrillar myopathy. Biopsy section from a patient with a desmin gene mutation. **A,** H&E stain shows granulomatous accumulations *(black arrow)* and basophilic fibers. **B,** Immunolabeling with antidesmin demonstrates protein surplus myopathy.

TABLE 3-5. PATHOGENESIS OF TOXIN- AND DRUG-INDUCED MYOPATHIES

MYOPATHY TYPE	CLINICAL SIGN	DRUGS e.g.
Rhabdomyolysis, acute/subacute proximal myopathy	Direct myotoxicity	Alcohol, statins
	Hypokalemia	Diuretics
	Inflammation	Penicillamine
	Mitochondrial injury	Azidothymidine
Chronic painless proximal myopathy	Protein catabolism	Steroids, alcohol
	Lysosomal autophagia	Chloroquine
	Microtubular dysfunction	Vincristine

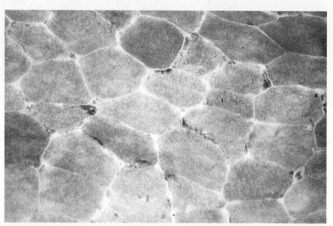

Fig. 3-52. Ragged red fibers in a modified Gomori trichrome–stained biopsy section from a patient with mitochondrial myopathy. The subsarcolemmal accumulations of mitochondria produce an even red staining in the fiber periphery.

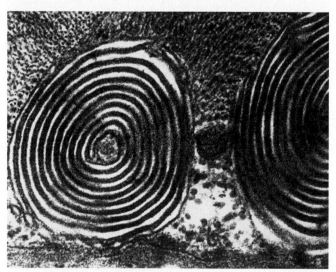

Fig. 3-53. Mitochondrial myopathy. EM showing whorled mitochondria.

Hypokalemia, caused by diuretics, purgatives, and licorice derivatives, can also precipitate a painful myopathy, as well as a chronic painless proximal myopathy.

Drug-induced inflammatory myopathy is rare but can be caused by a variety of drugs, most commonly penicillamine, although this drug more often induces myasthenia (see later). Finally, several drugs, notably azidothymidine, used in the treatment of HIV infection, can cause mitochondrial dysfunction, with pathologic features similar to those of mitochondrial myopathy.

Chronic Painless Proximal Myopathy
Alcohol is the most common cause of chronic painless proximal myopathy; indeed, alcoholic myopathy is the most common of all muscle diseases, although commonly insidious and unrecognised). Steroid myopathy can pose a taxing clinical problem, as it is often

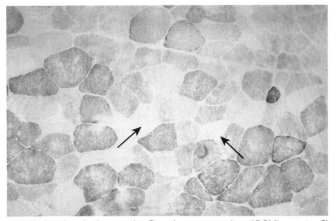

Fig. 3-54. Mitochondrial myopathy. Cytochrome c oxidase (COX)-negative fibers (arrows), and normally stained (COX-positive) fibers.

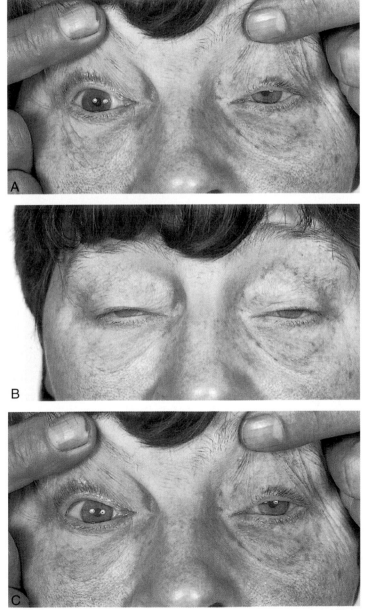

Fig. 3-55. External ophthalmoplegia in a patient with chronic progressive external ophthalmoplegia, "CPEO plus." There is marked bilateral ptosis and almost complete external ophthalmoplegia. **A,** Looking to the right. **B,** Looking straight ahead. **C,** Looking to the left.

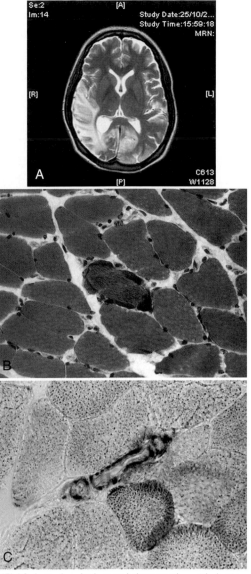

Fig. 3-56. MELAS (mitochondrial encephalomyopathy with lactic acidosis and strokelike episodes). **A,** T-2-weighted MRI brain scan showing ischemic infarction in the right middle and right and left occipital lobes. The patient presented with left hemifield neglect and developed bilateral cortical blindness. **B,** Muscle biopsy. H&E section showing accumulations of abnormal mitochondria (equivalent to 'ragged red' fibres). **C,** Succinate dehydrogenase staining showed diagnostic, abnormal accumulations of mitochondria in endomysial blood vessels.

on biopsy (Fig. 3-87). Chronic hypokalemia, caused by diuretics or liquorice and its derivatives can produce a similar clinical and pathological picture.

Drugs that interact with muscle membrane systems (notably the microtubular system and lysosomes), such as chloroquine, colchicine, and vincristine, can also cause this syndrome, but the pathologic feature here is a vacuolar myopathy (Fig. 3-88). These drugs inhibit microtubule polymerization, which is thought to result in impaired lysosomal transport. Colchicine can cause a subacute painful myopathy with raised CK levels, but more often it induces a chronic painless myopathy.

MYASTHENIA GRAVIS AND OTHER NEUROMUSCULAR TRANSMISSION DISORDERS

The term myasthenia denotes fatigable muscle weakness—weakness that increases disproportionately with repetitive activity. Myasthenia gravis (MG) is a clinical syndrome that results from defective neuromuscular transmission caused by antibodies to proteins of the neuromuscular junctions on the postsynaptic membranes. The most commonly targeted proteins are the nicotinic acetylcholine receptors (AChRs), but in a small proportion of cases, antibodies are directed

difficult to distinguish weakness due to steroid myopathy from a myopathy intrinsic to the condition being treated. It is probably over-diagnosed, but iatrogenic steroid myopathy has features that are identical to those of the myopathy of Cushing's syndrome (see earlier). It is characterized by selective type 2 muscle fiber atrophy

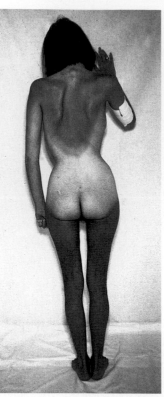

Fig. 3-57. Acid maltase deficiency presenting as limb-girdle syndrome.

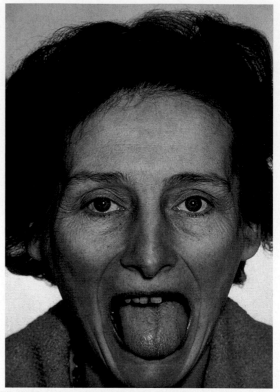

Fig. 3-58. Acid maltase deficiency presenting with macroglossia.

against muscle-specific kinase (MuSK). Lambert-Eaton myasthenic syndrome (LEMS) is caused by antibodies to the neuronal presynaptic voltage-gated Ca^{2+} channels.

Neuromyotonia is clinically distinct from myasthenia and LEMS and is mediated by antibodies to voltage-gated presynaptic K^+ channels (VGKC Abs).

The Neuromuscular Junction

A neuromuscular junction comprises the presynaptic nerve terminal, containing synaptic vesicles of acetylcholine (ACh), and the postsynaptic membrane of the muscle fiber, which is thrown into many folds that increase its surface area (Fig. 3-89). Acetylcholine receptors are concentrated at the entrances to the clefts. These receptors are non–voltage gated sodium channels, comprising several subunits surrounding an ion pore, supported by several proteins, notably rapsyn and MuSK, that are involved in the regulation of receptor clustering (Fig. 3-90). ACh interaction with the receptor results in opening of the pore and depolarization of the postsynaptic membrane. The action potential then invades the myofiber via the T-tubular system, the first stage in excitation–contraction coupling.

Particular neuromuscular junction disorders result from defective function at each stage of this sequence. They can be classified as presynaptic or postsynaptic and may be genetic or acquired (Box 3-6).

Myasthenia Gravis

Myasthenia gravis is a common disorder with a prevalence of around 10 per 100,000. It has two peaks of incidence: early onset, most commonly affecting females, and late onset, more commonly in males. There is epidemiologic evidence that the disease is increasing in frequency and may be underdiagnosed, particularly in the elderly.

Patients with MG generally present with fatigable weakness, particularly of the cranial musculature. Fluctuating ptosis, which may be unilateral or asymmetrical, is the most common manifestation (Fig. 3-91). Sustained upward gaze results in a slow fall of the affected eyelids. Cogan's sign is elicited by asking the patient to look downward for 10 to 20 seconds and then return the eyes rapidly to the primary position. In patients with MG, the affected lids tend to overshoot and then droop quickly, or twitch repetitively.

BOX 3-6 CLASSIFICATION OF NEUROMUSCULAR JUNCTION DISORDERS

Presynaptic Neuromuscular Disorders
- Acquired
  - Neuromyotonia (mediator: VGKC antibodies)
  - Lambert-Eaton myasthenic syndrome (mediator: VGCC antibodies)
  - Botulism (mediator: *Botulinum* toxin)
- Genetic
  - Familial infantile myasthenia

Synaptic Disorders
- Genetic
  - Acetylcholinesterase deficiency

Postsynaptic Neuromuscular Disorders
- Acquired
  - Myasthenia gravis (mediators: AChR antibodies, MuSK antibodies)
- Genetic
  - AChR deficiency
  - Slow channel syndrome
  - Low affinity fast channel syndrome

AChR, acetylcholine receptor; MuSK, muscle-specific kinase; VGCC, voltage-gated Ca^{2+} channel; VGKC, voltage-gated K^+ channel.

Diplopia is also frequent. A variety of eye movement abnormalities can occur (Fig. 3-92) and may be complex (Fig. 3-93). Some 10% of MG cases are purely ocular, both on clinical and neurophysiologic grounds (ocular myasthenia). If the symptoms remain confined to the eyes for more than 3 years, progression to the generalized form is unlikely.

Facial muscle weakness may be found, leading to failure of complete eyelid closure and a characteristic posture of the lips (Fig. 3-94).

Other common symptoms include progressive jaw weakness affecting chewing, and neck weakness involving flexion or extension and often both. Like polymyositis, MG is part of the differential diagnosis of dropped head syndrome. Bulbar symptoms may also occur in isolation (bulbar myasthenia), and MG should always be considered in the differential diagnosis of dysphagia and dysphonia. Involvement of the diaphragm and intercostal muscles may cause type 2 respiratory failure. A triple-furrowed tongue is a rare but characteristic feature (Fig. 3-95). In the limbs, proximal weakness, especially of the

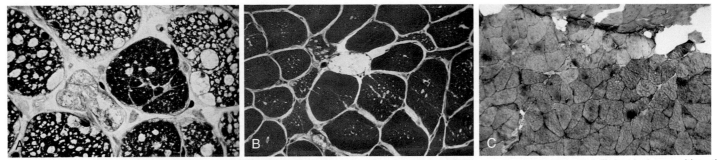

Fig. 3-59. Muscle biopsies stained with H&E. **A,** Infantile Pompe's disease. **B,** Adult acid maltase deficiency. The vacuoles are lysosomes stuffed with glycogen. Note the greater glycogen accumulation in the younger patient. **C,** Increased PAS staining in acid maltase deficiency in an adult patient, reflecting glycogen accumulation.

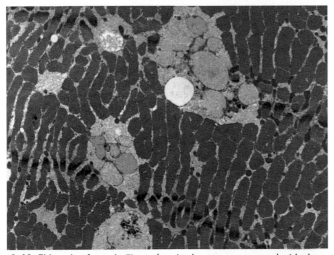

Fig. 3-60. EM study of muscle fibers showing lysosomes engorged with glycogen.

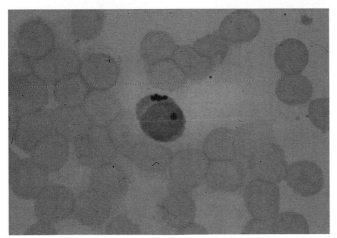

Fig. 3-61. Excess glycogen storage in lysosomes may also be seen on a blood film stained with PAS, or by electron microscopy.

triceps, is usually evident, and fatigability can often be demonstrated at the bedside. The reflexes are preserved.

The clinical diagnosis of MG is usually confirmed by the demonstration of AChR antibodies in the blood, which are present in about 85% of patients with generalized MG and in about 50% of those with purely ocular MG. Of the remaining "seronegative" cases, about half have anti-MuSK antibodies (see later); anti-MuSK antibodies are virtually never found in seropositive MG cases. Most of the remaining patients also have AChR antibodies, but the antibodies are of low affinity in the standard immunoassay and can be detected only with solid-phase assays. There is no direct relationship between the AChR antibody titer and the clinical state of the patient, and titers may remain high even in asymptomatic patients after treatment, although there is a slow reduction over time. Presumably, this represents a positive shift in the balance between AChR regeneration and destruction as a result of treatment. The antibodies cross the placenta, and

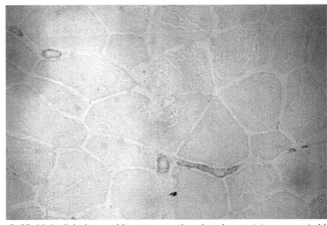

Fig. 3-62. McArdle's disease. Negative myophosphorylase staining except in blood vessels (the mutation affects only the muscle isoform).

10% to 15% of infants of mothers with MG will develop self-limiting neonatal myasthenia.

Myasthenia gravis may be associated with antibodies to a number of other muscle proteins, including antistriational (anti-titin) and antimyosin antibodies. The serum CK level is usually normal.

The Tensilon (intravenous edrophonium hydrochloride) test is still helpful if performed with suitable controls and observed by independent observers, not least for the psychological boost from the dramatic improvement the patient experiences for a short period (Fig. 3-96).

In seronegative cases particularly, neurophysiological studies are crucial. There is usually excessive decrement of the action potential amplitude on repetitive stimulation at 3 Hz, but the most sensitive test for neuromuscular junction dysfunction is single-fiber EMG, which in patients with MG shows increased jitter and blocking of potentials (Fig. 3-97).

Pathogenesis. The thymus is key to the pathogenesis of MG. AChR proteins are present on myoid cells in the normal thymus, and the gland is a source of AChR-reactive T cells and AChR antibodies (Fig. 3-98). Thymic hyperplasia is common in early-onset MG. Thymoma, sometimes malignant, is present in some 10% of MG patients, and such cases are more likely to have antistriational antibodies (see later). CT or MRI of the mediastinum is an essential part of the investigation (Fig. 3-99).

The motor endplates show dramatic simplification of the postsynaptic junctional folds (Fig. 3-100). The density of the AChRs is reduced by a number of processes, including cross-linking of adjacent receptors by antibodies, followed by complement-mediated degradation with lysis of postsynaptic membrane, and in some instances direct blockade of the AChR by antibody (Fig. 3-101).

The etiology of MG is unknown, but it is clearly an autoimmune disease and may be associated with other autoimmune diseases, notably hypothyroidism. Antithyroid and other autoantibody species may be detectable in blood. Immunogenic drugs, such as penicillamine and procainamide, can also induce antibody-positive MG (Fig. 3-102). More commonly, certain drugs that can interfere with the function of neuromuscular junctions, such as aminoglycoside antibiotics, can unmask latent myasthenia.

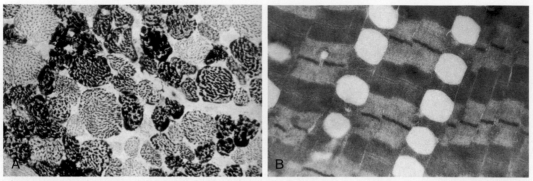

Fig. 3-63. Muscle biopsy from a patient with carnitine deficiency. **A,** Sudan black stain showing excess accumulation of lipid within muscle fibers. **B,** EM of biopsy from this patient demonstrating lipid droplets between myofibrils.

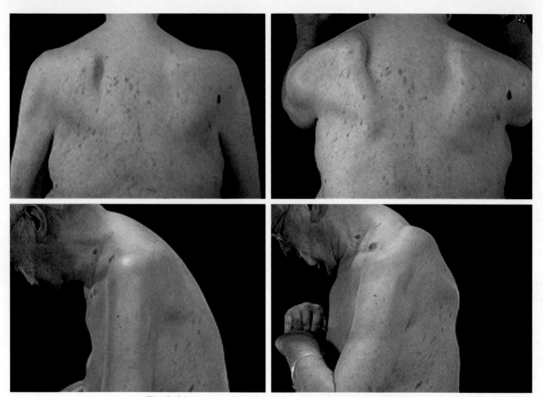

Fig. 3-64. Limb-girdle phenotype in chronic polymyositis.

MuSK MG. Myasthenia gravis associated with MuSK antibodies is a distinct condition with characteristic clinical features. It typically affects young females, who present with marked facial, neck, bulbar, and respiratory muscle weakness. Thymic pathology is much less common, and MuSK-positive patients are more resistant to conventional treatment and less likely to achieve remission than AChR antibody positive patients. Initial response to conventional treatment may also be suboptimal, but plasma exchange is very effective.

Lambert-Eaton Myasthenic Syndrome. Lambert-Eaton myasthenic syndrome is caused by antibodies to voltage-gated Ca^{2+} channels (VGCCs) in the presynaptic membrane. The antibodies cross-link the channels, altering the normal arrays of active zones for ACh release (Fig. 3-103). This results in the characteristic clinical feature of the condition: reduced or absent tendon reflexes that increase in amplitude after muscle contraction against resistance, as increased neural drive overcomes the reduced transmitter release. This may be associated with temporary improvement in strength.

LEMS is strongly associated with underlying malignancy, particularly small cell lung cancer, which is found in some 40% of cases. The neuromuscular syndrome can antedate the discovery of the tumor by several years. The condition may also be associated with other malignancies and other autoimmune disorders such as celiac disease.

The presentation is more suggestive of a myopathy than myasthenia, with gradually progressive proximal weakness, most prominent in the legs.

There may be myalgia and muscle tenderness. Fatigability is rarely prominent, and cranial and bulbar musculature is affected in only a minority of cases, and then usually mildly. Respiratory involvement is rare.

On direct inquiry, patients usually complain of a dry mouth with an unpleasant metallic taste. This is caused by muscarinic receptor involvement, and other symptoms of autonomic dysfunction may also occur.

The neurophysiologic findings in patients with LEMS are diagnostic. During nerve conduction tests, the evoked compound action potential is of low amplitude and falls further at low rates of stimulation. Higher rates of stimulation produce a striking augmentation. The resting evoked response amplitude is also increased after a brief period of sustained contraction (Fig. 3-104).

Serial imaging, particularly chest CT and whole-body PET, is required to screen for tumor. VGCC antibodies are detected in some 95% of cases of LEMS. Small cell lung cancer is thought to originate from neural crest cells, and these tumors may express VGCC that might act as autoantigens.

Neuromyotonia

Acquired neuromyotonia (Isaac's syndrome) is not a form of myasthenia but has a similar immunopathogenesis. The main clinical features are cramps, muscle stiffness, and widespread myokymia that can be triggered by muscle contraction. Other features such as pseudomyotonia, muscle hypertrophy, excess sweating, and paresthesia

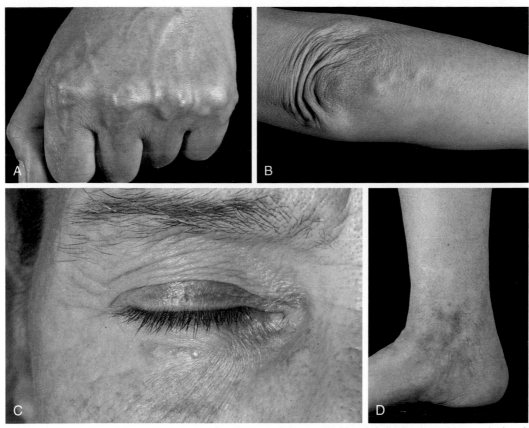

Fig. 3-65. Overlap myositis. In addition to typical myopathic features of polymyositis, this patient exhibited rheumatoid nodules over the knuckles and elbows **(A)** and telangiectasia around the eyes and ankles **(B)**.

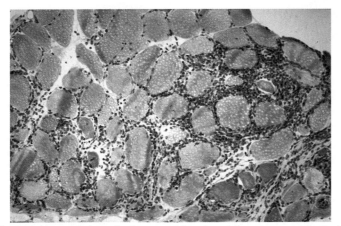

Fig. 3-66. Histopathology of polymyositis. There is an inflammatory reaction in the endomysium, with fiber necrosis and regeneration

may occur. Neuromyotonia results from hyperexcitability of the motor nerves, particularly the terminal branches of the neuromuscular junctions, caused by voltage-gated potassium channel (VGKC) antibodies that inhibit repolarization of the axons after an action potential. This leads to a state of continuous muscle fiber activity. Again, EMG is diagnostic. The resting trace shows irregular bursts of high-frequency discharges, each comprising groups of single motor units firing as doublets, triplets, or multiples. The CK level may be increased, reflecting the muscle fiber hyperactivity.

Botulism
The toxins of Clostridium botulinum, the most potent neurotoxin known, have strong affinity for presynaptic membranes, where they block exocytosis of ACh at the neuromuscular junctions and in the autonomic nervous system. Food-borne botulism is now uncommon, but wound botulism is seen among parenteral drug users, particularly in relation to "skin popping." In addition to gastrointestinal symptoms, which can include severe constipation, there is generalized weakness with ptosis, extraocular impairment, and signs of autonomic dysfunction, characteristically pupillary paralysis. Gastroparesis and pseudo-obstruction are also common features. The neurophysiologic findings are similar to those of LEMS.

Botulinum toxin has also found an important role in the treatment of movement disorders and cosmetic surgery.

Congenital Myasthenic Syndromes
Congenital myasthenic syndromes are very rare disorders that result from genetic defects of presynaptic, synaptic, and postsynaptic neuromuscular junction transmitter and receptor proteins. They therefore can be classified as presynaptic (e.g., familial infantile myasthenia), synaptic (acetylcholinesterase deficiency), and postsynaptic (AChR deficiency, slow-channel syndrome, low-affinity fast-channel syndrome). Symptoms start at birth or in infancy, with the exception of slow-channel syndrome, which may begin in adult life as a myopathy.

Postsynaptic disorders are the most common. Acetylcholine receptor deficiency syndrome results from mutations coding for proteins that constitute the AChR subunits. The most common is ε-subunit deficiency. Affected infants may present with severe weakness, including oculomotor, cranial, and bulbar muscle weakness, and arthrogryposis is common. Other mutations cause alterations in AChR function, resulting in shortening or prolongation of channel opening times. Slow-channel syndrome is characterized by prolonged channel opening time. Mild cases can begin in adult life with generalized weakness, bulbar dysfunction, and limb-girdle weakness. Breathing may be affected. On EMG, there is a decrement on repetitive stimulation, typical of myasthenia, but two or more motor potentials are elicited by a single stimulus.

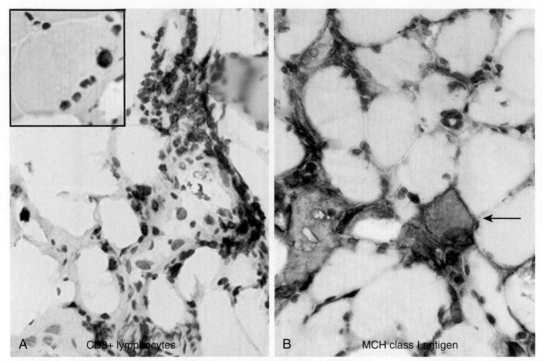

Fig. 3-67. Immunopathology of polymyositis. The inflammatory infiltrate stains positively with a CD8 lymphocyte marker *(left)*. The nonnecrotic fiber in the *inset* is being invaded by a lymphocyte *(arrow)*. There is a generalized upregulation of MHC class I antigens on the surface of the muscle fibers *(arrow) (right)*.

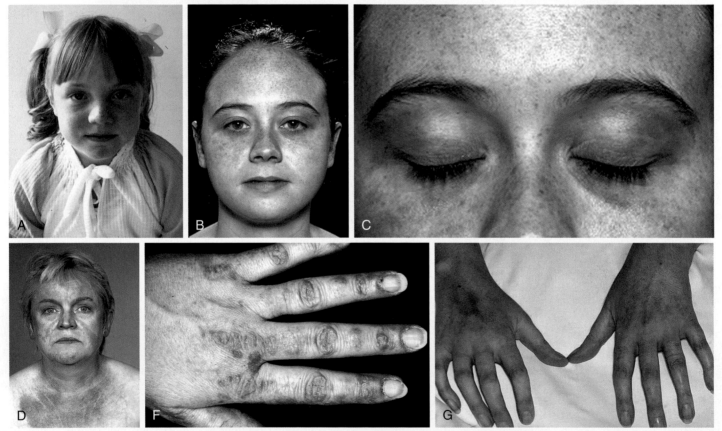

Fig. 3-68. Skin rashes in dermatomyositis. The facial rash tends to affect the periorbital skin, malar areas, and supraorbital ridges. It may be subtle, as in this child **(A)** and young girl **(B)**. The rash is prominent in this woman **(C)** and also affects the light exposed area of her chest. In dark-skinned patients **(D)**, there may be skin depigmentation. Changes in the hands include rash over the knuckles, Gottron's papules, and dilated nail-fold capillaries **(E)**.

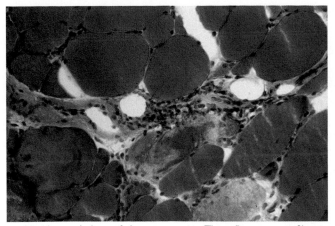

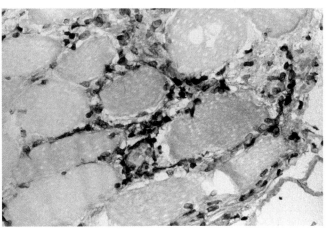

Fig. 3-69. Histopathology of dermatomyositis. The inflammatory infiltration is mainly perivascular and perifascicular.

Fig. 3-70. Immunohistochemistry of muscle in dermatomyositis. The inflammatory infiltrate is mainly CD4 lymphocytes.

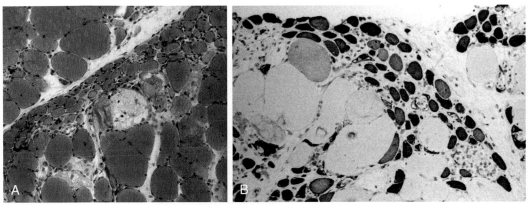

Fig. 3-71. Perifascicular atrophy in dermatomyositis. Fibers at the periphery of fascicles are significantly smaller.

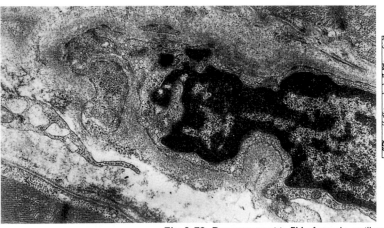

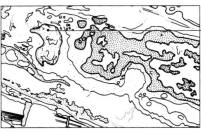

tubuloreticular structure

Fig. 3-72. Dermatomyositis. EM of muscle capillary with tubuloreticular structure.

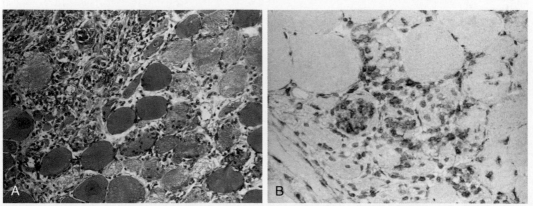

Fig. 3-73. Necrotizing myopathy may be a manifestation of underlying malignancy. **A,** Widespread fiber necrosis and degeneration with marked inflammatory infiltration. **B,** However, the CD68 marker (section from another area of biopsy) shows that much of this reaction is the result of macrophage accumulation, not lymphocytes.

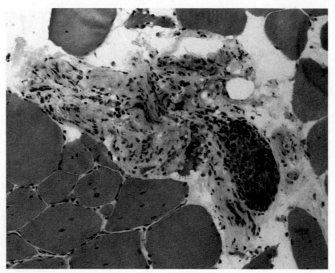

Fig. 3-74. Noncaseating granuloma in muscle in a case of systemic sarcoidosis.

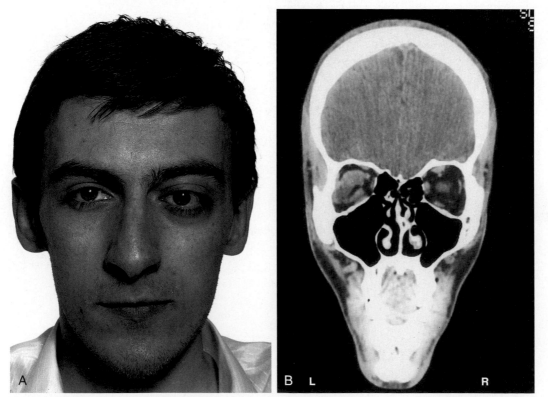

Fig. 3-75. Orbital pseudotumor. Left-sided proptosis *(left).* A complete external ophthalmoplegia of the left eye was found. Coronal CT brain scan *(right).* There is gross thickening and enlargement of the extraocular muscles in the left orbit.

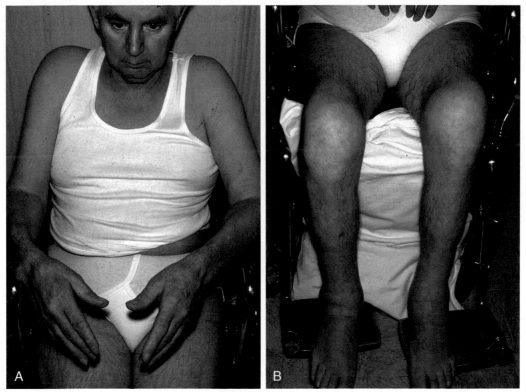

Fig. 3-76. Inclusion body myositis. **A,** Scalloping of the forearm muscles. **B,** Selective quadriceps wasting.

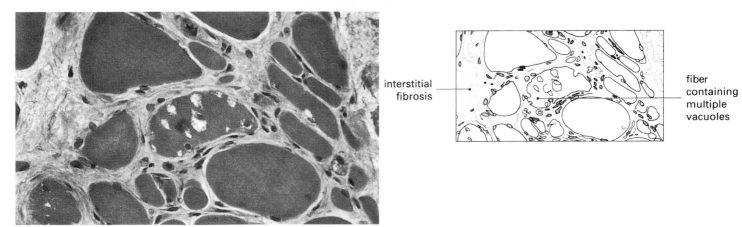

interstitial fibrosis

fiber containing multiple vacuoles

Fig. 3-77. Inclusion body myositis. Rimmed vacuoles in some of the fibers demonstrate basophilic material on the walls of the vacuoles. Some fibers are hypertrophied, and there is marked interstitial fibrosis.

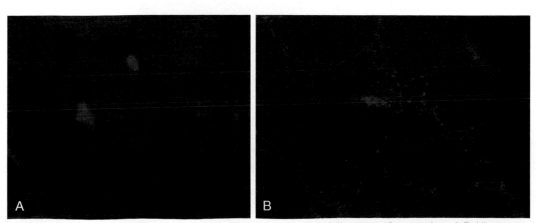

Fig. 3-78. Aberrant protein accumulation in muscle fibers in inclusion body myositis. **A,** Amyloid deposition (Congo red stain). **B,** Ubiquitinated phosphorylated tau.

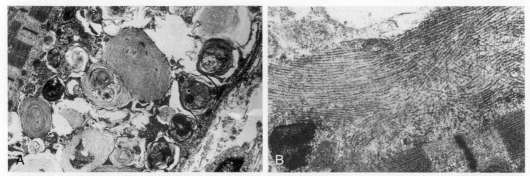

Fig. 3-79. Ultrastructural findings in inclusion body myositis. **A,** The walls of the vacuoles are lined by accumulations of pseudomembranous "myelinoid" whorls. **B,** Characteristic 15- to 18-nm paired helical filament accumulations in the cytoplasm.

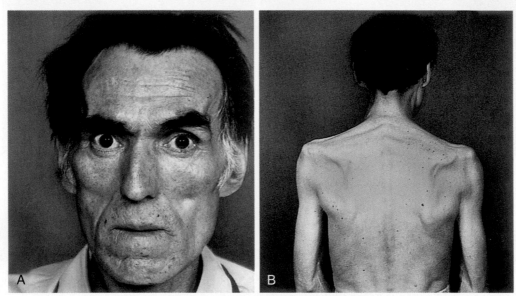

Fig. 3-80. Facial appearance and proximal muscle wasting in thyrotoxic myopathy.

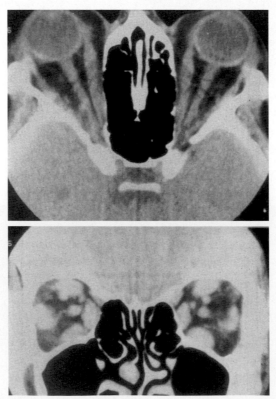

Fig. 3-81. CT scan of the orbits in patient with Graves' ophthalmopathy shows bilateral enlargement of extraocular muscles.

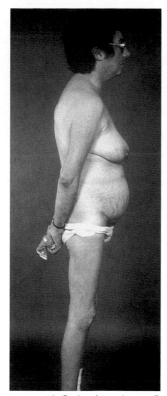

Fig. 3-82. Adrenal carcinoma with Cushing's syndrome. Gross limb-girdle wasting and abdominal striae.

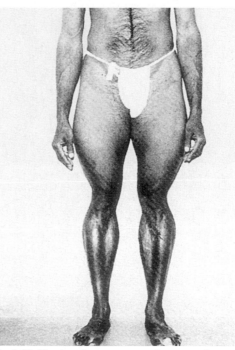

Fig. 3-83. Muscle enlargement secondary to cysticercosis.

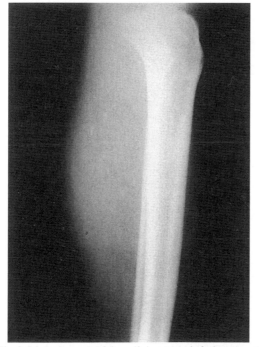

Fig. 3-84. Radiograph of the calf showing calcified cysticerci.

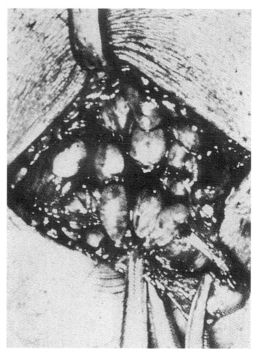

Fig. 3-85. Cysticerci in muscle on biopsy.

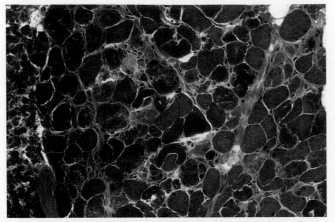

Fig. 3-86. Necrotizing myopathy caused by a statin. Severe myalgia and proximal weakness began within a week of starting the drug, and the creatine kinase level was markedly increased. The biopsy shows multifocal fiber necrosis with regeneration (basophilic fibers) and macrophage infiltration.

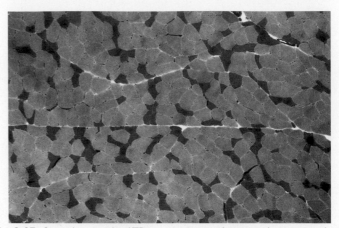

Fig. 3-87. Steroid myopathy. ATPase preparation showing selective atrophy of dark-staining type 2 fibers.

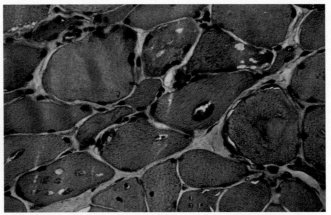

Fig. 3-88. Vacuolar myopathy resulting from colchicine. The patient was being treated for familial Mediterranean fever. The vacuoles are lined with whorled membranous and spheromembranous bodies.

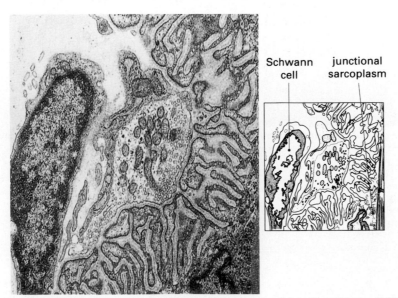

Schwann cell junctional sarcoplasm

Fig. 3-89. Normal neuromuscular junction. EM study showing the axon terminal containing synaptic vesicles of acetylcholine (ACh), covered by a Schwann cell. The postsynaptic membrane is thrown into many clefts and folds, and the ACh receptors are concentrated in the mouths of the clefts. The junctional sarcoplasm contains glycogen granules, ribosomes, and small tubular profiles.

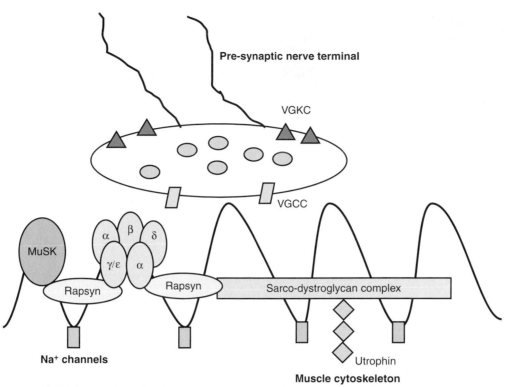

Fig. 3-90. Acetylcholine receptors (AChRs) are embedded in the postsynaptic membrane. They are made up of several subunits (α, β, γ, δ, γ/ε) and are associated with proteins that regulate AChR clustering, including rapsyn, MuSK, and perlecan. The receptor in the junctional membrane is shown in relation to the sarco-dystroglycan complex of the extrajunctional membrane. VGCC voltage-gated calcium channel; VGKC, voltage-gated potassium channel.

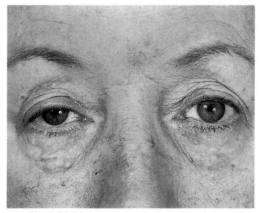

Fig. 3-91. Unilateral ptosis in myasthenia gravis.

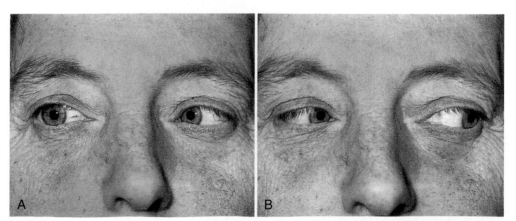

Fig. 3-92. Weakness of right lateral rectus muscle in myasthenia gravis **A,** Gaze to the right impaired in right eye. **B,** Normal gaze to the left.

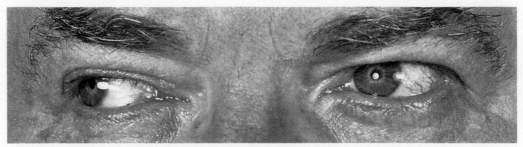

Fig. 3-93. Pseudo-internuclear ophthalmoplegia in a patient with myasthenia gravis.

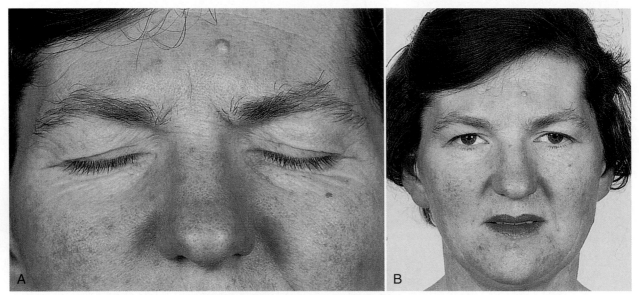

Fig. 3-94. Myasthenia gravis. **A,** Failure of complete eyelid closure. **B,** Characteristic configuration of the mouth.

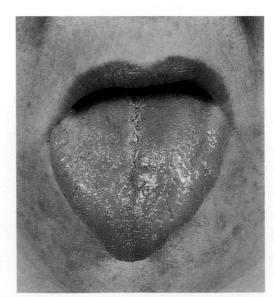

Fig. 3-95. Triple-furrowed tongue in a patient with myasthenia gravis.

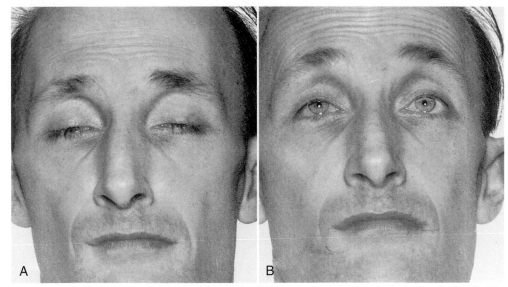

Fig. 3-96. Tensilon test in myasthenia gravis. Facial appearance before **(A)** and after **(B)** intravenous injection of edrophonium hydrochloride, a short-acting acetylcholinesterase inhibitor.

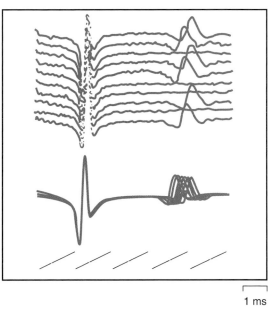

1 ms

Fig. 3-97. Single-fiber EMG in myasthenia gravis. The first fiber potential triggers the oscilloscope sweep *(upper).* The variation in timing of the second potential from a fiber innervated by the same axon is measured. Some of the second potentials are blocked. Averaged signals for 20 to 30 pairs show increased jitter *(lower).*

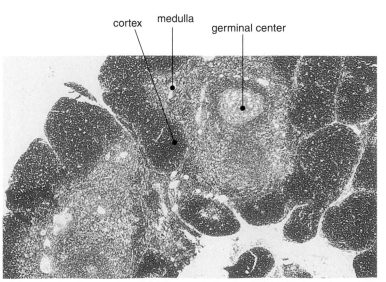

Fig. 3-98. The thymus in myasthenia gravis. Section showing the relative increase in the size of the medulla to the cortex, and one prominent germinal center.

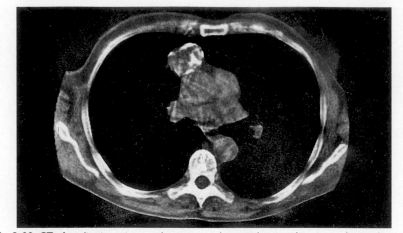

Fig. 3-99. CT of mediastinum in myasthenia gravis, showing thymic enlargement due to thymoma.

synaptic
space

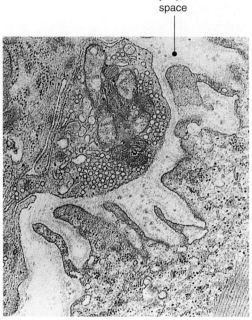

Fig. 3-100. Endplate region in myasthenia gravis. Simplification of the postsynaptic region and widening of the synaptic space.

IgG deposit on
degenerate
material in the
synaptic space

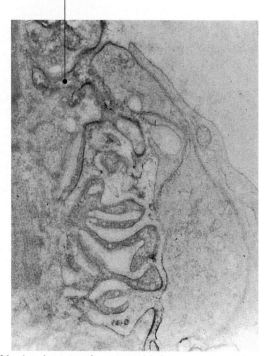

Fig. 3-101. Localization of anti-acetylcholine receptor IgG antibody by immuno–electron microscopy in myasthenia gravis. Deposits appear on short segments of some junctional folds and on degenerate material in the synaptic space.

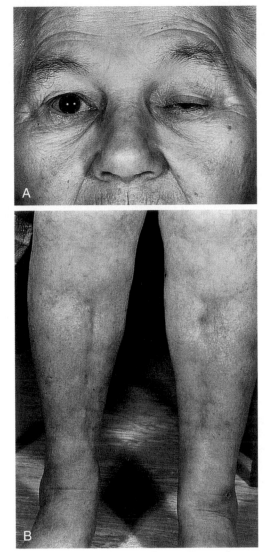

Fig. 3-102. Myasthenia gravis induced by D-penicillamine during treatment of scleroderma. **A,** Unilateral ptosis. **B,** Characteristic skin changes of scleroderma.

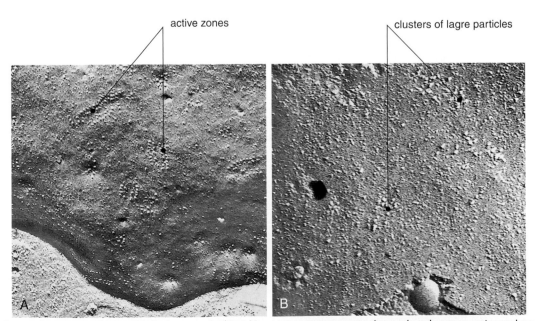

Fig. 3-103. A, Freeze-fractured neuromuscular junction from a normal subject. Numerous active zones are clustered on the presynaptic membrane. **B,** Presynaptic membrane from a patient with Lambert-Eaton myasthenic syndrome. The number of active zones is reduced and the organization is disrupted, with clusters of large particles.

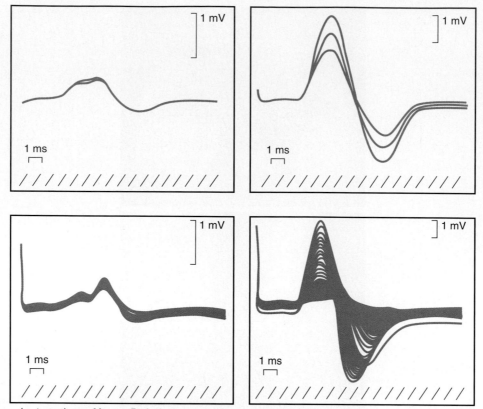

Fig. 3-104. Lambert-Eaton myasthenic syndrome. **Upper:** Evoked motor potential at rest *(left)* increases in amplitude after muscle contraction *(right)*. **Lower:** Augmentation of motor potential amplitudes during repetitive stimulation at 10 Hz *(left)* and at 50 Hz *(right)*.

CHAPTER

CEREBROVASCULAR DISEASE: CEREBRAL INFARCTION

4

ANATOMY

The common carotid artery bifurcates in the neck to form the external and internal carotid arteries. The internal carotid artery has no branches before entering the skull through the foramen lacerum. Flow through the external carotid artery assumes importance for the brain only if the internal carotid artery is occluded. Then, increased flow through the facial and superficial temporal branches can feed intracranial structures via anastomoses with the ophthalmic artery. The ophthalmic artery arises anteriorly from the carotid siphon. Beyond this point, the internal carotid artery pierces the dura and gives off two further branches, the posterior communicating and anterior choroidal arteries, before terminating in the anterior and middle cerebral arteries (Fig. 4-1).

The vertebral artery arises from the subclavian artery. It enters the transverse foramen of the fifth or sixth cervical vertebra, passes upward in the vertebral canal, and then winds posteriorly around the atlas to pierce the dura mater at the level of the foramen magnum. The major intracranial branch of the vertebral artery is the posterior inferior cerebellar artery. The two vertebral arteries unite at the junction of the pons and medulla to form the basilar artery. The major branches of the basilar artery are the paired anterior inferior and superior cerebellar arteries. Circumferential branches from the basilar artery invest the brainstem and supply it with perforating paramedian vessels. At its termination, the basilar artery forms the paired posterior cerebral arteries (Fig. 4-2).

The distribution of the branches of the anterior, middle, and posterior cerebral arteries is illustrated in Figures 4-3 and 4-4.

Variation in the size and distribution of individual cerebral vessels is considerable. The vertebral artery may originate from the aortic arch or even from the carotid system. An asymmetry in size of the vertebral arteries is prominent in about 10% of individuals, the left usually being larger (Fig. 4-5).

Variations from the classic configuration of the circle of Willis have been demonstrated in up to 50% of individuals, consisting of differing calibers, or absence or reduplication of one or more of the component vessels (Fig. 4-6). After occlusion of one internal carotid artery, cross-flow through the circle of Willis may suffice to maintain filling in the middle cerebral artery distal to the occlusion (Fig. 4-7).

Multiple anastomoses exist between the individual cerebral veins. The surface veins drain into the intradural venous sinuses, including the superior sagittal, lateral, and cavernous sinuses. The deeper veins largely converge on the internal cerebral veins that drain into the straight sinus via the vein of Galen (Fig. 4-8). The straight sinus runs posteriorly and drains into the transverse sinus that is not continuous (or is only tenuously continuous) with the superior sagittal sinus. The transverse sinuses begin at the internal occipital protuberance, the right usually continuous with the superior sagittal sinus, and the other with the straight sinus. Eventually, they form the sigmoid sinuses, which in turn drain into the internal jugular veins.

CLASSIFICATION

Stroke is the consequence either of infarction, in which death of brain tissue follows interruption of its blood supply, or of hemorrhage, in which bleeding takes place in the brain substance. The stroke arising in some patients with subarachnoid hemorrhage incorporates one or both of these mechanisms.

CEREBRAL INFARCTION

Cerebral infarction is most commonly either the result of embolic occlusion of an intracranial vessel from material derived from an extracranial source or, less often, the result of thrombus formation within an intracranial vessel. Primary atherosclerotic thrombosis is rare in the larger intracranial vessels, with the exception of the basilar artery and its branches (Fig. 4-9). Occlusion of the microscopic intracerebral vessels is common, but how frequently this manifests as a stroke syndrome remains uncertain. In such vessels, a combination of connective tissue infiltration with fibrinoid material and subintimal foam cells causes obliteration of the lumen (Fig. 4-10). Probably many of the bright signal areas identified on T2-weighted MR images in older individuals are the consequence of this pathologic process, or they simply represent état criblé (Fig. 4-11). The area of brain supplied by these occluded vessels contains small cavities (lacunes), the majority of which are less than 1 cm in diameter, and within which is found a meshwork of gliotic tissue (Fig. 4-12). The distinction of expanded perivascular spaces (état criblé) from lacunes can be difficult on MR scanning. État criblé spaces are usually less than 3 mm in diameter and are homogeneous and well demarcated on T2-weighted images. Lacunes are generally larger, are irregularly shaped, and are nonhomogeneous on the same images. Pathologically, the spaces around vessels with état criblé contain a small artery and are often partially filled in by fibrous tissue. Lacunes do not contain fibrous tissue or a single central vessel (although larger ones may have some capillaries), and they may contain some macrophages.

Cerebral emboli are principally derived from the heart and the major extracranial vessels (Fig. 4-13). Those originating from the neck arteries are most commonly formed of a platelet–fibrin mixture or cholesterol. Atheromatous disease in the carotid tree predominates at the carotid bifurcation and then in the siphon (Fig. 4-14). Initially, fatty streak deposits are found, followed by a fibromusculoelastic plaque containing intimal smooth muscle cells and macrophages filled with lipid. The cells are surrounded by extracellular lipid and by fibrotic tissue. A sudden expansion of the plaque occurs if hemorrhage takes place in it, with resulting damage to the endothelium to which fibrin and platelets adhere (Fig. 4-15). Hemorrhages causing plaque rupture lead to acute embolic occlusions upstream from the rupture site. In the posterior circulation, atheroma is largely confined to the origins of the vertebral and posterior cerebral arteries, along with the intracranial vertebral arteries and the proximal sections of the basilar artery. In some patients with a history of cerebral ischemia, postmortem examination reveals cerebral vessels occluded by material containing cholesterol crystals, presumably of embolic origin (Fig. 4-16).

The heart is an important source of emboli, not only to the intracranial vessels but also, in the case of large emboli, to the major neck vessels (Fig. 4-17). Cerebral emboli occur in up to 10% of patients with akinetic heart muscle after myocardial infarction. Patients with mitral stenosis and atrial fibrillation are susceptible to both systemic and cranial embolization from thrombus in the left atrium (Fig. 4-18). Mitral valve prolapse is relatively innocuous hemodynamically but can act as a source of microemboli to the brain (Fig. 4-19). Infective endocarditis most commonly forms on the mitral and aortic

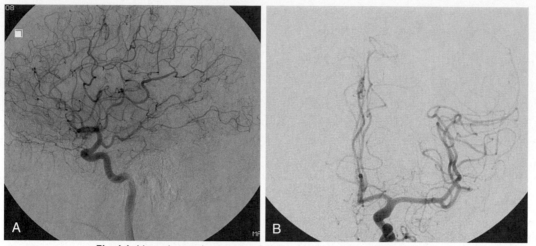

Fig. 4-1. Normal carotid angiogram. **A,** Lateral view. **B,** Anteroposterior view.

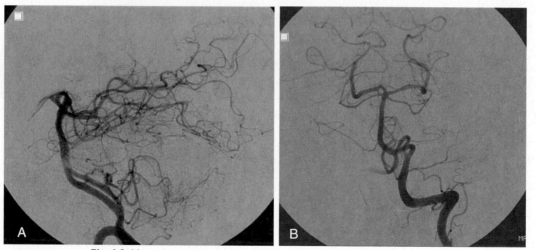

Fig. 4-2. Normal vertebral angiogram. **A,** Lateral view. **B,** Anteroposterior view.

LATERAL SURFACE

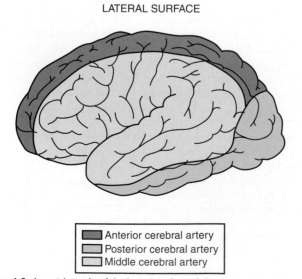

Anterior cerebral artery
Posterior cerebral artery
Middle cerebral artery

Fig. 4-3. Arterial supply of the lateral surface of the cerebral hemisphere.

AXIAL AND CORONAL SECTIONS

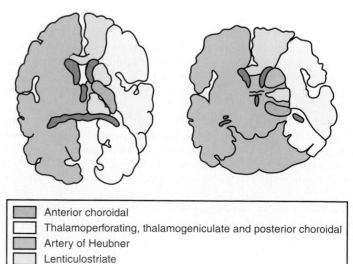

Anterior choroidal
Thalamoperforating, thalamogeniculate and posterior choroidal
Artery of Heubner
Lenticulostriate

Fig. 4-4. Arterial territories in horizontal and coronal sections.

valves. The disease is now more commonly associated with prosthetic valves than with rheumatic heart disease. Many cases occur in older patients without clinical or pathologic evidence of rheumatic valvular lesions (Fig. 4-20). Marantic endocarditis (nonbacterial thrombotic endocarditis) tends to occur in association with carcinoma, but at times it appears in young individuals without an apparent precipitating cause (Fig. 4-21). A large patent foramen ovale is likely to present with a hemodynamic disturbance of cardiac function (Fig. 4-22). Smaller defects of at least 7 mm in diameter have been reported in some 6% of autopsies. The lesion may be associated with an atrial septal aneurysm. Whether such lesions are more common in the stroke population than the general population remains unsettled, but in at least some cases a patent foramen is associated with paradoxical embolization from venous sources to the cerebral circulation, with resultant stroke.

Protruding atheroma of the thoracic aorta has been linked, via an embolic process, to the occurrence of perioperative stroke in patients undergoing coronary artery bypass graft. Various techniques have been used, including intraoperative surface aortic ultrasonography to detect atherosclerosis of the ascending aorta with a view to modifying operative technique if there are positive findings.

Cerebral infarction can also occur if there is a massive failure of cerebral perfusion, the consequence usually of either severe myocardial infarction or profound hypotension due to blood loss. In such

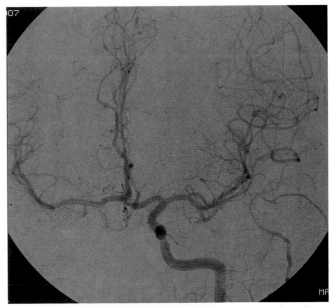

Fig. 4-7. Filling of the middle cerebral artery from the contralateral internal carotid system, subsequent to a carotid artery occlusion.

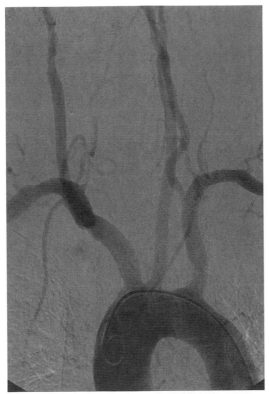

Fig. 4-5. Arch angiogram showing asymmetrical vertebral arteries.

THE CIRCLE OF WILLIS

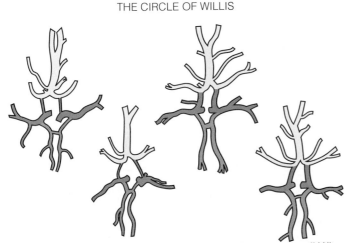

Fig. 4-6. Anatomic variants of the constituent vessels of the circle of Willis.

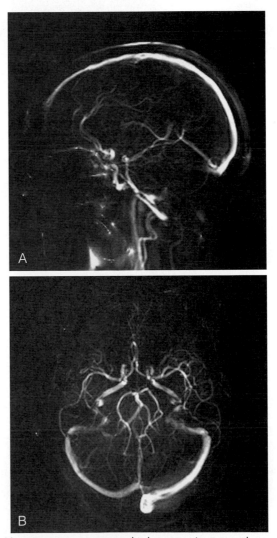

Fig. 4-8. Magnetic resonance venography demonstrating a normal venous system. **A,** Lateral view. **B,** Anteroposterior view.

cases, the infarction is not confined to the distribution of a single vessel but is more likely to be found in the border-zone (watershed) areas at the margins of supply of the major cerebral vessels (Fig. 4-23) or in vulnerable regions such as the hippocampus and cerebellar cortex (Fig. 4-24). In some cases, there is widespread neocortical damage in laminar or pseudolaminar patterns.

PATHOLOGIC AND PHYSIOLOGIC CONSEQUENCES OF CEREBRAL INFARCTION

Soon after the onset of cerebral infarction, swelling of both gray and white matter appears, with the former sometimes showing petechial hemorrhages (Fig. 4-25). When the infarct is the consequence of cerebral embolism, breakup of the occluding embolus allows restoration of blood flow to the ischemic region. Leakage of blood through damaged blood vessels within the infarct leads to hemorrhagic infarction (Fig. 4-26).

Subsequently, infarcts evolve with waves of inflammatory cells (polymorphonuclear granulocytes, then macrophages, then lymphocytes) and with formation of granulation tissue with proliferation of capillaries (Fig. 4-27). Ultimately, gliotic scars wall off and fill in small infarcts. Larger infarcts show cystic degeneration with shrinkage of the affected hemisphere and dilatation of the ipsilateral lateral ventricle. If the infarct involves the motor strip, destruction of pyramidal fibers or their parent Betz cells causes Wallerian degeneration

of the distal pyramidal pathways. Consequently, in the spinal cord, degeneration appears in the uncrossed anterior and crossed lateral corticospinal tracts (Fig. 4-28).

Autoregulation suffices to maintain cerebral blood flow despite wide variation in perfusion pressure. The arterial tension of carbon dioxide is critical in the regulation of cerebrovascular resistance, and vasodilation occurs with rising P_{CO_2} levels. Mean cerebral blood flow tends to fall in areas of acute cerebral infarction; however, more meaningful information is derived from measurement of regional flow.

A syndrome of luxury perfusion, in blood-flow terms, is an area adjacent to an infarct with inappropriately high blood flow compared with the analogous area in the uninfarcted hemisphere. During the first few days after infarction, luxury perfusion reflects dysregulation in blood flow. Later-occurring luxury perfusion, beginning at about 3 days after infarction, is the consequence of capillary sprouting (neovascularization). Luxury perfusion, defined metabolically, is an area in which there is a greater reduction of metabolic activity than of flow.

The ischemic penumbra around an area of cerebral infarction is defined as a volume of brain tissue that has suffered an ischemic process that is still, at least partially, reversible. Studies using PET have defined such areas by the presence of low cerebral blood flow (CBF), relatively preserved cerebral oxygen metabolic rate, and a high oxygen

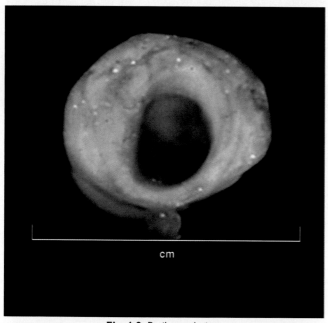

Fig. 4-9. Basilar occlusion.

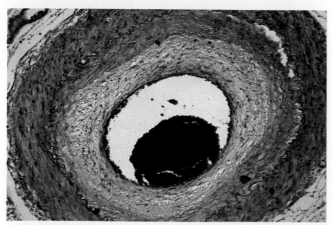

Fig. 4-10. Section of an artery from within the cavity of an old occipital infarct. The thick-walled artery has an atherosclerotic expansion of the intima with arteriosclerotic fibrosis of the media and adventitia (Luxol fast blue, H&E, ×10).

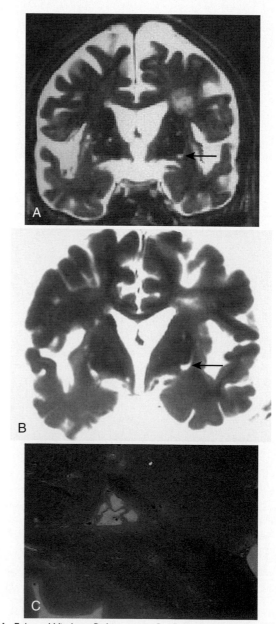

Fig. 4-11. Enlarged Virchow-Robin space. **A,** Coronal MR image before death (*arrow*). **B,** Coronal MR of same image after death and subsequent formalin fixation. **C,** Pathologic section (H&E).

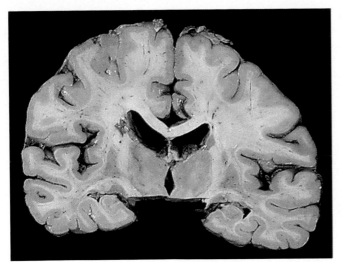

Fig. 4-12. Lacunar infarct in the medial portion of the posterior limb of the left internal capsule.

SOURCES OF EMBOLI

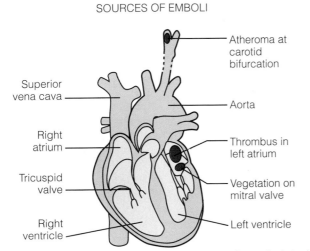

- Superior vena cava
- Atheroma at carotid bifurcation
- Aorta
- Right atrium
- Thrombus in left atrium
- Tricuspid valve
- Vegetation on mitral valve
- Right ventricle
- Left ventricle

Fig. 4-13. Potential sources of embolic material passing into the cerebral circulation.

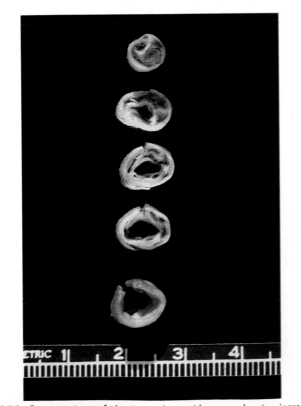

Fig. 4-14. Cross-sections of the internal carotid artery showing increasingly severe stenosis associated with plaque hemorrhage.

extraction fraction. Such areas can be identified by PET scanning some hours after the onset of an ischemic stroke, with a liability then to evolve into areas of frank infarction (Fig. 4-29). These areas are more difficult to define histopathologically, although in experimental models they appear to be represented by zones of vacuolation from acute edema containing apparently normal neurons in which special techniques can demonstrate double-stranded DNA damage.

Cerebral edema is an important complication of both cerebral infarction and hemorrhage. In the case of infarction, the edema is both vasogenic and cytotoxic (i.e., both intracellular and extracellular). Edema reaches a maximum about 4 to 5 days after cerebral infarction, leading to obscuration of the cortical gyral pattern and, with large infarcts, the development of midline shift and subfalcine herniation (Fig. 4-30). In addition to the midline shift, transtentorial or uncal herniation may occur, leading to ischemia and hemorrhage in the rostral brainstem (Figs. 4-31 and 4-32).

The inflammatory cell reaction that occurs in the acutely ischemic brain is associated with the expression of inflammatory cytokines, such as tumor necrosis factor. In the experimental animal, interventions that inactivate cytokines reduce ischemic damage. After ischemia, there is induction of a nitric oxide isoform (iNOS) not normally present in most cells, with evidence that this agent can contribute to the degree of ischemic damage. Elevated levels of cyclooxygenase-2, triggered by ischemia-induced inflammation, may also contribute to the tissue damage.

INVESTIGATION

Investigation of the patient with cerebrovascular disease, particularly when embolization is considered likely, will involve the heart as well as the major cerebral vessels. Echocardiography is not justified in the absence of any evidence incriminating the heart as a source of embolization, at least in older patients. Transthoracic two-dimensional echocardiography is the initial investigation of choice. Transesophageal studies are indicated if cardiac embolism is strongly suspected, or if the left atrium, left atrial appendage, and interatrial septum require evaluation. Rarer cardiac pathology sometimes detected includes atrial myxoma and tumor invasion of the heart (Fig. 4-33). In patients with stroke and patent foramen ovale, risk factors associated with stroke recurrence include the demonstration of a right-to-left shunt on the basis of the passage of more than 20 microbubbles to the left atrium during contrast echocardiography (Fig. 4-34).

Computed Tomography Scanning

Computed tomography remains of major importance in the assessment of the stroke patient in the acute phase. It allows differentiation of cerebral infarction from cerebral hemorrhage. The latter, if present, is always revealed if scanning has been performed at the correct time. By 10 days, and perhaps before, small hemorrhages will have become hypodense and no longer distinguishable from cerebral infarction. CT scanning identifies other pathologic processes mimicking stroke (e.g., tumor), and it indicates the distribution of

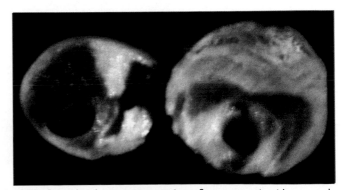

Fig. 4-15. Carotid endarterectomy specimen. Severe stenosis with recent plaque hemorrhage.

the pathologic process and whether there is evidence of unexpected ischemic change in other arterial territories. A plain CT scan may be normal within the first few hours of infarction, but by 24 hours, at least for larger infarcts, the scan is virtually always abnormal. On the other hand, only about 40% of patients with lacunar infarction or with small cortical infarcts will have an abnormal scan at 48 hours. Between 10 days and 3 weeks after stroke, the infarct becomes isodense in comparison to normal brain and, therefore, is invisible. Contrast enhancement is found in about 70% of cases, reaching a maximum intensity after about 2 weeks (Fig. 4-35). Sometimes, the

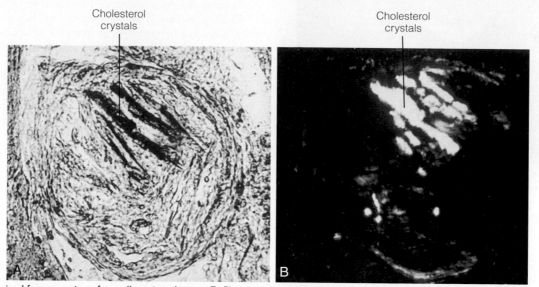

Fig. 4-16. A, Unstained frozen section of a small meningeal artery. **B,** Photograph with illumination through crossed Polaroid screens to show cholesterol clefts.

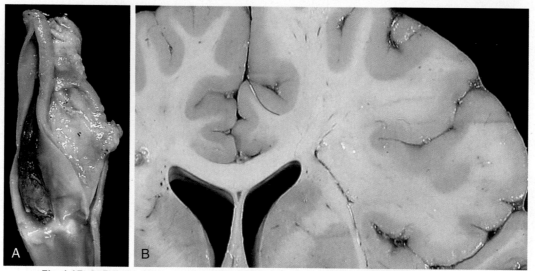

Fig. 4-17. A, Embolus filling a carotid artery. **B,** Resulting right middle cerebral artery territory infarct.

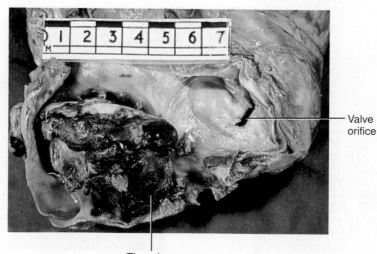

Fig. 4-18. Mitral stenosis with a large thrombus occupying the left atrium.

enhancement shows a ring pattern mimicking that seen in tumor or abscess (Fig. 4-36). Secondary hemorrhagic change in an infarction appears as a lesion of mixed density, with the higher density usually lying centrally (Fig. 4-37).

The development of functional (perfusion) CT (PCT) through whole-brain perfusion or dynamic perfusion techniques has made available data that allow appraisal of the ischemic penumbra surrounding a cerebral infarct. Dynamic PCT requires the intravenous administration of N-iodinated contrast material. The penumbra, based on the area around the infarct with increased regional cerebral

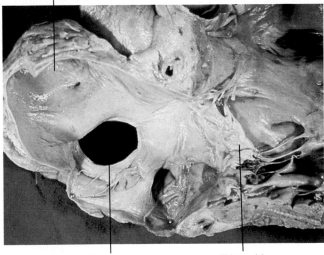

Fig. 4-22. Patent foramen ovale. There is a large defect in the atrial septum.

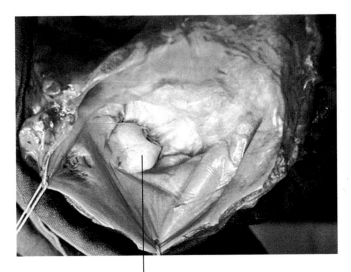

Fig. 4-19. Prolapsed mitral valve viewed from the left atrium.

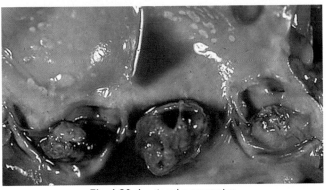

Fig. 4-20. Aortic valve vegetation.

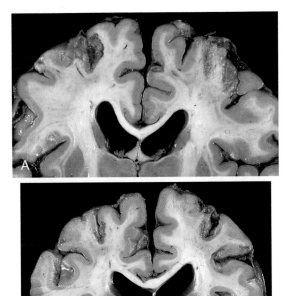

Fig. 4-23. Coronal sections of a brain showing border-zone infarcts at different levels (**A** and **B**).

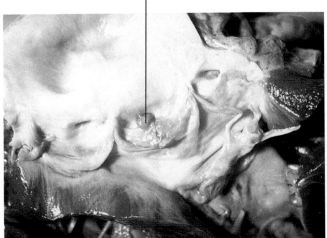

Fig. 4-21. Aortic valve with vegetations occupying the middle cusp of the valve.

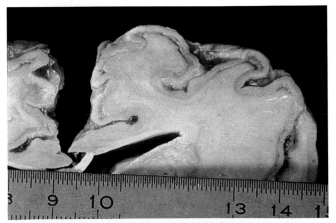

Fig. 4-24. Coronal brain section showing extensive laminar necrosis in a patient who had survived a severe hypoxic episode several months previously.

blood flow, can be defined with an accuracy similar to that obtained by acute and delayed diffusion-weighted MR techniques (Fig. 4-38). It is now possible to obtain a CT, a CT angiogram, and CT perfusion data in a few minutes in the setting of an acute stroke that allows assessment of the brain (for hemorrhage), the carotid vessels, and areas of core infarct and ischemic penumbra. With PCT, in an area of prolonged mean transit time (MTT) (or time to peak [TTP]), an area of reduced cerebral blood volume indicates core infarct, and an area of reduced CBF represents tissue at risk (ischemic penumbra).

Magnetic Resonance Imaging

Conventional MRI is more sensitive than CT for detection of acute cerebral infarction. An abnormal signal is apparent within the first hour of using diffusion-weighted imaging (DWI). Any associated edema is hyperintense on T2-weighted images after a few hours (Fig. 4-39). As the infarct matures, it may assume the same signal characteristics as the surrounding normal brain on some sequences (pseudo-normalization). In long-standing infarcts, cystic changes show signal characteristics of CSF surrounded by a zone of increased signal on T2-weighted images, corresponding to areas of gliosis.

MRI is more sensitive than CT in the detection of brainstem infarcts and acute lacunes (Fig. 4-40). It is particularly useful in demonstrating new infarcts in the presence of preexisting vascular disease (Fig. 4-41). In acute stroke, the combination of conventional imaging, MR angiography, DWI, and perfusion-weighted imaging (PWI) shows great promise for differentiating between core infarct and ischemic penumbra. PWI involves the collection of data after administration of an IV bolus of gadolinium-based contrast. Using certain assumptions, it is possible to estimate TTP, MTT, cerebral blood volume, and CBF values. With PWI MRI, the values obtained are not absolute but relative. In general, although there are exceptions, DWI lesions are said to represent areas of core infarction (irreversible ischemia) and CBF is said to represent ischemic penumbra (potentially reversible ischemic areas). Areas with MTT abnormalities are generally larger than those shown on CBF and are best thought of as areas that have a reduction in blood flow (not all of which is threatened) (Fig. 4-42).

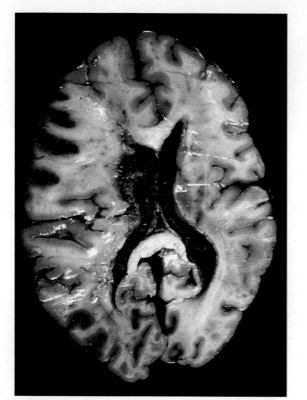

Fig. 4-25. Large acute infarct in middle cerebral territory with focal hemorrhage and subfalcine herniation.

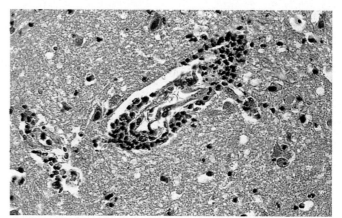

Fig. 4-27. Acute cerebral infarct. Dead hypereosinophilic neurons and an infiltrate of polymorphonuclear granulocytes around a cortical blood vessel.

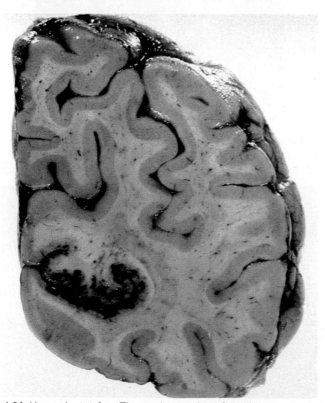

Fig. 4-26. Hemorrhagic infarct. The visual cortex has infarcted as a result of compression of the posterior cerebral artery after parahippocampal herniation.

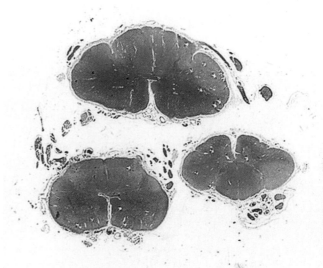

Fig. 4-28. Three sections of spinal cord showing Wallerian degeneration of one lateral column (*pink*) consequent to an old right middle cerebral artery infarct.

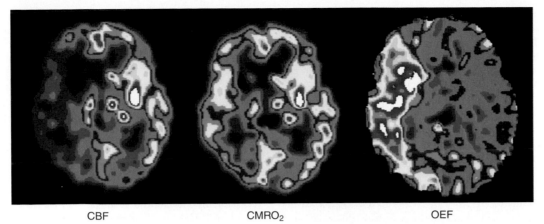

CBF   CMRO₂   OEF

Fig. 4-29. PET scan demonstrating an ischemic penumbra on the left side, characterized by reduced cerebral blood flow (CBF) and relatively preserved oxygen consumption (CMRO₂), resulting in a markedly increased oxygen fraction (OEF) throughout the whole middle cerebral artery territory.

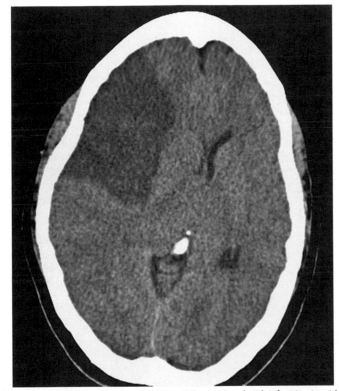

Fig. 4-30. CT showing edema and midline shift associated with infarction in middle cerebral artery territory.

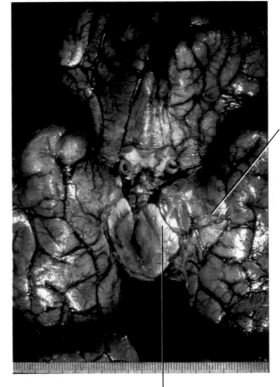

Swollen mesial temporal structures

Compressed midbrain

Fig. 4-31. Marked herniation of medial temporal structures compressing the left side of the midbrain.

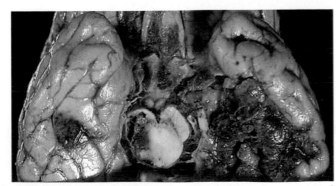

Fig. 4-32. Substantial left uncal herniation with acute hemorrhagic necrosis of the right cerebral peduncle (Kernohan's notch phenomenon).

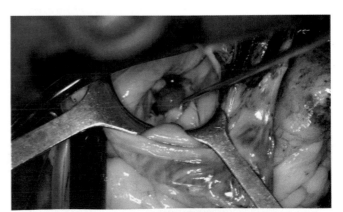

Fig. 4-33. Myxoma. The lesion had been identified on echocardiography as a mobile mass arising from the ventricular aspect of the anterior mitral leaflet.

Noninvasive Screening of the Neck Vessels
Carotid artery flow can be measured with continuous wave bidirectional Doppler, and plaques in the wall can be imaged by real-time B-mode ultrasonography. The most accurate noninvasive screening technique in the carotid vessels combines B-mode ultrasound imaging with a pulsed Doppler flow detector (Duplex scanner). A pulse of ultrasound is transmitted to the neck, and the reflected signal is measured at varying time intervals to allow assessment of structures at different depths. The Doppler system analyzes flow patterns in those vessels identified by the B-mode image. A color-coded system enables direction of flow to be visually presented.

After identification of the common carotid artery, the region of the bifurcation is scanned for any evidence of stenosis or occlusion. Calcified plaques can be identified (Fig. 4-43), as can more severe disease or occlusion (Fig. 4-44). The technique can be used to evaluate asymptomatic carotid stenosis and to assess any re-stenosis occurring after carotid endarterectomy. Vertebral duplex is of more limited value. Variation of vertebral artery caliber is common; the vertebral artery origins are not visualized, and abnormalities that are detected—for example, reversal of vertebral flow—may be asymptomatic.

Transcranial Doppler directs an ultrasound beam through a variety of skull base foramina to assess flow in the terminal internal carotid and the first segments of the anterior, middle, and posterior cerebral arteries. In addition, it permits detection of asymptomatic embolization (Fig. 4-45).

Angiography
Conventional angiography for the investigation of suspected cerebrovascular disease is fast becoming redundant. In the past, arch angiography with subtraction views was used to visualize the major neck vessels, and selective angiography of carotid or vertebral vessels to visualize more distal structures.

Two-plane views are carried out of the carotid bifurcation, because plaques can readily be missed if a single-plane view is performed (Fig. 4-46). Disease in the carotid siphon can also act as an embolic source. Occasionally, the stenosis is suggested by a bruit confined to the ipsilateral orbit (Fig. 4-47). Atheroma of the middle cerebral artery is a fairly uncommon cause of transient ischemic attacks. A middle cerebral artery stenosis or occlusion (Fig. 4-48) is not amenable to direct surgery, nor are its effects ameliorated by an intracranial–extracranial bypass graft. Vertebral angiography is seldom undertaken. The finding of a subclavian steal syndrome is often incidental (Fig. 4-49).

Computed Tomography Angiography. Computed tomography angiography (CTA) can be used to accurately assess the carotid bifurcation, and this can be done in the same setting as conventional CT (Fig. 4-50).

Magnetic Resonance Angiography. Originally based on time-of-flight (TOF) techniques, MR angiography (MRA) is now being replaced by contrast-enhanced MRA. This is a more rapid procedure, reducing movement artifact, and it allows a larger area to be imaged. Gadolinium is the contrast medium. For the evaluation of carotid stenosis, studies suggest that lesions of 30% stenosis and greater are detected with high sensitivity and specificity, but overestimation of stenosis may occur if the narrowing is severe. In the posterior circulation, the procedure is less successful for detecting severe stenosis or occlusions at the origin of the vertebral arteries. Currently, three-dimensional TOF MRA is most commonly the procedure of choice for the evaluation of previously coiled intracranial aneurysms, two-dimensional TOF MRA is used to assess carotid bifurcation disease, and contrast-enhanced MRA is used when assessment of the origins of the vessels from the aortic arch is needed (Figs. 4-51 and 4-52).

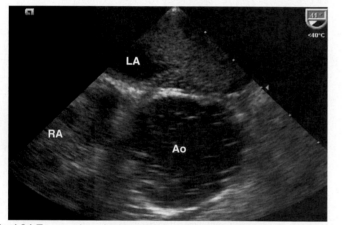

Fig. 4-34. Transesophageal echocardiogram of the right atrium (RA) with contrast, showing a dense puff of contrast material in the left atrium (LA) due to a patent foramen ovale. Contrast can also be seen in the aorta (Ao).

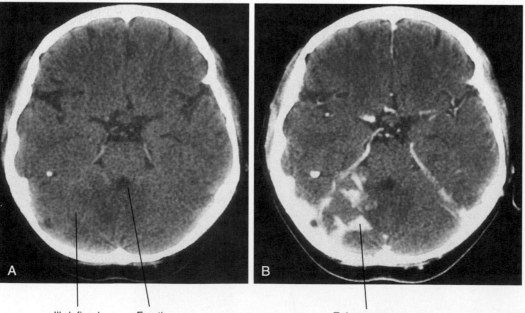

Ill-defined   Fourth
low density   ventricle   Enhancement
Fig. 4-35. Cerebellar infarct. CT showing enhancement, **A,** Before contrast. **B,** After contrast.

Single-Photon Emission Computerized Tomography

Single-photon emission CT (SPECT) is performed using either a multidetector or a rotating gamma camera system. Assessment of regional flow is obtained using either intravenous radioactive tracers or by gas inhalation.

After an infarction, a perfusion defect is identified that corresponds to the distribution of the affected vessel. An area of increased uptake may be seen around the margins of an infarct within the first 2 to 3 weeks of the event. Comparatives studies with CT indicate that the defect identified by SPECT is considerable larger, and is detected much sooner, than that obtained by CT scanning (Fig. 4-53).

Positron Emission Tomography

Positron emission tomography scanning combines the findings of CBF as measured with intravenous xenon, with simultaneous measurement of gamma ray emission with radioactive isotopes of oxygen and carbon dioxide. The results, analyzed by CT, are a summary of metabolic activity and blood flow in selected brain sections. The ischemic core is defined by a blood flow of less than 12 mL/100 g/m, and a cerebral metabolic rate for oxygen of less than 60 μmol/100 g/m. The penumbral region has a flow rate of between 12 and 22 mL/100 g/m and is characterized by an increased oxygen extraction fraction. Later, evolution of the penumbra into the infarcted state leads to a decline in its metabolic activity in relation to its blood flow (luxury perfusion state) (Fig. 4-54). As has been seen, the extent of the penumbra can be determined using misonidazole labeled with radioactive fluoride (^{18}F)—a marker of cellular hypoxia. Using the central benzodiazepine receptor ligand flumazenil as a marker of neuronal activity, scanning between 3 and 16 hours after symptom onset predicts the location and extent of the final infarct as identified by scanning 2 to 3 weeks later with CT or MRI (Fig. 4-55).

CLINICAL SYNDROMES

In transient ischemic attacks, usually the consequence of an embolic interruption of blood flow, resolution of symptoms occurs within 24 hours. A deficit persisting longer, resolving within 3 to 4 days, is defined as a reversible ischemic neurologic deficit, whereas a deficit persisting beyond this time is defined as a completed stroke. These clinical definitions do not necessarily define a specific pathologic substrate. Transient ischemic attacks lasting beyond 6 hours are not infrequently shown, on scanning, to be caused by infarction. On the other hand, some brain infarcts are silent. In many cases, the arterial territory involved in an ischemic event can be determined from the pattern of symptoms and signs associated with it.

Internal Carotid Artery Territory

Bifurcation Disease. The carotid bifurcation is a common site for atheromatous disease. Flow though a stenosis does not fall until the narrowing has reached some 90% of the lumen. Consequently, symptoms arising from atherosclerotic disease at this site are usually the result of embolic fragments detaching and entering the cerebral circulation. These fragments may be cholesterol based or a mixture of fibrin and platelets (Fig. 4-56).

Embolization to the central retinal artery, or one of its branches, leads to transient monocular blindness (amaurosis fugax). Examination of the fundus sometimes reveals cholesterol emboli even in the absence of persisting visual deficit (Fig. 4-57). Examples of hemisphere ischemia include dysphasia (when the dominant hemisphere is involved) and contralateral hemisensory or hemimotor disturbances. In the case of weakness, the leg is relatively spared unless the anterior cerebral artery territory is principally involved.

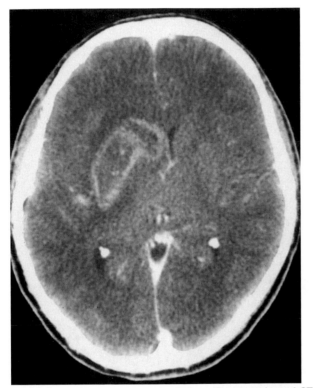

Fig. 4-36. Ring enhancement in a striatal infarct. Contrast-enhanced CT.

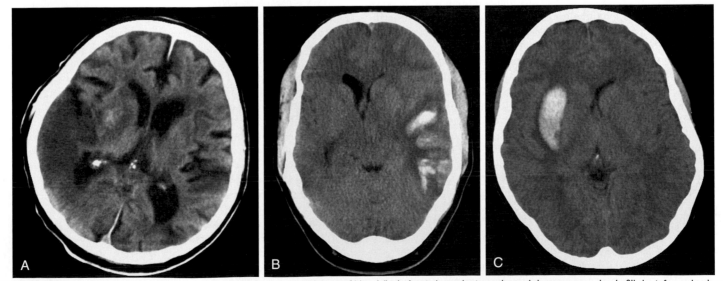

Fig. 4-37. CT scan showing hemorrhagic change in an infarct. The central zone of blood (high density) may be irregular and does not completely fill the infarcted volume. **A,** Basal gray matter. **B,** Cortical and subcortical. **C,** Primary bleed, for comparison, shows homogeneous hematoma.

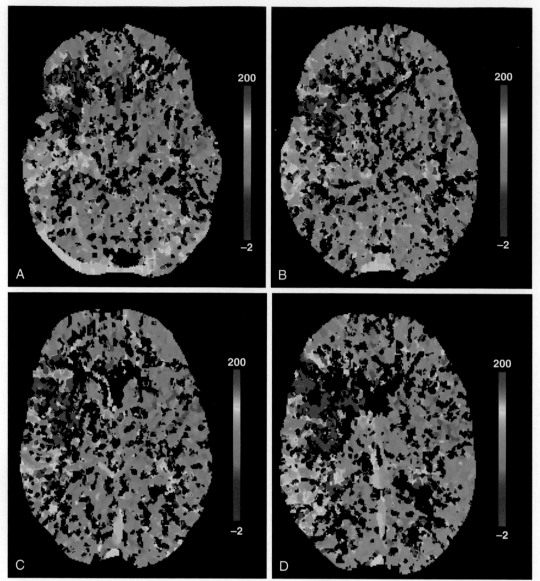

Fig. 4-38. Perfusion-weighted CT. Maps show large right hemisphere time-to-peak (TTP) and cerebral blood flow (CBF) defect with smaller cerebral blood volume (CBV) defect suggesting small core infarct with large tissue at risk. **A** to **D**, TTP map.

Stroke is usual, but not inevitable, after internal carotid occlusion. Flow in the anterior and middle cerebral arteries may be preserved via the circle of Willis. Alternatively, increased flow through the external carotid artery sometimes serves to maintain intracerebral flow via anastomoses between the superficial temporal artery and orbital branches of the ophthalmic artery (Fig. 4-58). The superficial temporal artery is prominent in such cases (Fig. 4-59). A low pressure state in the central retinal artery can lead to a venous stasis retinopathy in which there are dilated retinal veins associated with retinal hemorrhages (Fig. 4-60). The stroke associated with carotid occlusion may be embolic or caused by a low flow state. In the former, either the main stem or one of the middle cerebral branches is occluded; in the latter, watershed infarction occurs (Fig. 4-61). Sudden complete occlusion of the carotid artery from plaque rupture in the neck can result in infarction in both anterior and middle cerebral territories.

Intracranial Disease. Atheroma in the carotid siphon occurs less often than at the carotid bifurcation. Disturbance of retinal function depends on whether the disease is proximal or distal to the origin of the ophthalmic artery.

Anterior Choroidal Artery Territory

The anterior choroidal artery supplies the choroid plexus of the ipsilateral lateral ventricle and parts of the hippocampus, amygdala, uncus, internal capsule, basal ganglia, and part of the upper brainstem

(Fig. 4-62). Its occlusion results in an infarct in the basal ganglia and lateral geniculate body. The clinical picture includes contralateral motor and sensory loss associated with a hemianopia.

Anterior Cerebral Artery Territory

The anterior cerebral artery supplies the medial portion of the inferior frontal lobe and the medial surface of the frontal and parietal lobes (Fig. 4-63). On the lateral surface of the hemisphere, it supplies a narrow parasagittal strip in the frontal and parietal lobes. From the proximal segment of the anterior cerebral artery arise the medial lenticulostriate arteries, the largest of which is the recurrent artery of Heubner. Together they supply the anteromedial part of the basal ganglia.

Infarction within the territory of the anterior cerebral artery is usually the result of embolization from the internal carotid artery and can also follow a subarachnoid hemorrhage from an anterior communicating aneurysm, either as a result of vasospasm or as a consequence of surgical intervention (Fig. 4-64). It can also follow subfalcine herniation from any cause.

The neurologic deficit is largely determined by whether the occlusion is proximal or distal to the origin of the artery of Heubner. If distal, only the cortical branches of the artery are affected. There is weakness, principally of the lower limb and shoulder, with sensory loss over the lower limb. Apraxia of the left hand (in right-handed individuals) can occur with infarction in either hemisphere. If the

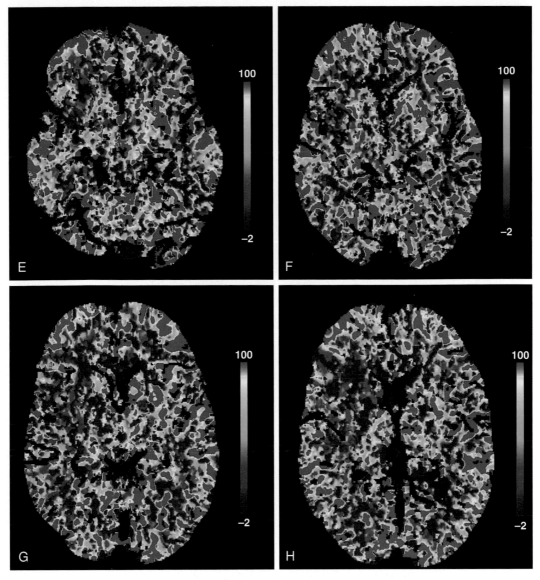

Fig. 4-38 cont'd, E to H, CBF map.

occlusion is proximal, the cortical lesion is accompanied by infarction of the corpus striatum, resulting in a more complete hemiplegia. With both levels of occlusion, there may be frontal lobe signs, including grasp and suckling reflexes, and a transcortical motor aphasia that combines a Broca-type aphasia with preserved repetition.

Middle Cerebral Artery Territory
The middle cerebral artery produces its anterior temporal and superior and inferior branches close to the sylvian fissure (Fig. 4-65). They supply a large part of the lateral surface of the frontal, temporal, and parietal lobes. Lenticulostriate branches arise from the first part of the artery and supply much of the corpus striatum and internal capsule and lateral portions of the thalamus. The vast majority of middle cerebral occlusions are embolic rather than thrombotic.

Patterns of infarction include those caused by occlusion of the artery close to its origin, occlusion of the deep perforating branches with relative preservation of cortical flow, occlusion of either the upper or lower trunk, and, finally, occlusion of cortical branches.

Main Stem Occlusion. The clinical disability of main stem occlusion is profound, with contralateral motor and sensory deficit, a homonymous hemianopia, and a global aphasia if the dominant hemisphere is affected. Anosognosia, spatial disorientation, and neglect of the affected limbs may be prominent. Imaging demonstrates an extensive infarct occupying most of the hemisphere, although in the very

early stages, the signs are subtle (Fig. 4-66). Angiography, performed early, demonstrates the occluded vessel (Fig. 4-67). In some cases, the occluded vessel can be identified on CT (Fig. 4-68) or by an absence of flow void on MRI. Many embolic occlusions break up within a week or so.

Occlusions of Deep Perforations. Infarction of the deep structures supplied by the middle cerebral artery (Fig. 4-69) usually is not the result of selective occlusion of the various lenticulostriate arteries but more often is the consequence of occlusion of the parent vessel with sparing of the cortical distribution due to collateral circulation. The contralateral deficit is predominantly motor. Hemorrhagic change in infarcts is more commonly seen with MRI than CT, particularly with gradient echo T2 sequences, and is more common with gray matter infarcts than white matter infarcts.

Occlusion of the Frontoparietal Branch. Infarction occupies the frontal and anterior/superior parietal lobes with sparing of the posterior/inferior parietal lobe and the temporal lobe (Fig. 4-69). There is a contralateral motor and sensory deficit with relative sparing of the leg. If the dominant hemisphere is involved, a nonfluent aphasia appears.

Occlusion of the Parietotemporal Branch. The deficit in the parietotemporal branch occlusion is subtler, particularly if the nondominant hemisphere is involved. A superior quadrantic hemianopia is

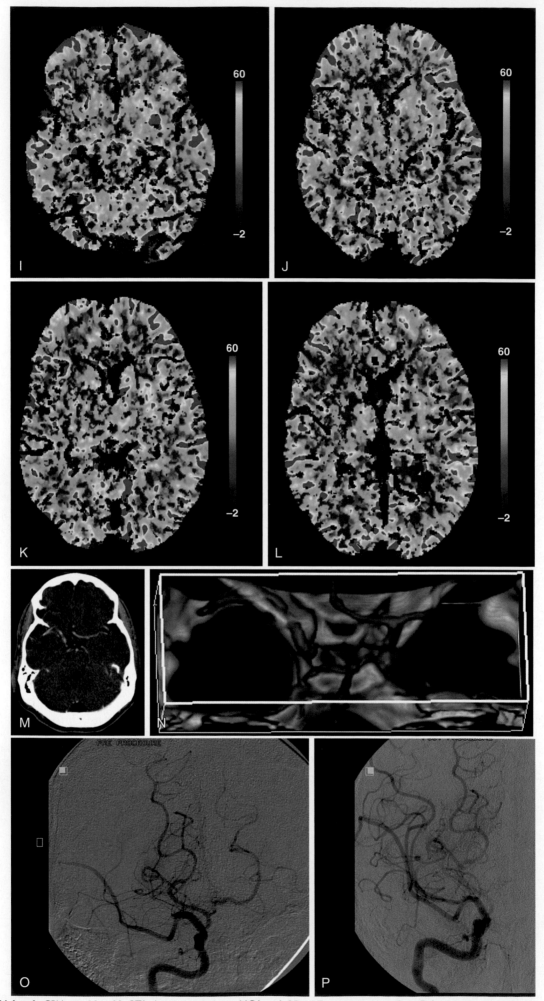

Fig. 4-38 cont'd, I to L, CBV map. **M to N,** CTA showing embolus in MCA with 3D VRT reconstruction. **O to P,** Angiogram pre and post intra arterial TPA.

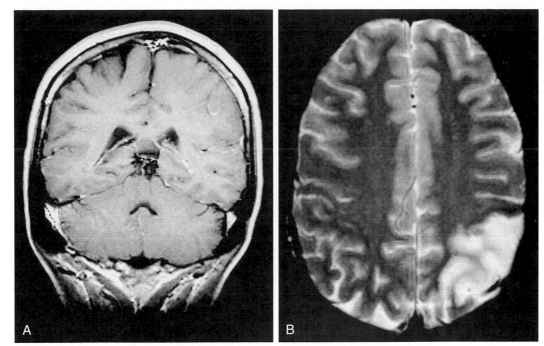

Fig. 4-39. MRI scan of recent cerebral infarct. **A,** T1-weighted image. There is obliteration of the sulci on the left and slight distortion of the ventricle. **B,** T2-weighted axial image. The parieto-occipital infarct is hyperintense.

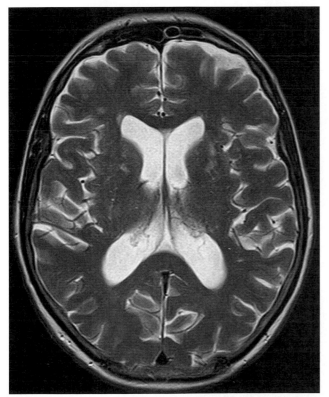

Fig. 4-40. Axial T2-weighted MRI. Lacunar infarcts in both lentiform nuclei.

accompanied, in a nondominant hemisphere infarct, by visuospatial problems, and in a dominant hemisphere infarct by a Wernicke-type aphasia resulting from ischemia of the posterior part of the superior temporal gyrus (Fig. 4-70).

Occlusion of Cortical Branches.   These occlusions are almost always embolic, although the vasculitides and vasospasm secondary to a subarachnoid hemorrhage may produce a similar picture. The deficit is determined by the area of cortex affected (Fig. 4-71).

Posterior Circulation Territory
Subclavian Artery Disease.   Severe stenosis or occlusion of the subclavian artery proximal to the origin of the vertebral artery can lead

to reduced flow in both vessels. Theoretically, reversed flow from a higher-pressure system (i.e., the basilar artery filled by the contralateral vertebral) may occur to maintain flow in the relevant arm, particularly when it is exercised. In the subclavian steal syndrome, patients present either with symptoms resulting from reduced flow to the upper limb (e.g., a cold hand) or with symptoms such as diplopia or circumoral paresthesia, considered to be the result of blood being stolen from the basilar territory.

Radiologic evidence of the phenomenon is far more common than its clinical declaration. Examination reveals reduced blood pressure and pulses in the relevant arm, often with a bruit over the subclavian artery. The existence of the phenomenon can be confirmed either by noninvasive studies or by angiography (Fig. 4-72).

Vertebral Artery Disease.   Occlusion of a single vertebral artery near its origin is unlikely to be significant unless the contralateral vertebral artery is atretic (Fig. 4-73). Stenotic disease of the vertebral artery can be a source of emboli to the posterior circulation. Intracranial vertebral artery occlusion is potentially more serious. Possible consequences include impaired flow in the posterior inferior cerebellar artery, resulting in lateral medullary infarction, infarction of the cerebellum, or embolization to parts of the basilar system.

Lateral Medullary Infarction (Wallenberg Syndrome).   The clinical picture of lateral medullary infarction includes, ipsilateral to the infarct, a Horner's syndrome, facial spinothalamic loss, palatal paresis, and limb cerebellar signs with contralateral limb and trunk spinothalamic loss of varying distribution. The gait is ataxic (Figs. 4-74 and 4-75).

Cerebellar Infarction.   Cerebellar infarction is commonly the consequence of an intracranial vertebral artery occlusion and is sometimes accompanied by infarction of the lateral medulla. Headache, dizziness, and ipsilateral cerebellar signs are accompanied by ipsilateral cranial nerve signs, particularly a gaze paresis and a facial palsy if the brainstem is compressed. Obliteration of the fourth ventricle by a swollen cerebellum results in hydrocephalus (Fig. 4-76).

Basilar Artery Disease.   Basilar artery occlusion is not necessarily fatal, although many patients are left with substantial neurologic deficit. Proximal occlusions are usually atheromatous, distal ones more often the result of embolization from either the vertebral artery

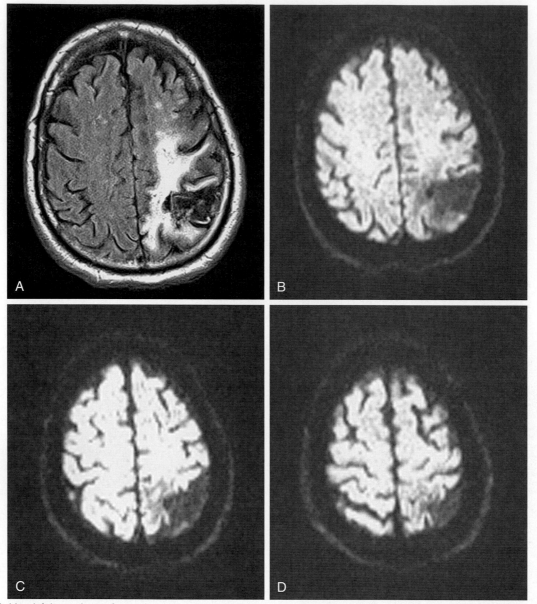

Fig. 4-41. New left-hemisphere infarcts adjacent to a mature infarct seen only on diffusion-weighted imaging (DWI). **A,** FLAIR. **B** to **D,** DWI.

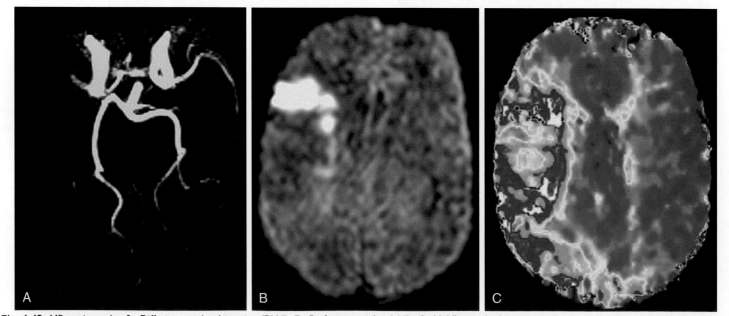

Fig. 4-42. MR angiography. **A,** Diffusion-weighted imaging (DWI). **B,** Perfusion-weighted MR. **C,** Middle cerebral artery occlusion with small core infarct with large ischemic penumbra (at-risk tissue).

or the heart (Figs. 4-77 and 4-78). The pons is particularly affected by the ischemia consequent to a basilar occlusion (Fig. 4-79). Clinical findings include a tetraparesis, cranial nerve involvement either at a nuclear or supranuclear level, and oculomotor signs, including gaze paresis or an internuclear ophthalmoplegia. If the ischemia affects both the pontine gaze center on one side and the medial longitudinal fasciculus from the contralateral side, an ophthalmoplegia occurs in which the only eye movement remaining is abduction away from the side of the lesion (Fig. 4-80) (the one-and-a-half syndrome). Larger pontine infarcts may lead to a "locked-in" state. If the basilar occlusion is distal, then physical signs consequent to midbrain ischemia emerge, including pupillary abnormalities, abnormalities of vertical

gaze, and an altered consciousness state. Bilateral infarction in posterior cerebral artery territory can occur with occlusion of the terminal portion of the basilar artery. Cortical blindness is likely and may be accompanied by amnesic syndromes. In addition, a "top of the basilar" syndrome can result in infarction of the midbrain bilaterally with involvement of the superior cerebellum and the thalamus.

Posterior Cerebral Artery Disease. The posterior cerebral artery, via its cortical branches, supplies the inferior and medial surfaces of the temporal and occipital lobes, together with a small area on the lateral surface of the hemisphere. It also gives rise to the thalamoperforating vessels. Most posterior cerebral artery occlusions are embolic (Fig. 4-81). Others may result from unilateral (uncal) or central transtentorial herniation. Proximal occlusions lead to infarction of the occipital lobe, and of the medial and inferior aspects of the temporal lobe, together with parts of the thalamus and midbrain. More distal occlusions spare the deeper structures. Occipital infarction results in a contralateral homonymous hemianopia, which may be complete, quadrantic, or paracentral. Macular sparing is seen in some cases (Fig. 4-82). Thalamic infarction leads to contralateral sensory loss, sometimes with spontaneous pain and hypersensitivity to contact (the thalamic syndrome).

Various abnormalities of higher cortical function occur as a result of either left or right posterior cerebral artery occlusions. Combined infarction of the left occipital lobe and of the splenium of the corpus callosum produces the syndrome of alexia without agraphia. Speech, repetition, and writing are preserved. The patient can spell out the individual letters of a word but is unable to read fluently, even script that he has just written. There is usually a deficit of color naming, but color matching is preserved. In some patients with left posterior cerebral territory infarction, there is a visual agnosia. In right posterior cerebral territory infarction, a difficulty in recognizing familiar faces is sometimes encountered (aprosopagnosia).

Bilateral posterior cerebral artery occlusion, usually resulting from embolization to the bifurcation of the basilar artery, leads to bilateral occipital infarction (Fig. 4-83). Cortical blindness ensues, sometimes accompanied by denial of visual loss (Anton's syndrome). A state of agitated delirium is described with infarction of the hippocampus and fusiform and lingual gyri. Infarction of the mesial temporal lobes bilaterally produces a profound disorientation of memory function resembling Korsakoff's psychosis.

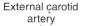

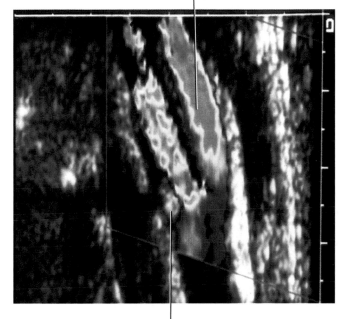

Fig. 4-43. Calcified plaque at the carotid bifurcation. Duplex scan.

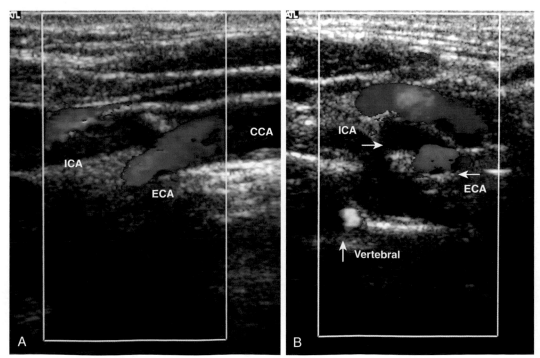

Fig. 4-44. Carotid artery occlusion. **A** and **B,** Duplex scan in two planes.

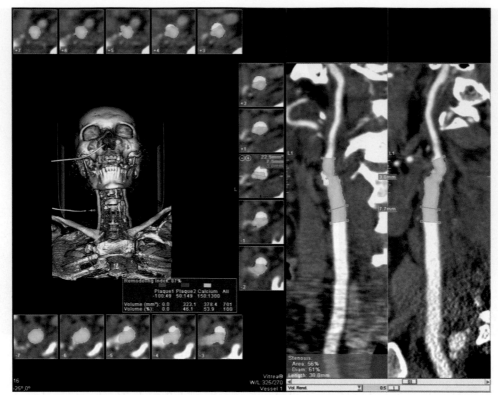

Fig. 4-50. CT angiography data can be reconstructed in any plane and viewed as a 3D structure. Semiautomated software can calculate cross-sectional areas.

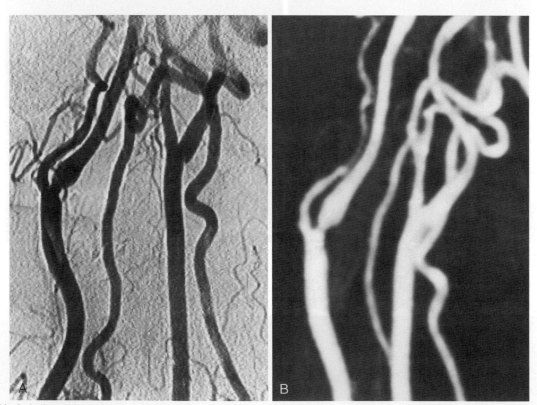

Fig. 4-51. A, Arch angiogram revealing a 50% stenosis of the right internal carotid artery origin. **B,** Comparable magnetic resonance image.

a long stenotic channel (string sign), and pouching or pseudo-aneurysm formation. MR angiography can reveal a similar picture, and MR allows identification of abnormal signal from the relevant segment (Fig. 4-93).

Vertebrobasilar Dissection.   Vertebrobasilar dissection may be either extracranial or intracranial. Extracranial dissections tend to be distal and are often bilateral. They predominate in women. Pain is characteristically referred to the region of the mastoid process. Intracranial dissections predominate near to the origin of the posterior inferior

cerebellar artery and sometimes produce a lateral medullary syndrome. They may also appear, however, as a subarachnoid hemorrhage. Basilar dissections are rare; trauma and neck manipulation are important risk factors. Imaging produces an appearance similar to that seen with carotid dissections (Fig. 4-94).

Cerebral Vasculitis
Vasculitis is seen with the collagen vascular diseases, as an idiopathic phenomenon, and as a drug-induced syndrome (Fig. 4-95). Cerebral vasculitis (primary angiitis) is a vasculitic disorder characterized by

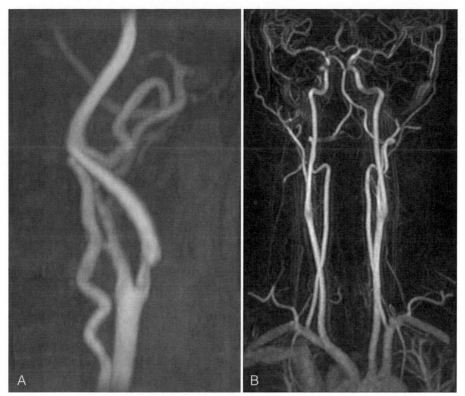

Fig. 4-52. A, Noncontrast-enhanced 2D time-of-flight (TOF) MR angiography showing internal carotid artery (ICA) origin stenosis. **B,** Contrast-enhanced MRA reconstruction. Frontal view showing increased volume of coverage and origins of vertebral artery and common carotid artery.

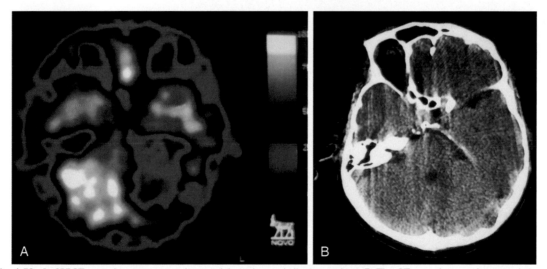

Fig. 4-53. A, SPECT scan showing gross ischemia of the right cerebellar hemisphere. **B,** The CT scan shows only minimal change.

headache, confusion, intellectual impairment and focal neurologic events. The CSF often shows a lymphocytosis with a moderately raised protein concentration. Angiography may reveal focal areas of stenosis alternating with segments of dilatation (Fig. 4-96). An association exists in many cases with infection with herpes zoster (varicella-zoster) virus, especially with zoster of the ophthalmic division of the trigeminal nerve. Virus has been demonstrated by immunohistochemistry and electron microscopy in the walls of affected cerebral arteries in biopsies and autopsies of patients with primary cerebral angiitis. Often, the inflammation is granulomatous. Treatment is with corticosteroids and cyclophosphamide.

Amphetamines and other potent sympathomimetic drugs can trigger stroke, sometimes hemorrhagic, at other times ischemic, the result of vasculitis or vasospasm (Fig. 4-97). A similar picture is seen with phenylpropanolamine, and cocaine abuse can trigger either hemorrhagic or ischemic stroke.

Antiphospholipid Syndrome

Clinical features that have been attributed to the presence of antiphospholipid antibodies include a migraine like condition, retinal ischemia and an encephalopathic condition with strokelike events. Other features include venous thrombosis, multiple spontaneous abortions, and livedo reticularis. Imaging abnormalities have been described (Fig. 4-98).

CADASIL

Cerebral autosomal dominant arteriopathy with subcortical infarcts and leukoencephalopathy (CADASIL) has been mapped, in terms of the causative gene, to chromosome 19. It usually appears in the third decade, with attacks of migraine with aura. Within 10 years, recurrent ischemic events, often in the form of lacunar infarcts, may appear, followed by dementia. The vascular process principally affects leptomeningeal and perforating arteries, with infiltration of

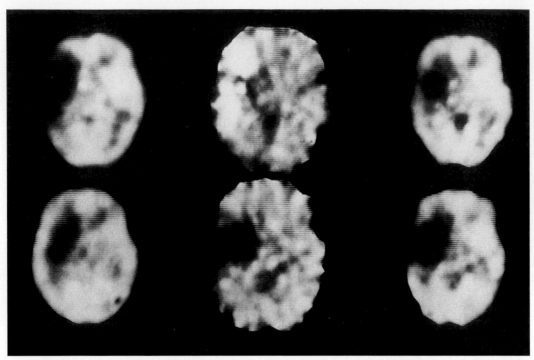

Fig. 4-54. PET scan showing a left temporoparietal infarct at 8 hours *(upper)* and 4 days *(lower)*. The scans on the *left* indicate cerebral blood flow; those on the *right* show metabolic activity, and the *middle* scans indicate the oxygen extraction ratio.

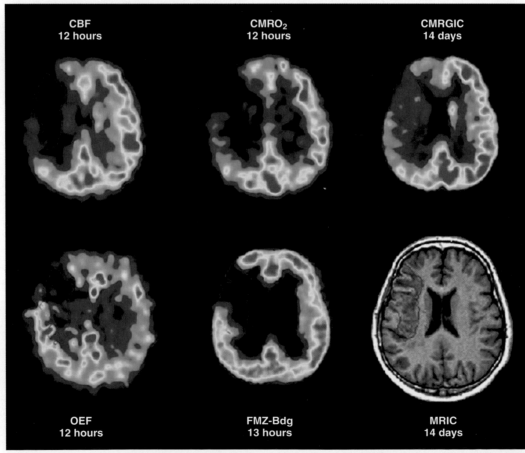

Fig. 4-55. Co-registered transaxial PET images at the caudate/ventricular level of cerebral blood flow (CBF), steady-state FMZ binding (Bdg), and oxygen extraction fraction (OEF) at 12 hours and CMRGIC and MRI at 2 weeks after moderate left hemiparesis and hemihypesthesias of acute onset. The large defect is visible in all PET modalities, and its cortical outline is defined on the MRI. FMZ binding precisely predicts the extension of the final infarct, whereas CBF delineates a considerably larger volume of disturbed perfusion.

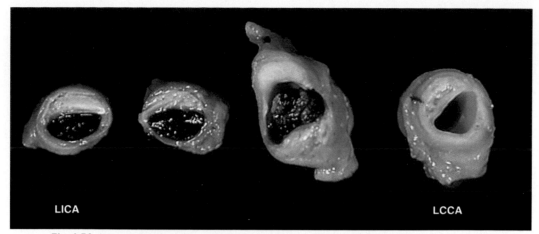

Fig. 4-56. Acute carotid occlusion. Cross-section showing atherosclerotic vessel filled with thrombus.

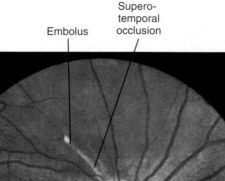

Fig. 4-57. Cholesterol embolus with occlusion of the superior temporal branch of the central retinal artery.

the media by a material of unknown origin. The deposits are periodic acid–Schiff positive and electron dense. Diagnosis can be established by punch biopsies of the skin, with demonstrations by electron microscopy of deposits in the walls of arterioles and capillaries. MRI reveals multiple subcortical infarcts with diffuse white matter change (Fig. 4-99). Pathologically, the white matter damage resembles that seen in Binswanger's disease.

Takayasu's Disease

Takayasu's disease is a granulomatous aortitis of unknown cause resulting in the occlusion of the major vessels arising from the aortic arch. The condition predominates in Asian women. An initial inflammatory phase is followed by later complications resulting from vessel occlusions, particularly of the carotid vessels. The erythrocyte sedimentation rate is often elevated. In the later stages, imaging demonstrates the occlusive process (Fig. 4-100).

Thrombotic Thrombocytopenic Purpura

In thrombotic thrombocytopenic purpura, microaggregates form in the arteries of, particularly, the kidney and the central nervous system. Cerebral infarction is a potential consequence (Fig. 4-101).

HYPERTENSIVE ENCEPHALOPATHY

Hypertensive encephalopathy is characteristically triggered by a sudden elevation of blood pressure, often in a previously normotensive individual. The brain becomes edematous with fibrinoid necrosis in the medium-sized and small cerebral vessels. The posterior hemisphere is particularly affected. Clinical features include headache, vomiting, visual disturbances, and alteration of the conscious level. Seizures occur and are sometimes focal.

CT scanning reveals areas of low attenuation, and MRI shows areas of increased signal intensity that resolve once the blood pressure is satisfactorily controlled (Fig. 4-102). Acute hypertension is one of the causes of posterior reversible edema syndrome.

CLINICAL EXAMINATION

In addition to defining the neurologic deficit, examination of the stroke patient includes assessment of the cardiovascular system, the neck vessels, and the presence or absence of hypertension. Those patients with evidence of a hyperlipidemic state (Fig. 4-103) usually have a previous history of myocardial infarction or peripheral vascular disease.

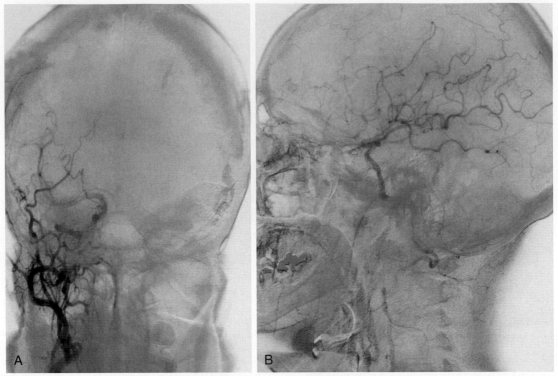

Fig. 4-58. Internal carotid artery occlusion with filling of the intracranial circulation via the ophthalmic artery. Carotid angiogram. **A,** Anteroposterior view. **B,** Lateral view.

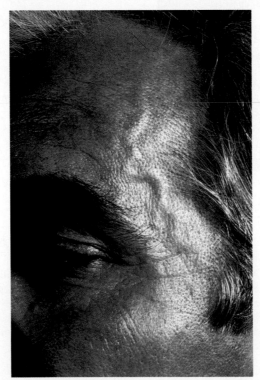

Fig. 4-59. Distended superficial temporal artery in a patient with an internal carotid occlusion.

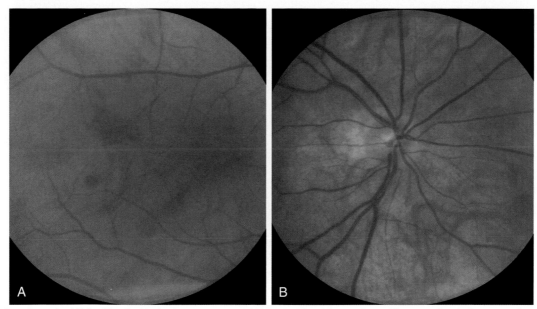

Fig. 4-60. Venous stasis retinopathy. Mildly dilated retinal veins are accompanied by peripheral hemorrhages. The central retinal artery collapsed with minimal digital pressure on the globe.

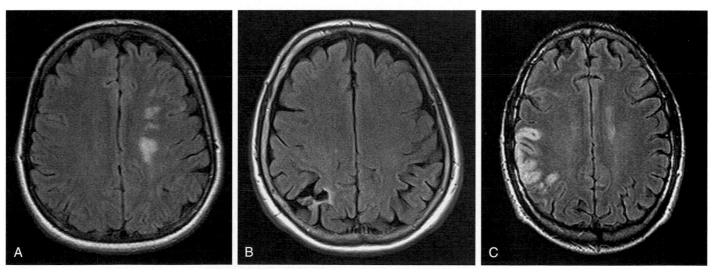

Fig. 4-61. Carotid occlusion with patterns of watershed infarction on MRI. **A,** Deep white-matter infarct (perforator watershed). **B,** Parietal infarct (middle [MCA], anterior [ACA], and posterior [PCA] cerebral artery cortical watershed). **C,** Laminar cortical infarct (MCA watershed).

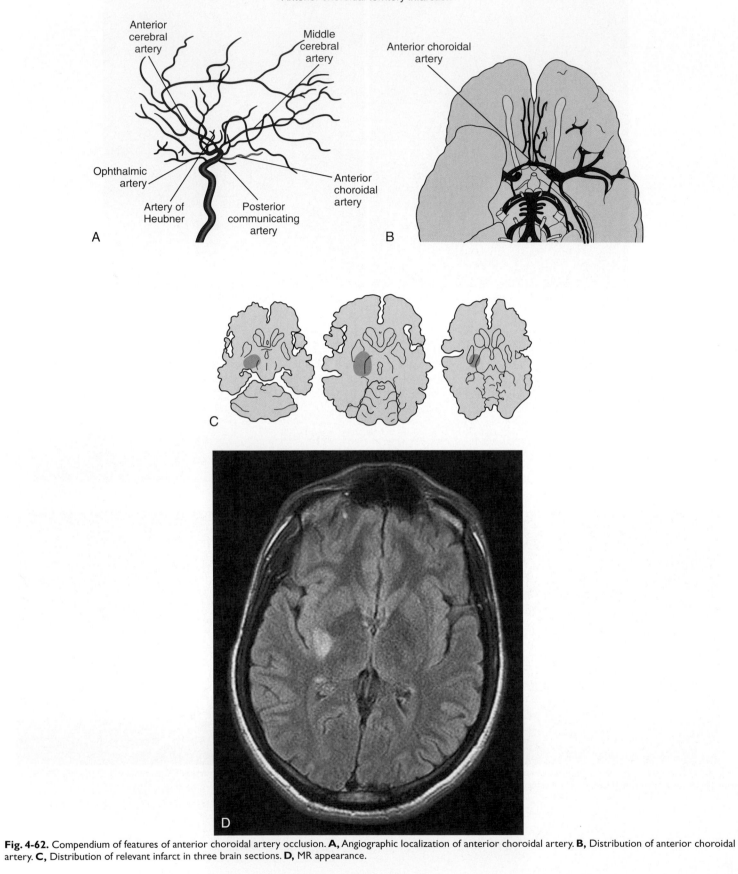

Fig. 4-62. Compendium of features of anterior choroidal artery occlusion. **A,** Angiographic localization of anterior choroidal artery. **B,** Distribution of anterior choroidal artery. **C,** Distribution of relevant infarct in three brain sections. **D,** MR appearance.

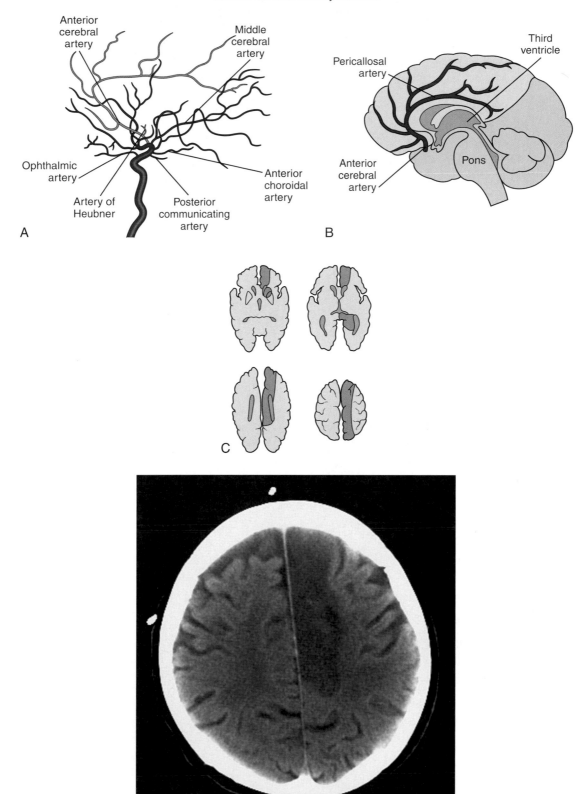

Fig. 4-63. Compendium of features of anterior cerebral artery occlusion. **A,** Angiographic localization of anterior cerebral artery. **B,** Distribution of the anterior cerebral artery along the medial aspect of the hemisphere. **C,** Distribution of relevant infarct in four brain sections. **D,** CT appearance before contrast enhancement.

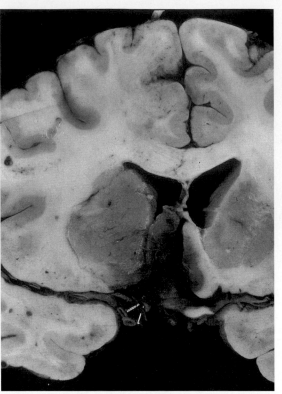

Fig. 4-64. Infarction of the cerebral cortex and underlying white matter, and anterior inferior striatum after clipping of the anterior cerebral artery in a patient with subarachnoid hemorrhage.

Middle cerebral territory infarction

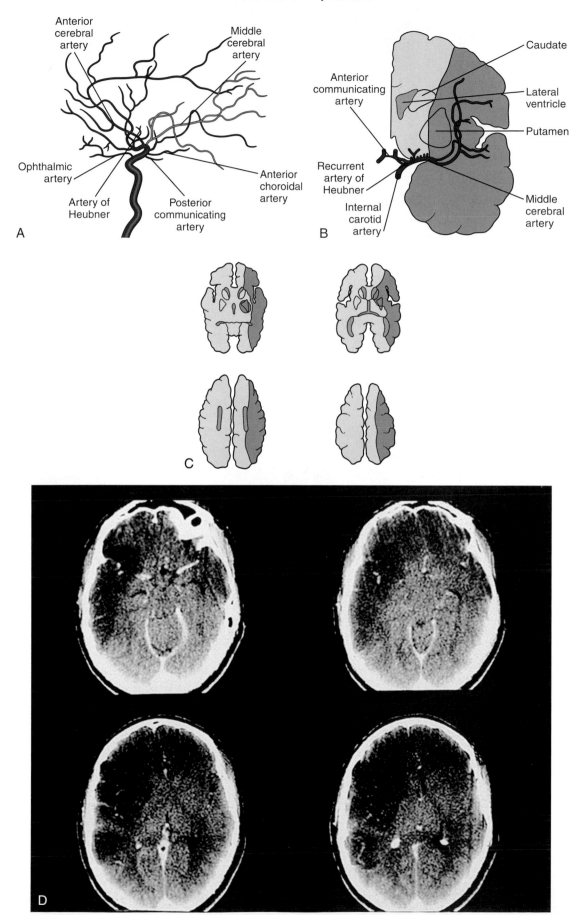

Fig. 4-65. Compendium of features of middle cerebral artery (MCA) occlusion. **A,** Angiographic localization of the MCA. **B,** Distribution of the MCA (coronal section). **C,** Distribution of relevant infarct in four brain sections. **D,** CT appearance.

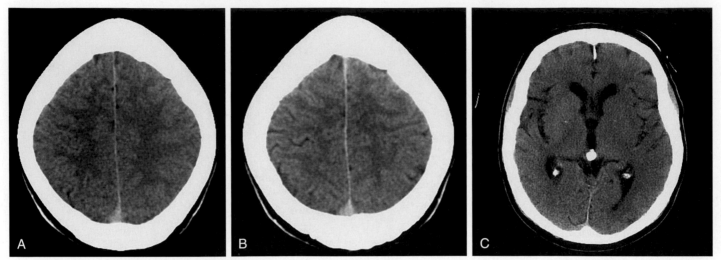

Fig. 4-66. Early signs of infarction on plain CT include sulcal effacement (**A** and **B**) and loss of the lentiform nucleus and external capsular ribbon (**C**).

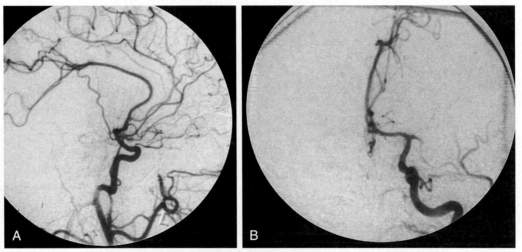

Fig. 4-67. Conventional angiography of middle cerebral artery occlusion (lateral, AP).

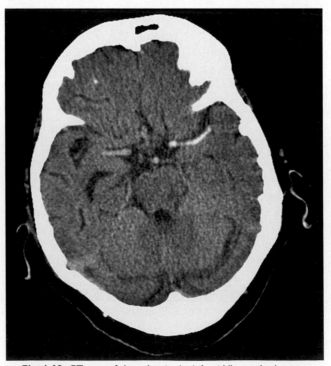

Fig. 4-68. CT scan of thrombus in the left middle cerebral artery.

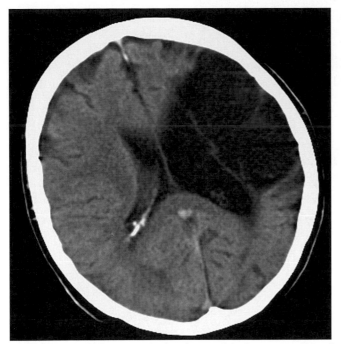

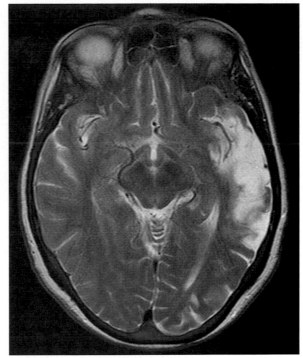

Fig. 4-69. CT scan of infarction in the distribution of the frontoparietal branch of the middle cerebral artery.

Fig. 4-70. MR image of infarction in the distribution of the parietotemporal branch of the middle cerebral artery.

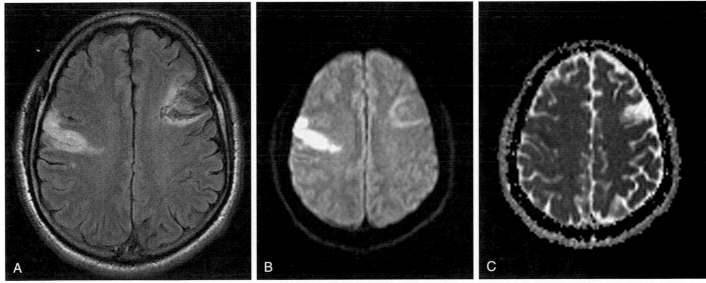

Fig. 4-71. Wedge-shaped cortical infarcts: mature on *left*, acute on *right*. **A,** FLAIR. **B,** Diffusion-weighted imaging. **C,** Apparent diffusion coefficient map.

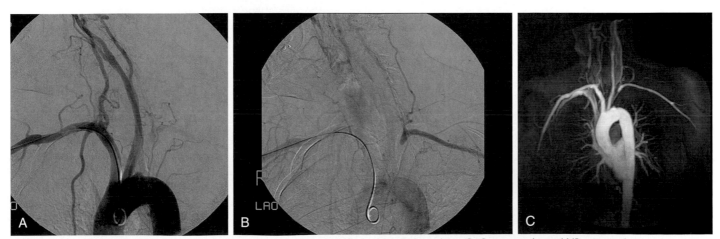

Fig. 4-72. Arch angiogram of subclavian steal syndrome. **A,** Early phase. **B,** Late phase. **C,** Contrast-enhanced MR angiography.

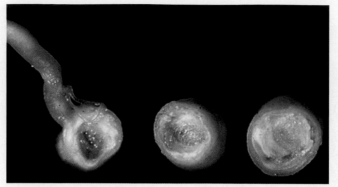

Fig. 4-73. Occluded left vertebral artery.

LATERAL MEDULLARY INFARCTION

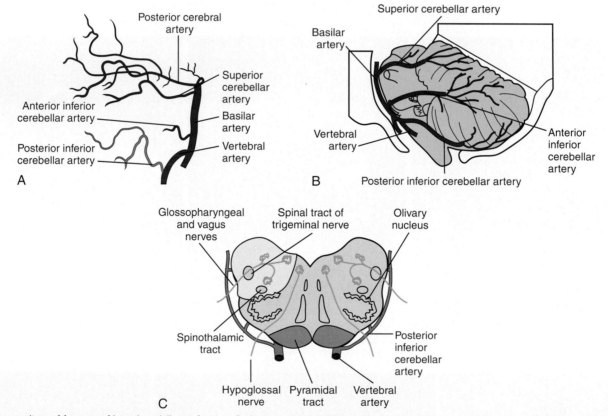

Fig. 4-74. Compendium of features of lateral medullary infarction. **A,** Angiographic localization of posterior inferior cerebellar artery. **B,** Distribution of the posterior inferior cerebellar artery. **C,** Distribution of infarct.

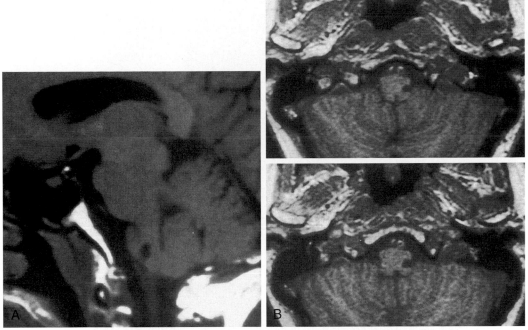

Fig. 4-75. Lateral medullary infarct. T1-weighted MRI. **A,** Sagittal section. **B,** Axial section.

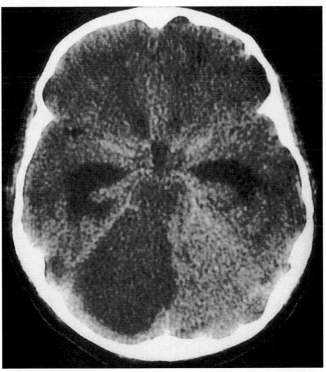

Fig. 4-76. CT of cerebellar infarction with secondary hydrocephalus.

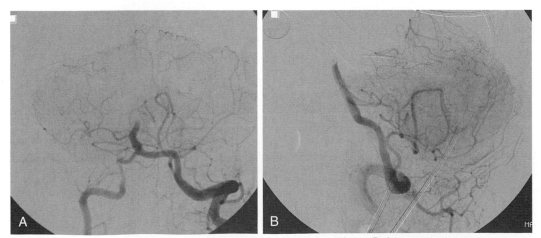

Fig. 4-77. Angiogram of a mid-basilar artery occlusion. **A,** Lateral view. **B,** Anteroposterior view.

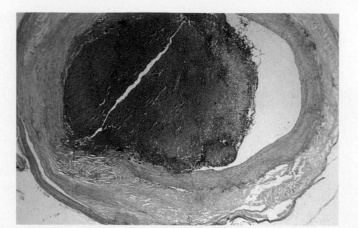

Fig. 4-78. Basilar occlusion. Plaque rupture into lumen associated with thrombosis (Luxol fast blue, H&E, ×25)..

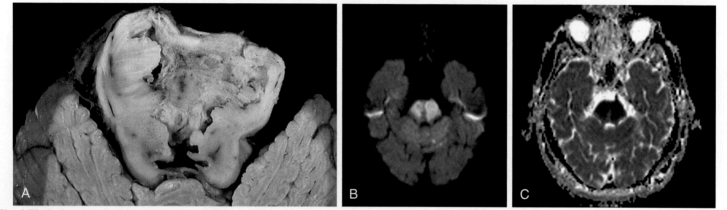

Fig. 4-79. A, Brainstem infarct with pontine cavitation. The patient had survived in a virtually locked-in state for 6 weeks. **B,** Brainstem infarct secondary to basilar occlusion. Diffusion-weighted imaging. **C,** Apparent diffusion coefficient map.

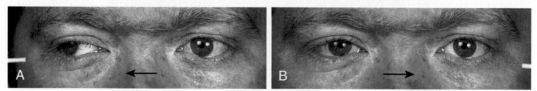

Fig. 4-80. One-and-a-half syndrome. There is a left internuclear ophthalmoplegia **(A)**, with a left gaze paresis **(B)**.

POSTERIOR CEREBRAL TERRITORY INFARCTION

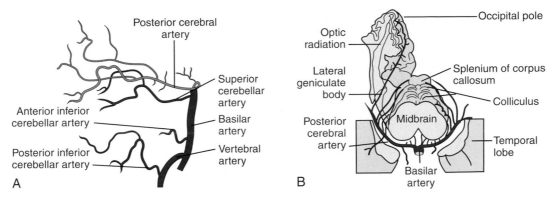

A

Posterior cerebral artery

Superior cerebellar artery

Anterior inferior cerebellar artery

Basilar artery

Posterior inferior cerebellar artery

Vertebral artery

B

Optic radiation

Lateral geniculate body

Posterior cerebral artery

Occipital pole

Splenium of corpus callosum

Colliculus

Midbrain

Temporal lobe

Basilar artery

POSTERIOR CEREBRAL TERRITORY INFARCTION

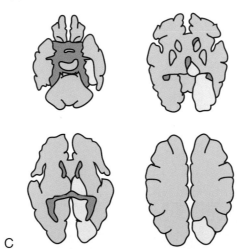

C

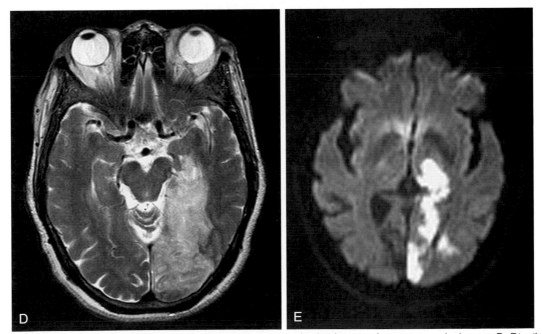

D

E

Fig. 4-81. Compendium of features of posterior cerebral artery occlusion. **A,** Angiographic localization of posterior cerebral artery. **B,** Distribution of the posterior cerebral artery. **C,** Distribution of infarct in four brain sections. **D** and **E,** MR (FLAIR and diffusion-weighted imaging) appearance. Note involvement of the thalamus and medial temporal lobe as far forward as the hippocampus.

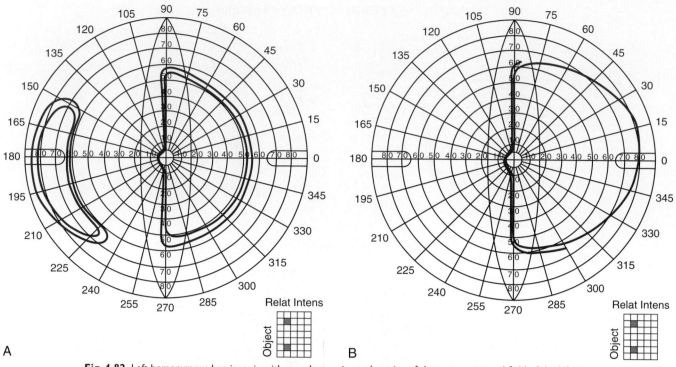

A

B

Fig. 4-82. Left homonymous hemianopia with macular sparing and sparing of the outer temporal field of the left eye.

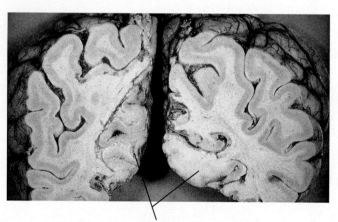

Infarcts

Fig. 4-83. Bilateral infarction in posterior cerebral artery territory involving gray and white matter.

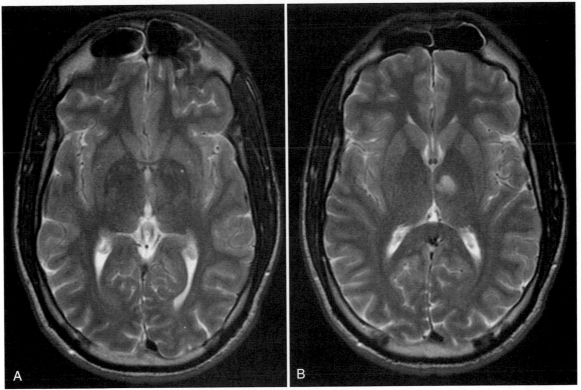

Fig. 4-84. Acute infarct on MR affecting left mammillothalamic tract giving rise to inability to form new memories.

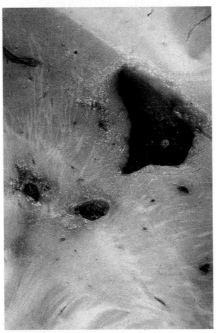

Fig. 4-85. Multiple lacunes in the right putamen.

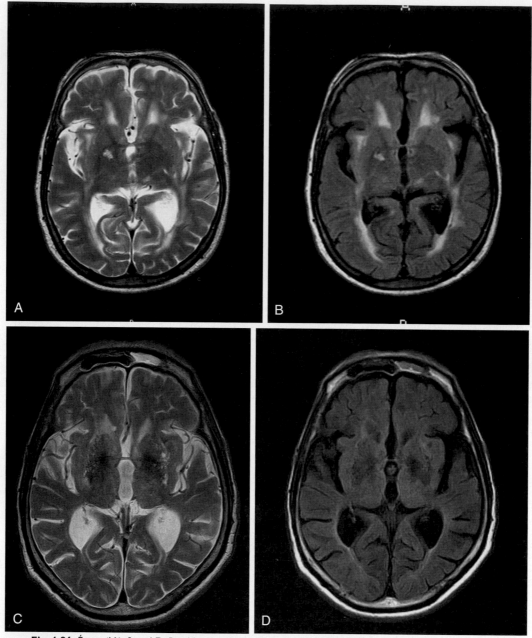

Fig. 4-86. État criblé. **A** and **B,** Basal lacunes (high signal on FLAIR). **C** and **D,** Dilated Virchow-Robin spaces.

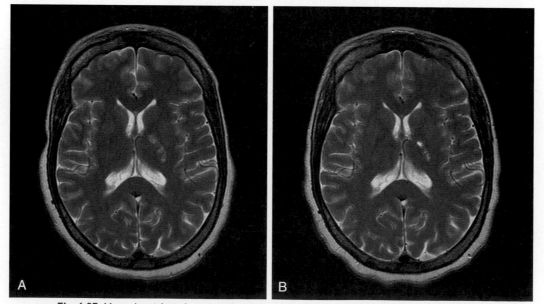

Fig. 4-87. Motor hemiplegia. Lacune in the internal capsule. T2-weighted MRI. **A,** Acute. **B,** Mature.

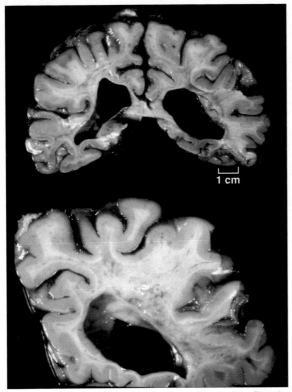

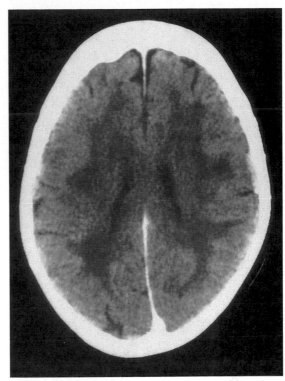

Fig. 4-88. Binswanger's encephalopathy. **A,** Coronal brain slice. Discoloration of the white matter, particularly that overlying the ventricular roof. **B,** Coronal slice of right parieto-occipital region. The affected white matter is somewhat granular; note the preservation of the subcortical ∪ fibers.

Fig. 4-89. Binswanger's encephalopathy. CT demonstrating bilateral periventricular lucencies.

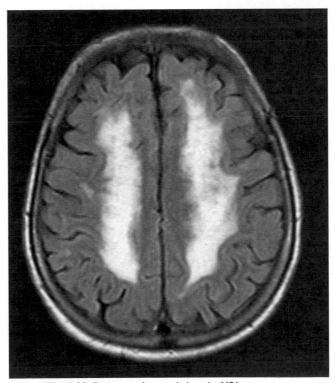

Fig. 4-90. Binswanger's encephalopathy. MRI appearance.

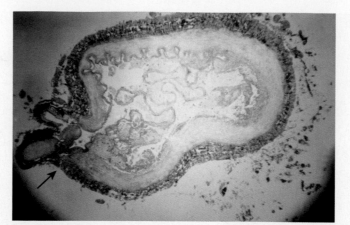

Fig. 4-91. Dissection of the internal carotid artery that had propagated to the middle cerebral artery. The site of dissection can be seen as an intimal flap *(arrow)*.

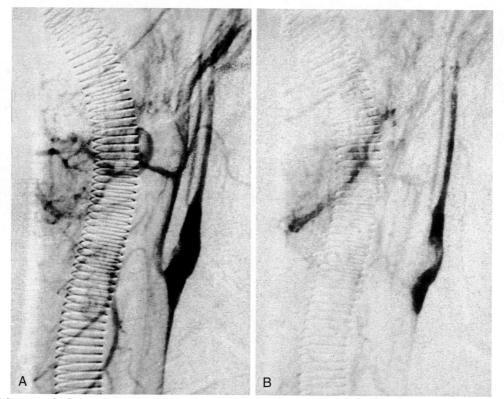

Fig. 4-92. Carotid dissection. **A,** Contrast material remains in the proximal segment of the internal carotid artery. **B,** It then progressively tapers distally.

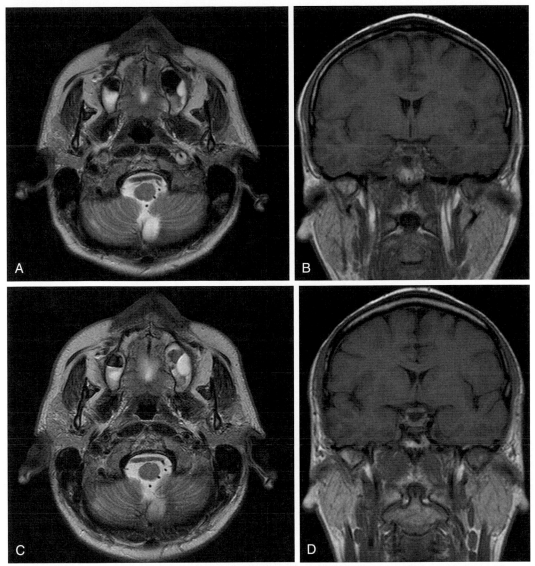

Fig. 4-93. Early and late images of bilateral internal carotid artery (ICA) dissection. **A** and **C,** Axial T2-weighted images. **B** and **D,** Coronal T1-weighted images. High signal is seen surrounding both ICAs on the acute images, with subsequent resolution and return of the normal flow voids.

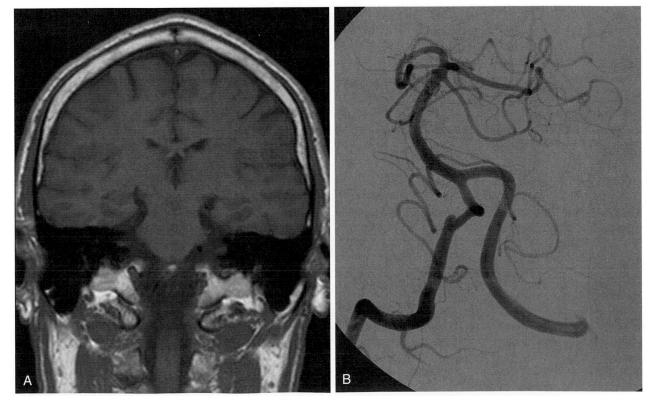

Fig. 4-94. Vertebral dissection. Acute, coronal T1-weighted MRI. **A,** A focal dissection (area of high signal intensity) in the prepontine right vertebral artery (VA). **B,** Follow-up angiogram showing persistent wall irregularity.

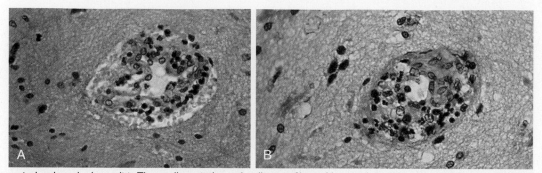

Fig. 4-95. A and **B,** Acute isolated cerebral vasculitis. The small cortical vessel walls are infiltrated by mostly lymphocytic and histiocytic cells, along with occasional polymorphonuclear leukocytes. The endothelial cells are reactive, with enlargement and enlarged nuclei.

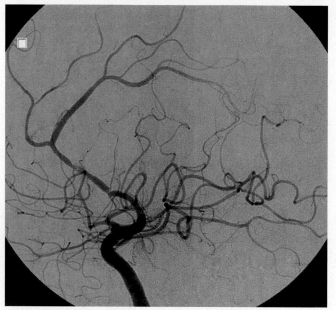

Fig. 4-96. Angiographic appearance of CNS vasculitis.

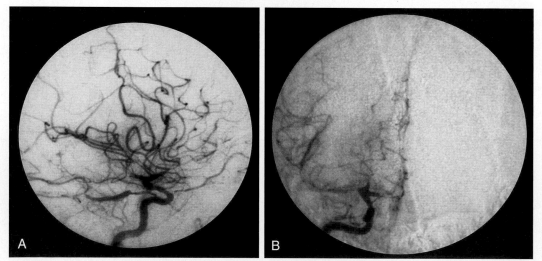

Fig. 4-97. Amphetamine-induced cerebral infarction. Angiography demonstrating anterior and middle cerebral artery occlusions. **A,** Lateral view. **B,** Anteroposterior view.

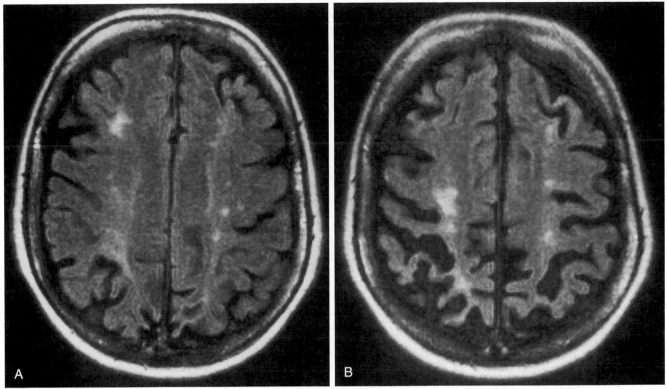

Fig. 4-98. Antiphospholipid syndrome. **A** and **B**, MRI in two cases showing characteristic hemispheric signal changes.

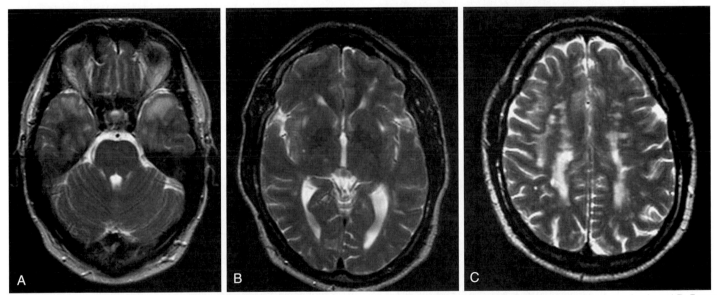

Fig. 4-99. CADASIL (cerebral autosomal dominant arteriopathy with subcortical infarcts and leukoencephalopathy). MRI. **A,** Typical anterior temporal pole, and **B,** External capsule involvement. **C,** Widespread leukoaraiosis.

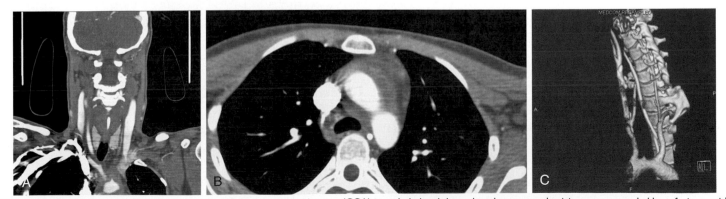

Fig. 4-100. Takayasu's disease. CT angiography. The left common carotid artery (CCA) is occluded and the arch and great vessel origins are surrounded by soft tissue with narrowing of the arch lumen. **A,** Core CT angiography, maximum intensity projection. **B,** Axial CT angiography. **C,** Three-dimensional volume reconstruction.

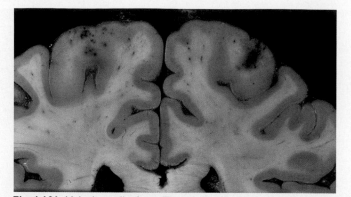

Fig. 4-101. Multiple small infarcts. Thrombotic thrombocytopenic purpura.

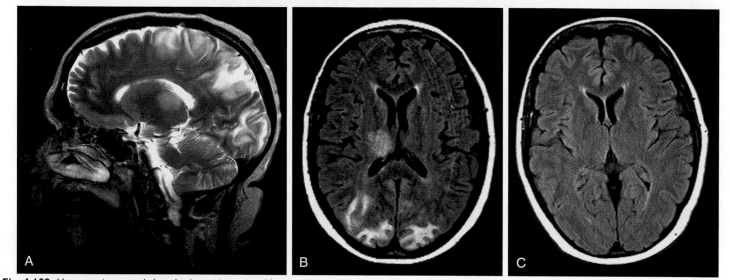

Fig. 4-102. Hypertensive encephalopathy (posterior reversible encephalopathy syndrome). **A** and **B,** Early MR images showing predominantly posterior white matter involvement, although the basal ganglia can be involved. **C,** Subsequent resolution.

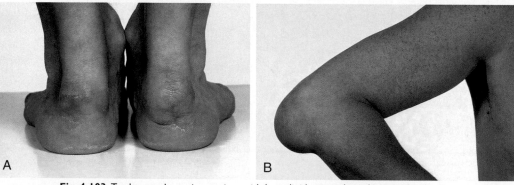

Fig. 4-103. Tendon xanthoma in a patient with hyperlipidemia and cerebrovascular disease.

CEREBRAL HEMORRHAGE AND OTHER CEREBROVASCULAR DISORDERS

CEREBRAL HEMORRHAGE

Cerebral hemorrhage is responsible for approximately 10% of all strokes. Its incidence is lessening, probably because of improvement in the management of hypertension, with which it is closely associated. Additional risk factors include previous cerebral infarction, coronary artery disease, diabetes mellitus, and, intriguingly, low serum cholesterol levels.

When the brains of hypertensive individuals are examined at autopsy, smaller intraparenchymal arteries and arterioles are found to be thick walled. The thickening is principally collagenous (arteriosclerotic and arteriolosclerotic) without much lipid deposition (i.e., not atherosclerotic) (Fig. 5-1). Deep penetrating vessels in the basal ganglia and thalamus, and vessels in the white matter, are more affected than cortical vessels. The affected vessels frequently have hemosiderin deposits in their walls and in the surrounding perivascular spaces (Virchow-Robin spaces) (Fig. 5-2). They also become tortuous and may even coil on themselves, producing an appearance in tissue section previously misinterpreted as aneurysms (Charcot-Bouchard aneurysms). In more advanced disease, the vessel wall appears split by lipid-laden macrophages (lipohyalinosis), and the intima and media may have fibrinoid necrosis (Fig. 5-3). Classically, hypertensive hemorrhages are most associated with vessels with fibrinoid deposits, although in individual cases this may be difficult to demonstrate, as the affected vessels may be destroyed in a large hemorrhage.

When seen in the acute phase either by scanning or at autopsy, cerebral hemorrhages are space-occupying lesions that largely displace rather than destroy tissue, a significant difference from cerebral infarcts. However, a certain amount of tearing of fiber tracts occurs, so that hemorrhages in or crossing the posterior limb of the internal capsule result in hemiparesis.

As a cerebral hemorrhage resolves, it leaves a slit-like cavity surrounded by hemosiderin, with comparative preservation of surrounding structures (Fig. 5-4). Again, this differs from infarction, in which the necrotic tissue is either liquefied (leaving a large cavity) or remains as a "mummified" coagulum.

It is now recognized that subclinical hemorrhage can occur in the cerebral substance. After such hemorrhages (microbleeds, or petechial hemorrhages), hemosiderin deposition occurs and can be detected by gradient echo T2-weighted MRI images (Fig. 5-5). These hemorrhages, initially described in patients who had presented with a hematoma, are now recognized to occur in the normal aging population and even in those who are normotensive. In general, however, microbleeds correlate both with elevated levels of mean systolic and mean diastolic blood pressure and with the presence of lacunes and confluent ischemic white matter change (Fig. 5-6).

Cerebral hemorrhages from chronic hypertension tend to occur at particular sites, especially in the deep gray matter. In descending order of frequency, they occur in the basal ganglia (particularly putamen), thalamus, cerebellum, pons, and deep central white matter.

Superficial lobar hemorrhages are more likely to be related to a vascular malformation, a bleeding diathesis, or amyloid angiopathy.

CLINICAL FEATURES

Certain clinical features, particularly headache, loss of consciousness, seizures, and vomiting, were once considered so characteristic of intracerebral hemorrhage that their absence was thought to cast doubt on the diagnosis. Headache, however, is often lacking in patients with small intracerebral bleeds and is sometimes conspicuous in patients with cerebral infarction. An early reduction of the consciousness level in a patient with a hemispheric stroke suggests that the causative lesion is a hemorrhage, yet many patients with small cerebral hematomas remain alert. Seizures often occur in both hemorrhage and infarction, but vomiting is more suggestive of an intracerebral hematoma. Hemorrhage at certain sites can certainly be located to that region, even if the underlying pathology is not necessarily suspected.

Hemorrhages in the Putamen and Internal Capsule
Bleeding in the putamen and internal capsule most commonly begins in the putamen as a consequence of rupture of one of the lateral lenticulostriate arteries. Extension of the hematoma occurs anteroposteriorly in the putamen, superficially (i.e., laterally toward

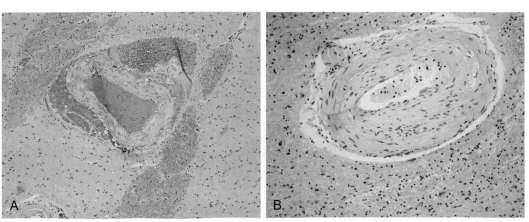

Fig. 5-1. Hypertensive changes in deep cerebral vessels. **A,** Putaminal artery with arteriosclerotic thickening of the intima and media. **B,** A similar vessel with surrounding scattered hemosiderin deposits in the perivascular space (Luxol fast blue, H&E).

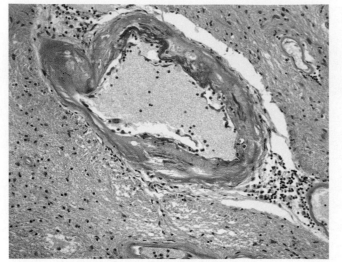

Fig. 5-2. Severe hypertensive changes in a cerebral artery include (in addition to the changes described in Fig. 5-1) intimal deposition of fibrinoid and a mild perivascular mononuclear cell infiltration.

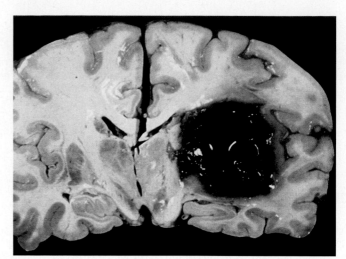

Fig. 5-3. Recent putamen hematoma with compression of the right lateral ventricle, and midline shift.

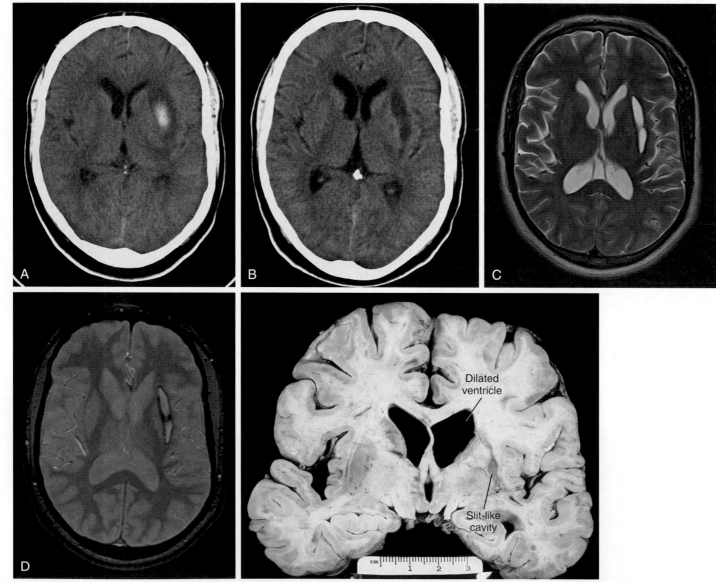

Fig. 5-4. Right putaminal hemorrhage. **A,** Acute CT. **B,** Late CT. Mature appearance on MR T2-weighted image **(C)** and on gradient echo T2-weighted image **(D)**, demonstrating slitlike cavity with hemosiderin walls, better seen on **D. E,** Coronal brain section. The right putamen is replaced by a hemosiderin-discolored area with a slitlike cavity, the residuum of an old hypertensive hemorrhage.

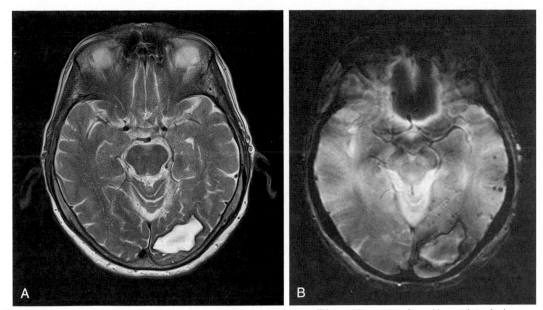

Fig. 5-5. Conventional T2-weighted spin echo image **(A)** and gradient echo T2-weighted image **(B)**, revealing areas of signal loss only in the latter, representing hemosiderin deposits in a subacute hematoma in the occipital lobe.

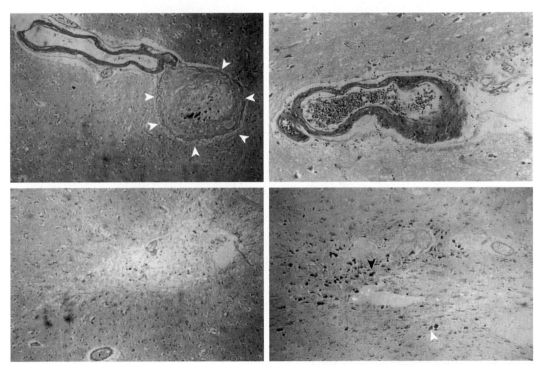

Fig. 5-6. Autopsy specimens from a 50-year-old man with hypertension. An organized miliary pseudoaneurysm *(upper left)* is connected to an arteriosclerotic vessel (H&E, ×200). Another microvessel *(upper right)* is also markedly arteriosclerotic with fibrinoid changes (H&E, ×200). A small infarct is evident where macrophages have accumulated and cystic changes have occurred around the pseudoaneurysm *(lower left)* (H&E, ×200). Hemosiderin pigment contained in the macrophages is abundant around the arteriosclerotic microvessels *(lower right)* (Berlin blue, ×120).

the insula), or deeply (i.e., eventually, across the internal capsule into the caudate or thalamus) in some cases, with rupture into the lateral ventricle (Fig. 5-7). Clinical features include progression over minutes or hours of contralateral motor and sensory deficits together with conjugate ocular deviation to the side of the lesion. Speech or visuospatial disturbances can occur, depending on whether the dominant or nondominant hemisphere is involved.

The predominant limb signs include contralateral sensory loss and a variety of involuntary movements, including dystonia and chorea. Alteration of the consciousness state is common.

Thalamic Hematoma

Many of the initial symptoms of thalamic hematoma are similar to those of putamenal hemorrhages, including headache, alteration of the consciousness state, and contralateral limb weakness, especially

if the posterior limb of the internal capsule is torn by a hemorrhage extending laterally toward the putamen from a primary site in the thalamus. Rupture medially can cause bleeding into the third ventricle; rupture superiorly can extend to the lateral ventricle (Fig. 5-8). A number of oculomotor disturbances occur. If the hemorrhage affects the medial thalamus, the eye may deviate away from the side of the lesion. A common combination of findings is deviation of the eyes, convergence, and constricted pupils. Convergence spasm can mimic the effects of a sixth-nerve palsy.

Pontine Hematoma

Large pontine hemorrhages, which are often rapidly fatal, tend to occupy the central part of the pons, sometimes extending into both the midbrain and the fourth ventricle (Fig. 5-9). Typically, the patient is comatose with a tetraparesis, decerebrate rigidity, paresis of horizontal eye movement both to the doll's head maneuver and caloric stimulation, and small, or very small, but reactive pupils. Smaller pontine hematomas are lateralized. Hematomas placed basally produce a contralateral hemiparesis, sometimes with ataxia. Spread to the tegmentum results in cranial nerve palsies. Lateral tegmental hematomas produce oculomotor disturbances, including internuclear ophthalmoplegia, the one-and-a-half syndrome, and gaze paresis (Fig. 5-10).

Cerebellar Hematoma

Most cerebellar hematomas occur in the region of the dentate nucleus (Fig. 5-11). Clinical features include headache, vomiting, ipsilateral cerebellar signs, and a tendency to deviate to the affected side when walking. As the hematoma expands, secondary brainstem

compression occurs. The patient becomes increasingly drowsy, and additional signs appear including an ipsilateral gaze paresis, facial weakness, and extensor plantar responses.

INVESTIGATION OF SUSPECTED HEMATOMA

CT Scanning

CT scanning identifies all symptomatic hematomas but provides little information about the contiguous vasculature. Adjacent edema is likely in the first few days (Fig. 5-12). Large hemispheric hematomas may rupture into the lateral ventricle, and cerebellar hematomas into the fourth ventricle. Enhancement occurs in a proportion of hematomas and is often ring shaped (Fig. 5-13). In some cases, the scan returns to normal, but in others an area of low attenuation persists.

MRI Scanning

Cerebral hematomas can be detected by appropriate MR techniques as soon as 30 minutes after the onset of the lesion. The appearance of the hemorrhage is critically dependent on the age of the lesion. Initially, the hematoma consists of intact red cells with intracellular oxyhemoglobin (hyperacute hematoma, isointense with T1 weighting,

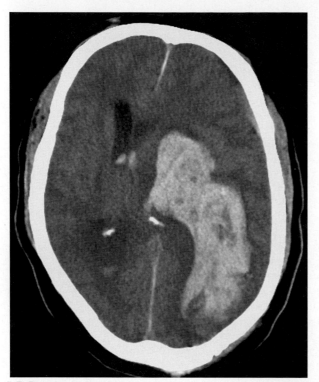

Fig. 5-7. Deep hemisphere hematoma with rupture into the ventricular system.

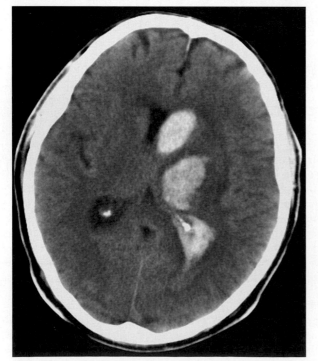

Fig. 5-8. CT scan of thalamic hematoma with rupture into lateral ventricle.

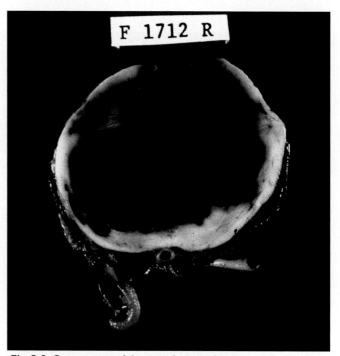

Fig. 5-9. Cross-section of the pons showing a hypertensive hemorrhage.

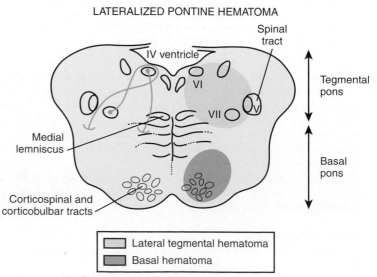

Fig. 5-10. Basal and lateral tegmental pontine hematomas.

hyperintense with T2 weighting). Within 6 to 12 hours, deoxyhemoglobin has formed in the red cells, leading to hypointensity on T2-weighted images (acute hematoma). After 2 to 3 days, the deoxyhemoglobin has been converted to intracellular methemoglobin, leading to increased signal on T1- and decreased signal on T2-weighted images, which spreads centrally from the periphery of the hematoma, early subacute hematoma (Figs. 5-14 and 5-15). This is followed by extracellular methemoglobin, which is of high signal on T2- and T1-weighted images (Fig. 5-16). The increased signal can persist over several months. Eventually, hemosiderin accumulates in the margins of the hematoma, producing a rim of hypointensity on T2-weighted images that can persist indefinitely (Fig. 5-17). More than 50% of patients with primary intracerebral hemorrhage show focal areas of signal loss at other sites on gradient echo T2-weighted MRI, indicative of past microbleeds.

Angiography

Angiography is usually not performed if the hematoma is at a site typical of a hypertensive bleed, although MR angiography (MRA) allows visualization of adjacent vessels without risk to the patient.

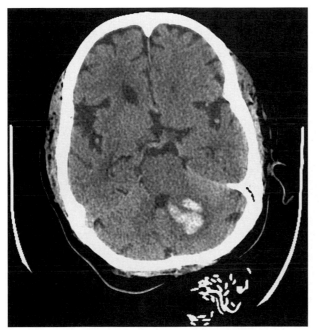

Fig. 5-11. CT scan of cerebellar hematoma.

NONHYPERTENSIVE INTRACEREBRAL HEMORRHAGES

VASCULAR MALFORMATIONS

Vascular malformations of the brain are classified according to the type of vessel involved in the communication. Capillary telangiectases are common but usually clinically silent. Venous angiomas (synonymous with developmental venous anomalies [DVAs]) contain multiple low-pressure channels linked to a single vein that usually then drains peripherally (Fig. 5-18). They are best regarded as anomalous venous drainage channels and are not pathologic. Cavernous hemangiomas contain thin-walled sinusoidal spaces and are most commonly located in the subcortex. There are no dilated feeding arteries or distended veins. They may be multiple or familial, or both. They may bleed repetitively with time, with most bleeds being subclinical. They often appear with epilepsy because of the cortical location of the lesions, and because they bleed repetitively they may contain blood products of different ages, giving a characteristic appearance on MRI. Fifteen percent are multiple, and they are more readily identified using gradient, rather than spin, echo sequences on MRI (Fig. 5-19). A particular form of pial venous abnormality is found in Sturge-Weber syndrome. This results in localized cortical venous hypertension with secondary atrophy and often cortical calcification. (Fig. 5-20)

Arteriovenous malformations (AVMs) contain arteries and dilated veins without intervening capillaries (Fig. 5-21). The nidus of the AVM is the primary abnormality, but the largest volume of the lesion is usually the tortuous thick-walled veins. AVMs have the capacity to enlarge by progressive recruitment of vessels, which become more muscular (arterialized) and tortuous under the influence of the high pressure and high flow from the arterial feeders. It seems likely that a developmental disorder is the mechanism in at least some AVMs. The veins, or associated arterial or venous aneurysms, are, presumably, the sites of rupture. In sites of turbulent flow, the vessels may undergo atherosclerotic change, with intimal plaques showing all the features of conventional atherosclerosis; this is the case even in young individuals whose other arteries show no atherosclerosis. The majority remain asymptomatic, with larger AVMs being less likely to rupture than small ones. The hemorrhage risk is calculated to be 2% to 4% per annum, but it rises substantially in those who have already bled. Besides size, other factors predisposing to hemorrhage include exclusive deep venous drainage, high intranidal pressures, and AVM-related aneurysms, which are found in about 10% of cases. The bleeding is usually less

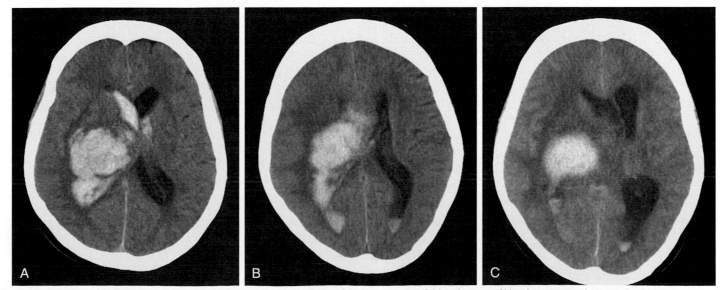

Fig. 5-12. Right hemisphere hematoma with intraventricular extension. **A,** Day 0. **B,** Day 2. **C,** Day 5. Note layering of blood in posterior horns at day 2, and clot retraction at day 5 but increased shift caused by edema and hydrocephalus (effaced sulci).

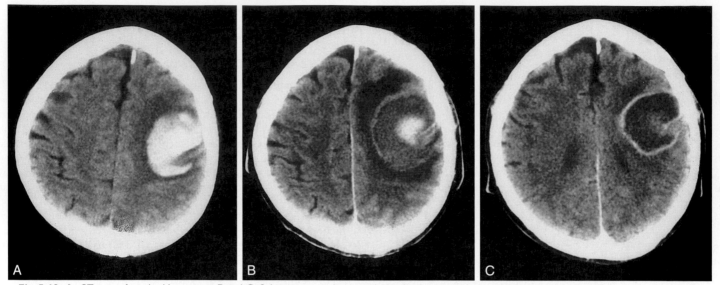

Fig. 5-13. A, CT scan of cerebral hematoma. **B** and **C,** Subsequent resolution with the development of a low-density area associated with ring enhancement.

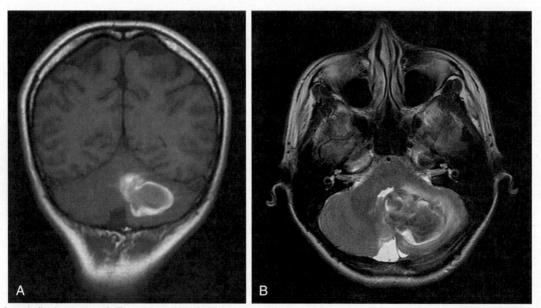

Fig. 5-14. MR image of cerebellar hematoma. **A,** T1-weighted MRI. **B,** T2-weighted MRI. Early sub-acute hematoma (i.e., intact red blood cells, intracellular deoxyhemoglobin).

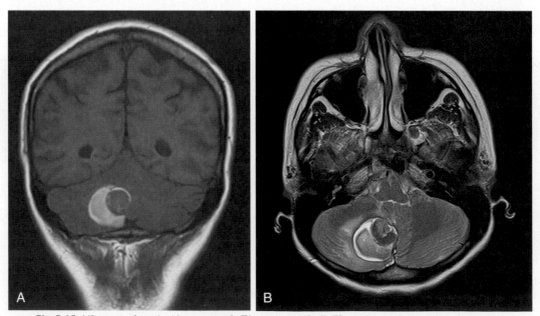

Fig. 5-15. MR image of cerebral hematoma. **A,** T1-weighted MRI. **B,** T2-weighted MRI. Mixed age hematoma.

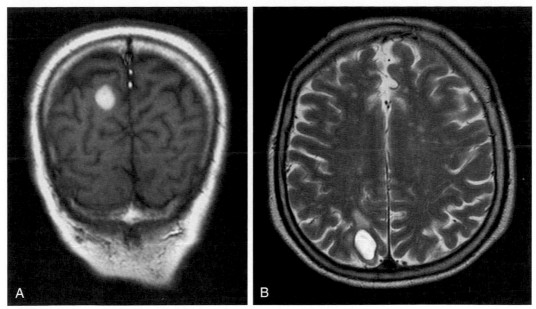

Fig. 5-16. MR image of cerebral hematoma. **A,** T1-weighted MRI. **B,** T2-weighted MRI. Mixed-age hematoma. Late sub acute hematoma.

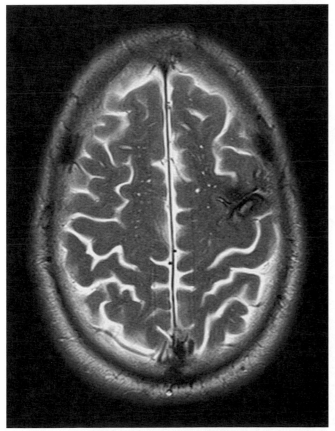

Fig. 5-17. T2-weighted MR image of cerebral hematoma, chronic. Hemosiderin lines the old hematoma cavity and the adjacent sulci (because there was localized subarachnoid hemorrhage).

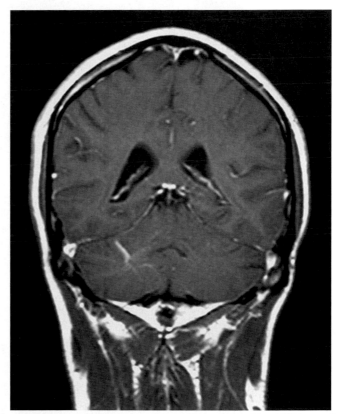

Fig. 5-18. Right cerebellar venous angioma. Coronal T1-weighted MR image after contrast enhancement.

paroxysmal than that after rupture of a berry aneurysm, with a correspondingly better prognosis.

AVMs are rarely found in children, except for the special case of so-called vein of Galen malformations, which are arteriovenous fistulas draining directly into the internal cerebral veins, the basal veins of Rosenthal or the vein of Galen itself. These are congenital malformations that may be detected in utero but are otherwise usually found early in infancy.

Seizures in patients with cerebral hemisphere AVMs are relatively common and often focal. Whether AVMs produce recurrent

headache alone is debated. A steal phenomenon has been identified, in which exaggerated flow through the malformation steals blood from the adjacent brain. Cognitive changes may be seen as a consequence.

Dural arteriovenous fistulas (dAVFs) are thought to be acquired lesions in which there is an abnormal connection between an artery (usually a dural branch) and a cerebral venous sinus (or its wall). As a result, there is rapid shunting of blood into the sinus, with an increase in the pressure in the sinus. Over time, more vessels are recruited and the fistula increases in size. Occasionally, the fistulas undergo spontaneous obliteration. As the pressure in the sinus increases, normal venous drainage is impaired, and patients may present with epilepsy (secondary to cortical dysfunction), symptoms of raised intracranial

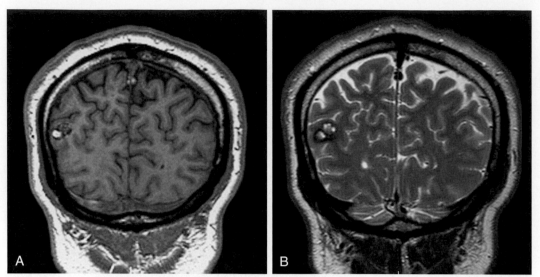

Fig. 5-19. Right parietal cavernous hemangioma, coronal view. **A,** T1-weighted MRI. **B,** T2-weighted MRI. Note mixture of acute and chronic blood products.

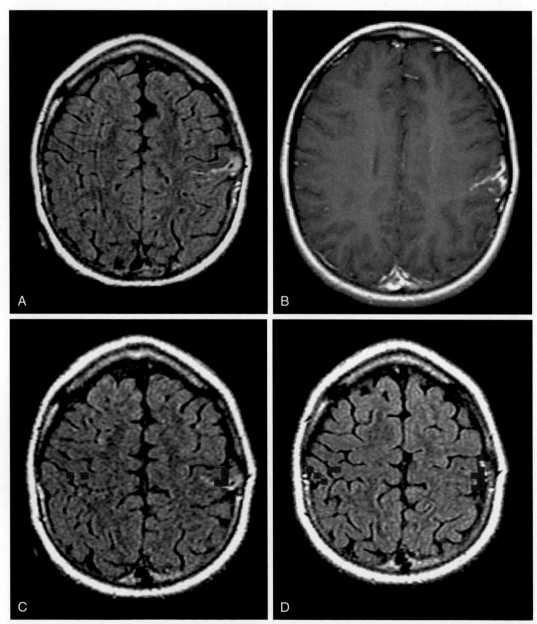

Fig. 5-20. A, Anatomic MRI showing an enhancing pial angioma of Sturge-Weber type in the left perirolandic region. **B** to **D,** Functional MRI showed functional activation for the hand, located directly beneath the pial angioma. Invasive stimulation mapping confirmed the location of hand function identified by functional MRI.

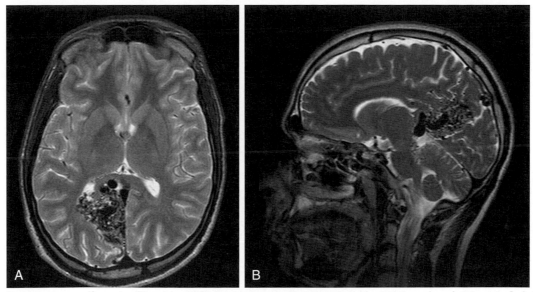

Fig. 5-21. Right occipital arteriovenous malformation. T2-weighted MRI showing multiple dilated arteries and a single large deep draining vein. **A,** Axial view. **B,** Sagittal view.

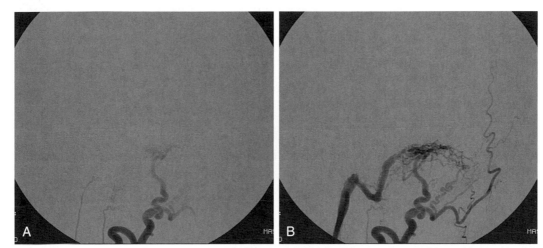

Fig. 5-22. A, Lateral angiogram showing multiple branches off a dilated occipital artery feeding a dural fistula in the wall of the transverse sinus. **B,** The jugular vein fills early.

pressure, hemorrhage (if there is rupture), tinnitus, or visual distur-bance (in the case of caroticocavernous fistulas, which are dAVFs located in the cavernous sinus wall) (Fig. 5-22).

Investigation and Treatment of Vascular Malformations

Arteriovenous Malformations. Precontrast CT usually shows a mixed-density lesion (Fig. 5-23), sometimes with areas of calcification, although some AVMs are undetectable on unenhanced CT (Fig. 5-24). Enhancement identifies the nidus and the dilated draining veins. In a patient with an intracerebral hematoma, an AVM may be suspected if the hematoma does not appear in one of the sites classically associated with hypertensive bleeds (Fig. 5-25). With MRI, there is prominence of the abnormal vessels, best seen on T2-weighted imaging as multiple serpiginous areas of low-signal intensity (flow voids.)

The pattern of signal on MR images is influenced by whether pre-vious hemorrhage has occurred. In the acute setting, abnormal signal from the hematoma dominates the picture. With resolution of the hematoma, hemosiderin staining is visible on MRI with flow voids, unless the AVM has been destroyed by the rupture.

Formal angiography remains the primary technique for imaging AVMs, particularly in terms of vascular supply and drainage and treatment rationalization. The risk of angiography in this context, at 0.3% to 0.8% morbidity, is lower than in individuals being evaluated for transient ischemic attack or stroke (3% to 3.7%). Both internal and external carotid injection may be necessary, the latter to find the dural feeding vessels to the malformation. Typically, there are mul-tiple feeders and multiple draining veins (Fig. 5-26).

MANAGEMENT OF ARTERIOVENOUS MALFORMATIONS. The three main tech-niques are surgery, embolization, and stereotactic radiosurgery (highly focused radiotherapy). Most commonly, a combination of treatments is used, often embolization (Fig. 5-27) to reduce the size, followed by either surgery or stereotactic radiosurgery (STRS). Ste-reotactic radiosurgery or radiation (gamma knife) aims to obliterate the nidus of the lesion, thereby destroying its own arterial supply. Two-year obliteration rates range from 40% to 80%. Success is more likely with small lesions, a small number of draining veins, hemi-sphere location, and younger age. Morphologic change during the 6 to 18 months after the irradiation period appears to predict a favor-able outcome (Fig. 5-28). Adverse effects include radiation necrosis, irradiation stenosis of intracranial vessels, and cranial nerve palsies. Inevitably, the hemorrhage risk remains until the lesion is obliterated.

The aim of treatment is the complete obliteration of the nidus, as partial treatment confers no reduction in hemorrhage risk (unless there is an obvious bleed point, such as an aneurysm).

Developmental Venous Anomalies and Cavernous Angiomas.
Devel-opmental venous anomalies are detectable by CT or MRI. When they are small, it may be necessary to use contrast-enhanced sequences to see them, and it is important to recognize them as normal variants not needing further investigation. Cavernous angiomas on CT appear as slightly hyperdense lesions but without significant displacement of adjacent structures (Fig. 5-29). Some may enhance with contrast. MRI demonstrates a central nucleus that appears hyperintense on T1- and T2-weighted images, with a surrounding hypointensity on T2-weighted

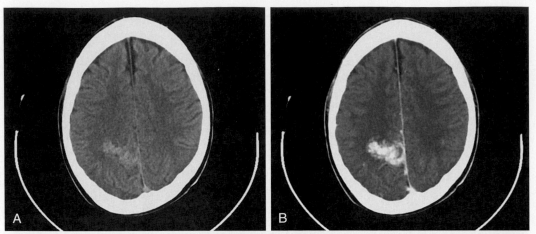

Fig. 5-23. CT scans of arteriovenous malformation. **A,** Before contrast, there is subtle irregular hyperdensity. **B,** After contrast, there is enhancement.

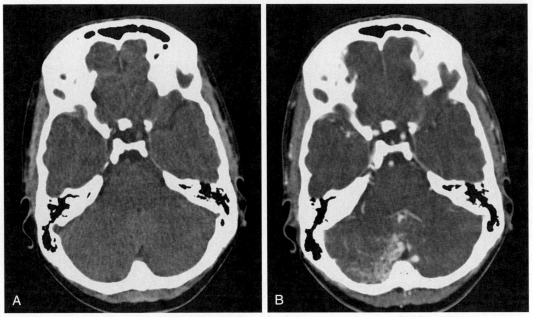

Fig. 5-24. CT scans of arteriovenous malformation. Normal precontrast scan. **B,** After contrast.

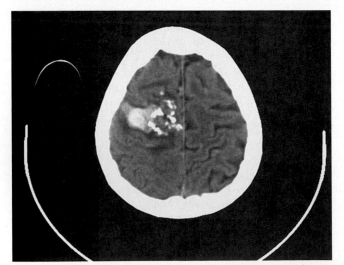

Fig. 5-25. Calcification in arteriovenous malformation with adjacent acute hematoma.

images reflecting the accumulation of hemosiderin in the surrounding brain tissue. Pathologically, cavernous hemangiomas consist of back-to-back thin-walled vessels of variable but usually increased diameter without arterial feeders and with occasional large draining veins. The lack of brain parenchyma between the vessels is the crucial pathologic characteristic distinguishing them from capillary telangiectases (Fig. 5-30).

MANAGEMENT OF DEVELOPMENTAL VENOUS ANOMALIES AND CAVERNOUS ANGIOMAS. Developmental venous anomalies require no treatment. There is no endovascular treatment for cavernous angiomas, as they are angiographically invisible. They do not respond to stereotactic radiosurgery. Surgical resection is the only therapeutic option and is usually reserved for those lesions in noncritical cortical locations that are causing intractable epilepsy.

Dural Arteriovenous Fistulas. Dural arteriovenous fistulas may be very large at presentation. Their arterial supply is derived from branches of the external carotid artery, with drainage into one of the large sinuses. Some bleed, resulting in subdural hemorrhage; others, particularly the large ones, can present with raised intracranial pressure. In some cases, the symptoms are determined by the anatomic location of the malformation.

Malformations of the cavernous sinus may drain anteriorly via one or other ophthalmic vein, or posteriorly via the petrosal sinuses. Those draining anteriorly produce mild proptosis with dilatation of conjunctival vessels, often accompanied by a sixth-nerve palsy (Fig. 5-31). A venous stasis retinopathy can occur, sometimes resulting in central retinal vein occlusion. If the fistula is close to the temporal bone, the patient often complains of a high-pitched noise or bruit. Similar malformations are found on the tentorium cerebelli and in the posterior fossa.

Evidence of a caroticocavernous fistula may be visible on CT scan or MR imaging as a dilated superior ophthalmic vein (Fig. 5-32),

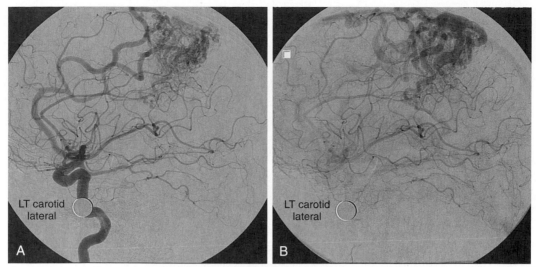

Fig. 5-26. Angiograms of arteriovenous malformation showing dilated feeding arteries and early filling of superior sagittal sinus. **A,** Early arterial phase. **B,** Late arterial phase.

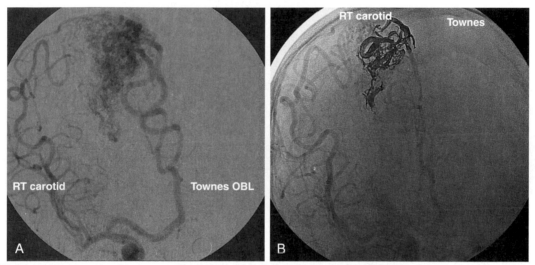

Fig. 5-27. Subtraction angiogram showing cast of embolic material. **A,** Before embolization. **B,** Unsubtracted angiogram after embolization.

although they are often seen only with angiography. When a supratentorial arteriovenous fistula is being sought, angiography must include injection of both the internal and external carotid arteries (Fig. 5-33).

MANAGEMENT OF DURAL ARTERIOVENOUS FISTULAS. Dural arteriovenous fistulas may close spontaneously or after angiography, and some will close with repeated manual vascular compression of the feeding artery if this is feasible. Treatment aims to reduce the risk of intracranial hemorrhage or to eliminate symptoms. Therefore, patients with no risk of intracranial hemorrhage from their dAVF (risk of hemorrhage can be assessed only by catheter angiography) are not usually offered treatment unless they have intractable symptoms (e.g., tinnitus that prevents sleep). Surgical intervention and endovascular treatment are both feasible for dural fistulas (Fig. 5-34), with the preferred option varying according to the anatomy and location of the lesion. There is no role for stereotactic radiosurgery. Successful closure leads to regression of the physical signs (Fig. 5-35). Spinal dAVFs are considered elsewhere.

CEREBRAL AMYLOID ANGIOPATHY

Cerebral amyloid angiopathy is characterized by the deposition of congophilic amyloid Aβ in cerebral cortical and leptomeningeal vessels. Rare familial forms have been associated with amyloid of various origins, including gelsolin and cystatin C, but the most common form of amyloid deposited is amyloid Aβ. Sporadic (nonfamilial) amyloid angiopathy is associated only with amyloid Aβ deposition.

Secondary degeneration of the arterial wall can lead to fibrinoid necrosis (Fig. 5-36). Sporadic amyloid angiopathy correlates with age and is said to occur in up to 50% of individuals over the age of 80. Very commonly, there are accompanying amyloid (senile) plaques of the type found in patients with Alzheimer's disease. Indeed, over 90% of patients with pathologically confirmed Alzheimer's disease have coexisting cerebral amyloid angiopathy. Patients with familial amyloid angiopathy generally present with cerebral hemorrhage in the fourth or fifth decade of life.

There is a significant association between the possession of apolipoprotein-ε4 and the occurrence of cerebral amyloid angiopathy. In addition, an association exists with the possession of apolipoprotein-ε2.

Cerebral amyloid angiopathy is a recognized cause of cerebral hemorrhage in elderly persons, in the absence of hypertension or coagulopathy. The hemorrhages are lobar (Fig. 5-37), occurring in the cerebral cortex or subcortical white matter. Recurrent hemorrhages are characteristic (Fig. 5-38). The parietal, temporal, and occipital lobes are particularly affected. Recurrence of lobar hemorrhage is more likely if the individual possesses apolipoprotein-ε4 or ε2.

COAGULATION DISORDERS

Intracerebral hemorrhage is a recognized hazard of anticoagulant therapy and can occur in patients with thrombocytopenia from any cause. In patients with factor VIII or IX deficiency, hematomas may

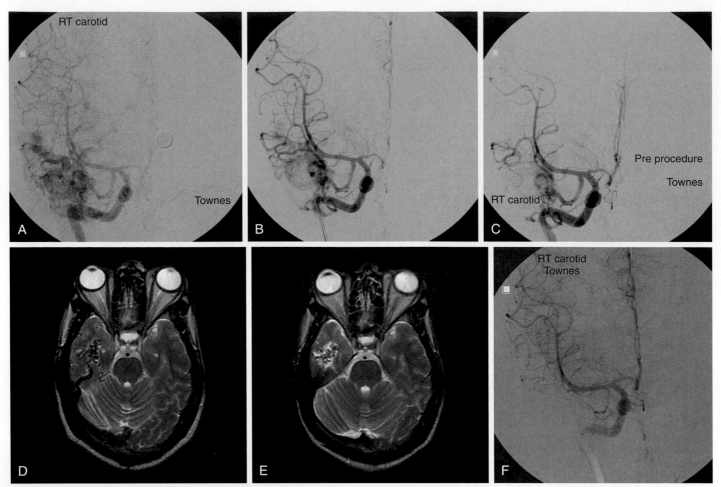

Fig. 5-28. Stages of treatment of arteriovenous malformation. **A,** Initial angiogram. **B,** After first embolization. **C,** After second embolization. **D,** MRI after second embolization. **E,** MRI 1 year after stereotactic radiosurgery (STRS), showing high signal change around nidus. **F,** Angiogram 2 years after STRS, showing complete obliteration.

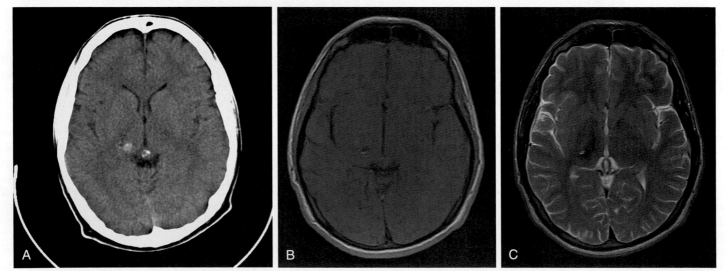

Fig. 5-29. Cavernoma. **A,** CT scan. **B,** Axial T1-weighted MRI image. **C,** T2-weighted MRI image. Note hyperdensity on CT. The hypointense rim on T2-weighted MRI is the result of hemosiderin, and the variable signal intensity in the center is caused by blood products of different ages.

occur spontaneously or as a consequence of minor head injury (Fig. 5-39). Hematomas in patients with clotting disorders may appear slightly more heterogeneous because of inability of the blood to clot. However, other causes of intracerebral hemorrhage, including rupture of a berry aneurysm, substance abuse (especially cocaine, amphetamines, and other sympathomimetics), and bleeding into a cerebral tumor (e.g., metastatic melanoma, or lung or ovarian carcinoma) should also be considered.

ANEURYSMS

Saccular (berry) aneurysms are found at the bifurcations of the major cerebral arteries at the base of the brain. About 85% arise in the anterior circulation, at the junction of either anterior cerebral artery with the anterior communicating artery, at the bifurcation of the middle cerebral artery, or at the junction of the posterior communicating and internal carotid arteries (Fig. 5-40). The remaining 15% occur at

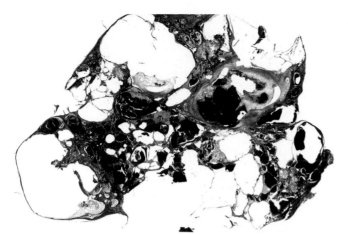

Fig. 5-30. Cavernous angioma. Previous embolization with occlusion of some of the lumina by embolic material (H&E).

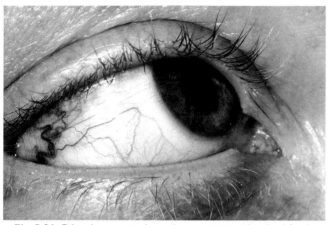

Fig. 5-31. Dilated conjunctival vessels in a patient with a dural fistula.

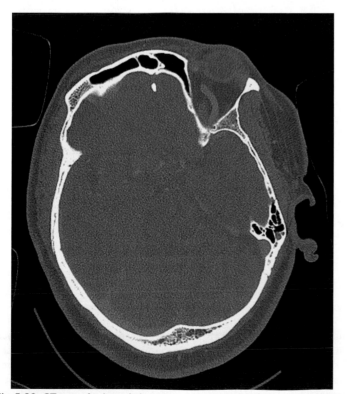

Fig. 5-32. CT scan of a distended superior ophthalmic vein in the left orbit draining a dural fistula.

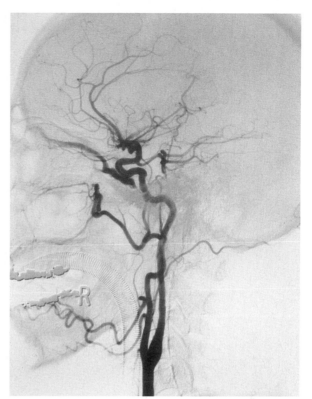

Fig. 5-33. Carotid angiogram of a caroticocavernous fistula. The fistula has filled and is draining anteriorly into the orbit.

various sites in the posterior circulation. Microscopic analysis reveals that the smooth muscle coat and elastic lamina of the intracranial artery end abruptly at the neck of the aneurysm, the wall of which is composed of fibrous tissue (Fig. 5-41). In some cases, the aneurysm is an incidental postmortem finding. Some 20% of aneurysms are multiple.

In some cases, the aneurysm is placed so critically that its enlargement, without rupture, can compromise adjacent structures. In this way, a posterior communicating aneurysm can present with a third-nerve palsy, which inevitably affects the pupil if it is complete in other respects (Fig. 5-42). In some patients with subarachnoid hemorrhage (SAH), careful history taking reveals previous episodes of paroxysmal head and neck pain, probably the consequence of small leaks from the aneurysm (sentinel bleeds).

More substantial bleeding leads to the characteristic clinical features of SAH. Mortality for those admitted to hospital approaches 50% over the first 3 months but is nearly immediate if the hemorrhage is massive (Fig. 5-43). Indeed, it is suggested that mortality may be as high as 50% in the first 24 hours, as many of those individuals either die immediately or before they can be taken to hospital. Typical symptoms include severe headache, neck pain with stiffness, vomiting, and loss of consciousness. The sudden increase in intracranial pressure can lead to hemorrhage into the preretinal space (subhyaloid hemorrhage) (Fig. 5-44). Focal neurologic signs appearing soon after the onset, and not explicable by pressure effects of the aneurysm itself, are caused by extension of the hemorrhage into the cerebral substance.

Investigation. Development of blood-stained CSF with xanthochromia is virtually inevitable after subarachnoid hemorrhage (Fig. 5-45). The mean duration of persisting red cells in the CSF after SAH is 9 days, with a range of 4 to 19 days. Hemolysis of red cells starts after approximately 12 hours. Spectrophotometry can identify heme breakdown products in the supernatant fluid even when visual inspection has been normal (Fig. 5-46).

CSF examination in this setting is not without risk. Consequently, CT is the first investigation of choice in suspected SAH. It demonstrates blood in 90% of patients who are scanned within 24 hours

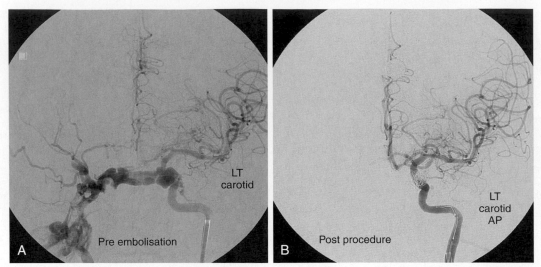

Fig. 5-34. Angiograms of caroticocavernous fistula. **A,** Before embolisation. **B,** After embolisation. Note immediate filling of cavernous sinuses on both sides, which resolves after treatment.

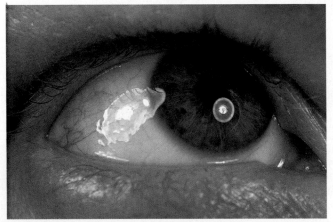

Fig. 5-35. Right eye of the patient seen in Figure 5-31, after successful embolization of the fistula.

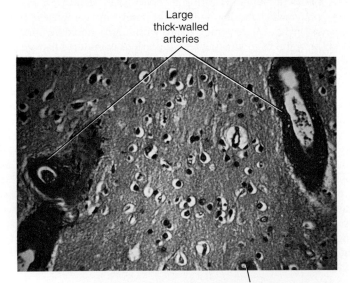

Fig. 5-36. Cerebral amyloid angiopathy. Thick-walled large arteries and small intraparenchymal arterioles and capillaries (Congo red, ×25).

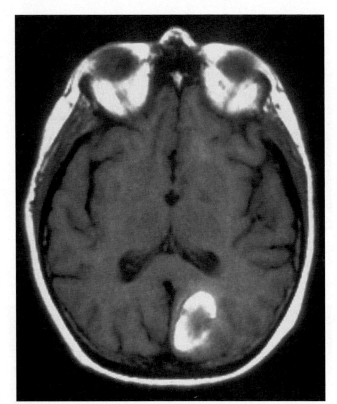

Fig. 5-37. T1-weighted MRI of cerebral amyloid angiopathy with a lobar occipito-parietal hemorrhage of 3 days' duration. Central dark area of deoxyhemoglobin with peripheral bright methemoglobin.

of onset (Fig. 5-47). In some cases, the blood is diffusely distributed (Fig. 5-48), but in others its localization suggests the site of the ruptured aneurysm (Fig. 5-49). Subsequent focal ischemia secondary to vasospasm is more likely if the CT demonstrates thick clot rather than thin sheets of subarachnoid blood. There is some indication that severe symptomatic hemisphere infarcts from vasospasm are predicted by thick accumulations of clot in the sylvian fissures around the major branches of the middle cerebral artery.

The sensitivity of CT for acute SAH is 90%, but as there is a false-negative rate, lumbar puncture is mandatory if SAH is suspected and the CT is normal. CT angiography (CTA) is often performed at the same time as the CT and detects more than 90% of 2-mm aneurysms and 99% of those greater than 3 mm (Fig. 5-50). MR scanning is not performed routinely in patients with subarachnoid hemorrhage, as it has proved less sensitive for the detection of subarachnoid blood. Angiography is performed if there is proven (or high clinical suspicion of) SAH, and if no aneurysm is demonstrated on CTA. Causes of negative angiograms include aneurysms that have disintegrated at the moment of hemorrhage, and vasospasm. Identification of the relevant aneurysm, in such cases, is simplified if local vasospasm is found. Vasospasm seldom appears in the first 72 hours after hemorrhage (Fig. 5-51).

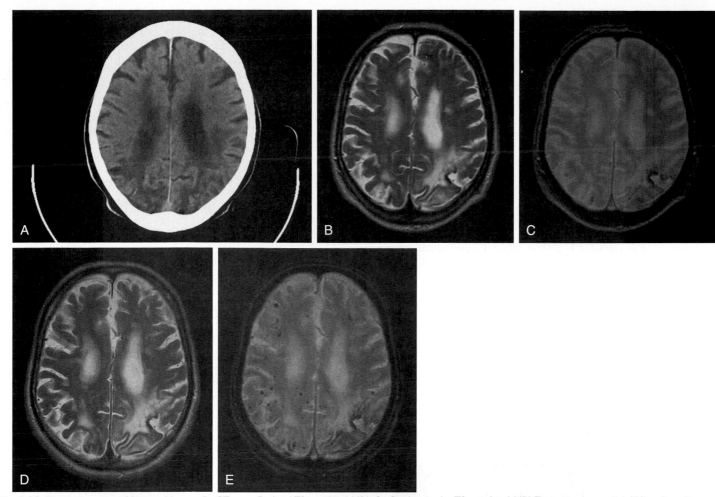

Fig. 5-38. The patient is an 80-year-old man. **A,** CT scan. **B,** Axial T2-weighted MRI. **C,** Gradient echo T2-weighted MRI. Two years later, axial **(D)** and gradient echo **(E)** T2-weighted MRIs were repeated. Note evidence of mature biparietal lobar hemorrhages, and multiple small microbleeds (visible only on the gradient echo sequences), which have dramatically increased in number.

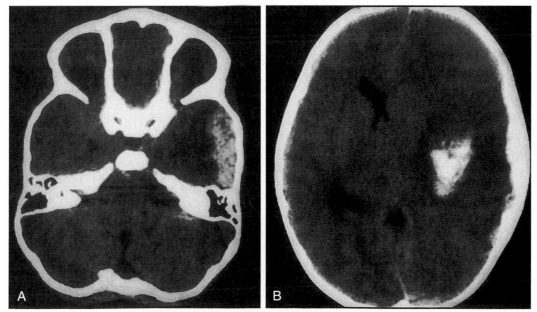

Fig. 5-39. CT scan of a patient with factor IX deficiency. **A,** Subdural hematoma. **B,** Intracerebral hematoma.

Management. Most aneurysms are now treated endovascularly. This involves catheterization of the aneurysm, usually via a femoral arterial puncture and the placement of platinum coils into the aneurysm sac to prevent blood from flowing into the aneurysm (Fig. 5-52). This causes thrombosis and in some cases endothelialization across the neck. There is a small but appreciable neck recurrence rate with endovascular treatment, but this does not seem to be matched by an equivalent rebleed rate. Neck recurrences can be retreated if necessary. Some new coils have a bioactive component that encourages clot stabilization, with the aim of reducing recurrence rates. Other new coils have a swellable coating that increases the volume filled in the aneurysm and reduces coil compaction and recurrence rate. Coiling can be achieved in wider-necked aneurysms using balloon assistance techniques or with an adjunctive stent.

Surgical clipping is increasingly reserved for those patients who cannot be coiled, usually because of unfavorable anatomy. Patients are given nimodipine to reduce the risk of spasm and may need an external ventricular drain (or shunt) or repeated lumbar puncture to treat hydrocephalus (Fig. 5-53).

CTA and MRA can be used to visualize intracranial aneurysms as small as 2 mm. These procedures have replaced angiography in screening high-risk populations (in some cases, berry aneurysms are familial), and for reappraisal of patients who have had endovascular therapy (MRA, not CTA), which has been necessary as a recanalization rate of up to 10% occurs with this procedure (Fig. 5-54).

Arteriosclerotic Aneurysms

Ectatic intracranial vessels occasionally become diffusely dilated in a fusiform manner as a result of atheromatous changes in a hypertensive individual (Fig. 5-55). The basilar artery is particularly affected. The changes can be detected by CT or MRI. Ectatic vessels, if sufficiently large, can obstruct the CSF pathway or compress adjacent nerve tissue.

Giant Aneurysms

Giant aneurysms exceed 25 mm in diameter. They represent about 5% of all intracranial aneurysms. They rupture infrequently, more often appearing either as a space-occupying lesion or with distal embolization from thrombus contained in their lumen (Fig. 5-56).

Some giant aneurysms are saccular, others are fusiform, arising in degenerative basilar or internal carotid vessels. Calcification of the aneurysm may be visible on plain CT. They are thought to be different from berry aneurysms and may be secondary to small microdissections of the arterial wall with repeated cycles of repair and rebleed. The wall may enhance, and there is frequently lamellated thrombus in the periphery. After injection of contrast agent, there may be little filling of the aneurysm because of the presence of thrombus. The characteristic features are displayed by MRI (Fig. 5-57). Large basilar aneurysms may distort the brainstem, leading to secondary hydrocephalus. Cavernous aneurysms are liable to compress the nerves in the sinus, including cranial nerves III, IV, and VI, the first and second divisions of the trigeminal nerve; and the ocular sympathetic fibers.

CEREBRAL VENOUS THROMBOSIS

Isolated cortical vein thrombosis is rare. In most patients, variable involvement of the cortical veins is accompanied by occlusion of one or more of the major sinuses (Fig. 5-58). The condition can be idiopathic, but recognized risk factors include disease processes affecting the vessel wall (e.g., Behçet's syndrome), an alteration of blood flow, local sinus–based infection, and pregnancy or the use of an oral contraceptive. Conditions that induce thrombophilia (e.g., deficiencies of antithrombin III, protein C, protein S, heparin, cofactor 2, and factor V Leiden mutation) can lead to cerebral venous thrombosis.

Pathologic changes in the brain include cerebral edema and either hemorrhage or hemorrhagic infarction (Fig. 5-59). With superior sagittal sinus thrombosis, there is headache, raised intracranial pressure, and seizures—features that may also be encountered in thrombosis of the deeper veins (Fig. 5-60). In a proportion of patients, particularly those with superior sagittal sinus thrombosis, presentation mimics that of benign intracranial hypertension.

Investigation

With CT, venous infarcts become hypodense and edematous more rapidly than arterial infarcts, frequently with central hemorrhagic components.

Precontrast CT may also reveal evidence of thrombosed venous sinuses (Fig. 5-61), with postcontrast films displaying filling defects. The presence of an empty triangular shape (the delta sign) in the posterior aspect of the superior sagittal sinus on postcontrast CT is considered particularly characteristic.

MRI and MR venography are the imaging techniques of choice, as they usually identify the affected sinus, as well as displaying any parenchymal change (Fig. 5-62). CT venography is also very useful for nonocclusive thrombus. Formal venography is now seldom undertaken. The imaging manifestations of venous thrombosis are extremely variable, and often both CT and MR are necessary for diagnosis. Care must be taken not to place too much reliance on the MRV.

Although management of this condition remains controversial, most patients are heparinized and then later switched to warfarin, even in the presence of hemorrhagic infarcts. Steroids are without value. The role of direct thrombolysis achieved by infusing thrombolytics directly into the affected sinus remains unresolved. Seizures are commonplace and are managed symptomatically.

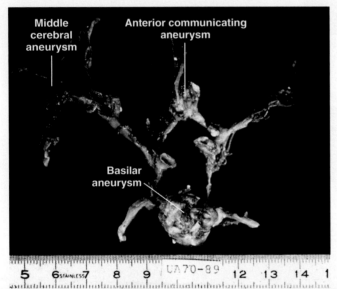

Fig. 5-40. Circle of Willis. Aneurysms are seen at the basilar tip, two along the right middle cerebral artery, one on the anterior communicating artery, and a fifth on the first segment of the right anterior cerebral artery.

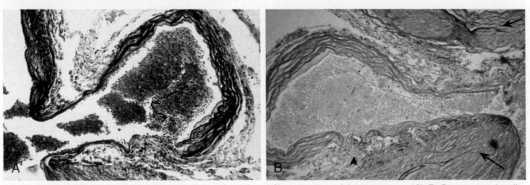

Fig. 5-41. Saccular (berry) aneurysm. **A,** Fibrous collagen stains blue; muscle, red; and fibrin, bright red (azocarmine, ×10). **B,** Parent vessel wall contains an elastic lamina *(arrows),* which becomes broken *(arrowhead)* and disappears as it enters the neck of the aneurysm (elastic stain, ×10).

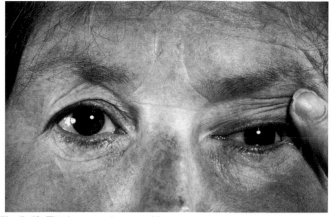

Fig. 5-42. Third-nerve palsy caused by a posterior communicating aneurysm.

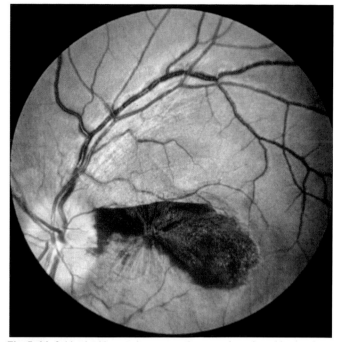

Fig. 5-44. Subhyaloid hemorrhage secondary to subarachnoid hemorrhage.

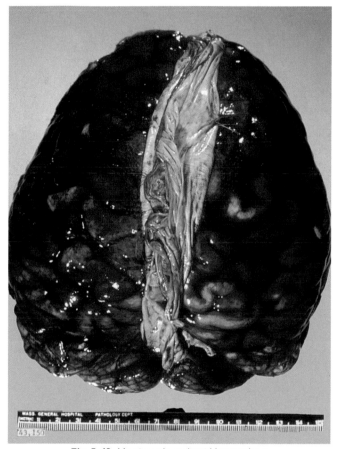

Fig. 5-43. Massive subarachnoid hemorrhage.

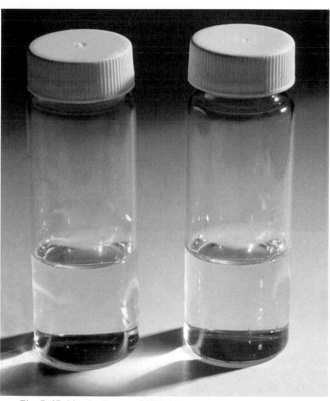

Fig. 5-45. Xanthochromic CSF *(left)* compared with normal *(right)*.

Moyamoya Disease

Moyamoya disease predominates in women of Asian origin. Younger patients typically present with ischemic events, adults with intracerebral or subarachnoid hemorrhage. Stenosis, congenital hypoplasia, or occlusion is found in the terminal parts of both internal carotid arteries and in their main branches (Fig. 5-63). Alongside this occlusive process, multiple small anastomotic channels are found in the region of the circle of Willis and the pia mater (Fig. 5-64).

MRI reveals the collaterals as flow voids in the basal ganglia (Fig. 5-65). Angiography identifies both the occlusive disease and the abnormal anastomotic channels. The etiology of the condition is unknown, but a similar picture is seen in children with sickle cell disease. Surgical treatments used for progressive ischemia include extracranial and intracranial bypass to one or both middle cerebral arteries. Follow-up angiography suggests the anastomoses remain patent and that subsequent ischemic events are reduced in frequency. There is no firm evidence that the procedure reduces the risk of subsequent cerebral hemorrhage.

Intravascular Lymphoma

Intravascular lymphoma results in the invasion of cerebral arteries, veins, and capillaries by neoplastic lymphoid cells, with relative sparing of the adjacent parenchyma (Fig. 5-66). Typically, strokelike episodes, which may be hemorrhagic or ischemic in origin, occur. Associated features include neuropathies, either cranial or peripheral, and dementia. Imaging is likely to reflect the mixed pathologic process. Distinction from a cerebral vasculitis may be achieved only at postmortem examination.

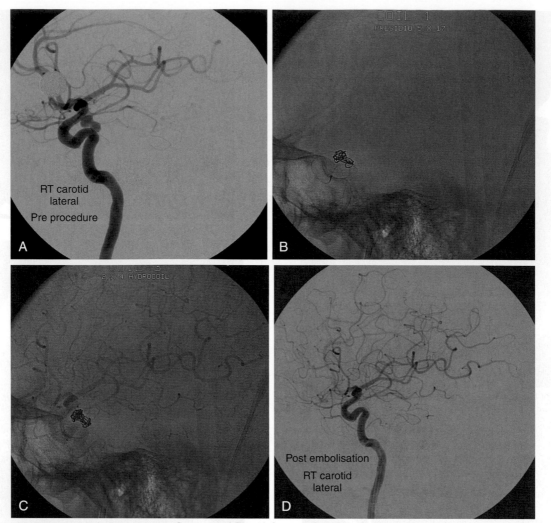

Fig. 5-52. Bilobed posterior communicating artery aneurysm. **A,** untreated, **B,** with first coil, **C,** and **D,** after final coil unsubtracted and subtracted images demonstrating no residual filling of the aneurysm.

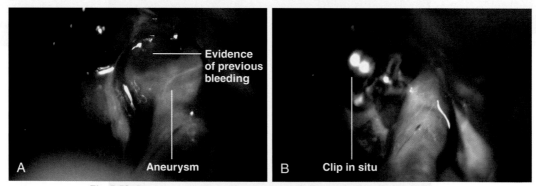

Fig. 5-53. Posterior communicating aneurysm. **A,** Before clipping. **B,** After clipping.

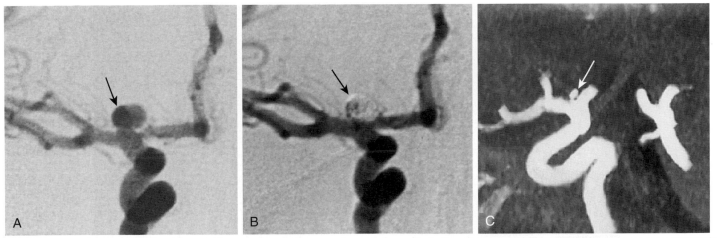

Fig. 5-54. Unruptured aneurysm of the right carotid termination. **A,** Aneurysm *(arrow)* before embolisation. Digital subtraction angiography image, anteroposterior view. **B,** Remnant aneurysm cavity *(arrow)* is seen 4 months after treatment. **C,** MR angiogram demonstrating remnant cavity *(arrow)*.

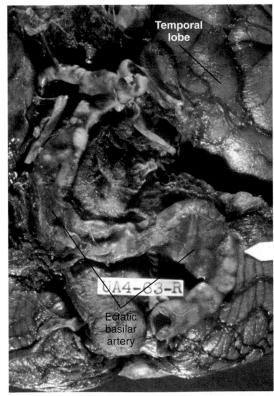

Fig. 5-55. Ectasia of the basilar artery.

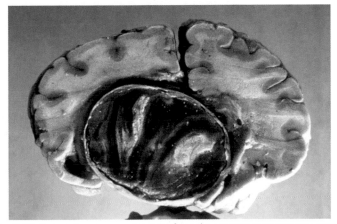

Fig. 5-56. A giant 6-cm aneurysm arising from the anterior communicating artery and causing frontal lobe compression. There is extensive central and peripheral calcification.

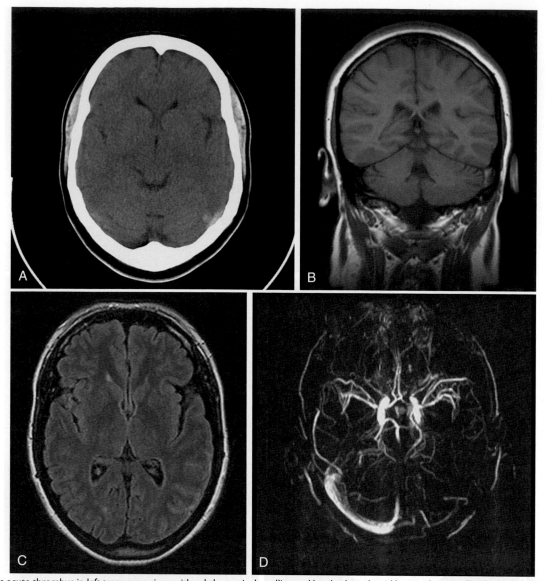

Fig. 5-61. Hyperdense acute thrombus in left transverse sinus with subtle cortical swelling and local subarachnoid hemorrhage on FLAIR. Coronal T1-weighted image demonstrates large left transverse sinus with acute thrombus. No flow is seen on MR venography. **A,** CT, **B,** Coronal T1-weighted MRI. **C,** Axial FLAIR MRI. **D,** MR venography.

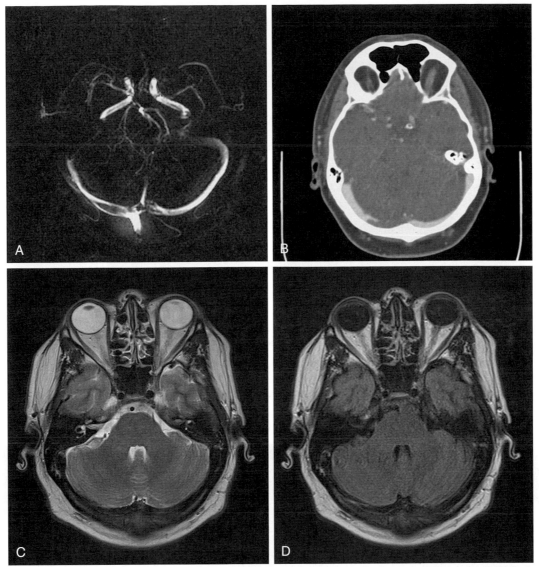

Fig. 5-62. Nonocclusive thrombus best seen on CT venography. **A,** MR venography. **B,** CT venography. **C,** Axial T2-weighted MRI. **D,** Axial FLAIR MRI.

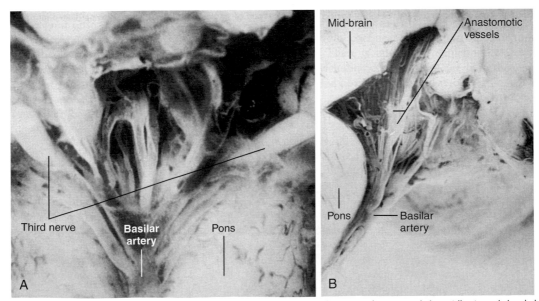

Fig. 5-63. Moyamoya disease. Termination of the basilar artery with hypertrophic arterial branches extending toward the midbrain and the thalamus. **A,** Anterior view. **B,** Lateral view.

patients are depressed, but treatment of the depressive illness appears to have no effect on cognitive function.

INVESTIGATION

CT scanning is commonly the first investigative technique used, principally to exclude other pathologic processes rather than to define specific imaging changes that might be linked to Alzheimer's disease. Only rarely does CT identify a reversible cause of a dementia syndrome. It has proved disappointing when attempts have been made to correlate the degree of dementia with certain radiologic characteristics. A relatively poor correlation exists between measures of cortical atrophy and the results of psychometric evaluation. Measurement of ventricular size has provided a better correlation, although there is disagreement about the best index of ventricular dilation. Serial scanning may help by providing evidence of progressive ventricular dilatation (Fig. 6-4).

MRI scanning provides more specific information than CT. A reduction in volume of the hippocampal formation and the parahippocampal gyrus on MRI are predictive for the development of Alzheimer's disease. Atrophy in the medial temporal region correlates

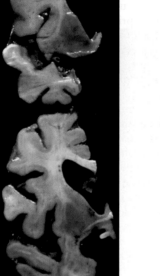
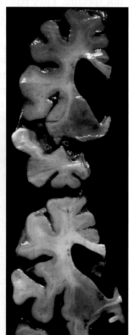

Fig. 6-1. Alzheimer's disease. Moderate to severe gyral atrophy with narrow gyri and wide sulci, along with marked ventricular dilation reflecting loss of white matter.

with neuropsychological performance in Alzheimer's disease (Fig. 6-5). Atrophy of the corpus callosum is a prominent feature of Alzheimer's disease, the severity of the dementia correlating mainly with atrophy of the rostral and mid sections.

Regional cerebral blood flow studies, using single-photon emission computed tomography (SPECT), are of limited value in the diagnosis of Alzheimer's disease. Flow in the posterotemporal and inferoparietal areas correlates with the severity of dementia and shows progressive decline on serial studies (Fig. 6-6).

Positron emission tomography scanning demonstrates a bilateral reduction of oxygen use and glucose uptake principally in the parietal and temporal lobes in the early stages, with later involvement of the frontal lobes. Impaired metabolism as measured by ^{18}F-fluorodeoxyglucose PET appears predictive of cognitive decline in Alzheimer's disease.

Various CSF markers have been studied for their possible role in diagnosis. CSF tau protein levels are higher, and amyloid-β-peptide levels lower, in Alzheimer's disease than in controls. In addition, CSF levels of neuronal thread protein tend to be elevated.

TREATMENT

Cholinesterase inhibitors have proved to have a limited role in the treatment of Alzheimer's disease. Agents available include donepezil, rivastigmine, and galantamine. Patients so treated show significant improvement in terms of global function and on some measures of cognitive function, but then they continue an inevitable decline.

DEMENTIA AND LEWY BODIES

Dementia and Lewy bodies are increasingly recognized as a cause of dementia. Alternative terms for the condition include cortical Lewy body disease and diffuse Lewy body disease. In many cases, the pathologic changes include those of Alzheimer's disease, particularly senile plaques (tangles may be absent in cases of dementia with Lewy bodies). The condition is characterized by, in addition to dementia, substantial fluctuations in the degree of cognitive impairment and visual hallucinations. Frequent falls are typical, and the patients are often excessively sensitive to neuroleptic medication. Clinical diagnosis can be difficult, however, and many cases go unrecognized until postmortem examination.

The brainstem changes of the disease mirror those of Parkinson's disease. Lewy bodies are found in the cerebral cortex, principally in the small neurons of the deeper cortical layers (Fig. 6-7).

FRONTOTEMPORAL DEMENTIA AND LOBAR ATROPHIES

Although once considered synonymous with Pick's disease, the frontotemporal dementias are a diverse group of conditions, with similar clinical features but different pathologic substrates. Frontal lobe

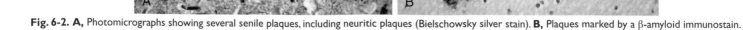

Fig. 6-2. A, Photomicrographs showing several senile plaques, including neuritic plaques (Bielschowsky silver stain). **B,** Plaques marked by a β-amyloid immunostain.

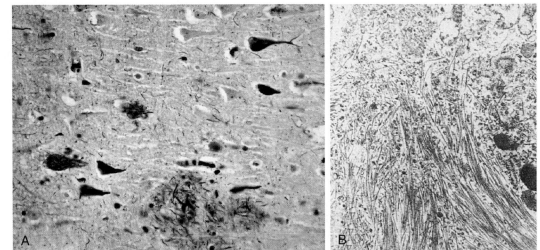

Fig. 6-3. Alzheimer's disease. **A,** Neuro-fibrillary tangles (Bielschowsky stain). **B,** Electron micrograph showing part of a neurofibrillary tangle (×3000).

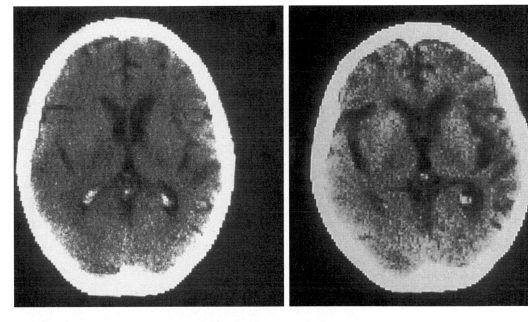

Fig. 6-4. Alzheimer's disease. Serial CT scans showing the progression of cortical atrophy and ventricular dilatation over a 2-year period.

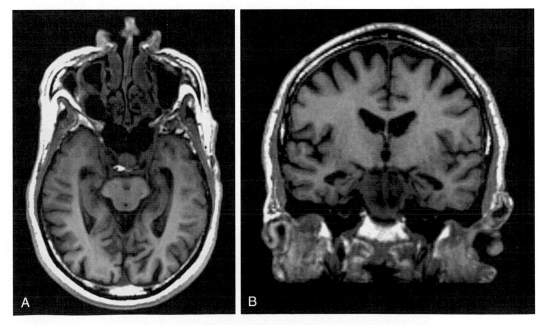

Fig. 6-5. Alzheimer's disease. Axial **(A)** and coronal **(B)** T1-weighted MRI demonstrating hippocampal atrophy.

deficits are often prominent, with alteration of social behavior and personality coupled with impaired judgment and insight. Speech output falls eventually to a state of mutism. Various behavioral disturbances occur, including agitated depression and excess alcohol intake. Extrapyramidal signs may be found, coupled with frontal lobe release signs. The diseases under this umbrella include the following:
Frontotemporal lobar degeneration (FTLD) with tau pathology
Pick's disease
Familial tauopathies
FTLD with ubiquitin-only immunoreactive change
FTLD with motor neuron disease (MND)
FTLD with neurofilament inclusions

FRONTOTEMPORAL LOBAR DEGENERATION WITH TAU PATHOLOGY

This group includes Pick's disease and the familial frontotemporal dementia with Parkinsonism (see Chapter 7).

PICK'S DISEASE

Pick's disease is rare. It occurs sporadically or as a familial disorder inherited as an autosomal dominant. It generally appears in the sixth decade. The atrophy principally involves the frontotemporal lobes typically producing "knife-edge" gyri (Fig. 6-8).

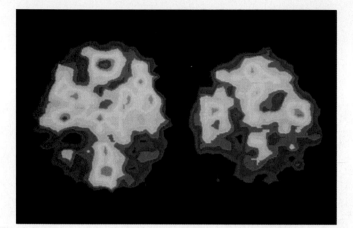

Fig. 6-6. Alzheimer's disease. SPECT scan showing reduction of temporoparietal blood flow.

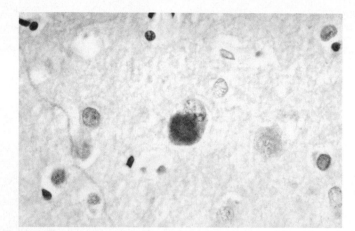

Fig. 6-7. Cortical Lewy body disease. Cortical neuron containing a Lewy body (immunoperoxidase anti-ubiquitin, hematoxylin).

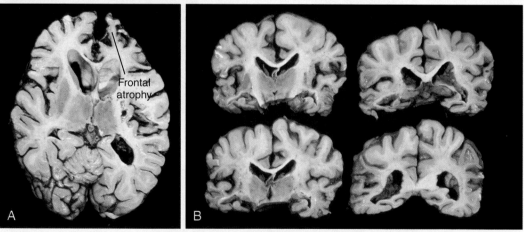

Fig. 6-8. Pick's disease. **A,** Axial plane section. There is severe frontal lobe gyral atrophy. **B,** Grouping of four coronal slices showing temporal atrophy with "knife-edge" gyri.

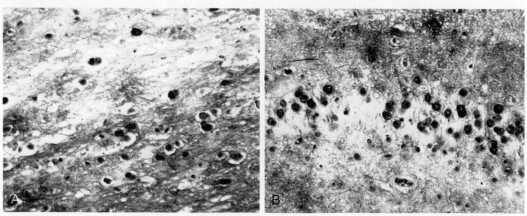

Fig. 6-9. Pick's disease. Pick bodies in cortical neurons and in hippocampal dentate gyral neurons (Bielschowsky stain).

The essential microscopic finding is the Pick body, a neuronal cell inclusion that takes up silver stain (Fig. 6-9). Pick bodies are found in pyramidal neurons and dentate granule cells in the hippocampus, and in the affected areas of the neocortex. Tau protein is present in the Pick body but differs from that found in other tau disorders. Neuronal loss is severe in the affected areas, along with astrocytic gliosis. Swollen neurons are found, again taking up silver stain.

Clinical features include disturbance of mood and personality with inappropriate behavior. Disturbances of memory, intellect, and visuospatial function appear later. Many patients have perseverative speech, with repetition of particular words or phrases.

Scanning demonstrates the distribution of the atrophic process (Fig. 6-10). SPECT scanning shows reduction of flow in the anterior aspect of the hemisphere (Fig. 6-11).

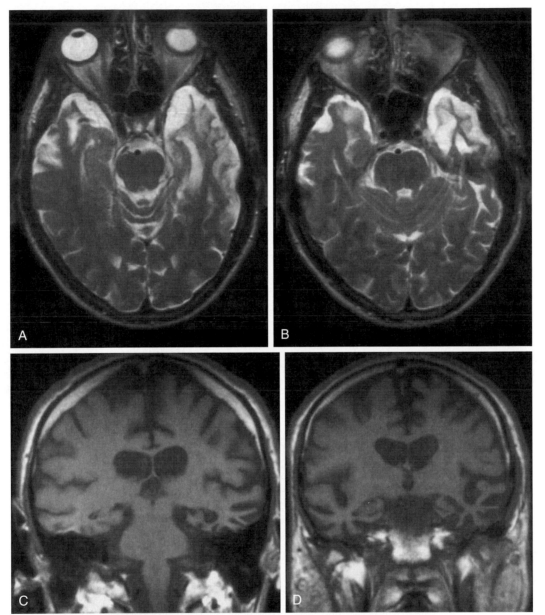

Fig. 6-10. Pick's disease. T2-weighted axial slices (**A** and **B**) and T1-weighted coronal slices (**C** and **D**).

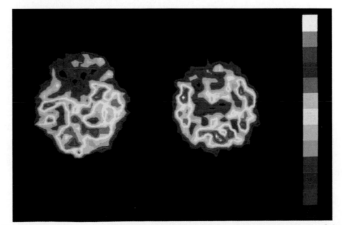

Fig. 6-11. Pick's disease. SPECT scan showing reduction of flow in the anterior aspect of the hemispheres.

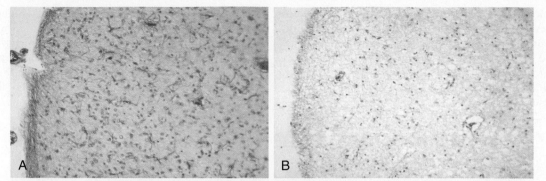

Fig. 6-12. Frontotemporal dementia. **A,** Mild to moderate cortical gliosis (H&E, ×100). **B,** Spongiotic changes (phosphotungstic acid hematoxylin, ×100).

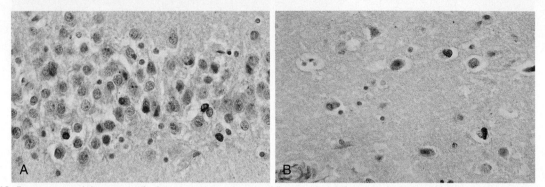

Fig. 6-13. Frontotemporal dementia with ubiquitin immunoreactivity. Ubiqinated cytoplasmic inclusions in hippocampal dentate granule cells.

FAMILIAL TAUPATHIES

Frontotemporal degeneration and Parkinsonism linked to chromosome 17 are discussed in Chapter 7.

FRONTOTEMPORAL LOBAR DEGENERATION WITH UBIQUITIN-ONLY IMMUNOREACTIVE CHANGES

Patients with FTLD with ubiquitin-only immunoreactive changes have the clinical characteristics of frontotemporal dementia. There is appropriately distributed neuronal loss with swollen neurons and, in severe cases, status spongiosus (Fig. 6-12). Neuronal inclusions are found and are identical to those found in patients with dementia associated with MND, and they show ubiquitin immunoreactivity (Fig. 6-13).

Other frontotemporal degenerations include those associated with motor neuron disease and those with neurofilament inclusions.

The clinical patterns associated with the frontotemporal dementias (FTDs) fall into several categories. The pattern already referred to is defined as the frontal variant of FTD. In addition, there are semantic dementia, which is associated with loss of memory for words, impaired comprehension, and word substitution, and primary progressive aphasia characterized by a slowly progressive nonfluent aphasia.

ARTERIOSCLEROTIC DEMENTIA

The criteria for making the diagnosis of arteriosclerotic or vascular dementia have limitations. The underlying pathology is not uniform. Some patients have diffuse small vessel disease, others have multiple infarcts relating to large vessel disease, and still others have dementia because of a global perfusion failure. Furthermore, vascular changes

in the brain may coexist with other pathologies—for example, those of Alzheimer's disease. Neuroimaging is of critical importance in making the diagnosis, although certain clinical features may suggest the possibility.

Typically, patients tend to have a history of strokelike events and may show an abrupt or stepwise deterioration in cognitive function. Focal symptoms or signs are likely, gait apraxia is common, and nocturnal confusion is often conspicuous. Varying scoring systems have been devised (e.g., the Hachinski score) to further the diagnosis, but they are prone to error. Vascular dementia accounts for perhaps 10% of cases of dementia overall.

In small vessel disease (subcortical arteriosclerotic encephalopathy, Binswanger's disease), there is hyalinization of small arteries and arterioles resulting in rarefaction of the deep white matter, particularly of the frontal and temporal lobes. There is commonly coexisting lacunar infarction, typically concentrating in the basal ganglia, thalamus, and pons. In addition, some patients display granular cortical atrophy, the result of widespread cortical microinfarcts.

Macroinfarcts, even when multiple, seldom produce a global cognitive decline. Global perfusion failure is liable to result in watershed infarction, typically with ischemic damage to the hippocampus.

IMAGING

CT or MRI demonstrates either multiple infarcts or diffuse white matter disease (Fig. 6-14). SPECT or PET can help distinguish multi-infarct dementia from Alzheimer's disease. In the former, patchy reduction of flow is found scattered throughout the hemispheres (Fig. 6-15). In the latter, metabolic activity, assessed with ^{18}F-fluorodeoxyglucose scanning, reveals asymmetrical cortical and subcortical changes.

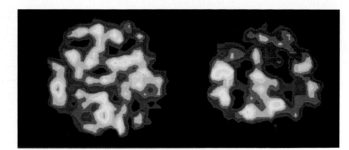

Fig. 6-15. Multi-infarct dementia. SPECT showing patchy blood flow reduction in both hemispheres.

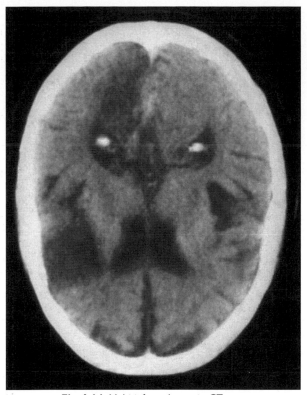

Fig. 6-14. Multi-infarct dementia. CT scan.

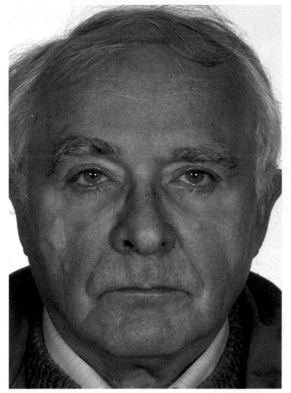

Fig. 7-25. Facial appearance of patient with progressive supranuclear palsy.

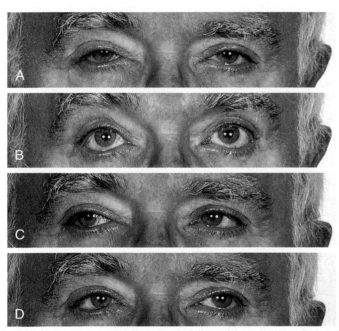

Fig. 7-26. Progressive supranuclear palsy. A, Failure of downward gaze. B, Relative preservation of upward gaze. C and D, Relative preservation of horizontal gaze.

MULTISYSTEM ATROPHY

In its fully developed form, multisystem atrophy (MSA) represents a combination, in varying degrees, of olivopontocerebellar degeneration, striatonigral degeneration, and degeneration of the intermediolateral column of the thoracic and lumbar spinal cord.

Olivopontocerebellar atrophy can occur in isolation and is usually sporadic, and its diagnosis prone to error. It accounts for a substantial proportion of sporadic, late-onset cases of cerebellar ataxia as well as some cases that demonstrate autosomal dominant inheritance. Patients present with an ataxia of gait and limbs, accompanied by dysarthria and abnormalities of extraocular movement. Corticospinal tract signs may emerge. Pathologically, there is neuronal loss and gliosis in the brainstem and cerebellum (Fig. 7-34). PET studies

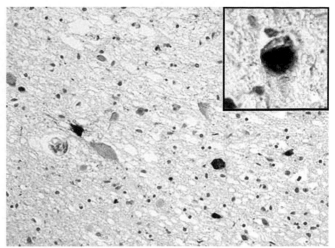

Fig. 7-27. Tau pathology in locus caeruleus is composed of dystrophic neuritis and globose tangle-like inclusions. *Inset:* High-power magnification of neuronal inclusions (anti-tau monoclonal antibody AT8).

reveal hypometabolism in the cerebellum and brainstem (Fig. 7-35). A proportion of these patients later develop the features of MSA. The figure amounted to a third of such cases, followed over a period of 14 years in one study. The development of MSA has a substantial, adverse effect on survival in such cases.

Striatonigral degeneration has distinctive features that separate it from idiopathic Parkinson's disease. There is striking nerve cell loss in the putamen, with lesser changes, accompanied by gliosis, in the caudate and globus pallidus. The substantia nigra and locus caeruleus both show depigmentation and cell loss. Lewy bodies are usually absent, as are neurofibrillary tangles (Fig. 7-36). In its pure form, the condition can be difficult to distinguish from idiopathic Parkinson's disease. Certain features suggest the diagnosis, however, including the absence of tremor, the presence of unexplained falls, and a failure to respond to levodopa.

A profound autonomic failure, associated with loss of cells in the intermediolateral column of the thoracic and lumbar spinal cords, may occur in isolation (Shy-Drager syndrome), in association with a parkinsonian syndrome due to degenerative changes in the substantia nigra and elsewhere, identical to those of idiopathic Parkinson's disease, or, as part of multisystem atrophy. The pathologic correlate of the autonomic failure is neuronal loss from the intermediolateral cell column of the thoracolumbar spinal cord (Fig. 7-37). Various tests have been devised to analyze the autonomic failure in greater detail. The pressor response to infusion of tyramine reflects noradrenaline stores in the sympathetic nerve endings, and to noradrenaline measures the degree of α-adrenoreceptor sensitivity (Fig. 7-38).

Urinary symptoms and studies of bladder function may allow distinction to be made between Parkinson's disease and MSA. The striated muscle of the external anal and urethral sphincter is innervated in part by fibers originating from Onuf's nucleus in the sacral spinal cord. Neuronal loss in Onuf's nucleus leads to signs of denervation and reinnervation in anal and urethral sphincter muscle as seen with electromyography (EMG). Sphincter muscle abnormalities are described in 90% or so of patients, whereas such changes are absent in idiopathic Parkinson's disease. Whereas patients with MSA with sympathetic neurocirculatory failure have normal cardiac sympathetic innervation, patients with Parkinson's disease have evidence of cardiac sympathetic denervation as shown by SPECT studies utilizing metaiodobenzylguanidine (MIBG), a guanidine analogue that shares the same neuronal transport and storage mechanism with noradrenaline. Such changes may be evident before symptomatic development of a parkinsonian state.

Brain imaging can reveal characteristic changes. Striatal abnormalities include putaminal atrophy and putaminal hypointensity relative to the pallidum on T2-weighted images, as well as slit-like signal changes at the posterolateral putaminal margin. Infratentorial

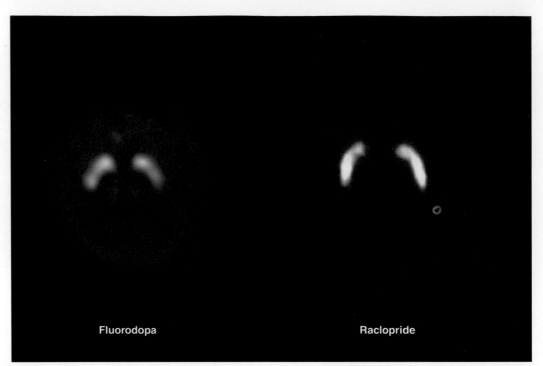

Fluorodopa   Raclopride

Fig. 7-28. PET scan. Frontotemporal dementia. Reduced fluorodopa uptake and increased raclopride binding in the striatum.

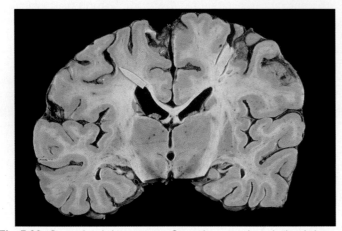

Fig. 7-29. Corticobasal degeneration. Coronal section through the thalami and red nuclei showing atrophy around the rolandic fissure *(arrow)*.

changes include atrophy and signal change in the pons and middle cerebellar peduncles. A "hot-cross bun" sign has been described in the pons on T2-weighted MR images (Fig. 7-39).

The cellular pathology of MSA is characterized by the abnormal accumulation of the protein α-synuclein. Various cytoplasmic inclusions are described, involving glial cytoplasm, neuronal cytoplasm, neuronal and glial nuclei, and neuropil threads (Fig. 7-40).

Patients present with varying combinations of autonomic failure, parkinsonism, and cerebellar ataxia. Onset is most commonly in the sixth decade, with men being rather more frequently affected than women. Other features include severe dysarthria, stridor, and dystonia. Generally, response to dopa is poor, but a small proportion of patients respond well, at least initially, and may develop dopa-induced dyskinesias affecting the axial muscles.

OTHER PARKINSONIAN SYNDROMES

Hallervorden-Spatz disease is now described under the title of pantothenate kinase–associated neurodegeneration. There is deficiency of the relevant gene, and the condition is usually inherited as a recessive. The condition generally starts before the mid teens with a combination of dystonia, tremor, and rigidity. Pyramidal signs and dementia

follow. Later onset occurs typically with an extrapyramidal syndrome with dementia. MR images, using T2-weighting, reveal signal change in the globus pallidus with a central hyperintensity ("eye of the tiger") (Fig. 7-41). The globus pallidus is atrophic and discolored. It shows neuronal loss and gliosis with pigment deposition. The pigment is a mixture of lipofuscin, neuromelanin, and iron (Fig. 7-42).

ARTERIOSCLEROTIC PARKINSONISM

The concept of arteriosclerotic parkinsonism, introduced by Critchley, has been revived. The vascular substrate is usually in the form of lacunar infarction and arteriosclerotic leukoencephalopathy (Fig. 7-43). Rigidity and bradykinesia predominate, with an emphasis on the lower limbs. Rest tremor is uncommon. There may be additional signs declaring this not to be idiopathic Parkinson's disease, including pyramidal signs, pseudobulbar palsy, and cerebellar signs. Imaging reveals multiple lacunar infarction, with or without Binswanger changes. Dopa therapy is usually ineffective.

DYSTONIA

Dystonia is defined as a syndrome of sustained muscle contractions, usually producing twisting and repetitive movements or abnormal postures. Classification is complex and based on age of onset, etiology, and distribution. Genetic factors are incorporated into the classification scheme where possible (Box 7-2). Early-onset dystonia tends to begin in one or more limbs before eventually spreading to the trunk. Adult-onset dystonia initially affects cranial-, cervical-, or brachial-innervated muscles and tends to remain localized.

PRIMARY DYSTONIA

Early-onset primary torsion dystonia was originally termed dystonia musculorum deformans. It is inherited as an autosomal dominant and in many families, whether Ashkenazi Jews or not, is linked to the 9q34 chromosome. The DYT1 gene encodes a novel 332–amino acid protein, torsin A. Phenotypic variation is recognized both within and between affected kindreds. Accordingly, focal manifestations or craniocervical presentations are recognized. Other forms of generalized dystonia have been mapped to chromosome 8p and chromosome 1p.

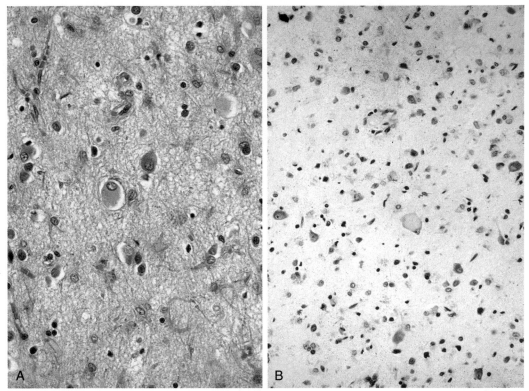

Fig. 7-30. Corticobasal degeneration. Cerebral cortex showing severe gliosis with an achromatic neuron. **A,** Stained with Luxol fast blue, H&E (×250). **B,** Stained with cresyl violet (×250).

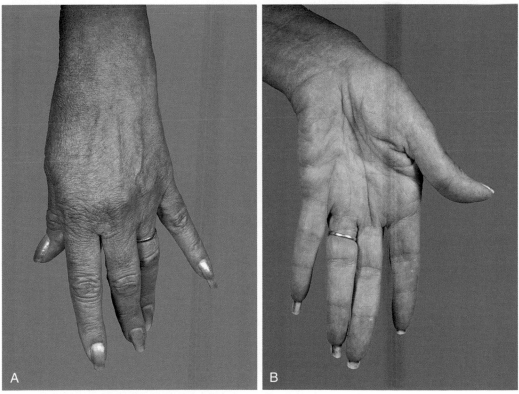

Fig. 7-31. Corticobasal degeneration. Dystonic posturing of the left hand.

Primary Focal Dystonia
This the commonest form of dystonia. Although it is usually sporadic, autosomal dominant inheritance is described.

Spasmodic Torticollis
In spasmodic torticollis, intermittent or sustained contraction of the neck muscles produces abnormal head posturing, most often rotational. Some patients enter a period of remission, only to relapse at a later date (Fig. 7-44). Retrocollis may accompany the torticollis.

In long-standing cases, pain, sometimes secondary to degenerative disease of the cervical spine, is likely.

Selective peripheral denervation procedures have been used in the past for torticollis and still have a role if the patient has become resistant to botulinum toxin (Fig. 7-45). Results are unsatisfactory, however, if the patient has substantial cervical spine degenerative disease.

Botulinum toxin, either type A or type B, acts by inhibiting release of acetylcholine at the neuromuscular junction. The injections need

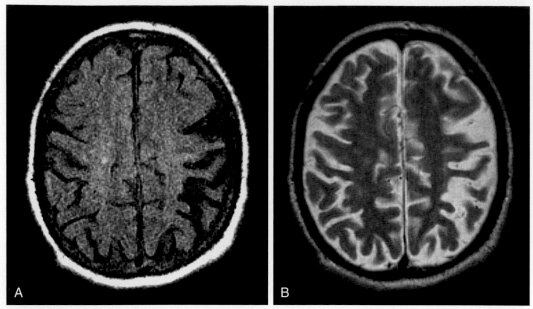

Fig. 7-32. Corticobasal degeneration. Flair and T2-weighted MRI demonstrating predominant left cortical atrophy.

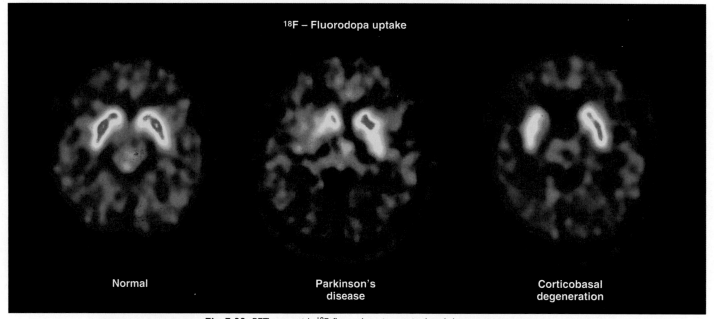

Fig. 7-33. PET scan with ¹⁸F-fluorodopa in corticobasal degeneration.

to be repeated every 3 to 4 months, and the effects may diminish with time, partly because of antibody formation.

For refractory dystonia, various forms of deep brain stimulation have been devised that particularly target the posteroventral globus pallidus internus. The procedure has been applied to cases of both generalized and focal dystonia. The procedure is often helpful in terms of pain control, but its long-term role in management remains unsettled.

Blepharospasm

Blepharospasm, initially intermittent, can eventually be so persistent that the patient is effectively blind. In the early stages, episodic clonic contraction of the lids occurs, sometimes triggered by certain physical activities. In some patients, the spasm can be relieved by touching either eyelid (Fig. 7-46).

Oromandibular Dystonia

The oromandibular type of focal dystonia results in involuntary movements of the tongue and mouth, typically triggered by attempts to eat or speak. Dysphagia and dysarthria are inevitable. Tongue trauma is frequent (Fig. 7-47).

Spasmodic (Spastic) Dysphonia

By affecting the laryngeal muscles, spasmodic dysphonia imparts a strained, strangulated quality to the voice.

All these forms of cranial dystonia can occur in isolation, or be accompanied by an essential tremor or a dystonic limb tremor.

Writer's Cramp

Many focal dystonias affect the dominant upper limb. The most common is writer's cramp. Patients describe a discomfort in the hand, associated with the use of excessive force. Abnormal posturing is typical (Fig. 7-48). The writing correspondingly deteriorates (Fig. 7-49). Sometimes, abnormal posturing spreads to proximal muscles. In most patients, other skilled activities remain unaffected. Treatment is often unsuccessful. Patients may be best advised to learn to write with the other hand, although this may then succumb to the same problem. Selective injection of botulinum toxin into affected muscles can produce short-term improvement, but the effect tends to be poorly sustained after multiple injections. Other occupational cramps affect musicians, keyboard operators, and hairdressers.

SECONDARY DYSTONIAS

A vast array of conditions can cause secondary dystonia. Dopa-responsive dystonia is a childhood-onset-dystonia with limb involvement. Typically, there is a diurnal variation in symptoms, with the condition worsening toward the end of the day. Additional features include hyperreflexia and parkinsonism. A dramatic response occurs to low-dose dopa and sometimes to anticholinergic therapy. The gene responsible, mapped to chromosome 14, is associated with mutations of GTP-cyclohydrolase 1. Hemidystonia is associated with lesions, predominantly vascular, in the contralateral thalamus, putamen, or caudate (Fig. 7-50). Postanoxic dystonia is usually the result of a prenatal insult but is sometimes seen after an anesthetic disaster in adult life (Fig. 7-51).

Wilson's Disease

Wilson's disease has an estimated worldwide prevalence rate of 1 in 30,000 live births. It is inherited as an autosomal recessive. A defect of copper metabolism leads to the accumulation of copper in various organs, particularly the liver and the brain. The responsible gene has been located to q14.3 on chromosome 13. The gene codes for a copper-transporting P-type ATPase. Many mutations have been described.

Increased copper deposition occurs in the liver, brain, Descemet's membrane of the cornea, and kidneys. Pathologic changes include cirrhosis of the liver (Fig. 7-52) and atrophy of the putamen, where cavitation may appear (Fig. 7-53). Histology reveals neuronal loss, fibrillary astrocytes, and lipid- and pigment-laden macrophages. Alzheimer type II astrocytes are found. Opalski cells, round cells with a small central nucleus and eosinophilic cytoplasm, are found, particularly in the globus pallidus (Fig. 7-54).

Serum ceruloplasmin levels are depressed, but the pathogenetic role of this is not clear. Urinary excretion of copper is increased.

Some 50% of patients with Wilson's disease have manifestations of liver disease before the onset of neurologic dysfunction. Features of this include poor growth, jaundice, ascites, and hematemesis.

The neurologic picture is dominated by a variety of movement disorders. Tremor, more often a fine-action tremor than the classic wing-beating movement, dystonia, and choreoathetoid movements are all seen (Fig. 7-55). Dysarthria and dysphagia are often prominent, typically accompanied by drooling of saliva.

A particular facial expression is described, associated with retraction of the upper lip (risus sardonicus) (Fig. 7-56). Psychiatric manifestations include behavioral and mood disturbances. A Kayser-Fleischer ring, resulting from copper deposition in Descemet's membrane, is virtually inevitable in patients with neuropsychiatric symptoms, although slit lamp microscopy may be necessary to detect it (Fig. 7-57).

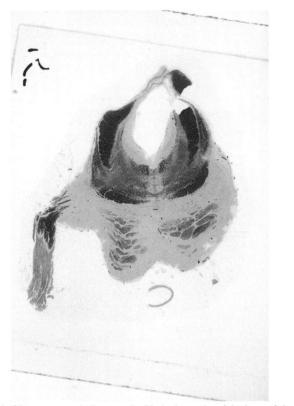

Fig. 7-34. Olivopontocerebellar atrophy. Marked atrophy of the base of the pons with loss of transverse pontine fibers. The superior cerebellar peduncles are preserved.

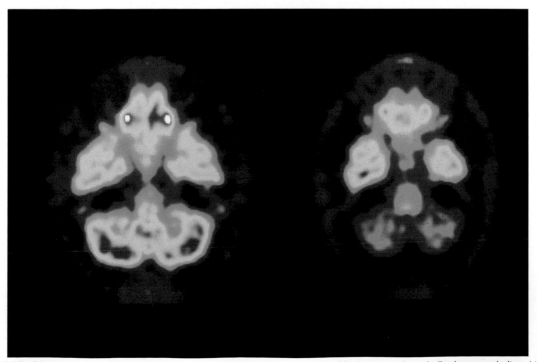

Fig. 7-35. Olivopontocerebellar atrophy. PET scan demonstrating control *(left)* and brainstem and cerebellar hypometabolism *(right)*.

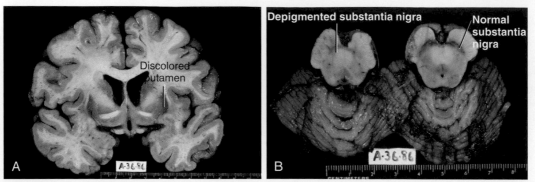

Fig. 7-36. Striatonigral degeneration. **A,** Bilateral symmetrical discoloration and degeneration of the putamen. **B,** Transverse section of midbrain showing pallor of each substantia nigra *(left)* compared with control *(right)*.

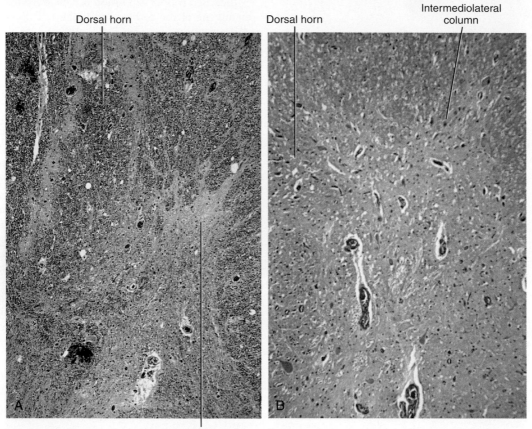

Fig. 7-37. Multisystem atrophy. **A,** Transverse section of thoracic spinal cord with almost total depletion of intermediolateral cell column neurons. **B,** Normal subject (Luxol fast blue, H&E).

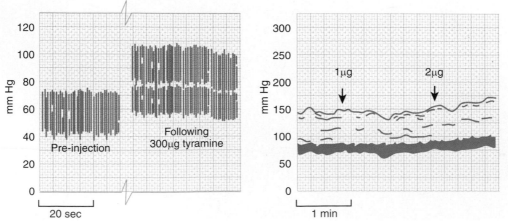

Fig. 7-38. Multisystem atrophy. Blood pressure tracings showing hypersensitivity to infusion of **A,** tyramine and **B,** noradrenaline.

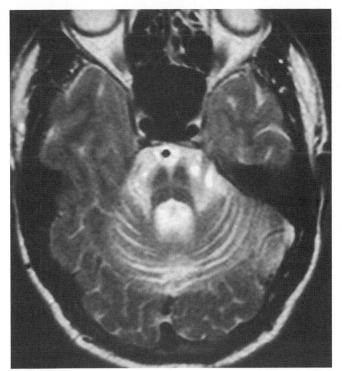

Fig. 7-39. Multisystem atrophy. T2-weighted MR image of the pons showing the "hot-cross bun" sign.

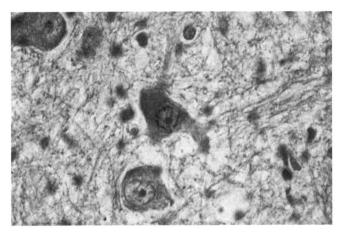

Fig. 7-40. Multisystem atrophy. Neuronal nuclear inclusion appearing as a delicate web of argyrophilic intranuclear filaments (Gallyas silver impregnation).

Biochemical markers for the diagnosis include increased urinary copper and depressed serum total copper and ceruloplasmin levels.

CT demonstrates ventricular dilatation and cortical atrophy with hypodensities in the basal ganglia (Fig. 7-58). MR is more sensitive, demonstrating increased signal in T2-weighted images in the thalamus or basal ganglia (Fig. 7-59).

Later-onset Wilson's disease (clinical manifestations beginning between 20 and 40 years of age) manifests with predominant neurologic and psychiatric symptoms. Early treatment can prevent the development of neurologic abnormalities, but if they are already present, complete remission (i.e., of the neurologic signs) occurs in only 20%. It has been suggested that patients with predominant dystonia fare less well than those with predominant tremor.

Agents capable of reducing the abnormal copper load include D-penicillamine, trientine, tetrathiomolybdate, and dimercaprol. Agents also exist that can reduce intestinal copper absorption.

Liver transplantation is recommended when there is severe liver disease, and it can apparently, at least in some cases, reverse neurologic dysfunction.

CHOREIFORM AND BALLISTIC MOVEMENTS

Sydenham's (Rheumatic) Chorea

Rheumatic chorea is rare in the West but is seen in up to 10% of patients after streptococcal infection in endemic areas (e.g., Kuwait). The preceding streptococcal infection generally occurs within the previous 1 to 6 months. Recurrences occur in up to 20% of cases. It is largely confined to the 5- to 15-years age group. The condition is considered to be the result of cross-reacting antibodies affecting the caudate nucleus. The condition is generally bilateral but sometimes unilateral. Although recovery is the rule, a mild persisting chorea, tremor, or neuropsychological deficit is well recognized. Patients with a history of Sydenham's chorea are subsequently more susceptible to chorea induced by drugs—for example, oral contraceptives.

Huntington's Disease

Huntington's disease is inherited as an autosomal dominant. The relevant gene, located to the short arm of chromosome 4, encodes a cytoplasmic protein, huntingtin. The pathologic changes predominate in the medium-sized GABAergic projection neurons of the basal ganglia, which are severely depleted. There is an associated gliosis. Atrophy of the caudate and putamen is characteristic (Fig. 7-60). Immunohistochemical staining for ubiquitin or huntingtin reveals accumulation of huntingtin in intranuclear inclusion bodies or in neurites (Fig. 7-61).

The relevant gene displays a trinucleotide repetition of over 39, compared with between five and about 36 repetitions in normal

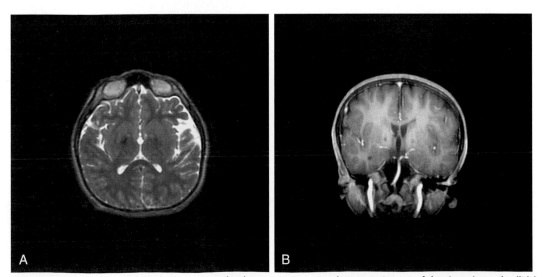

Fig. 7-41. Hallervorden-Spatz. T2-weighted axial and T1-weighted coronal MR images demonstrating eye-of-the-tiger sign and pallidal cavitation.

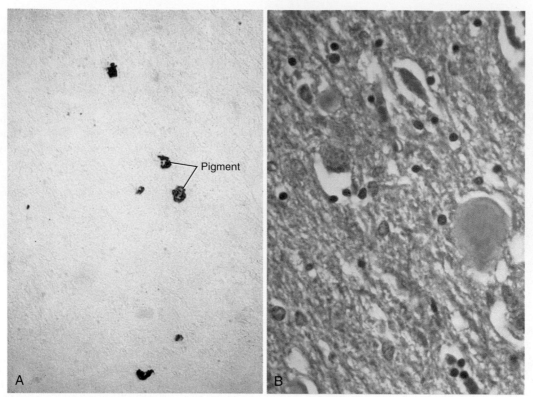

Fig. 7-42. Pantothenate kinase–associated neurodegeneration. **A,** Pigment deposition in the globus pallidus (Perls Prussian blue reaction, ×62.5). **B,** Axonal swelling (H&E, ×250).

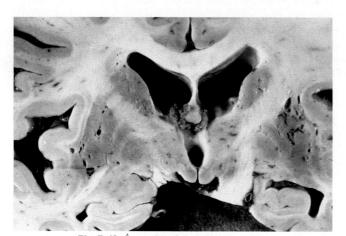

Fig. 7-43. État criblé. Coronal brain section.

BOX 7-2   CLASSIFICATION OF DYSTONIAS

By Age of Onset
- Early-onset. Tends to start in a limb
- Late-onset. Tends to start in cranial-, cervical-, or brachial-innervated muscles, and remain localized

By Distribution
- Focal (e.g., torticollis, blepharospasm)
- Segmental: contiguous body regions (e.g., face and jaw)
- Multifocal (e.g., arm and leg)
- Generalized: both legs and at least one other body region

By Cause
- Primary (idiopathic)
  - Childhood or adolescent limb onset (dominant; penetrance 30%, many resulting from DYT1 GAG deletions)
  - Mixed phenotype, child or adult onset; may begin in limb, neck, or cranial innervated muscles (autosomal dominant with incomplete penetrance; mapped to chromosome 8 [DYT6] in some families)
  - Adult cervical-, cranial-, or brachial-innervated onset (autosomal dominant with very reduced penetrance)
- Secondary
  - Genetically determined conditions (e.g., dopa-responsive dystonia, Wilson's disease, homocystinuria, neuroacanthocytosis)
  - Environmental causes (e.g., head injury, stroke, tumor, peripheral injury)
  - Dystonia as part of parkinsonism
  - Psychogenic dystonia

---

individuals. The expanded gene fragment can be detected by a polymerase chain reaction–based assay.

The disease occurs in all races, with a prevalence of 2 to 7 in 100,000 although regional clustering occurs. All patients harboring the gene eventually develop the disease. In most, onset is in the third or fourth decade of life, but about 10% of cases develop before the age of 20, and a further 10% beyond the age of 60. Age of onset inversely correlates with the length of the trinucleotide repeat expansion.

Anticipation occurs—that is, the disease tends to manifest earlier in later generations. Juvenile cases are more likely to show paternal transmission. In such cases, (the Westphal form) chorea may be inconspicuous, with a predominance of akinesia and rigidity, sometimes coupled with dystonia, myoclonus, ataxia, and seizures (Fig. 7-62).

In more typical cases, the onset of the movement disorder is subtle with slight restlessness of, say, the fingers, mouth, or tongue before more generalized movements appear. Later, dystonia, rigidity, and akinesia become more prominent. Other features include a general motor clumsiness, dysarthria, and dysphagia.

Subtle personality changes in the form of paranoia, anxiety, or antisocial behavior can precede the movement disorder by years. Later, overt cognitive decline is apparent, with particular emphasis on defects of initiation, psychomotor speed, and efficiency in attention, planning, and learning.

Investigative findings, although often suggestive, do not provide specific confirmation of the disease and are now generally irrelevant. The electroencephalogram tends to be featureless and of low voltage. Measurements of caudate atrophy, using the ratio of the intercaudate to the frontal horn span, incompletely differentiate the condition from Alzheimer's disease.

MRI allows some differentiation of the choreic and rigid forms. In the former, caudate atrophy is present, but there is seldom abnormal signal intensity in the caudate or putamen. In the rigid form, caudate atrophy is equally prominent, but, in addition, T2-weighted images demonstrate increased signal intensity in the caudate and putamen (Fig. 7-63).

SPECT demonstrates a reduction in regional blood flow compared with controls, using 2-fluoro-2-deoxy-D-glucose labeled with radioactive fluoride (^{18}F). PET scanning demonstrates depressed striatal metabolism in affected individuals (Fig. 7-64).

Therapy is severely limited. Some psychiatric symptoms and the hyperkinesias may respond to relevant drug therapy. Fetal transplantation to the striatum has been attempted with only modest benefit.

OTHER CHOREIFORM DISORDERS

Chorea is a recognized complication of systemic lupus erythematosus and may be a presenting feature. A predominantly unilateral chorea is an occasional complication of oral contraceptive therapy and may

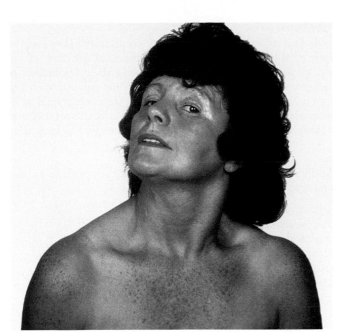

Fig. 7-44. Spasmodic torticollis. A characteristic head posture. Contraction of the left sternomastoid is particularly prominent.

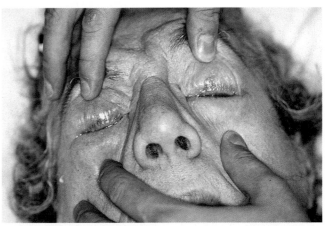

Fig. 7-46. Blepharospasm.

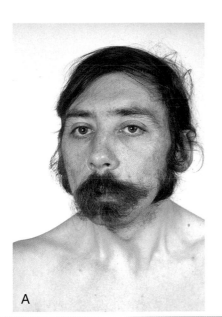

A

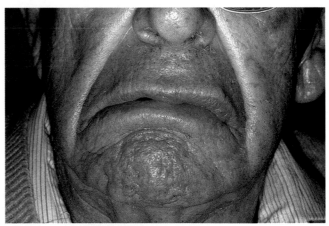

Fig. 7-47. Oromandibular dystonia.

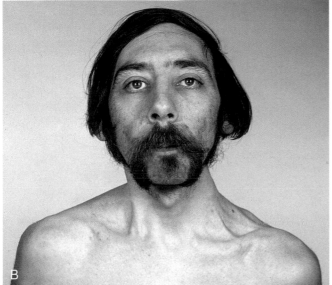

B

Fig. 7-45. Spasmodic torticollis. Neck posture before **(A)** and after **(B)** cervical rhizotomy and accessory nerve division.

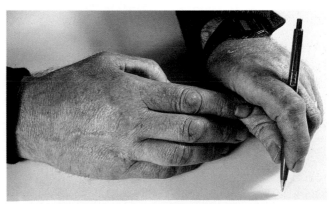

Fig. 7-48. Writer's cramp. Abnormal hand posture.

occur in pregnancy. Infective processes causing chorea include HIV infection and variant Creutzfeldt-Jakob disease. Chorea has been described in polycythemia rubra vera and thyrotoxicosis. Chorea is occasionally seen after an acute stroke. The problem, usually associated with lesions of the basal ganglia and adjacent white matter, tends to remit.

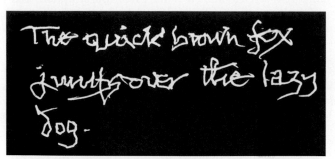

Fig. 7-49. Writer's cramp. An example of the patient's script.

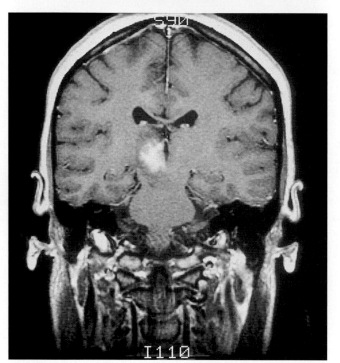

Fig. 7-50. MRI scan demonstrating gadolinium enhancement in a thalamic tumor. The patient had presented with hemidystonia.

Hemiballismus

Ballistic movements are wild and flinging in quality. They have been considered as part of a continuum with chorea at the other extreme, partly because ballistic movements, during their resolution, may evolve into a typical choreiform picture. Most patients with hemiballismus have a lesion, usually vascular, in the contralateral subthalamic nucleus. The condition usually resolves spontaneously and is best controlled in the acute stages by dopaminergic blocking agents.

Tremor

A classification system for tremor has been developed and no doubt will be subject to further revision.

Enhanced physiologic tremor
Classical essential tremor
Primary orthostatic tremor
Task- and position-specific tremors
Dystonic tremor
Parkinsonian tremor
Cerebellar tremor
Holmes's tremor (rubral or midbrain tremor)
Palatal tremor
Drug-induced and toxic tremor
Peripheral neuropathic tremor
Psychogenic tremor

Essential tremor is inherited as an autosomal dominant, although many cases appear sporadically. The movement principally affects the upper limbs but sometimes involves the head or voice. Misdiagnosis is common. Its prevalence is reported to lie between 0.4% and 3.9%. Alcohol is capable of temporarily abolishing the tremor in about 50% of cases.

Primary orthostatic tremor has a frequency of 14 to 18 Hz. The predominant complaint is of a feeling of unsteadiness while standing, although the tremor can be detected in other situations—for example, when exerting an active isometric force from a supine position. The underlying source of the tremor is central, but it has not been identified. Drug treatments include primidone, valproate, clonazepam, and gabapentin.

Some of the distinguishing features of psychogenic tremor include abrupt onset, fluctuating course, onset in one extremity, and distractibility.

Myoclonus

Myoclonus consists of shocklike involuntary movements, usually the result of brief bursts of muscle activity. Myoclonus can originate from the cortex, subcortex, brainstem, or spinal cord.

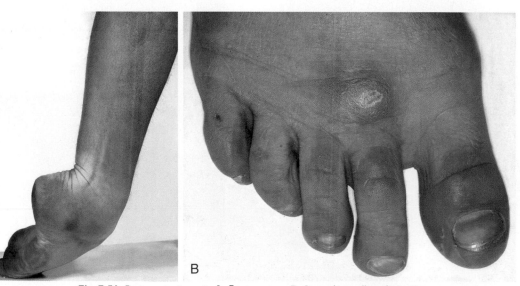

Fig. 7-51. Postanoxic dystonia. **A,** Foot posture. **B,** Secondary callous formation.

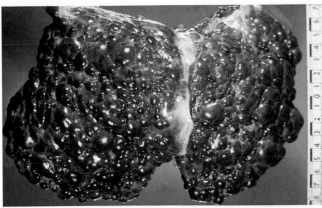

Fig. 7-52. Wilson's disease. Postnecrotic cirrhosis.

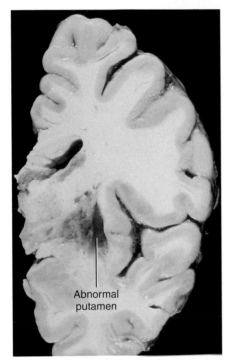

Abnormal
putamen

Fig. 7-53. Wilson's disease. Coronal brain slice showing cavitation and discoloration of the putamen, with lesser changes in the caudate and globus pallidus.

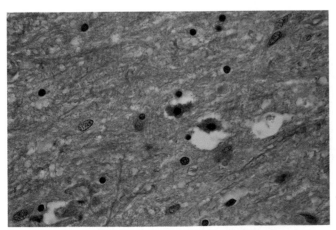

Fig. 7-54. Wilson's disease. Opalski cells *(arrows)*.

Cortical myoclonus is the consequence of an abnormal discharge in the sensorimotor cortex with propagation in the corticospinal tract. Epileptic myoclonus may be confined to single muscle jerks or to repetitive focal jerking (epilepsia partialis continua), or it may be part of an epileptic syndrome in which other seizure types occur.

Brainstem myoclonus usually results in generalized jerks rather than focal discharges. Palatal myoclonus, or tremor, manifests as a rhythmic palatal movement. The condition may be essential, causing an ear click because of rhythmic contraction of tensor veli palatini and not associated with focal brainstem pathology, or symptomatic, in which a focal brainstem lesion is present, typically affecting a circuit between the red nucleus, inferior olivary nucleus, and dentate nucleus. The consequent hypertrophy of the contralateral inferior olive can be detected on imaging. In this situation, the myoclonus is caused by contraction of levator veli palatini.

Spinal myoclonus may be segmental or multisegmental. Focal myoclonus is usually the consequence of an underlying structural lesion, but multiple level spinal myoclonus is commonly idiopathic. Here, there are repetitive axial jerks, typically beginning in the abdominal muscles and then spreading. The diagnosis can be confirmed using EMG.

Psychogenic myoclonus is recognized, often accompanied by an abnormal psychological state and evidence of non organic motor or sensory deficit.

Tics

Isolated tics are quite common in childhood, usually remitting within a year or so of onset. Motor tics are brief, rapid, jerking movements of individual muscles, groups of muscles, or whole body parts. Examples include facial grimacing, abdominal jerking, and limb movement. Complex motor tics produce patterned and coordinated movements. Tics are triggered by stressful situations and are, at least temporarily, suppressible.

Tourette's syndrome is characterized by the presence of multiple motor and vocal tics, usually appearing between the ages of 4 and 11. Both simple and complex movements materialize. Additional features include echolalia and coprophenomena. Accompanying psychological disturbances include obsessive–compulsive disorder and attention deficit hyperactivity disorder. The prevalence is estimated at 5 in 10,000 with a male-to-female ratio of 4:1. It seems most likely that the condition is inherited as an autosomal dominant with incomplete penetrance, but other genetic models have been suggested. Structural neuroimaging has proved unhelpful, and data from imaging and neurochemical studies regarding the dopaminergic system have been contradictory. Dopaminergic blocking agents, particularly haloperidol, remain the drugs of choice in management.

Tardive Dyskinesia

Tardive dyskinesia encompasses a range of involuntary movement disorders (choreiform, athetoid, or dystonic) encountered during the course of neuroleptic treatment. A minimum of 3 months' exposure to the agent is required, with the persistence of movements beyond 1 month of drug withdrawal. The most common movements are orofacial and lingual (Fig. 7-65). Other movements include blepharospasm and involvement of the proximal limbs and trunk. Dystonic posturing is sometimes the predominant feature and tardive dystonia is sometimes classified separately. Other movements include akathisia and various respiratory dyskinesias.

The prevalence of tardive dyskinesia among psychiatric patients has been reported to be as high as 20%, but the figure appears to be significantly lower for those individuals treated with atypical agents—for example, risperidone. Older patients and women are more liable to be affected.

Treatment of the problem is complex and is influenced by the type of movement disorder. Early recognition and withdrawal, or reduction, of neuroleptic medication are preferable, if feasible.

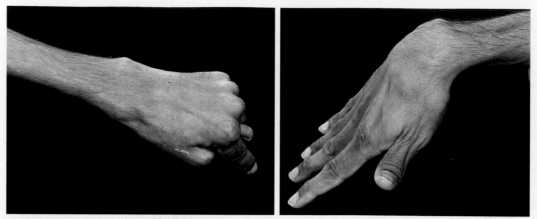

Fig. 7-55. Wilson's disease. Abnormal hand postures.

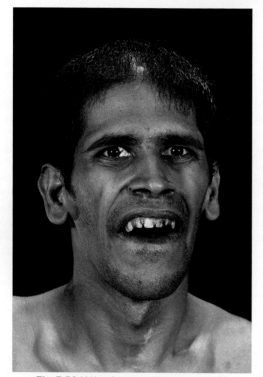

Fig. 7-56. Wilson's disease. Risus sardonicus.

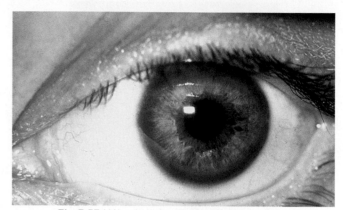

Fig. 7-57. Wilson's disease. The Kayser-Fleischer ring.

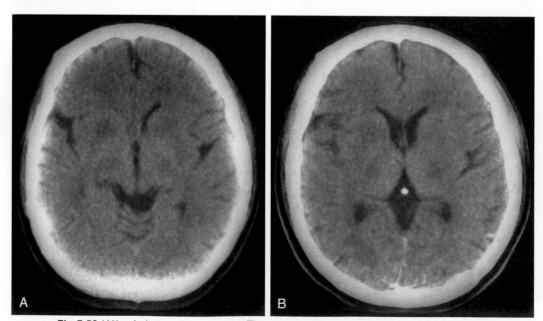

Fig. 7-58. Wilson's disease. CT appearance. There are ill-defined hypodensities in both basal ganglia.

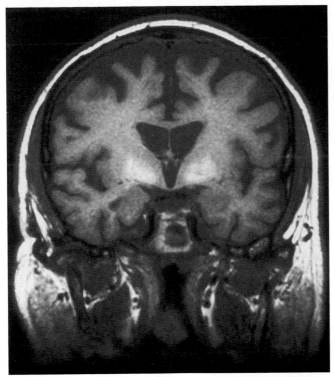

Fig. 7-59. Wilson's disease. Putaminal signal change on T1-weighted MR images.

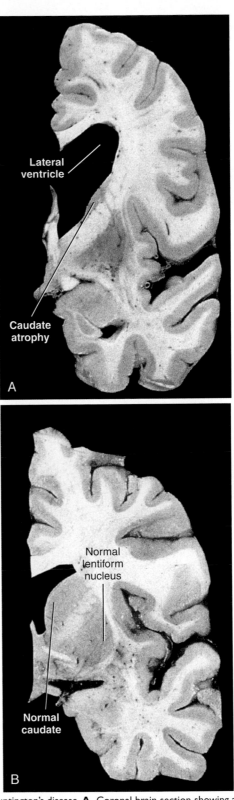

Fig. 7-60. Huntington's disease. **A,** Coronal brain section showing a dilated lateral ventricle with atrophy of the caudate and lentiform nuclei. **B,** Control section.

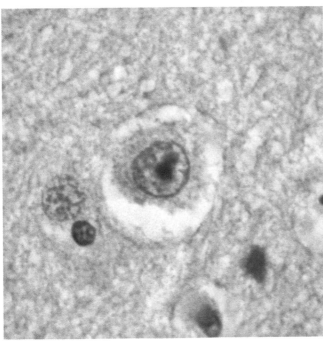

Fig. 7-61. Intranuclear inclusion in Huntington's disease.

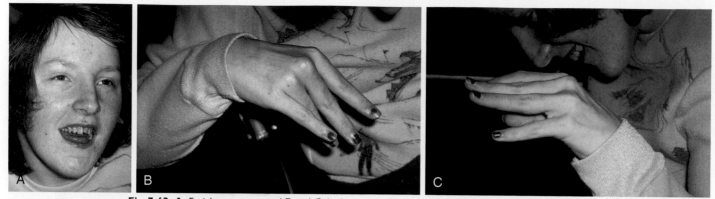

Fig. 7-62. A, Facial appearance and **B** and **C,** limb postures in a patient with juvenile Huntington's disease.

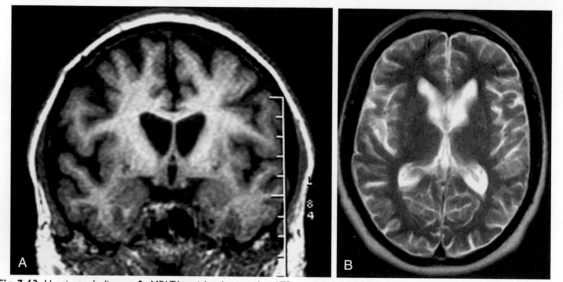

Fig. 7-63. Huntington's disease. **A,** MRI T1-weighted coronal and T2-weighted axial, **B,** demonstrating caudate and cortical atrophy.

HUNTINGTON'S DISEASE

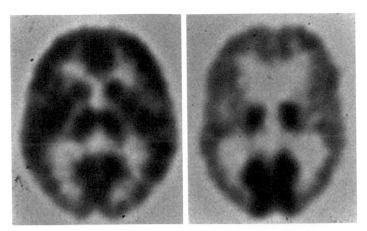

Control   HD

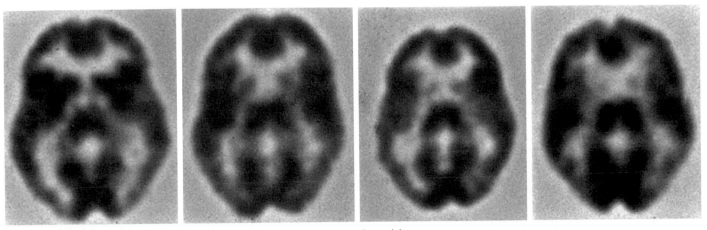

Asymptomatic: at-risk

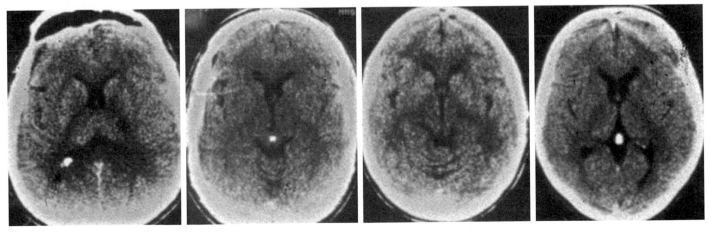

XCT

Fig. 7-64. Huntington's disease. PET scans. Reduced caudate flow compared with control *(upper)*. Comparison of CT and PET scans in detecting changes in asymptomatic, at-risk individuals *(lower)*.

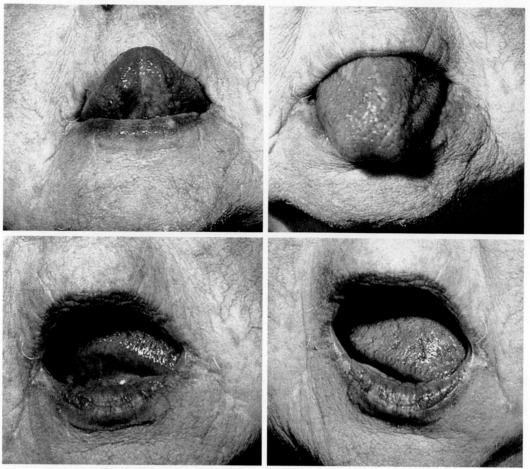

Fig. 7-65. Tardive dyskinesia. A variety of involuntary tongue movements.

INTRACRANIAL TUMORS: PARANEOPLASTIC (NONMETASTATIC) NEUROLOGIC SYNDROMES

Intracranial tumors can be classified as intraaxial or extraaxial. The former are mostly malignancies and include the gliomas, embryonal tumors, lymphomas, and germ cell tumors, as well as metastatic tumors that have spread to the brain by hematogenous dissemination from primary sites elsewhere in the body. The latter are mostly benign and include meningiomas, nerve sheath tumors (mostly schwannomas), and tumors of the skull (mostly chordomas and chondrosarcomas). Some metastatic tumors are also extraaxial, although these are less common than intraaxial metastases. Tumors of the sella turcica and closely related anatomic sites include pituitary adenomas, germ cell tumors, and craniopharyngiomas. This general classification, and the more detailed ones that follow, are based primarily on histopathologic features; modern molecular genetic and other molecular biological studies are increasingly important adjuncts to improved classification with a better understanding of tumor origin and of tumor response to therapy and ultimate prognosis.

CLINICAL FEATURES OF INTRACRANIAL TUMORS

Intracranial tumors grow slowly compared with some other space-occupying intracranial lesions such as hematomas or even abscesses. Consequently, almost all such neoplasms have long periods of "silent" growth before they appear with neurologic symptoms or signs. The symptoms may have sudden onset, as with seizures or when hemorrhage in a tumor appears as a stroke, but more often the onset is insidious, and the clinical features represent the consequences of space occupation in the cranium and are recognized by localizing signs that reflect the site of the tumor. In some cases, as mass effects produce herniation with damage to or compression of adjacent structures, there may be false localizing signs.

Nonspecific Signs and Symptoms
Headache is probably the most common and least specific of all symptoms of brain tumors. It appears eventually in the large majority of patients with such tumors. The features of the headaches are generally nonspecific: an early morning predominance (headache on waking) is found in no more than 10% to 15% of cases. For tumors of the cerebral hemispheres or their coverings (i.e., supratentorial tumors), the headache is ipsilateral to the neoplasm in about 80% of cases, unless there is papilledema (a late sign in most cases).

Nausea or vomiting occurs in about half of patients with supratentorial tumors, and in a greater proportion of patients with infratentorial tumors. Nausea is more common than vomiting. These symptoms, especially in children, often lead to prolonged and fruitless evaluations and tests by gastroenterologists until an intracranial source is ultimately looked for by appropriate scans.

Seizures are more likely when the tumor is situated in the anterior rather than the posterior part of the cranium, but they are quite uncommon in patients with tumors limited to the posterior fossa. Over 50% of patients with frontal lobe tumors have seizures at some time before any neurosurgical procedure. In some, the seizures are the presenting feature. It is generally accepted that the new onset of

seizures (especially in adults or older children) requires imaging to rule out an intracranial neoplasm. Status epilepticus in an older patient is particularly suggestive of a frontal neoplasm. The type of seizure is also somewhat predictive of the site of a tumor, with a higher proportion of temporal lobe tumors found in patients with complex partial seizures.

Papilledema is more common with infratentorial than supratentorial tumors (Fig. 8-1). With the latter, it suggests either herniation with compression of the third ventricle and the foramina of Monro or the effects of tumors at the foramen of Monro, especially colloid cysts of the third ventricle. With infratentorial tumors, the presence of papilledema is probably the consequence of obstruction of CSF outflow at the foramen magnum or at the level of the aqueduct. This may occur relatively early in the clinical course, but, again, except for tumors arising in the lower fourth ventricle or in or immediately next to the aqueduct, the size of the tumors causing such obstruction is usually substantial, suggesting a considerable period of growth before the appearance of clinical symptoms or signs.

Although altered mentation is a particular feature of frontal lobe tumors, some degree of apathy and inertia is common to tumors arising from any site.

Focal Signs and Symptoms
The focal symptoms and signs of intracranial tumors reflect their anatomic location. Frontal lobe tumors are associated with alterations of mood and behavior, coupled with contralateral motor deficits and pyramidal tract signs. Incontinence may be prominent. As the tumor enlarges, and particularly if an intraaxial frontal tumor crosses the corpus callosum, profound inanition often appears, coupled with the emergence of primitive reflexes including spontaneous grasping or suckling (Fig. 8-2). This may closely resemble advanced dementia except for its more rapid progression.

Sensory signs and symptoms predominate in patients with parietal lobe tumors, along with contralateral motor or visual field abnormalities. Contralateral sensory or visual inattention (neglect) is particularly likely if the tumor is in the nondominant hemisphere. Dressing apraxia is typically associated with lesions of the nondominant parietal lobe (Fig. 8-3).

When the dominant temporal lobe is affected by tumor, speech disturbance is likely, either persistently or transiently associated with seizures (speech arrest). A superior quadrantic homonymous hemianopia is sometimes seen in such cases, as are contralateral pyramidal signs. As noted, complex partial seizures are particularly associated with temporal lobe lesions but sometimes result from tumors in the posterior frontal region. Visual field abnormalities are the most conspicuous feature of occipital neoplasms, again either as a fixed deficit or in the form of positive visual phenomena as the prodrome of a seizure.

Tumors of one cerebellar hemisphere result in ipsilateral cerebellar signs, whereas those predominantly involving the vermis lead to truncal ataxia. Brainstem tumors, especially pontine gliomas, are likely to present with cranial nerve signs (Fig. 8-4).

False localizing signs associated with supratentorial tumors include dysfunction of any of the third, fourth, fifth, or sixth cranial nerves. Unilateral or bilateral sixth-nerve palsies are the most common false

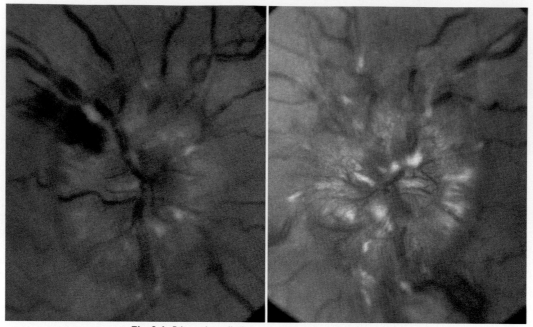

Fig. 8-1. Bilateral papilledema secondary to a cerebral tumor.

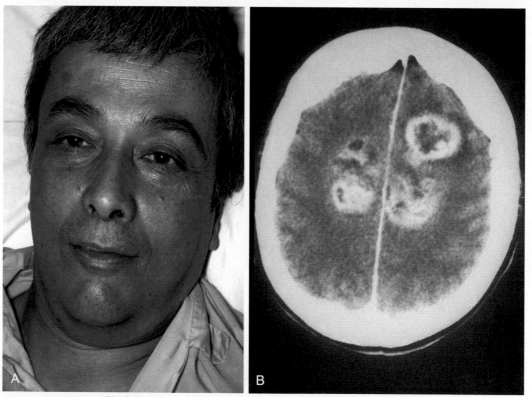

Fig. 8-2. Patient with callosal glioma. **A,** Clinical appearance. **B,** CT scan.

localizing sign encountered with cerebral tumors (Fig. 8-5). Uncal herniation may lead to compression of the contralateral cerebral peduncle against the tentorium, causing a hemiparesis ipsilateral to the side of the neoplasm (the Kernohan's notch phenomenon). Compression of either or both posterior cerebral arteries by the same herniation process can lead to occipital lobe infarction (Fig. 8-6).

THE INVESTIGATION OF INTRACRANIAL TUMORS

Plain skull radiographs and conventional angiography are no longer performed to establish a diagnosis of intracranial tumor. Angiography is still useful in some cases for surgical planning.

CT scanning revolutionized the investigation of intracranial tumors, although now it has been surpassed and replaced by MRI. The precontrast and postcontrast CT appearances of tumors are (in general, but with many specific exceptions) influenced by the degree of malignancy of the neoplasm, particularly with regard to intraaxial neoplasms. Although most low-grade gliomas are usually hypodense on CT scans, approximately half of hypodense intracerebral lesions found by CT are actually found to be higher-grade, more aggressive gliomas when surgically sampled or removed. Enhancement in a diffuse glioma of otherwise low-grade appearance suggests progression to a higher grade (because enhancement usually correlates with vascular hyperplasia, which is a correlate in turn of higher histopathologic and biological grade). This does not apply to certain specific types of tumors, such as pilocytic

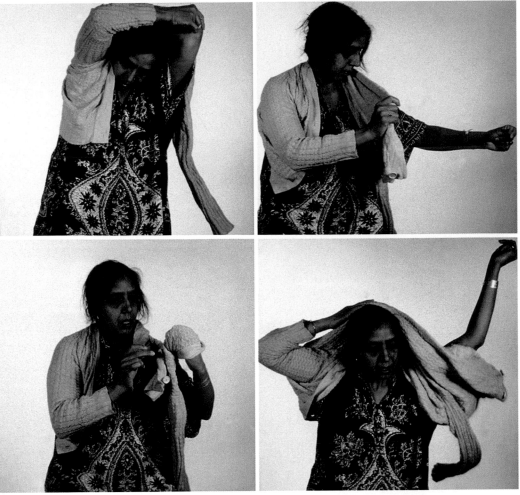

Fig. 8-3. Dressing apraxia.

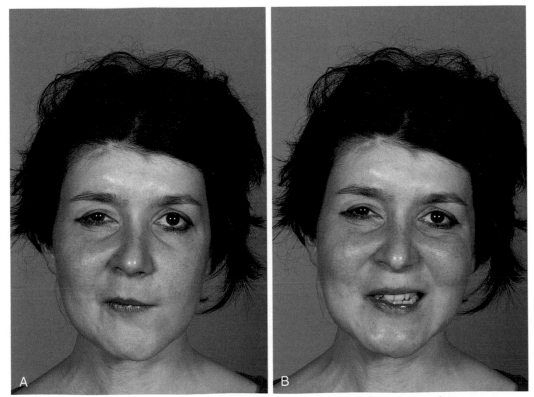

Fig. 8-4. Pontine glioma. **A,** Right facial myokymia. **B,** The associated right facial weakness.

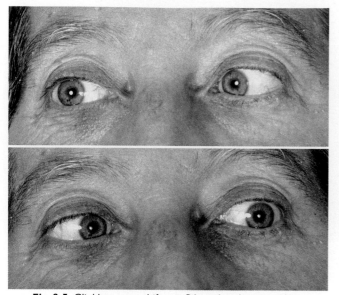

Fig. 8-5. Glioblastoma multiforme. Bilateral sixth nerve palsies.

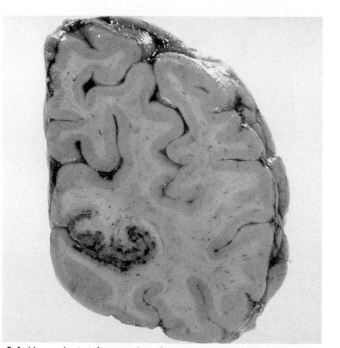

Fig. 8-6. Hemorrhagic infarct resulting from compression of the posterior cerebral artery after hippocampal herniation through the tentorial notch.

astrocytomas, nor is it true for diffuse low-grade intramedullary spinal cord gliomas.

High-grade gliomas, exemplified by glioblastoma multiforme, have a mixed-density CT appearance, reflecting the coexistence of solid tumor, tumor cysts, hemorrhage, necrosis, and edema. Enhancement after contrast administration is the norm, frequently in a ring pattern. Most such tumors have at least some mass effect, and deeper ones usually have substantial mass effect at presentation; only smaller more superficial tumors, found because the patients present with seizures, tend to have less mass effect. The CT appearance is often similar to that of cerebral abscess, certain stages of cerebral infarction, and some demyelinating diseases (e.g., tumefactive multiple sclerosis), and the true nature of the lesion may be demonstrable only by MRI, by following its evolution where clinically feasible, or by histopathologic examination. CT remains of value where bone destruction is being assessed (e.g., with clivus chordoma [Fig. 8-7]) and in preoperative planning (Fig. 8-8).

MRI is now the investigation of choice for the diagnosis and post-therapeutic assessment of brain tumors. Gliomas of different grades of malignancy can generally be distinguished by their imaging characteristics, more reliably than with CT. As with CT, low-grade diffuse gliomas are usually nonenhancing and are associated with little or no evidence of edema. They have low relative cerebral blood volume (rCBV) on perfusion imaging (Fig. 8-9): The T2 signal abnormalities of these tumors represent volumes of brain infiltrated by the tumor cells, not reactive edema. However, in the adult patient, 40% of nonenhancing tumors are grade 3 rather then grade 2. High-grade gliomas appear as high-signal-intensity lesions on T2 and fluid-attenuated inversion recovery (FLAIR), but with low-signal intensity on T1-weighted images and usually enhancing (Fig. 8-10). Diffuse infiltration shown as high T2 signal intensity resembling edema is a characteristic feature, and in some cases the tumors may appear to be multifocal by T1 but the separate lesions are usually connected by a single large confluent T1 or FLAIR abnormality. True multifocality and metastasis in the CNS can occur. Diffusion tensor imaging allows mapping of white matter pathways in the brain and can help determine whether they are significantly infiltrated by tumor (Fig. 8-11).

Diffusion-weighted MRI (DWI) appearances correlate to some extent with tumor malignancy. Furthermore, this technique allows fairly definitive distinction between necrotic gliomas and infarcts or abscesses: with DWI, the central core of an abscess or infarct exhibits high signal and the central component of high-grade tumors has a low signal. Hemorrhage into a tumor, or a cyst filled with proteinaceous fluid, may complicate this distinction (Fig. 8-12), because the resulting magnetic susceptibility alters signal characteristics.

Perfusion-weighted MRI techniques also correlate well with the histologic grade of a glioma, as high perfusion rates are found in tumors with high proliferative activity with concomitant rapid growth and aggressive clinical behavior. Perfusion-weighted MRI also helps

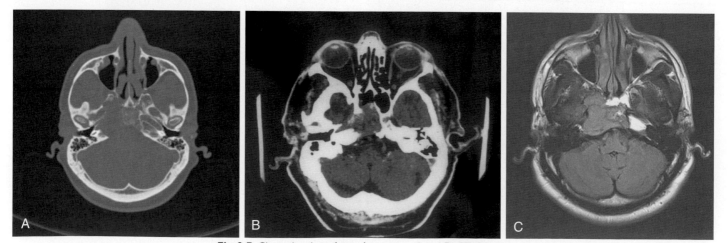

Fig. 8-7. Clivus chordoma bone destruction. **A** and **B,** CT. **C,** MRI.

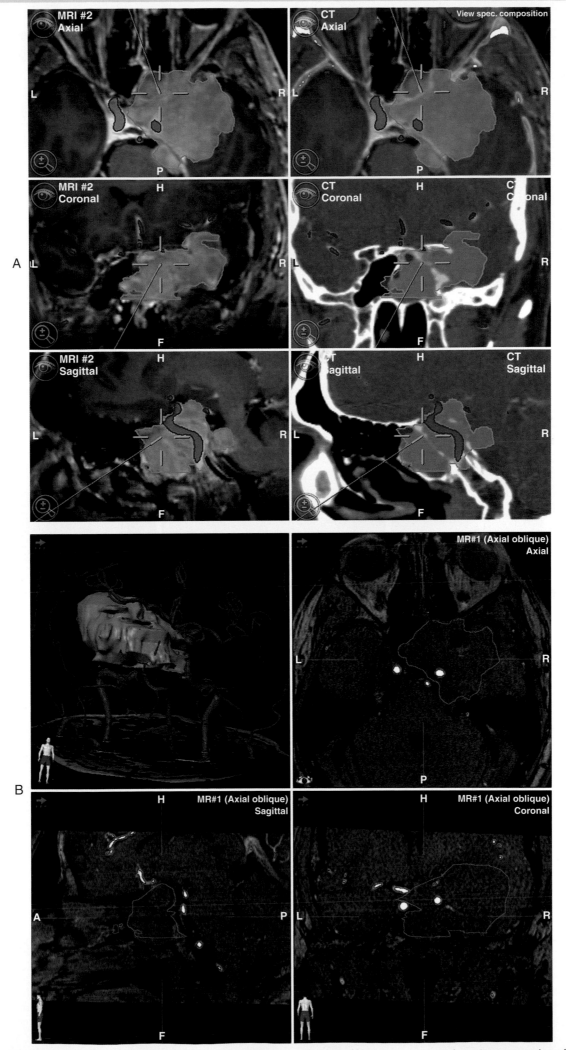

Fig. 8-8. Skull-base tumor with fused CT and MRI images displayed in three planes **(A)** and with tumor and arteries segmented out **(B)**.

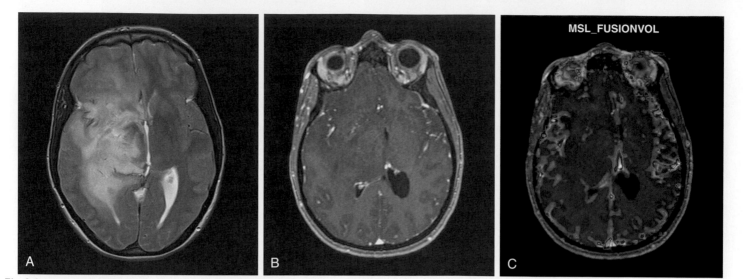

Fig. 8-9. Low-grade glioma. **A,** Axial T2-weighted MRI. **B,** Axial T1-weighted, gadolinium-enhanced MRI. **C,** Fused images of T1-weighted MRI and relative cerebral blood volume.

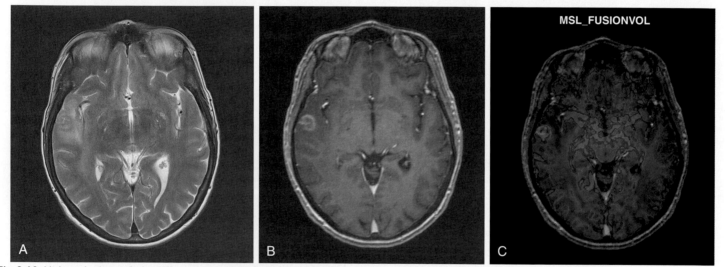

Fig. 8-10. High-grade glioma. **A,** Axial T2-weighted MRI. **B,** Axial T1-weighted, gadolinium-enhanced MRI. **C,** Fused images of T1-weighted MRI and relative cerebral blood volume.

discriminate neoplasms from mimics, including demyelinating disease, as the lesions of the latter are generally hypoperfused compared with hyperperfused neoplasms. In general, higher-grade gliomas have a higher rCBV than lower-grade gliomas, and oligodendrogliomas have higher rCBVs than astrocytomas. An increase in rCBV on follow-up may be the earliest marker for transformation from low to high grade.

Proton MR spectroscopy (MRS) has been suggested as a potential technique for improving preoperative grading of tumor malignancy, although this has not been shown to be superior to perfusion-weighted MRI. MRS assists in distinguishing gliomas from metastases. As the tumor grade increases, the ratio of choline to N-acetylaspartate (NAA) rises. Mobile lipids and lactate (indicators of necrosis) are generally not found in low-grade gliomas (Fig. 8-13).

Functional MRI can be used to assess the position of cortical function relative to a tumor. Loss of fractional anisotropy may indicate invasion of white matter tracts rather than displacement. White matter tracts can be visualized using mathematical algorithms in conjunction with diffusion tensor imaging (Fig. 8-14).

Pathologic investigation of brain tumors follows neurosurgical biopsies or excisions. Standard histopathologic methods using paraffin sections of formalin-fixed tissue samples remain an invaluable initial step in characterizing any tumor, and this is often the only pathologic investigation necessary. However, modern pathologic diagnosis also relies to a great extent on subsequent demonstration of more or less lineage-specific immunohistochemical markers, such

as glial fibrillary acidic protein (GFAP) intermediate filament expression in astrocytomas, or synaptophysin expression in neuronal tumor cells. Furthermore, immunostains are now used routinely to document proliferative activity in tumors, most commonly using antibodies to the nuclear cell-cycle–associated antigen Ki-67 (antibody MIB-1) to label all cells in G_1, G_2, S, or M phase of the cell cycle, and to then determine a labeling index, which is the ratio of labeled nuclei to all tumor cell nuclei in a representative sample of the tumor. Immunostains can also document abnormal expression of certain gene products, such as the p53 protein, the epidermal growth factor receptor, and tumor markers such as human chorionic gonadotropin (HCG), or the absence of normally expressed proteins, such as the CDKN2/p16 protein or the INI1 gene product. Similar techniques used on samples of metastatic tumors can help establish the likely primary site of such tumors when that may be in doubt because no primary site is known or because a patient has historically had more than one systemic malignancy.

TREATMENT OF BRAIN TUMORS: GENERAL CONSIDERATIONS

Treatment of a brain tumor almost always begins with a neurosurgical procedure. Symptoms of increased intracranial pressure are often relieved or at least ameliorated by preoperative steroid administration,

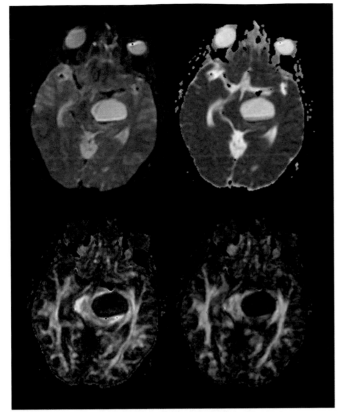

Fig. 8-11. Diffusion tensor (DT) imaging in a patient with a cystic ganglioglioma. The directions of white matter pathways are color coded in the DT image. Green, anterior/posterior; blue, inferior/superior; red, right/left. The corticospinal tracts are displaced posteriorly.

but definitive antitumor therapy is to a large extent dictated by the histopathologic diagnosis. Most extraaxial tumors are excised, and many such excisions are curative (meningiomas, cranial nerve schwannomas, some pituitary tumors). Intraaxial tumors are rarely surgically curable (with certain exceptions, such as most pilocytic astrocytomas), but there is increasing evidence that maximal surgical resection, where feasible without causing permanent important neurologic impairment beyond that already produced by the tumor, yields important benefits compared with biopsy alone.

After the diagnosis of a primary CNS malignancy such as a glioma, the conventional therapeutic options include external beam radiation therapy or chemotherapy (usually now delivered as multiagent combinations but not infrequently still using a single drug, such as temozolomide). Most patients with malignant gliomas are treated with a combination of radiation and chemotherapy. Other types of therapies, such as immunotherapy, remain experimental except in the treatment of specific tumor types, such as primary CNS B-cell non-Hodgkin's lymphoma, for which adjunctive therapy with an anti–B-cell monoclonal antibody is now common in combination with chemotherapy.

In certain situations, stereotactic radiosurgery may be used to treat small benign lesions, such as vestibular schwannomas or small meningiomas, or to treat small malignant lesions either when recurrence of a glioma is detected in surveillance MRI scans, or to control one or more lesions of documented metastatic character.

SPECIFIC TUMORS

METASTASES

Autopsies of patients with systemic cancer reveal that up to 20% have metastatic brain tumors, and unselected autopsy series suggest that up to 80% of all "brain tumors" are of metastatic origin. The proportion of metastatic tumors in clinical series of unselected brain tumors has been reported to be as high as 40%, however, so that at least 60%

of such tumors are likely to be primary in the CNS. In about two thirds of metastatic tumors, the lesions are multiple (Fig. 8-15), but detection of small metastatic deposits may require higher dosages of contrast (CT) or gadolinium (MRI) after an initial, apparently solitary lesion is detected.

The most common sources for brain parenchymal metastases are tumors of the lung, breast, skin (melanoma), and kidney. This reflects the high incidence of tumors of the lung and breast in the general population, but the proportion of patients with melanoma (still a relatively rare cancer, although one that has seen a steady increase in incidence) who have brain metastases at some point is reported to be as high as 50% (Fig. 8-16).

Metastatic deposits tend to occur at the junction of cortex and white matter, and more often in the distribution of the middle cerebral arteries. The lesions are usually more or less round, and they tend to be well demarcated from brain tissue as seen in CT scans or MR images when viewed by the neurosurgeon, and even histopathologically (Figs. 8-17 and 8-18). Many metastatic tumors have foci of necrosis or hemorrhage—especially those of lung origin or metastatic melanomas. Metastasis to the cerebellum is less frequent but is still more common than metastasis to the brainstem or spinal cord parenchyma. Another important pattern of metastatic spread of cancer in the nervous system is through cerebrospinal fluid spaces, producing a meningitis-like appearance that has been termed meningeal carcinomatosis (or lymphomatosis, as relevant) or even carcinomatous meningitis. Orbital metastases result in proptosis with limitation of extraocular movement (Fig. 8-19). Metastases sometimes grow from the dura and mimic meningiomas. Pituitary metastases, often an incidental finding, are reported in about 2% of patients with systemic malignancy. If invasive, they may result in visual deficits, or an ophthalmoplegia (Fig. 8-20).

Investigation

MRI is the investigation of choice. Often there is a striking contrast between a small tumor volume and a large area of adjacent edema (with a low T1 signal and a high T2 signal) (Fig. 8-21). Metastatic lesions on MRI may look like acute or subacute ischemic lesions (Fig. 8-22). Extradural metastases are less common. Extraaxial and intraaxial metastatic lesions may coincide (Fig. 8-23). In some patients with multiple lesions, the degree of associated edema may vary greatly from one lesion to another. Spread in the subarachnoid space may be seen well on FLAIR or postcontrast images.

Treatment

A single tumor may be of metastatic origin, or may be a new primary glioma, and if triple-dose contrast scans have failed to establish the presence of other lesions, biopsy may be required to establish the diagnosis. Gross total excision, wherever feasible, is a first step toward treatment of a single metastatic lesion. Excision of large metastases in patients with multiple lesions may be necessary to prevent herniation but is otherwise not generally important for antineoplastic treatment.

After a surgical procedure, most patients with brain metastases require radiation therapy. The best course for treating patients with an isolated single metastatic lesion is unclear. Patients with renal cell carcinomas (renal tubular adenocarcinomas) or with melanoma may benefit less from whole-brain radiation.

Depending on the type of cancer that has spread to the brain, certain chemotherapy regimens may also be of value as adjuncts in controlling the tumors, although many agents used to treat cancer in the rest of the body penetrate the blood–brain barrier poorly, if at all.

PRIMARY INTRAAXIAL BRAIN TUMORS

Classification

Although the medical literature is replete with classification systems for primary CNS tumors, the World Health Organization (WHO) classification is widely regarded as the best, and most alternatives have been abandoned. In part, this reflects the increasing tendency to

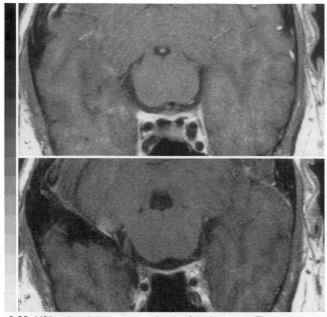

Fig. 8-23. MRI with gadolinium at two levels of the brainstem. There is an enhancing nodule of metastatic adenocarcinoma in the right cerebellopontine angle.

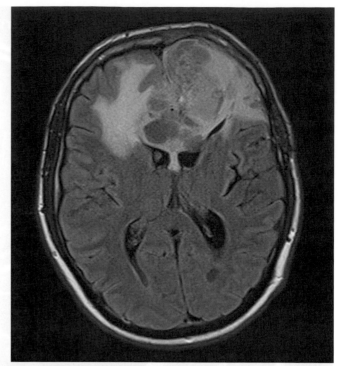

Fig. 8-25. Glioblastoma multiforme. MRI shows spread from one frontal lobe to the other across the corpus callosum.

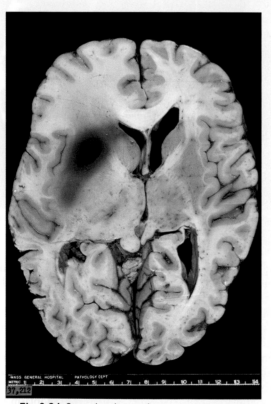

Fig. 8-24. Secondary hemorrhage in an astrocytoma.

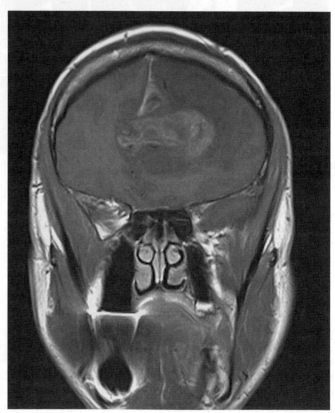

Fig. 8-26. Glioblastoma multiforme. MRI showing subependymal spread.

and become more anaplastic, contrast enhancement may be observed and the lesion becomes less circumscribed. Oligodendroglioma cells are usually GFAP negative, may be S100 positive, and often express other nonspecific neuroepithelial antigens such as Leu7/HNK1.

Mixed gliomas with oligodendroglial components and astrocytic components also may be low grade or anaplastic, using the same criteria used for pure oligodendrogliomas.

TUMORS IN OR ADJACENT TO THE VENTRICULAR SYSTEM

Ependymomas

Although ependymomas occur in all age groups, the majority are found in children. Most of these are in the posterior fossa, arising in the fourth ventricle, but some arise in or near the lateral ventricles or

third ventricle, and some are occasionally found quite far from any ventricle, or even, rarely, attached to the dura. Ependymomas also occur in the spinal cord, more in adults than in children.

Hazards of fourth ventricular tumors include obstruction of CSF flow with hydrocephalus, and dissemination along CSF pathways, although this is not as common as was once believed. These tumors may extrude into the subarachnoid space, especially in the posterior fossa, where they expand and extend through the foramina of Luschka toward the cerebellopontine angle. Such behavior strongly suggests a diagnosis of ependymoma rather than medulloblastoma. Subarachnoid extension may be downward, toward the foramen magnum alongside the medulla, or laterally into the cerebellopontine angle.

Histopathologically, the tumors are often highly cellular but are composed of monotonous regular bland cells with little pleomorphism. They tend to be well circumscribed, although a few have invasive borders like a diffuse glioma, and where the borders are sharp

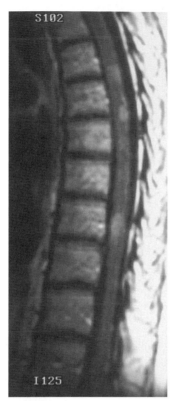

Fig. 8-27. Glioblastoma. Seedling deposits in the spinal cord. T1-weighted, gadolinium-enhanced MRI.

there is usually an adjacent gliotic reaction that may be quite intense. In almost all examples, there are focal perivascular radial arrangements of the tumor cells, with a circumferential zone of fibrillary processes around the vessels without tumor cell nuclei: perivascular pseudorosettes (Fig. 8-38). Some examples have distinctive central-lumen rosettes or larger more irregular canal-like spaces lined by epithelial tumor cells, but although these are definitive for the diagnosis of ependymoma, they are not always present. Both cystic and necrotic components may be conspicuous on MR images (Fig. 8-39). Contrast enhancement is essential to exclude seeding.

The best treatment for ependymomas starts with as near total surgical excision as is possible. Radiation therapy is standard adjunctive therapy, although it has been suggested that surgery alone may suffice for cerebral hemisphere ependymomas that have been totally excised.

Choroid Plexus Papilloma

Choroid plexus papillomas are rare benign tumors of the epithelium that lines the choroid plexus in the lateral, third, or fourth ventricles. In children, they predominate in the lateral ventricles; in adults, in the third ventricle. The macroscopic appearance is that of a granular polypoid growth, and microscopy reveals a papillary structure lined by cubical cells (Fig. 8-40). Papillomas enhance strongly on both CT scans and MR images (Fig. 8-41). These rare tumors may secrete CSF or may cause hydrocephalus by obstructing CSF flow. Treatment is by surgical excision.

Glioneuronal Tumors

It has long been recognized that some "gliomas" contain neuronal as well as glial elements. The best known of these is the ganglioglioma. Most gangliogliomas are low-grade neoplasms resembling low-grade fibrillary astrocytomas or pilocytic astrocytomas but containing, in addition to astrocytic tumor cells, large ganglion cells that are stained with neuronal immunostains, notably synaptophysin. Most respond favorably to surgical excision alone, although local recurrences are observed. Other glioneuronal neoplasms include the intraventricular ("central") neurocytoma, a tumor that most typically occurs in the lateral ventricles attached to the septum pellucidum and which

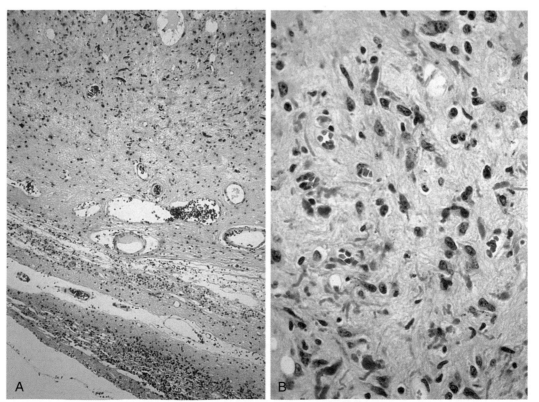

Fig. 8-28. A, Low-grade cerebellar astrocytoma. Edge of tumor *(above)* with compressed atrophic cerebellar folia *(below)* (H&E, ×80). **B,** Tumor cells with small ovoid nuclei and brightly eosinophilic cytoplasm surrounded by irregular rod-shaped eosinophilic structures (Rosenthal fibers) (H&E, ×320).

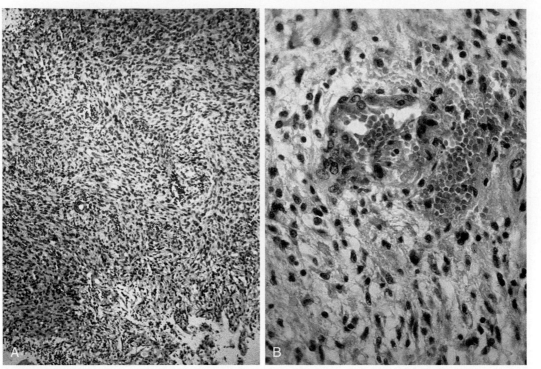

Fig. 8-29. Anaplastic astrocytoma. **A,** Cellular tumor with dark nuclei and solid fibrillary eosinophilic background (H&E, ×80). **B,** Evidence of vascular hyperplasia with proliferated endothelial and perithelial cells (H&E, ×320).

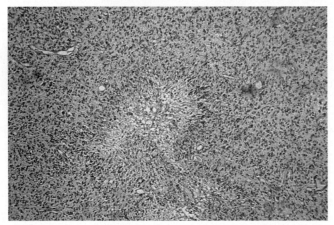

Fig. 8-30. Glioblastoma multiforme. Central necrotic zone surrounded by pseudopalisade of tumor cells (H&E, ×80).

histologically closely resembles oligodendroglioma. Radiologically, gangliogliomas are sharply demarcated, may be cystic, and may enhance. They predominate in the supratentorial region, particularly the temporal lobes.

EMBRYONAL CNS TUMORS

The embryonal CNS tumors arise from stem cells or progenitor cells—cells that are mostly undifferentiated but that retain a capacity to differentiate along glial (astrocytic, ependymal, oligodendrocytic) lines, along neuronal lines, and occasionally in other ways, such as to skeletal or smooth muscle. Traditional classifications have recognized distinctive tumors by their site of origin, although histologically these are more or less identical: medulloblastoma in the cerebellum, pineoblastoma in the pineal region, cerebral "neuroblastoma" in the cerebral hemispheres. The histopathologic similarities between these tumors of different sites prompted a classification of all of these as PNETs. More recent genetic data have suggested that at least some of the traditional separations by site reflect true differences in the cellular origins and differentiation potential of these neoplasms, particularly the cerebellar medulloblastoma. In addition, in recent years an additional tumor type, the atypical teratoid/rhabdoid tumor

(ATRT) has been recognized as being histopathologically, immunohistochemically, and genetically distinct.

Supratentorially, these tumors arise adjacent to the sylvian fissure and may be cystic as well as contrast enhancing.

Medulloblastoma

Medulloblastoma is the most common of the embryonal tumors or PNETs. More than half of cases occur in children younger than 10 years, although examples have been recorded in all ages including patients in their ninth decade. In younger patients, they typically arise from the region of the superior vermis of the cerebellum (Fig. 8-42). As with all PNETs, the histologic appearance is most often that of a highly cellular neoplasm packed with small "undifferentiated" cells, although immunostains frequently reveal some neuronal and glial marker expression (Fig. 8-43). The cells may be in patternless sheets in sections, may form distinctive neuroblastic central fibrillary rosettes as in adrenal and sympathetic neuroblastomas (Homer Wright rosettes) (Fig. 8-44), may form linear ("Indian file") arrangements, or may show more definitive signs of focal differentiation. The latter include ependymal rosettes and pseudorosettes (for which a diagnosis of ependymoblastoma was formerly suggested), and a distinctive follicular or nodular pattern in which much more mature neurocytoma-like cells form in the nodules with less well differentiated cells in the internodular zones (desmoplastic medulloblastoma) (Fig. 8-45).

These are aggressive, highly malignant neoplasms, which tend to spread widely via CSF pathways in many patients, some even before diagnostic surgery (Fig. 8-46). Hematogenous metastases to bone, liver, and lung are also recorded although less commonly (Fig. 8-47). CT or MRI demonstrates a tumor of mixed signal intensity with obliteration or lateral stretching of the fourth ventricle. As the tumor is densely cellular with a high nucleus-to-cytoplasm ratio, it is often dense on CT scans and shows restricted diffusion on MR images (Fig. 8-48). With gross or near gross total excision followed by craniospinal radiation therapy and systemic multiagent chemotherapy, 5-year survival is close to 80%.

Other Primitive Neuroectodermal Tumors

Survival for pineal PNET, cerebral PNET (supratentorial PNET), and brainstem PNET is less good than for medulloblastoma. In part this reflects less efficacious surgery with fewer gross total excisions,

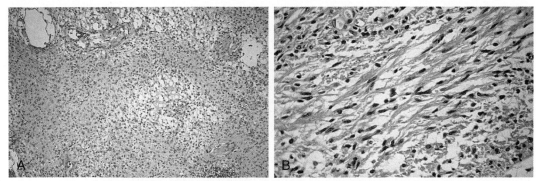

Fig. 8-31. Juvenile pilocytic astrocytoma. **A,** Relatively low cellularity, regular nuclei, and loose areas of spongy tissue alternate with more compact areas (H&E, ×80). **B,** Bipolar cells with eosinophilic cytoplasm and parallel cell processes (H&E, ×320).

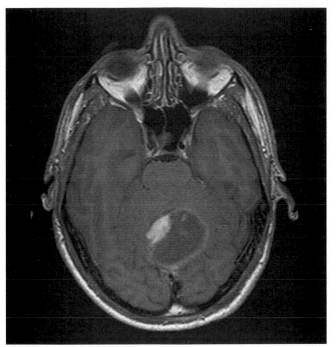

Fig. 8-32. Juvenile pilocytic astrocytoma. Axial T1-weighted, gadolinium-enhanced MRI.

but it also seems to reflect tumor biology as well. ATRTs are highly aggressive tumors that occur more often in children under the age of 18 months.

Pineal Region Parenchymal Tumors

Although pineal PNET (pineoblastoma) is not pathologically distinct from other PNETs, or genetically distinct from other supratentorial PNETs, the clinical presentation of a pineal region mass is often distinctive. Patients with these and other pineal-region tumors are liable to have hydrocephalus as a result of aqueductal compression, or they may present with visual signs (Parinaud's syndrome). The latter are the result of compression by the tumor of the quadrigeminal plate, which produces impairment of upward gaze, convergence-retractory nystagmus on attempted upward gaze, and light-near dissociated pupils.

In addition to pineal PNET, the pineal parenchyma may give rise to astrocytomas (said to be the second most common pineal tumor) or to tumors called pineocytomas. These are tumors of neuronal type in which the cells resemble those of central neurocytoma, with fairly regular round nuclei centrally placed in small to middle-sized cell bodies.

Imaging features in addition to hydrocephalus include distortion of the posterior third of the third ventricle and compression of the quadrigeminal cistern. Calcification is found in both pineocytomas and teratomas. Most of these tumors enhance after contrast injection. There are no specific features on MR images (Fig. 8-49).

NONNEUROEPITHELIAL INTRAAXIAL CNS TUMORS

Lymphoma

When systemic lymphoma involves the nervous system, it is almost always non-Hodgkin's lymphoma (NHL). As most NHLs are B-cell tumors, most CNS involvement from systemic NHL is also B-cell NHL. The most typical pattern of spread is a diffuse involvement of the subarachnoid space and leptomeninges, or lymphomatous meningitis. In contrast, primary CNS NHL, also mostly (>90%) of B-cell lineage, usually appears as single or multiple mass lesions in the brain parenchyma. These are infiltrative masses, often close to ventricular spaces, and thus may be found in the corpus callosum, thalamus, or basal ganglia (Fig. 8-50). Since the 1980s, the incidence of primary CNS NHL has increased to at least 3% of all newly diagnosed primary CNS neoplasms. Primary CNS NHL occurs in immunocompetent patients, but it also shows an increased incidence in immunosuppressed patients, including those with AIDS, those on immunosuppressive therapy, and those with certain congenital immune deficiency syndromes.

Primary CNS lymphoma is largely confined to the brain parenchyma (and the CSF) and rarely spreads to other organs. (In this context, ocular involvement is understood to be part of the CNS involvement.) Multifocality is observed in almost half of immunocompetent patients and is the rule in immunosuppressed patients. Given the propensity of the tumors to compress adjacent ventricles or to involve ventricular cavities and the subarachnoid space, it is not surprising that hydrocephalus from obstruction of CSF flow is common (Fig. 8-51).

CT scans or MR images will usually demonstrate the single or multiple lesions and these may appear well circumscribed. They typically enhance, and they are hypointense on T2-weighted images (Figs. 8-52 and 8-53). MRS may be useful by revealing elevated choline, depressed NAA, and the presence of lactic acid. Diagnosis may be established by finding B-cell NHL cells in CSF augmented by immunohistochemistry or flow cytometry. CSF cytology is positive in about 20% of patients with primary CNS NHL.

Steroids often have profound effects on CNS lymphomas, inducing dramatic shrinkage of lesions on MRI scans. For this reason, they should be avoided prior to biopsy, as the biopsies may then show only gliosis and nonspecific chronic inflammation. Unfortunately, the response to steroids is short-lived. Chemotherapy most often involves high dosages of methotrexate with leucovorin rescue. Addition of other conventional chemotherapy drugs has not shown benefit beyond the 4- to 5-year survivals currently achievable with methotrexate alone. Radiation usually produces a rapid reduction in tumor size, but there is usually an equally rapid recurrence of tumor. Recently, the addition of anti–B-cell (anti-CD20) antibodies has shown promise for patients who fail methotrexate therapy.

Germ Cell Tumors

Tumors with the histologic and immunohistochemical features of the germ cell neoplasias recognized in the gonads and mediastinum also occur as primary neoplasms in the CNS, most typically in the pineal

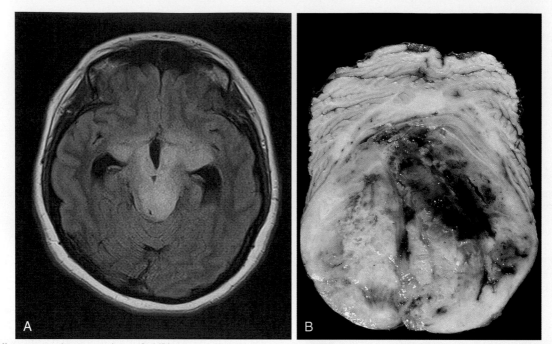

Fig. 8-33. Diffuse intrinsic brainstem glioma. **A,** MRI appearance. **B,** Expansion of the pons with a few crossing fibers detectable at the edges of the tumor.

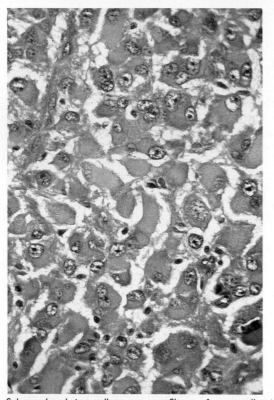

Fig. 8-34. Subependymal giant-cell astrocytoma. Sheets of tumor cells with eosinophilic, gemistocytic, astrocyte-like cytoplasm with large, pale nuclei and prominent nucleoli (H&E, ×320).

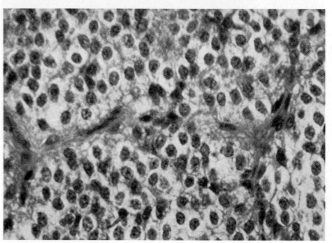

Fig. 8-35. Oligodendroglioma. A uniform honeycombed cellular pattern surrounding blood vessels (H&E, ×300).

aggressive tumors that respond less well to radiation and chemotherapy. These tumors have a considerable propensity for CSF dissemination.

Colloid Cysts of the Third Ventricle

These cystic masses have a wall with a fibrous outer layer and an inner single layer of cuboidal to columnar epithelial cells. They are found under the corpus callosum, attached to the septum pellucidum, between the pillars of the fornix, and hanging down into the foramina of Monro (Fig. 8-55). As they enlarge, they can be entrapped in and block the foramina, rapidly producing hydrocephalus. This may be posture dependent: The tumor may free itself from the foramina when the patient is upright but may fall back into an obstructive position when the patient is recumbent. This may account for the classic syndrome of morning headaches in patients with colloid cysts. Other clinical presentations include dementia, acute hydrocephalus, and atypical drop attacks.

The cysts exhibit high density on CT because of the high protein content of their colloid secretion (Fig. 8-56). MRI demonstrates no other specific features (Fig. 8-57), although the lesions are hypointense on T2-weighted images because of the elevated protein content. There may be rim enhancement. Complete excision is the treatment of choice; attempts to drain the cysts with stereotactic punctures provide immediate relief from symptoms but the cysts reaccumulate and symptoms recur unless the epithelium is resected.

and the suprasellar regions (Fig. 8-54). The most common tumor in this group is the germinoma. Others, conventionally grouped as nongerminoma germ cell tumors, include yolk sac tumor (endodermal sinus tumor), embryonal carcinoma, choriocarcinoma, and mature and immature teratomas.

Germinomas are best diagnosed by biopsy unless marker studies establish the diagnosis. The risk of substantial resections, particularly of suprasellar tumors that may jeopardize the optic nerves or chiasm, or of the pituitary stalk and hypothalamus, is unnecessary given the remarkable responsiveness of these tumors to either radiation therapy or chemotherapy (or combinations thereof). On the other hand, nongerminoma germ cell tumors, including all others except mature teratomas, are

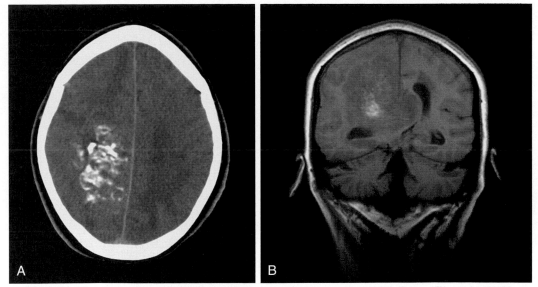

Fig. 8-36. Oligodendroglioma. **A,** Calcification demonstrated on conventional CT. **B,** Coronal T1-weighted MRI.

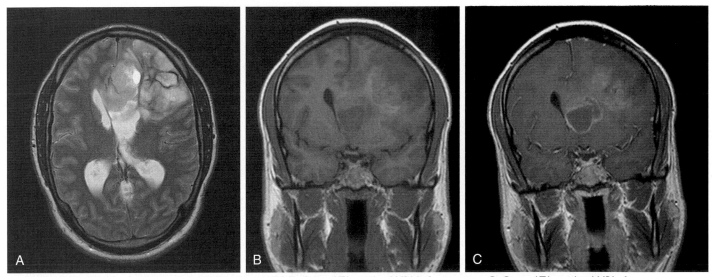

Fig. 8-37. Oligodendroglioma. **A,** Axial T2-weighted MRI. **B,** Coronal T1-weighted MRI, before contrast. **C,** Coronal T1-weighted MRI, after contrast.

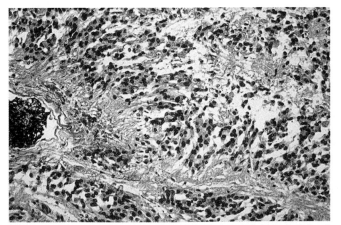

Fig. 8-38. Ependymoma. Cords of cells with oval vesicular nuclei radiating from the vessel wall (phosphotungstic acid–hematoxylin, ×350).

PRIMARY EXTRAAXIAL BRAIN TUMORS

Meningiomas

Meningiomas arise from the cells of the arachnoid layer of the leptomeninges, sometimes referred to as the arachnoid epithelium. These tumors, over 90% of which are benign, are more common in women from the age of puberty to the menopause, with a roughly equal sex distribution before and after that age range. Meningiomas are rare in children but do occur, especially after cranial radiation therapy. Syncytial (meningotheliomatous), transitional, and spindle cell (fibroblastic) forms are the most common. In the syncytial form, sheets of bland regular cells with epithelial features and convoluted nuclei with frequent cytoplasmic pseudoinclusions are found in lobulated masses (Fig. 8-58). There may be occasional cellular whorls, such as are sometimes also seen in normal arachnoid granulations. Whorls are more common in the transitional form (Fig. 8-59), where they coexist with spindle cells in fascicles; calcification of the whorls leads to the formation of psammoma bodies (Fig. 8-60). Meningiomas grow in the subdural space with broad dural attachments on their outer borders (against the skull) and push the arachnoid before them and the brain, so that they are encapsulated by these surrounding normal structures (Fig. 8-61). Invasion as fingers of adherent cells through the arachnoid and pia into the cortex or even the underlying white matter is a sign of a more aggressive neoplasm, and there is a strong tendency for local recurrence even after gross total surgical excision; such tumors are termed atypical meningiomas in the WHO classification (Fig. 8-62). Malignant meningiomas, which are rare, are defined as those with very high mitotic rates or those with particular histologic patterns, including papillary meningiomas, rhabdoid meningiomas, and clear cell meningiomas, as well as those with a

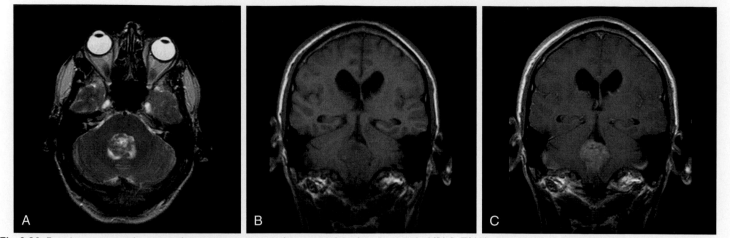

Fig. 8-39. Ependymoma: a partly cystic, enhancing mass occupies the region of the fourth ventricle. MRI **A,** T2 Weighted. **B,** T1 weighted. **C,** T1 weighted with gadolinium.

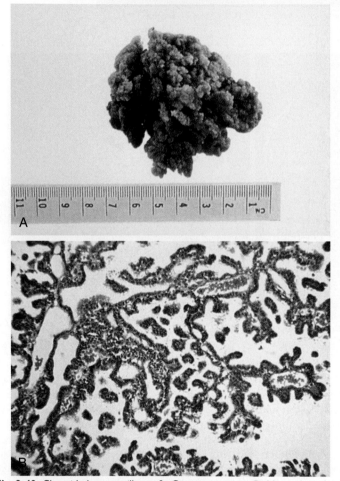

Fig. 8-40. Choroid plexus papilloma. **A,** Gross appearance. **B,** Microscopy showing papillary structures lined by cubical cells (H&E, ×60).

frankly sarcomatous appearance (Fig. 8-63). Malignant meningiomas have a capacity for distant metastasis, both by CSF pathways and by hematogenous dissemination. Multiple meningiomas are rare and usually occur in the context of neurofibromatosis type 2 (NF2) (see Schwannomas, later).

Meningiomas are found attached to the dura over the cerebral convexities (the most common site), between them on the falx, on the tentorium, at the skull base on the sphenoid wing, in the parasellar or suprasellar regions, at the olfactory groove, and, far less commonly, in the lateral or fourth ventricles, where they are thought to arise from arachnoidal nests in the tela choroidea (Fig. 8-64). The clinical features correspond to the sites at which the tumors are found. Sphenoid wing meningiomas usually occur with an ophthalmoplegia combined

with mild proptosis and evidence of involvement of the first division of the trigeminal nerve (Fig. 8-65). Tumors in the region of the olfactory groove can lead to anosmia, personality change, and visual loss, the last from optic nerve compression. Cerebral convexity tumors may provoke focal seizures; parasagittal tumors not only can cause seizures but also may cause focal neurologic deficits primarily affecting the lower extremities.

The typical CT appearance of a meningioma is of a hyperdense, well-demarcated mass in close contiguity to the falx, tentorium, or skull. In a small number of cases, the tumors are hypodense (some of these may be the microcystic or fatty lipomatous variant). The tumors enhance diffusely and densely. The adjacent brain edema may not be conspicuous (Figs. 8-66 and 8-67). Meningiomas frequently grow out through the dura and invade the overlying bone of the skull through the marrow spaces and haversian system, provoking hyperostosis, which may also occur in the absence of invasion. This does not imply malignancy or even atypicality. The bone changes are demonstrable by CT, and in unusual circumstances they appear as an externally evident deformity (Figs. 8-68 and 8-69). MR images show meningiomas as almost isointense to slightly hyperintense compared with brain on T1-weighted images, but the tumors are usually dark on T2 images, Enhancement after gadolinium administration is the norm (Fig. 8-70). They may be intensely vascular (Fig. 8-71), and there is often dural enhancement. Examination of bone is important, because in 3% of cases, interosseous involvement only is seen. On MRS, elevation of alanine may be seen, and on permeability studies, a rapid rise in contrast over time may be seen with no penetration into brain.

Benign meningiomas are treated by surgical excision; those few patients with inoperable residual tumor may require radiation therapy or radiosurgery. Whether to irradiate after excision of atypical meningiomas is uncertain. The benefit of radiation for malignant meningiomas is also uncertain.

Schwannomas (Neurilemmomas)

Schwannomas are tumors of peripheral nerves that are found throughout the body, but they come to neurologic attention most commonly when they grow on cranial nerves or spinal nerve roots. The most common site of origin for a schwannoma in the cranial cavity is the eighth cranial nerve, specifically the vestibular branch; the term *acoustic neuroma* is a double misnomer in that the tumor is neither from the acoustic branch nor is it a neuroma.

Patients with schwannomas of the eighth cranial nerve present with hearing loss, or, if the tumor is larger on presentation, there may be facial nerve weakness. Other symptoms include vertigo and tinnitus. With very large tumors, there may be hydrocephalus. With the wide availability of MRI, most such tumors are now found when small. They take origin most commonly at the junction of the peripheral and central components of the nerve close to the mouth

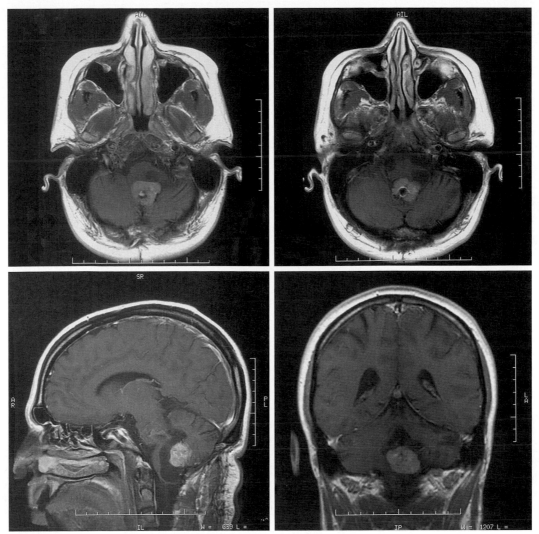

Fig. 8-41. Choroid plexus papilloma. MRI.

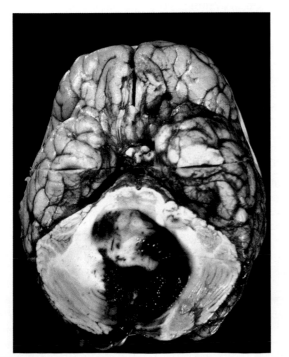

Fig. 8-42. Cerebellar primitive neuroectodermal tumor (medulloblastoma). The mass of dirty brown tumor has filled the fourth ventricle.

of the internal auditory meatus; with enlargement the internal auditory canal, the tumor extrudes into the cerebellopontine angle (Fig. 8-72). Histologically, these are encapsulated neoplasms that adhere to the nerve surface; they do not infiltrate or expand the nerves. However, larger lesions stretch the nerves to which they are attached, thinning them in the process. The tumors are composed of spindle cells organized in short compact fascicles, sometimes with distinctive rows of nuclei (i.e., nuclear palisades), with a second growth pattern of smaller, rounder cells in a loose fibrillary background with abundant extracellular space (Fig. 8-73). The compact tissues are called Antoni A tissue pattern, and the loose tissues Antoni B pattern. There are usually thick-walled vessels with hemosiderin deposits in and around their walls (Fig. 8-74). Mitotic figures are extremely rare and Ki-67/MIB-1 labeling indices are low (usually less than 3%).

Although sporadic schwannomas are usually unilateral, patients with NF2 tend to have bilateral eighth nerve schwannomas. Often, these are associated with schwannomas of other cranial nerves (especially the trigeminal) and of multiple spinal nerve roots, as well as of more peripherally placed peripheral nerves. There is also an increased incidence of meningiomas, which are often multiple, in patients with NF2, and there is an increased incidence of intramedullary spinal cord ependymomas. The NF2 gene maps to chromosome 22, and the region that carries the gene is generally deleted in the tumor cells of sporadic schwannomas, meningiomas, and many ependymomas as well. This is in contrast to the lesions of NF1, which include peripheral nerve neurofibromas (rarely intracranial, but found in some patients on spinal nerve roots); pilocytic astrocytomas and other low-grade astrocytomas of the optic nerves, chiasm, and hypothalamus;

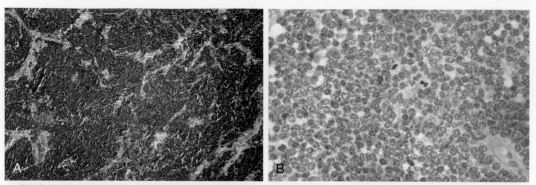

Fig. 8-43. Cerebellar primitive neuroectodermal tumor. **A,** High cell density (H&E, ×80). **B,** Mitotic figures (×320).

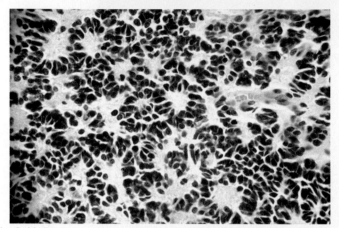

Fig. 8-44. Primitive neuroectodermal tumor. Central fibrillary rosettes (Homer Wright rosettes). Radial arrangement of small dark nuclei around central fibrillary structures (H&E, ×320).

and cerebral diffuse astrocytomas, all of which carry other chromosomal abnormalities without chromosome 22 deletions.

Investigations of eighth-nerve schwannomas include audiometry, which is abnormal in about 95% of cases, and examination of the stapedial reflex, which is abnormal in about 85%. Brainstem auditory evoked responses are also of value; a delay between the first potential (NI) and later components (particularly NII) is particularly suggestive. CT scanning reveals the expansion of the internal auditory meatus if the tumors are large enough, particularly if bone windows are used (Fig. 8-75). MRI with gadolinium, the imaging modality of choice, can be used to visualize small tumors, even those just a few millimeters in size that are still confined to the canal (Fig. 8-76). The effects of larger tumors in terms of distortion of the brainstem and cerebellum, and consequent hydrocephalus, are readily apparent (Fig. 8-77).

Treatment choices for small tumors include neurosurgical removal and stereotactic radiosurgery. Some neurosurgical approaches to very small tumors can spare hearing if it is preserved at the time of diagnosis. Larger tumors must be surgically excised; unless the tumor is very large, facial nerve function is now routinely preserved. After definitive surgery, recurrence is rare but is more likely with tumors with more obvious mitotic figures and higher MIB-1 rates.

Epidermoid and Dermoid Cysts

Epidermoid tumors are cystic growths originating from developmentally or traumatically displaced squamous epithelial cells. The epithelium, which grows on a fibrous wall facing the cyst, consists of stratified squamous epithelium that keratinizes, the keratin accumulating in the cyst. Dermoid cysts are similar but more complex, as they represent mature cystic teratomas with all of the elements of mature skin—epidermis, dermis, dermal adnexae (including hair follicles and sebaceous and eccrine glands), and erector pili muscles. Occasionally, other elements, most commonly cartilage, are also present.

Both dermoid and epidermoid cysts most commonly arise in the leptomeninges, with the cerebellopontine angles being a favored site for epidermoid tumors. They appear as gradually expanding cystic masses. If one ruptures, the spilled keratin (including hair in the case of dermoid cysts) evokes a chemical meningitis.

Investigation and Treatment. CT scanning demonstrates a low-density lesion that may have peripheral calcification (Fig. 8-78). On T1-weighted MR images, epidermoid tumors are hypointense, but they are hyperintense on T2-weighted images (Fig. 8-79). Epidermoids often resemble arachnoid cysts, but they show diffusion restriction (bright) on MRI.

Treatment is by excision.

Chordomas and Cartilaginous Tumors

Chordomas are tumors of notochordal remnants that arise principally in the base of the skull, especially the clivus, and in the bones of the sacrum. They sometimes involve the petroclinoid region more laterally. Other spinal (vertebral) sites are less common. Chordomas are more common in men and far more common in adults than in children. The tumors appear as lobulated masses with prominent bone destruction. Histologically, they are composed of trabecular cords of cells in a mucinous matrix; the cells are vacuolated, as they are filled with droplets of the mucinous myxoid matrix, which they secrete (Fig. 8-80). Most of these tumors grow slowly and have low mitotic rates; higher rates indicate a more aggressive tendency.

The clinical presentation of a clivus lesion reflects compression of the brainstem, its exiting nerves, the hypothalamus, or the region of the optic chiasm. The differential diagnosis can include pituitary adenoma for more anterior lesions. Bone destruction is best demonstrated by CT. The tumor appears hypointense on T1-weighted MRI, displacing the hyperintense bone marrow fat. On T2-weighted MRI, the tumors are usually hyperintense (Fig. 8-81). Calcification may be seen in up to 50% of cases. Contrast enhancement is common. Diagnosis is best established by surgical biopsy or partial excision; the role of radical surgical extirpation is limited by the tendency of the tumor to invade and destroy bone, so removal with margins is rarely possible. After surgery, most patients experience recurrent progressive growth, albeit at the same slow pace. The tumors are relatively radioinsensitive but may respond to high-dose focal irradiation with cyclotron-derived protons. Proton radiotherapy has a dosage cutoff that is measured by depth from skin, which gives rise to an unusual appearance after treatment (Fig. 8-82).

Chondrosarcomas of the skull base have similar presentations, imaging features, and clinical course. They pose similar therapeutic challenges but are often more aggressive than chordomas.

Hemangioblastoma

Hemangioblastomas are vascular neoplasms of uncertain cellular origin that arise most often in the cerebellar vermis or hemispheres but that also occur throughout the neuraxis in the leptomeninges, especially of the spinal cord. In the autosomal dominant genetic syndrome von Hippel–Lindau disease, there are usually multiple

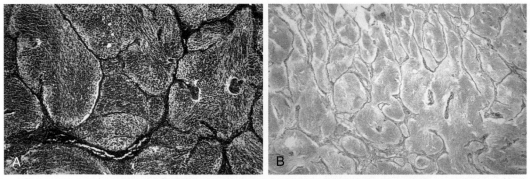

Fig. 8-45. Desmoplastic primitive neuroectodermal tumor. **A,** Cellular islands (staining red) bounded by glial and connective tissue borders (the latter staining blue) (azocarmine, ×80). **B,** Reticulin stain showing the reticulin fibers confined to the follicular borders (×20).

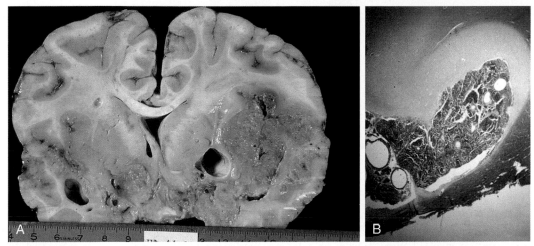

Fig. 8-46. A, Primitive neuroectodermal tumor with leptomeningeal dissemination. Coronal slice illustrating filling and distention of the sylvian fissures and the basal structures. **B,** From the same case, densely cellular mass of dark-staining tumor cells lying in the subarachnoid space above the corpus callosum (blue) and cingulate gyrus cortex (pink) (Luxol fast blue, H&E, ×10).

hemangioblastomas in the CNS and retina, accompanied by cysts of the kidneys, pancreas, and epididymis, and in some patients by renal cell carcinomas (renal tubular adenocarcinomas).

Hemangioblastomas are cystic lesions with a small mural nodule. Histopathologic examination shows macrophage-like stromal cells with pale, lipid-filled cytoplasm and large, often pleomorphic nuclei, associated with numerous small capillary-sized blood vessels (Fig. 8-83). The capillary proliferation is driven by secretion of vascular endothelial growth factor (VEGF) from the stromal cells. VEGF secretion is usually under the control of the *VHL* gene, and mutation of this gene in von Hippel–Lindau disease leads to the development of multiple tumors. In sporadic examples, the capillary proliferation is also driven by this mechanism because of somatic mutation or deletion of the VHL gene in the tumor stromal cells.

Presentation is either with hydrocephalus, a cerebellar syndrome, or (rarely) with polycythemia as a consequence of erythropoietin secretion by the tumor. CT scanning reveals a solid or (more usually) cystic lesion, and it will show the mural nodule in the latter case (Fig. 8-84). The nodule enhances intensely. Comparable findings are demonstrated by MRI (Fig. 8-85). Spinal MRI is necessary to exclude spinal spread. Angiography may be required to visualize small medullary lesions.

Therapy is by excision, sometimes following interventional neuroradiologic embolization of the tumor with beads of polyvinyl alcohol or similar particles. Small lesions may be treated by stereotactic radiosurgery.

Pituitary Tumors

Pituitary adenomas account for about 10% to 20% of intracranial neoplasms and occur more commonly in women. They reach a peak incidence between the third and sixth decades of life. Microadenomas are distinguished from adenomas solely on the basis of size; the former are less than 10 mm in diameter. Microadenomas come to attention when they produce endocrinologically active substances. Macroadenomas are often nonsecretory and are discovered because of the mass effect they exert.

Prolactinomas account for about 20% to 30% of those tumors removed at operation. Less common are the adenomas associated with adrenocorticotropic hormone (ACTH) and with follicle-stimulating hormone (FSH) or luteinizing hormone (LH) (each accounting for about 10% to 15%), and the growth hormone–producing adenoma (5%). Endocrinologically inactive adenomas represent a further 20%.

As they expand, the tumors spread upward into the suprasellar cistern. The more invasive varieties may extend downward into the sphenoid bone or laterally into one or both cavernous sinuses. Microscopically, a pattern of uniform cells is separated by a capillary network (Fig. 8-86). Immunohistochemical techniques differentiate the individual subtypes by hormonal content and allow a classification to be made according to the tumor's endocrine status.

The clinical presentation is determined by this status and partly by the extent of any local extension to adjacent structures. As the tumor expands, compression of these adjacent structures follows. The type of visual defect produced depends on the relationship of the pituitary fossa to the optic chiasm (Fig. 8-87). In the most common arrangement, compression of the chiasm from below produces a superior bitemporal field defect, which is typically asymmetrical (Fig. 8-88). An ophthalmoplegia occurs with extension into one or other cavernous sinus (Fig. 8-89). Prolactinomas in women produce amenorrhea and galactorrhea. Impotence and depressed libido are potential consequences in men. Growth hormone production results in gigantism or acromegaly depending on whether the tumor is active before or after epiphyseal closure (Fig. 8-90). Overproduction of ACTH leads to Cushing's disease. If the adrenal glands are removed in such

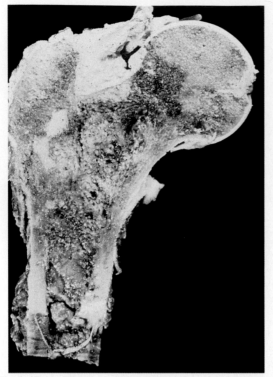

Fig. 8-47. Medulloblastoma. Metastasis in the head of the femur.

patients, on the mistaken assumption that they are the primary cause of the clinical picture, rapid further expansion of the pituitary adenoma occurs with compression of adjacent structures and hyperpigmentation (Nelson's syndrome).

Specific endocrine effects from thyroid-stimulating hormone (TSH) or FSH/LH-producing tumors are rare. Hypopituitarism results either from compression of the gland by an endocrinologically inert tumor, or acutely as a result of infarction of, or hemorrhage into, the gland (pituitary apoplexy). Typically, patients develop severe headache, ophthalmoplegia, and signs of subarachnoid hemorrhage if the underlying pathology is hemorrhagic.

Investigation. On CT scanning, pituitary macroadenomas are usually isodense or slightly hyperdense, with calcification in about a fifth and enhancement, usually of a homogeneous quality, in about three quarters (Figs. 8-91 and 8-92). In some cases, the tumors contain cystic areas or hemorrhage (Fig. 8-93). Pituitary microadenomas are more difficult to detect. With T1-weighted MRI sequences, microadenomas appear hypointense in comparison to the rest of the anterior lobe. They have well-defined margins and tend to lie laterally in the gland. They appear as focal areas of low signal intensity, displacing the pituitary stalk contralaterally and showing delayed enhancement compared with normal pituitary tissue (Fig. 8-94).

Macroadenomas are readily visualized, again preferably on T1-weighted sequences. Generally, the interface between the adenoma and the remnants of normal gland is not visible (Fig. 8-95). As the tumor increases in size, areas of hemorrhage, necrosis, or cystic degeneration commonly occur. Enhancement with gadolinium is likely but may be patchy (Fig. 8-96). A dynamic study to reveal gland enhancement over time can be helpful.

Treatment. Large tumors with suprasellar extension are treated surgically via the peritoneal or transfrontal approach. Postoperative radiotherapy reduces the risk of recurrence. Small tumors can be approached transsphenoidally via the nose.

For prolactinomas, a reduction in the size of the tumor is possible by the use of dopaminergic agonists. Primary treatment with bromocriptine is now considered for these tumors, surgery being reserved for those patients with rapidly deteriorating vision or for those women wishing to contemplate a further pregnancy. Serial fields eloquently demonstrate the treatment's effectiveness (Fig. 8-97). Drug therapies for growth hormone–secreting adenomas are also increasingly substituted for surgical excision.

Craniopharyngioma

Craniopharyngiomas represent about 3% of intracranial neoplasms and most commonly appear before the age of 20, although examples in older individuals are well known. Virtually all of them arise in close relationship to the sella. Cysts containing a cholesterol-rich oil are frequently found in the substance of the tumor (Fig. 8-98). Histologic examination reveals cystic spaces lined by neoplastic epithelial cells (Fig. 8-99) in a characteristic pattern. These tumors have a basal epithelial layer of small cells, sitting on either a fibrous capsule or a gliotic brain tissue capsule; growing in toward the cyst lumen is a multicellular layer of stellate cells, and at the cyst surface there is abrupt keratinization into stacks of large flat plates, so-called wet keratin. A less common papillary epithelial architecture is seen most commonly in adult patients. In children, presentation is with evidence of raised intracranial pressure or disturbances of hypothalamic function. In adults, visual failure is the more likely initial feature, leading in some cases to conspicuous optic atrophy (Fig. 8-100).

About 90% of the tumors calcify in childhood but much less commonly in adults. Papillary craniopharyngioma rarely calcifies. CT reveals either a solid or cystic mass, with the density characteristics of the cyst depending on the nature of its content, which may be calcified. Enhancement is either uniform or confined to the cyst margins. The MRI appearance is very variable, depending on the signal characteristics of the tumor and any cystic component (Fig. 8-101).

Resection is usually curative, although there is a substantial local recurrence rate. With incomplete resections, recurrence is virtually the rule. Other treatment choices include instillation of radioactive colloids into the cysts using stereotactic procedures, and radiation therapy, the latter using conformal techniques and for smaller lesions possibly stereotactic radiosurgery.

Osteoma

Osteomas of the skull may present neurologically as a result of the focal or generalized seizures that may be associated with them (Fig. 8-102).

THE NONMETASTATIC (PARANEOPLASTIC) CEREBRAL AND CEREBELLAR SYNDROMES

The nonmetastatic (paraneoplastic) cerebral and cerebellar syndromes involve central neurologic dysfunction occurring in patients with systemic cancers in whom there is no metastatic spread of the cancer to the CNS. Many of these syndromes are immune-mediated.

In limbic encephalitis, a subacute onset of memory impairment (sometimes episodic) occurs, with disorientation and agitation. Accompanying features variably include seizures, sleep disturbance, and hallucinations. Particularly affected are the medial temporal lobes, the hypothalamus, the amygdala, the hippocampus, and the cingulate gyrus (Fig. 8-103). Limbic encephalitis can be accompanied by lesions in the spinal cord, dorsal root ganglia, and brainstem.

Pathologic changes include neuronal loss, perivascular lymphocytic cuffing (Fig. 8-104), and microglial infiltration (Fig. 8-105), particularly in the hippocampi and medial temporal lobes. Signal changes are frequently found on MRI in the medial temporal lobes or the hippocampi (Fig. 8-106). Specific autoantibodies described in this syndrome include anti-Hu in lung cancer, anti-Ma2 in testicular tumors, and anti-CRMP5/CV2 in patients with thymomas. A form of limbic encephalitis unassociated with cancer appears in some cases to be related to voltage-gated potassium channel antibodies. Such antibodies can be shown to bind to hippocampal pyramidal neurons, but also to other neuronal populations, including the granular cell neurons of the cerebellum with sparing of Purkinje cells (Fig. 8-107).

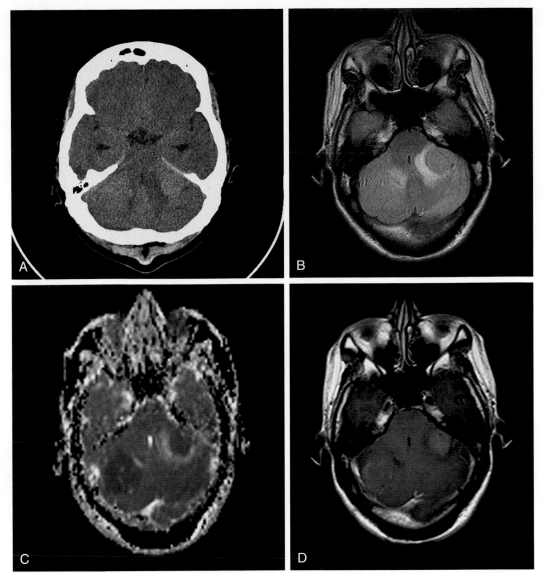

Fig. 8-48. Medulloblastoma. **A,** Unenhanced CT. **B,** MRI, fluid-attenuated inversion recovery (FLAIR). **C,** Apparent diffusion coefficient. **D,** T1-weighted MRI with contrast.

In some cases, immunotherapy both eliminates the antibody and improves the clinical syndrome.

Besides a cerebellar syndrome occurring in association with limbic encephalitis, a pure cerebellar syndrome of a noninflammatory type is recognized. It is particularly associated with carcinoma of the lung and ovary. The patients present with limb and gait ataxia, dysarthria, and various eye movement disorders. There is striking depletion of Purkinje cells in the cerebellum (Fig. 8-108). CT scanning performed serially may demonstrate evolving cerebellar atrophy (Fig. 8-109).

The syndrome may precede the malignancy by 3 years or appear up to 2 years after the malignancy has been diagnosed. Anti-Yo antibodies are usually found in breast and ovarian cancer. An anti-PCA-2 antibody directed at a 280-kD Purkinje cell cytoplasmic antigen occurs in small cell lung cancer associated with a cerebellar syndrome. An antibody reacting with the metabotropic glutamate receptor has been found in patients with Hodgkin's disease and a cerebellar syndrome.

Many of the tumors causing a paraneoplastic syndrome are occult at the time of presentation. In that circumstance, scanning with [18F] fluoro-2-deoxyglucose (FDG) PET may identify hypermetabolism suggestive of malignancy when conventional imaging has been negative (Fig. 8-110).

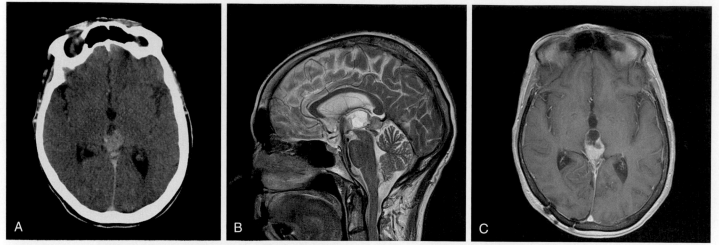

Fig. 8-49. Pinealoma. **A,** CT. **B** and **C,** MRI.

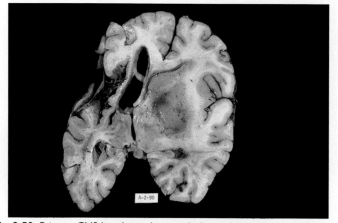

Fig. 8-50. Primary CNS lymphoma. Large right hemisphere tumor exerting mass effect. There is an old infarct in the left basal ganglia.

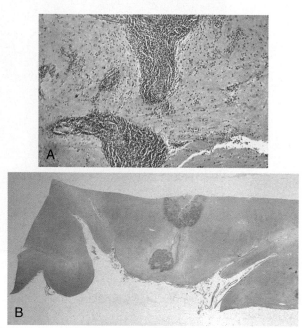

Fig. 8-51. Primary CNS lymphoma. **A,** Perivascular aggregation of small dark-staining cells with surrounding gliosis (H&E, ×80). **B,** Coronal section showing small-celled tumor surrounding the third ventricle (H&E, ×1).

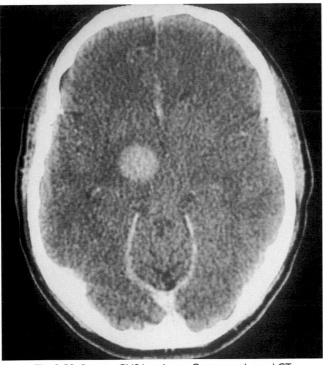

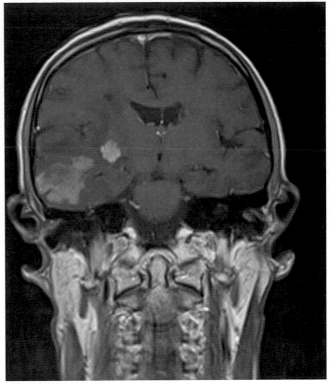

Fig. 8-52. Primary CNS lymphoma. Contrast-enhanced CT.

Fig. 8-53. Primary CNS lymphoma. MRI. Compared with gliomas, the enhancement is often more "solid" and may be multifocal.

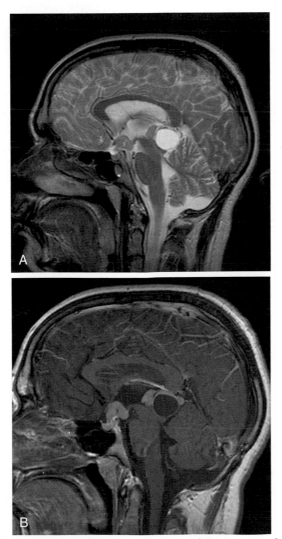

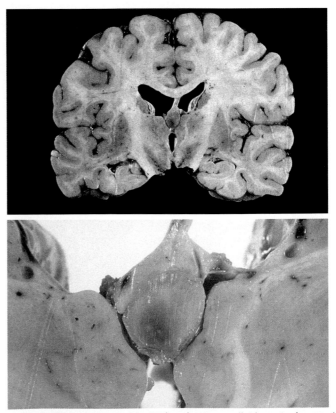

Fig. 8-54. Germinoma involving the suprasellar and pineal regions. **A,** Sagittal T2-weighted MRI. **B,** T1-weighted, gadolinium-enhanced MRI.

Fig. 8-55. Colloid cyst. Coronal brain slice showing a colloid cyst in the anterior part of the third ventricle, occluding the foramina of Munro.

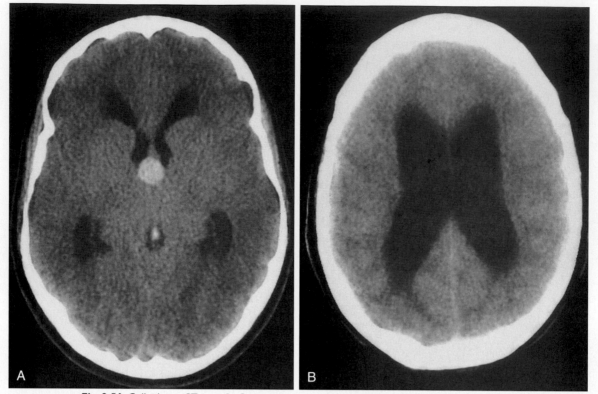

Fig. 8-56. Colloid cyst. CT scan. **A,** Cyst occupying the third ventricle **B,** Associated hydrocephalus.

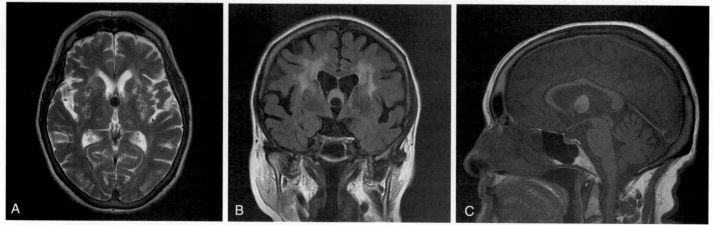

Fig. 8-57. Colloid cyst. **A,** Axial T2-weighted MRI. **B,** Coronal fluid-attenuated inversion recovery (FLAIR). **C,** Sagittal T1-weighted MRI.

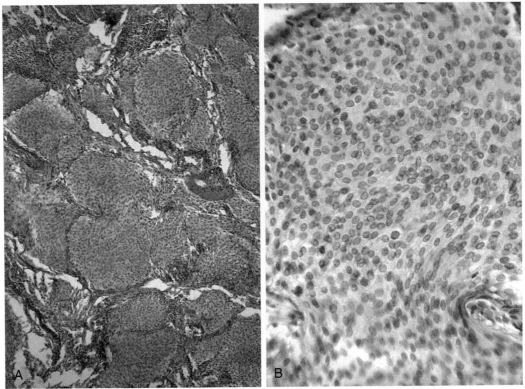

Fig. 8-58. Syncytial meningioma. **A,** Fine lobular architecture is apparent (H&E, ×80). **B,** Appearance of bland pale nuclei in syncytial lobule (H&E, ×320).

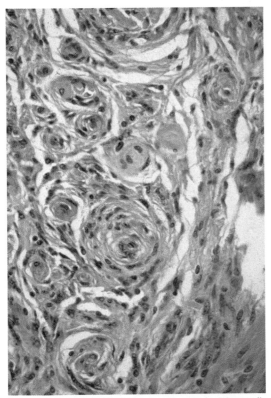

Fig. 8-59. Transitional meningioma. Whorls associated with spindly elongated "fibroblastic" cells (H&E, ×320).

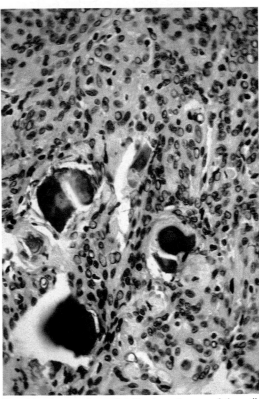

Fig. 8-60. Transitional meningioma. Calcification of some of the cellular whorls: psammoma bodies (H&E, ×320).

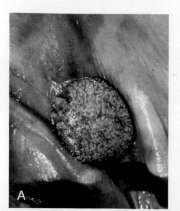

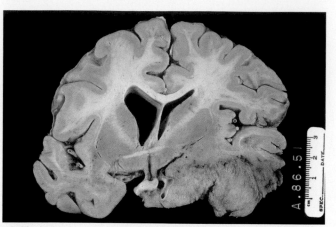

Fig. 8-62. Malignant meningioma. Subfrontal tumor surrounding the internal carotid and middle cerebral arteries, with a ragged interface between tumor and brain.

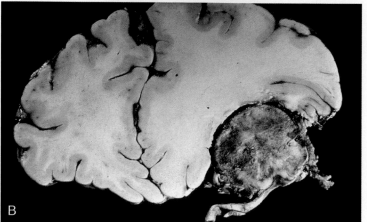

Fig. 8-61. Incidental meningioma found at postmortem. **A,** The patient had been jaundiced. **B,** Larger meningioma exerting mass effect.

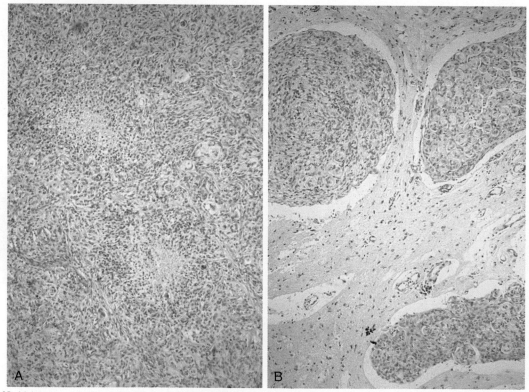

Fig. 8-63. Malignant meningioma. **A,** Two foci of necrosis. **B,** Fingers of moderately cellular tumor invading the white matter (H&E, ×80).

SITES OF MENINGIOMAS

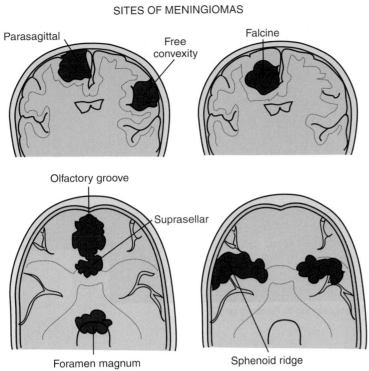

Parasagittal

Free convexity

Falcine

Olfactory groove

Suprasellar

Foramen magnum

Sphenoid ridge

Fig. 8-64. Distribution of intracranial meningiomas.

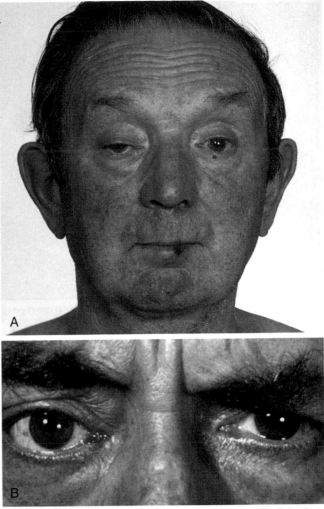

Fig. 8-65. A, Sphenoidal wing meningioma with right ptosis. **B,** Orbital meningioma with right proptosis.

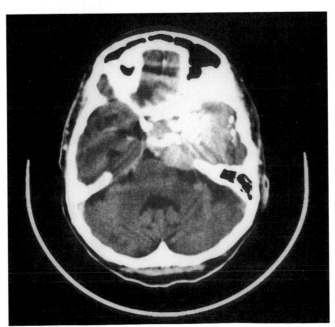

Fig. 8-66. Sphenoidal wing meningioma. Contrast-enhanced CT.

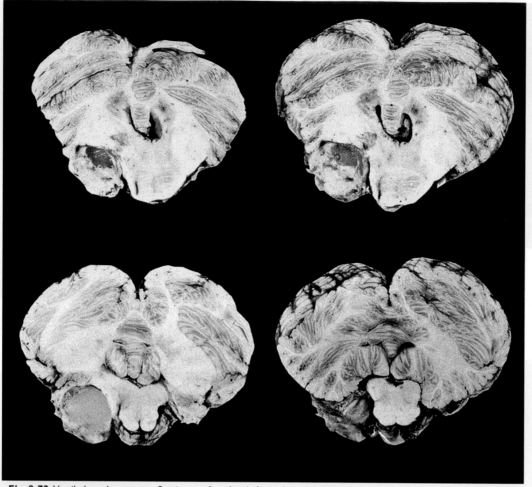

Fig. 8-72. Vestibular schwannoma. Sections at four levels from the medulla to the midbrain. The tumor is partly cystic.

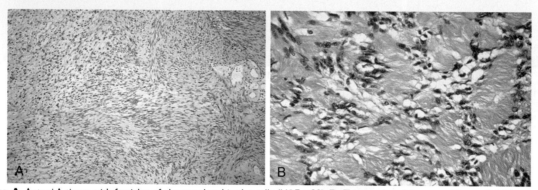

Fig. 8-73. Schwannoma. **A,** Antoni A tissue with fascicles of elongated or bipolar cells (H&E, ×80). **B,** Elongated nuclei arranged in parallel (Verocay body) (H&E, ×320).

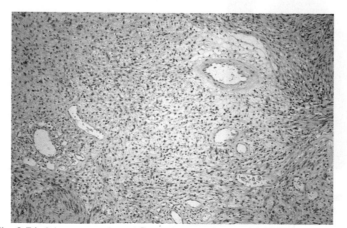

Fig. 8-74. Schwannoma. Antoni B area in central part of field. The tumor cells contain irregular round nuclei and lie in a spongy background (H&E, ×80).

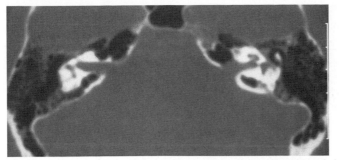

Fig. 8-75. Expansion of the left internal auditory meatus by a vestibular schwannoma. CT.

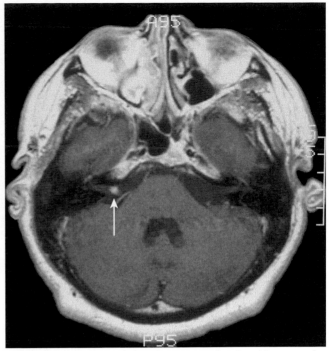

Fig. 8-76. Intracanalicular vestibular schwannoma enhancing with contrast *(arrow)*. T1-weighted MRI.

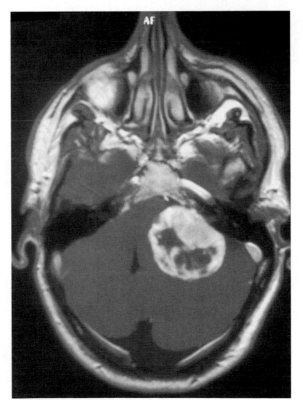

Fig. 8-77. Vestibular schwannoma. T1-weighted, gadolinium-enhanced MRI. Note substantial distortion of the fourth ventricle.

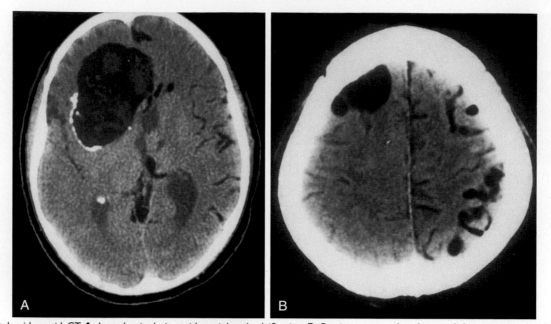

Fig. 8-78. Right frontal epidermoid. CT. **A,** Low-density lesion with peripheral calcification. **B,** Previous rupture has dispersed the contents over the surface of the contralateral hemisphere.

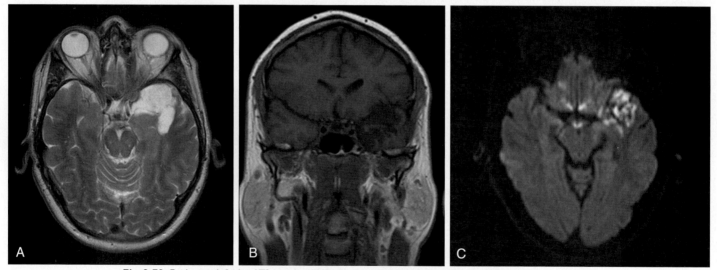

Fig. 8-79. Epidermoid. **A,** Axial T2-weighted MRI. **B,** Coronal T1-weighted MRI. **C,** Diffusion-weighted image.

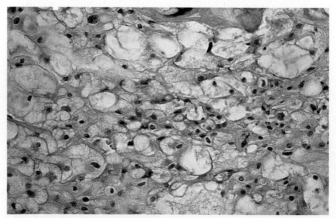

Fig. 8-80. Chordoma. Vacuolated cells (physaliferous cells). (H&E ×320)

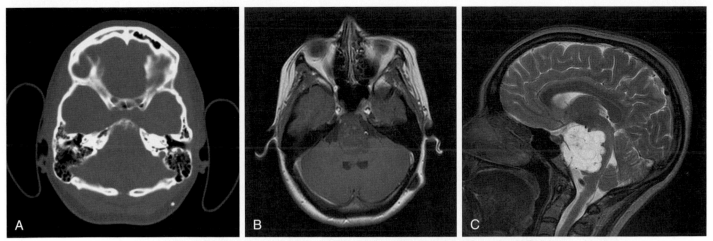

Fig. 8-81. Chordoma. **A,** CT. **B,** Axial T1-weighted MRI. **C,** Sagittal T2-weighted MRI.

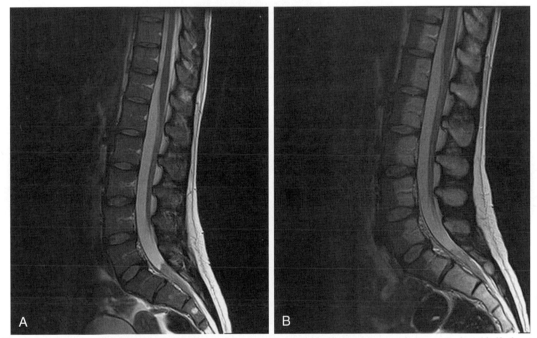

Fig. 8-82. Chordoma. **A,** Sagittal T2-weighted MRI. **B,** After proton radiotherapy. Note fatty marrow replacement in dorsal half of vertebral bodies.

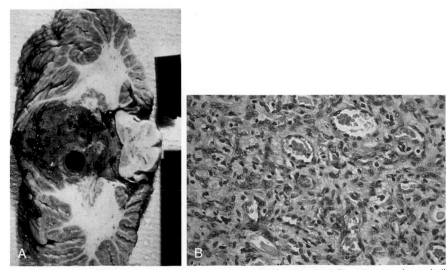

Fig. 8-83. Capillary hemangioblastoma. **A,** Macroscopic appearance. **B,** Numerous small capillary-sized vessels (H&E, ×320).

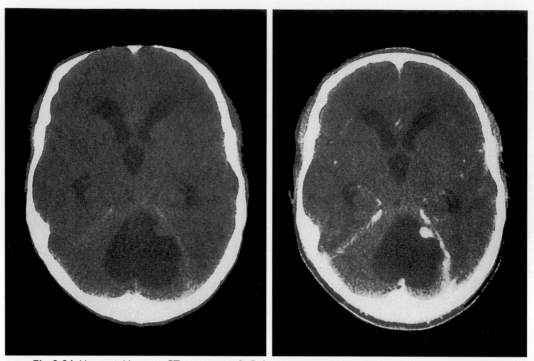

Fig. 8-84. Hemangioblastoma. CT appearance. **A,** Before contrast injection. **B,** With contrast enhancement.

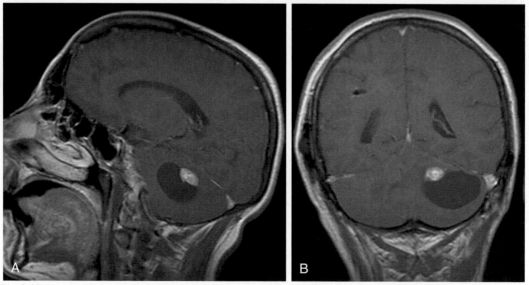

Fig. 8-85. Hemangioblastoma. Contrast-enhanced MRI showing cyst with enhancing mural nodule. **A,** Sagittal. **B,** Coronal.

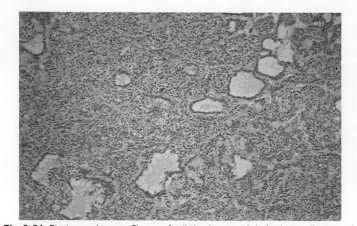

Fig. 8-86. Pituitary adenoma. Sheets of cells broken into lobules by capillaries, with duct formation (H&E, ×80).

RELATIONSHIPS OF THE CHIASM

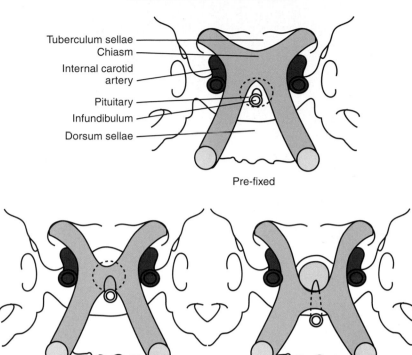

Tuberculum sellae
Chiasm
Internal carotid artery
Pituitary
Infundibulum
Dorsum sellae

Pre-fixed

Normal   Post-fixed

Fig. 8-87. The relationship of the chiasm to the pituitary fossa.

CHIASMATIC FIELD DEFECT

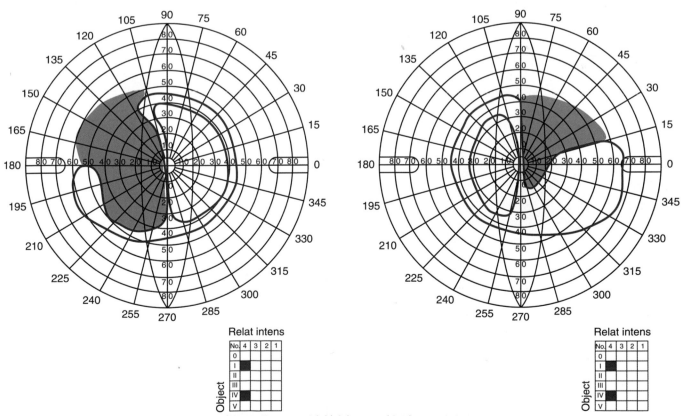

Relat intens

Object	No.	4	3	2	1
	0				
	I				
	II				
	III				
	IV				
	V				

Fig. 8-88. Superior bitemporal field defects resulting from a pituitary tumor.

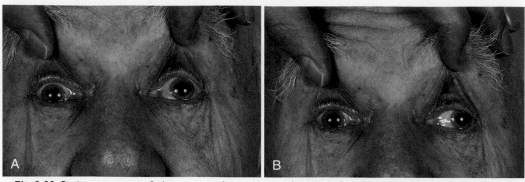

Fig. 8-89. Pituitary metastasis. **A,** Impairment of upward gaze of right eye. **B,** Impairment of adduction of right eye.

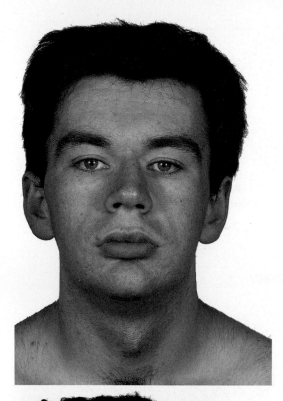

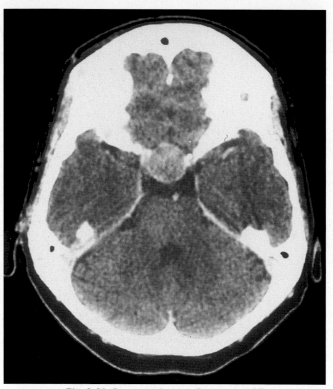

Fig. 8-91. Pituitary adenoma. Precontrast CT.

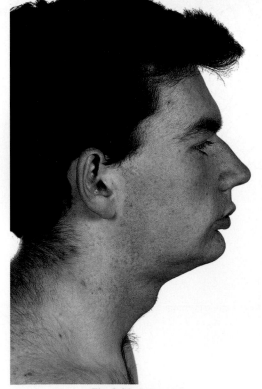

Fig. 8-90. Acromegaly.

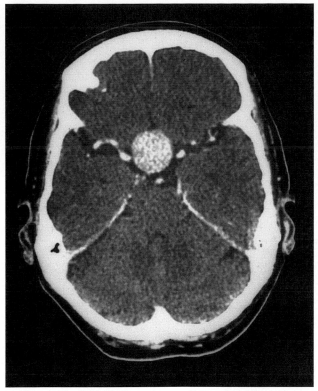

Fig. 8-92. Pituitary adenoma. Postcontrast CT.

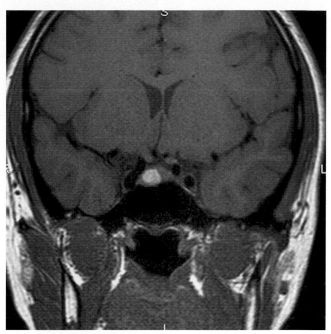

Fig. 8-93. Pituitary microadenoma with hemorrhage.

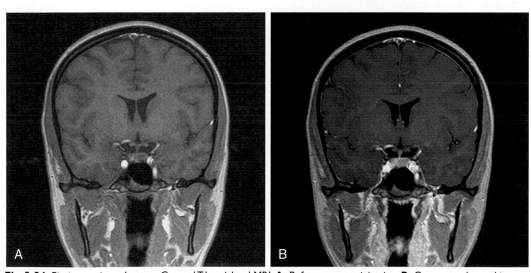

Fig. 8-94. Pituitary microadenoma. Coronal T1-weighted MRI. **A,** Before contrast injection. **B,** Contrast-enhanced images.

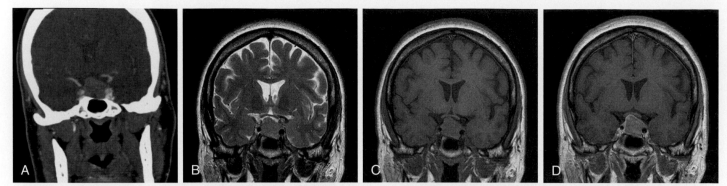

Fig. 8-95. Pituitary macroadenoma. **A,** CT. **B,** Coronal T2-weighted MRI. **C,** Precontrast T1-weighted MRI. **D,** Postcontrast T1-weighted MRI.

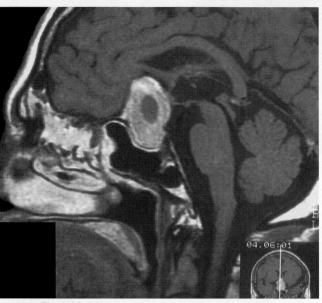

Fig. 8-96. Pituitary macroadenoma. Postcontrast MRI.

VISUAL FIELDS

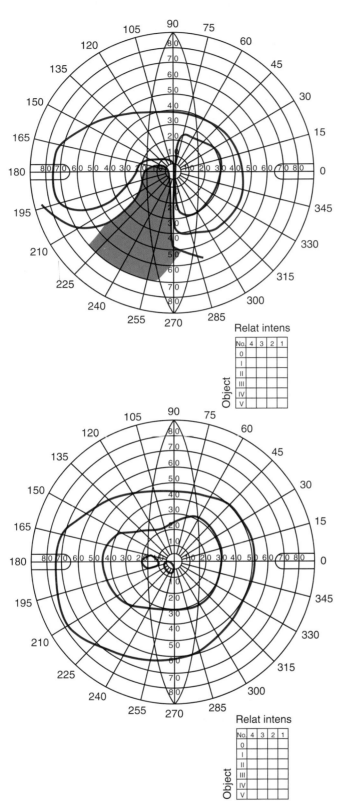

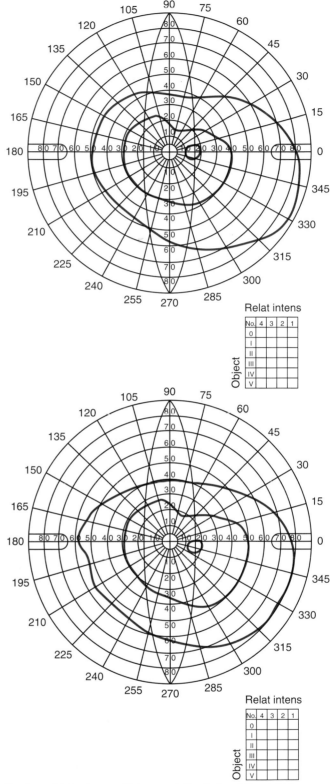

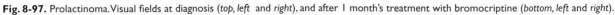

Fig. 8-97. Prolactinoma. Visual fields at diagnosis (*top, left* and *right*), and after 1 month's treatment with bromocriptine (*bottom, left* and *right*).

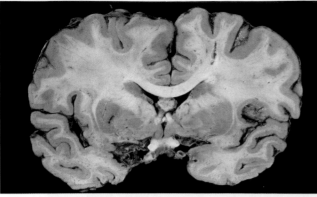

Fig. 8-103. Limbic encephalitis. Macroscopic features.

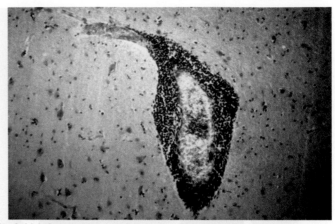

Fig. 8-104. Polioencephalitis. Perivascular lymphocytic cuffing at the junction of the cortex and white matter in the right temporal lobe (H&E, ×150).

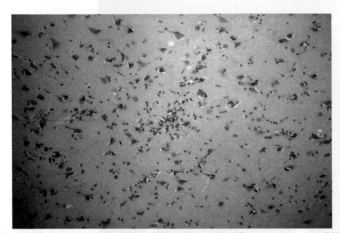

Fig. 8-105. Polioencephalitis. Microglial nodule in the left temporal cortex (H&E, ×130).

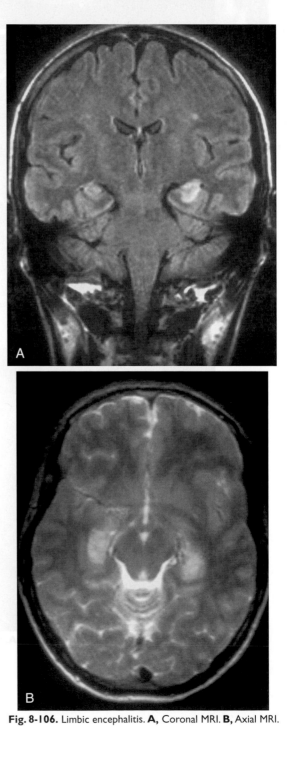

Fig. 8-106. Limbic encephalitis. **A,** Coronal MRI. **B,** Axial MRI.

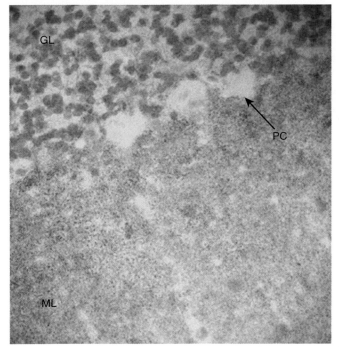

Fig. 8-107. Detection of voltage-gated potassium channel (PC) antibodies by indirect immunohistochemistry (×400).

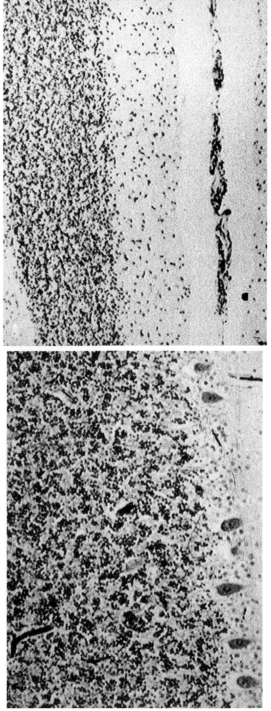

Fig. 8-108. Subacute cerebellar degeneration. **A,** Almost total absence of Purkinje cells in the cerebellar hemisphere (cresyl violet, ×80). **B,** Normal control (Luxol fast blue with cresyl violet counterstain, ×70).

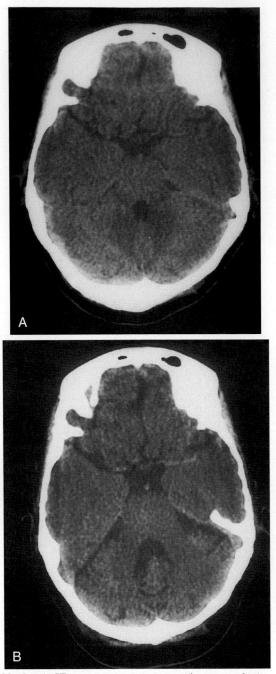

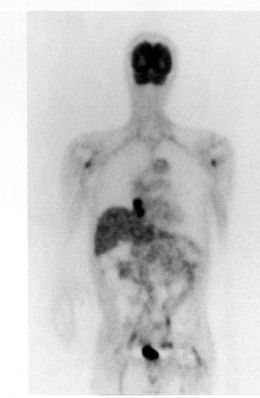

Fig. 8-110. PET scanning with [^{18}F]fluoro-2-deoxyglucose (FDG). Identifying a pulmonary lesion in a patient with a paraneoplastic syndrome.

Fig. 8-109. Serial CT scanning in a patient with paraneoplastic cerebellar syndrome, demonstrating evolving atrophy (A then B).

SPINAL TUMORS AND PARANEOPLASTIC DISORDERS

Spinal tumors arise in the cord substance, from the spinal meninges, the spinal roots, the epidural space or the spine itself. Most intramedullary tumors in adults are astrocytomas, ependymomas, or metastases; in children, astrocytomas are gangliogliomas, the most common intramedullary neoplasm. Astrocytomas occur both in a diffuse form and, less commonly, in a more circumscribed form, the pilocytic astrocytoma.

Ependymomas account for about 60% of primary tumors of the cord in adults and are predominantly found in the filum terminale. The most common meningeal neoplasm is the meningioma, which accounts for about a quarter of all primary intraspinal growths (Fig. 9-1). Less common tumors at this site are lipomas, hemangiopericytomas, and metastatic carcinomas or lymphomas. Schwannomas originate usually from dorsal nerve roots. Most occur in isolation rather than as a part of neurofibromatosis 1 (NF1) or neurofibromatosis 2 (NF2) (see Chapter 10). They are slightly more common than either meningiomas or intramedullary tumors. Spinal nerve root neurofibromas are uncommon and are almost always associated with NF1. A tumor infiltrating the epidural space is usually a metastatic carcinoma that has extended from the vertebral column, typically in the thoracic region. Other tumors occupying the epidural space include lymphomas, leukemic masses, and lipomas.

A number of primary bone tumors are liable to spread into the spinal canal and produce focal neurologic deficit. Examples include chordoma, multiple myeloma, and vertebral hemangioma.

CLINICAL FEATURES OF SPINAL TUMORS

The clinical features of a spinal tumor depend on its segmental location, on whether it is intramedullary or extramedullary, and on its speed of growth.

Foramen Magnum Lesions
Pain in association with a foramen magnum tumor, usually a schwannoma or meningioma, is liable to be referred to the neck and the occiput. Facial pain can coexist, the consequence of disruption of the spinal tract of the trigeminal nerve. A quadriparesis appears, often asymmetrical and sometimes associated with wasting of the small hand muscles. Horner's syndrome is more likely with intramedullary than with extramedullary tumors. Additional signs include disturbance of function of the eleventh and twelfth cranial nerves and down-beating nystagmus.

Cervical Lesions
At the level of the tumor, lower motor neuron signs appear, including wasting, weakness, and fasciculation. The biceps and supinator reflexes are depressed if the C5 and C6 segments are affected and the triceps reflex with C7 root involvement. If there is also cord compression, weakness and spasticity appear in the lower limbs together with altered sphincter function. Extramedullary tumors are likely to produce a radicular pattern of sensory loss, and intramedullary tumors to produce a disturbance of long-tract sensory function, either of pain and temperature or joint position sense. Sacral sparing

of spinothalamic loss is suggestive of an intramedullary tumor, but the same pattern is also sometimes seen with extrinsic tumors.

Thoracic Lesions
In thoracic lesions, there is a spastic paraparesis with a sensory level on the trunk to pain or temperature that tends to be slightly below the level of compression. Although radicular signs are likely with either a meningioma or schwannoma, the sensory or motor changes are often subtle. Radicular pain is prominent with these two tumors. The abdominal reflexes are absent in those segments at or below the level of compression.

Conus and Cauda Equina Lesions
Lesions at the levels of the conus and cauda equina result either in a mixture of lower and upper motor neuron signs in the lower limbs or in a purely lower motor neuron syndrome if the cauda equina is affected. In that case, a flaccid paraparesis develops with areflexia, segmental sensory loss, and a severe disturbance of sexual and sphincter function. With conus lesions that extend into the epiconus, an admixture of upper and lower motor neuron signs emerges, with reflex abnormalities determined by the site of the tumor.

Spinal Cord Clinical Syndrome
The clinical picture with cord compression tends to follow one of three patterns. In one, a transverse cord lesion disrupts all cord function below that level, with an appropriate sensory level, and a motor deficit involving either both upper and lower limbs, or the lower limbs alone, according to whether the cervical or thoracic cord is compressed. A hemicord (Brown-Séquard) syndrome is most often seen with extrinsic cord compression, but it can also develop with intramedullary tumors. Typically, ipsilateral to the compression there is a pyramidal deficit along with posterior column signs, with contralateral loss of spinothalamic function. Finally, intramedullary tumors can lead to a central cord syndrome in which a suspended level of pure spinothalamic loss is found, accompanied by pyramidal signs below the site of the lesion. If the cervical cord is involved, disruption of anterior horn cells produces focal lower motor neuron signs at the level of the lesion. Among intramedullary tumors, ependymomas above the filum tend to be located centrally, expanding more or less equally in all directions at any single level but at the same time occupying several contiguous cord levels. Patients with such tumors tend to have a predominance of sensory abnormalities, with weakness appearing later. By contrast, astrocytic tumors are more asymmetrical and tend to present with a combined motor and sensory deficit.

INVESTIGATION OF SPINAL TUMORS

Plain Radiography
Plain radiographs of the spine are seldom relevant in the investigation of suspected tumor. They are usually normal in the case of meningiomas unless the tumor is calcified or has eroded an intervertebral foramen. Some erosion is a particular characteristic of schwannomas and can be identified by either plain radiography or CT (Fig. 9-2).

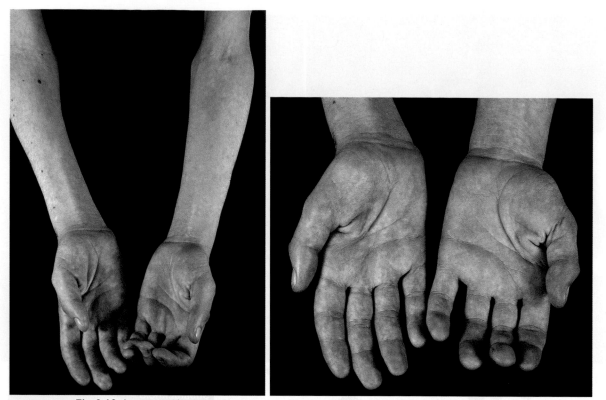

Fig. 9-19. A patient with a cervical astrocytoma. Distal upper limb wasting is more marked on the right.

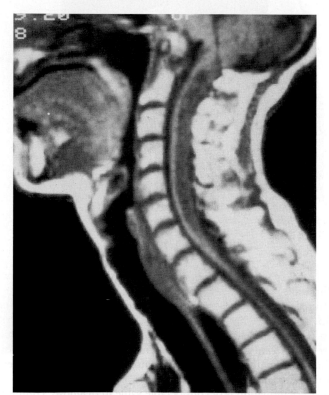

Fig. 9-20. Spinal astrocytoma. T1-weighted MRI.

Hemangiopericytoma

Hemangiopericytoma is a rare tumor that usually arises from the same sites in the cranial meninges at which meningiomas are found. Infrequently, it originates in the spine as a lobulated mass attached to the dura. These are highly vascular sarcomas that frequently recur locally after gross total excision, and they are also liable to metastasize. Imaging characteristics are similar to those of meningioma, but the rate of growth is much more rapid.

Nerve Sheath Tumors

Most schwannomas are isolated tumors arising from a dorsal root at any spinal level. Multiple tumors are usually a manifestation of neurofibromatosis 2 or infrequently of a syndrome called schwannomatosis. The peak incidence of presentation of sporadic schwannomas occurs in the fourth and fifth decades of life. Most remain confined to the intradural space, but some pass through an intervertebral foramen, forming a dumbbell-shaped mass. Whereas the plexiform neurofibroma is characterized by a diffuse expansion of the nerve root, the schwannoma is partly independent of it, with the nerve root draped over the surface of the tumor (Fig. 9-33).

Bone erosion is a particular feature of the schwannoma, identifiable either on plain radiograph or plain CT (Fig. 9-34). Lumbosacral neurofibromas appear with a root syndrome mimicking the effects of a prolapsed disc. A characteristic MRI signal pattern occurs with hyperintensity on T2-weighted images.

Although schwannomas are capable of malignant transformation, the vast majority are benign. Total excision is possible, but usually the associated nerve root has to be sacrificed. Nerve root neurofibromas are uncommon and then usually a part of NF1 (von Recklinghausen's disease). These are benign tumors, but they are more likely than schwannomas to undergo malignant transformation.

Lipomas

Lipomas in the dura occur mainly in the rostral portion of the spine. Those in the region of the filum terminale are associated with congenital spinal anomalies and are not true neoplasms. The lipoma is hyperintense on T1-weighted MR images (Fig. 9-35).

TUMORS OF THE EPIDURAL SPACE AND SPINE

Metastatic Carcinoma

The most common sources of extradural metastases are the breast, bronchus, prostate, and kidney. Metastases at this site are found at postmortem examination in up to 5% of patients with systemic cancer. About two thirds occur in the thoracic region. Pain, either confined to the spinal site or referred in a radicular distribution, is the

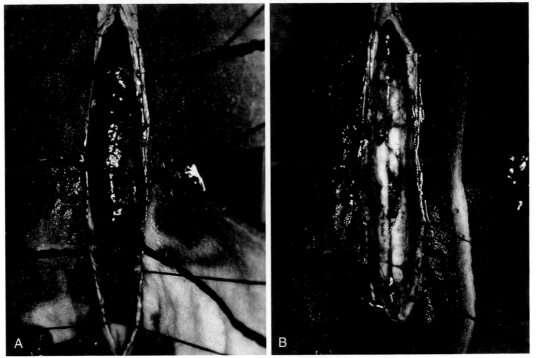

Fig. 9-21. Ependymoma. **A,** The tumor is seen as a dark, sausage-shaped mass fungating out of the midline dorsal myelotomy incision. **B,** After removal.

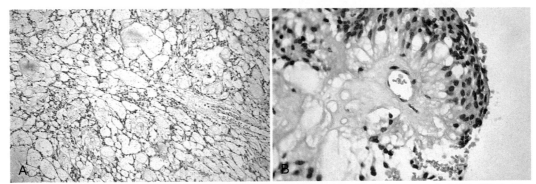

Fig. 9-22. Myxopapillary ependymoma. **A,** Lightly stained myxoid background substance containing strands of thin tumor cells (H&E, ×80). **B,** Characteristic papillary frond with central blood vessel surrounded by a radial array of tumor nuclei (H&E, ×320).

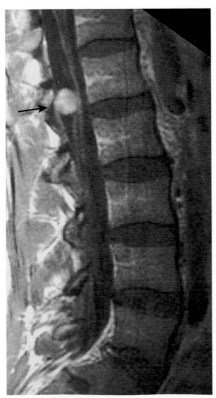

Fig. 9-23. Ependymoma of the filum terminale. Enhanced MRI.

usual presenting complaint and should alert the clinician to the need for imaging. By the first presentation, most patients have motor and sensory symptoms, and at least half have sphincteric disturbance. Typically, a lytic lesion in the vertebral body later infiltrates the extradural space. MRI is the investigation of choice, particularly for the identification of multiple metastases. Features include hypointensity on T1-weighted and hyperintensity on T2-weighted images, along with evidence of vertebral destruction and paravertebral extension. Enhancement is the norm. When the diagnosis is not established, CT-guided needle biopsy is the best way of obtaining tissue in most cases.

Corticosteroids are given immediately, although debate continues about the optimal dosage. Radiotherapy is the first line of treatment for radiosensitive tumors. Decompressive laminectomy has been largely abandoned, although its role alongside radiotherapy is being reevaluated.

Lymphoma and Leukemia

Lymphoma is more likely to cause cord compression than leukemia. Again, the mid-thoracic spine is the favorite site. Lymphoma usually invades the extradural space from a retroperitoneal paraspinal deposit via an intervertebral foramen, which is often unaltered by the process (Fig. 9-36). Radiotherapy is the treatment of choice, and the outcome is more favorable than that associated with metastatic carcinoma. Leukemic infiltration of the epidural space produces a similar picture.

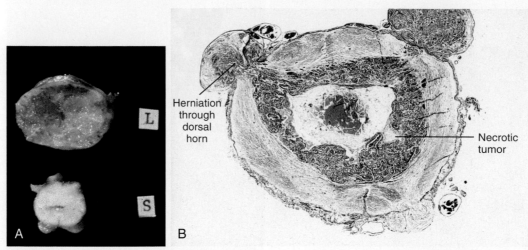

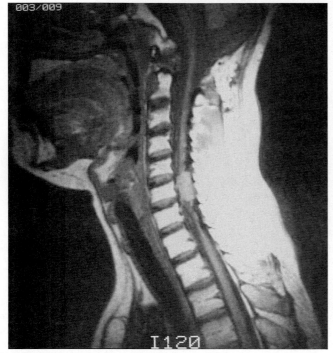

Fig. 9-24. Intramedullary metastasis. **A,** The lumbar cord (L) is largely replaced by tumor, with sparing of the sacral cord (S). **B,** The cord architecture is destroyed by necrotic tumor (cresyl violet, ×2.5).

Fig. 9-25. MRI. Intramedullary metastasis from primitive neuroectodermal tumor.

Lipomas
Spinal lipomas are usually found in the extradural space in the thoracic region. The histologic and MRI signal characteristics are similar to those of intradural lipomas.

Multiple Myeloma and Plasmacytoma
Solitary plasmacytoma and multiple myeloma have similar histologic features (Fig. 9-37). In some cases, an apparent solitary plasmacytoma is succeeded, years later, by serum electrophoretic evidence of multiple myeloma. The picture of spinal cord compression is similar to that seen with extradural metastases (Fig. 9-38). Bone scanning is often negative. MRI is the investigation of choice, revealing, on T1-weighted images, a hypointense area in comparison to adjacent bone marrow.

Hemangioma
Although hemangiomas are not uncommon at postmortem examination, patients rarely present with them. Symptoms include bone pain and evidence of nerve root or cord compression. The lesions can often be confidently diagnosed with plain radiography, when a pattern of vertical striations is seen associated with a lucent area. Typically, a hyperintense area is found on a T1-weighted MR image (Fig. 9-39).

Chordoma
The chordoma is thought to originate from notochordal remnants. In addition to the clivus chordoma (which represents some 40% of the total), spinal examples occur most often in the region of the sacrum (Fig. 9-40). Microscopy reveals features that are identical to those of clivus chordomas, with clusters, cords, and single neoplastic cells surrounded by a mucinous or myxoid connective tissue stroma. Some of the cells are vacuolated (Fig. 9-41). Bone destruction is prominent, and contiguous metastatic spread involves the lower cranial or sacral nerve roots. CT scanning reveals a mass lesion, sometimes partly calcified, with evidence of bone destruction (Fig. 9-42). A mixed signal pattern is evident on T2-weighted MR images.

Sacrococcygeal Teratoma
Sacrococcygeal teratomas are rare tumors, usually appearing in neonates or children. Posterior spread leads to invasion of the buttocks or the appearance of a subcutaneous mass. Anterior spread involves the pelvis. Histologically, an intermingling of tissues from ectoderm, mesoderm, and endoderm is typical. Despite their often extensive spread, the tumors are benign and capable of complete excision, although the capsule may be adherent to nervous tissue. Spillage of the teratoma contents at surgery can lead to arachnoiditis.

Paraneoplastic Spinal Syndromes
Subacute necrotizing myelopathy is a rare paraneoplastic disorder associated particularly with carcinoma of the bronchus. Axonal and myelin sheath degeneration is accompanied by a mild inflammatory cell reaction containing hemorrhagic foci (Fig. 9-43).

A spinal cord element is recognized as one component of encephalomyeloradiculitis. Historically, features include neuronal necrosis, microglial nodule formation, perivascular infiltration with mononuclear cells, and a reactive astrocytosis.

A motor neuron type of picture, sometimes resembling primary progressive sclerosis, has been identified in cancer patients and is sometimes associated with the presence of anti-Hu antibodies. An association of a paraneoplastic motor neuron disease with anti-Purkinje cell antibodies is recognized.

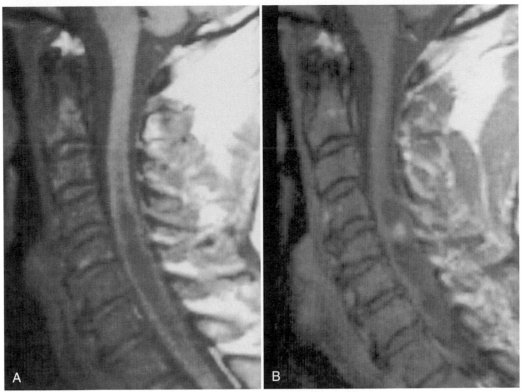

Fig. 9-26. Cervical hemangioblastoma. **A,** Before injection of contrast. **B,** With contrast enhancement.

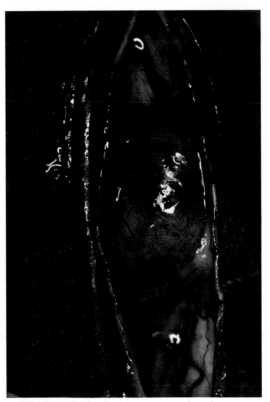

Fig. 9-27. Intradural spinal meningioma causing spinal cord compression.

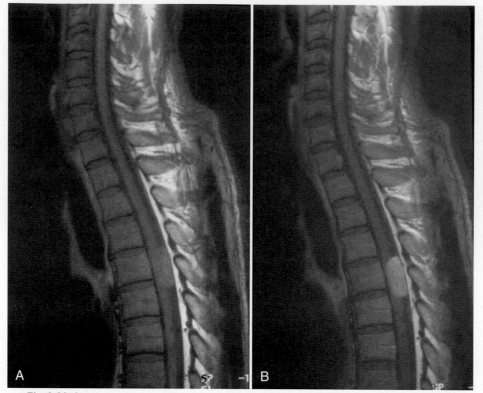

Fig. 9-28. Spinal meningioma. MRI. **A,** Before injection of contrast. **B,** With contrast enhancement.

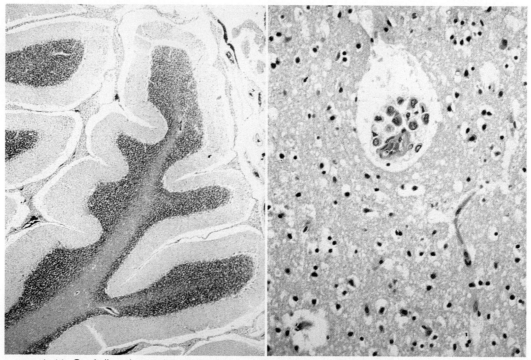

Fig. 9-29. Carcinomatous meningitis. Cerebellum showing leptomeningeal carcinomatosis and invasion along Virchow-Robin space (H&E, ×10 [left] and ×250 [right]).

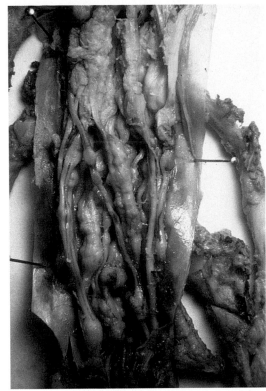

Fig. 9-30. Carcinomatous meningitis. Nodular thickening of cauda equina.

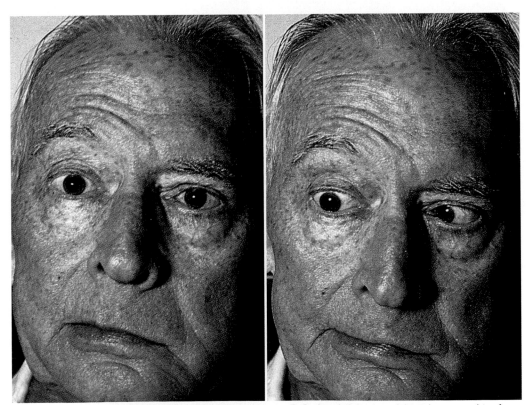

Fig. 9-31. Carcinomatous meningitis. **A,** Left lower motor neuron facial weakness. **B,** Reduced abduction of the right eye resulting from a sixth-nerve palsy.

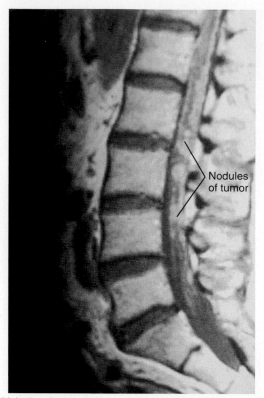

Fig. 9-32. Multiple enhancing nodules of leptomeningeal cancer, derived from the lung. T1-weighted lumbar MRI.

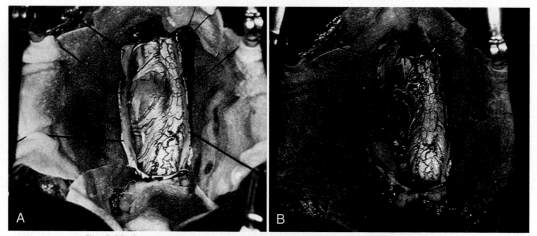

Fig. 9-33. Spinal schwannoma, operative views. **A,** Before removal. **B,** After removal.

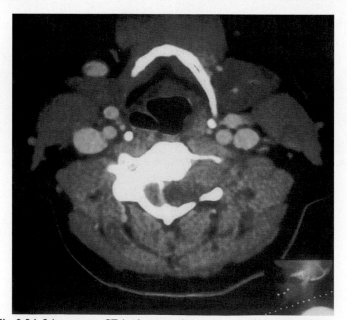

Fig. 9-34. Schwannoma. CT (with contrast) demonstrating bone erosion.

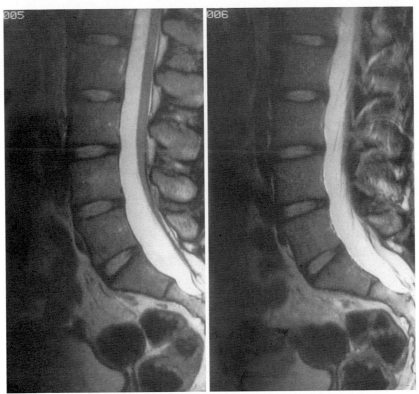

Fig. 9-35. Tethered cord associated with filum terminale lipoma. T2-weighted MRI.

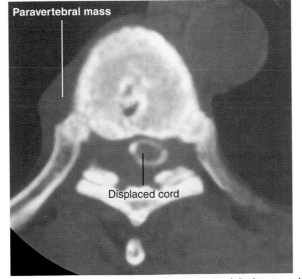

Fig. 9-36. Lymphoma. CT myelography demonstrating cord displacement. A paravertebral mass is visible.

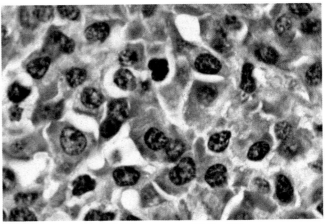

Fig. 9-37. Plasmacytoma (H&E, ×400).

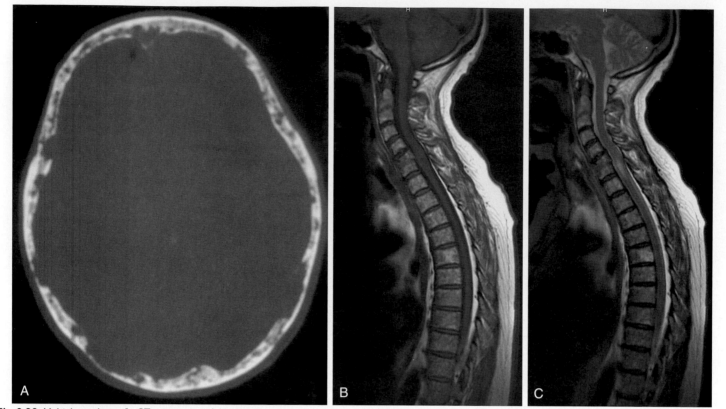

Fig. 9-38. Multiple myeloma. A, CT appearance of the skull. B and C, MRI of the cervical spine (T1-weighted and T2-weighted images). There is secondary cord compression with signal change.

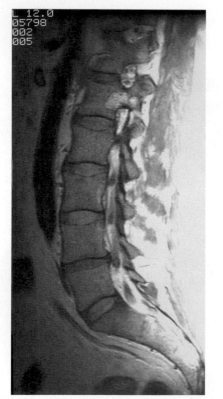

Fig. 9-39. MRI. Vertebral hemangioma. Increased signal on T2-weighted image.

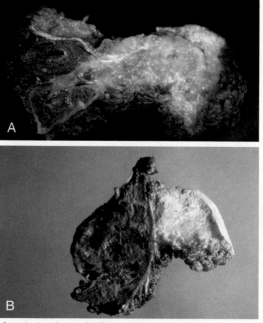

Fig. 9-40. Sacral chordoma. A, Typical lobulated architecture and mucoid cut surface. B, Chordoma extending from the peritoneum of the posterior pelvic wall (left) through to the subcutaneous tissue and skin (right).

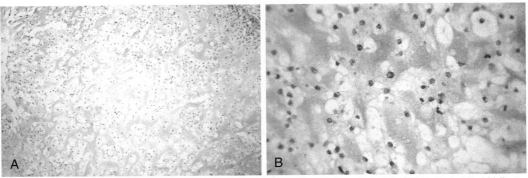

Fig. 9-41. Chordoma. **A,** Anastomosing cords of cells running through the myxoid, cartilage-like, matrix (H&E, ×25). **B,** Typical "bubbly" cytoplasm (H&E, ×100).

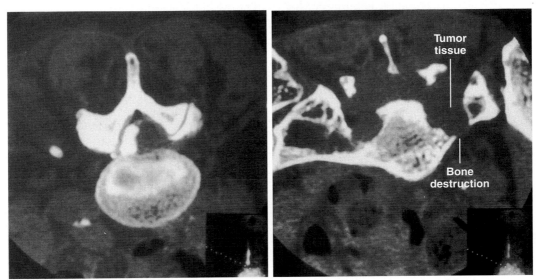

Fig. 9-42. Chordoma. CT myelogram. **A,** Displacement of thecal sac. **B,** Severe destruction of the sacrum.

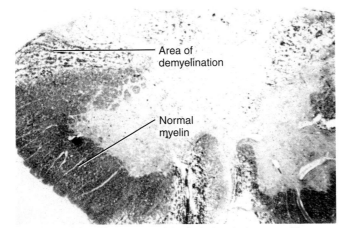

Fig. 9-43. Subacute necrotizing myelopathy. An area of demyelination containing fat is sharply demarcated from normal myelin (oil red O, Luxol fast blue, ×4).

Developmental abnormalities of the central nervous system can be divided into primary defects of development (Box 10-1) and secondary defects—the result of an injury to a previously normally developing brain. Most of the major primary brain malformations are the consequence of a failure to close part of the embryonic neural tube (neural tube defects) or of embryonic neural tube diverticulation. Less severe abnormalities often reflect defects in migration of cells from the periventricular germinal matrix to the cortex or other gray matter regions, resulting in abnormal gyral and sulcal formation or ectopic gray matter. Microcephaly describes a small cranium, usually the consequence of a small brain (micrencephaly). Macrocephaly describes an abnormally large cranium, which can result from megalencephaly. Sometimes, only one hemisphere is affected (hemimegalencephaly). Injuries causing secondary defects include ischemia (resulting in porencephaly). Sometimes the tissue loss is replaced by large, fluid-filled spaces (hydrancephaly).

NEURAL TUBE DEFECTS

Failure of cranial neural tube closure results in exencephaly, in which the brain is totally exposed or actually extruded through an associated skull defect. Abortion of the fetus is almost inevitable, but if it survives, the brain at birth consists predominantly of hindbrain that has degenerated to a spongiform mass—anencephaly (Fig. 10-1). Anencephaly is found in about 1 in 1000 live births. The failure to develop a calvarium in these cases results from the abnormal brain development. Much less commonly, anencephaly is associated with an extensive defect of spinal neural tube closure (rachischisis).

Cranioschisis consists of a skull defect through which various tissues protrude. The defect is usually in the midline region of the occiput or between the frontal and nasal bones. Herniation of the arachnoid alone produces a meningocele, whereas herniation of both brain tissue and arachnoid results in a meningoencephalocele (sometimes referred to as encephalocele).

Some encephaloceles contain duplications of portions of the brain, often the occipital lobes; others contain normal tissue displaced from their usual site. Depending on the size of the encephalocele, the intracranial contents may be significantly smaller than normal, resulting in microcephaly. The brain tissues in the encephalocele, being relatively unprotected, are often damaged during delivery or postnatally, and they are also susceptible to infection, resulting in meningitis.

Malformations that involve the caudal end of the neural tube and the overlying vertebral arches constitute the various forms of spina bifida (Fig. 10-2). These result from failure to close the posterior neuropore.

SPINA BIFIDA OCCULTA

In spina bifida occulta, the two halves of the vertebral arch fail to fuse. The lumbosacral junction is affected. The defect, which is asymptomatic, is sometimes revealed by the presence of a dimple or tuft of hair on the overlying skin surface.

SPINA BIFIDA CYSTICA

Protrusion of the meninges, and their contained CSF, through a vertebral defect constitutes a meningocele. If the spinal roots or cord are included, the lesion is a myelomeningocele. These defects, which appear most commonly in the lumbar region, are found in about 1 in 1000 births. In myeloschisis, the exposed spinal cord is unfolded as a result of a failure of fusion.

Diastematomyelia is a rare condition that can complicate spina bifida. The spinal cord is separated into two parts by either a bony spur or a fibrous band. Each part of the cord is invested by a dural sac (Fig. 10-3).

Meningocele and myelomeningocele are evident in infancy (Fig. 10-4). Although both are surgically repairable, the latter frequently results in substantial lower limb disability with motor and sensory disturbances and also with sphincter involvement. Wasting of the lower limbs is often prominent, with foot deformity (Fig. 10-5). Early surgery (often in the first week of life) may limit the disabilities and can reduce the risk of meningitis. Some disorders of midline fusion may not appear until adult life. Their presence is then sometimes suggested by the finding of a nevus or lipoma over the lumbosacral spine (Fig. 10-6). The skeletal abnormality is evident from plain radiographs (Fig. 10-7). Conditions associated with disorders of fusion include tethering of the cord or cauda equina, lipomata, and dermoid tumors. Intradural lipomas are likely to be adherent to adjacent structures, including the dura, the spinal cord, or its nerve roots, and cause tethering of the cord. Removal of lipomas and dermoids in children releases the tether and allows normal cord

---

BOX 10-1 CLASSIFICATION OF DEVELOPMENTAL DISORDERS OF THE BRAIN AND SPINAL CORD

Neural Tube Defects
- Exancephaly
- Anencephaly
- Meningoencephalocele
- Spina bifida occulta
- Spina bifida cystica
- Chiari malformation
- Dandy-Walker syndrome
- Agenesis of the corpus callosum

Disorders of Diverticulation
- Holoprosencephaly
- Septo-optic dysplasia

Disorders of Migration or Sulcation
- Ectopic gray matter
- Lissencephaly
- Focal gyral anomalies

Microcephaly

Megalencephaly

Hydrancephaly

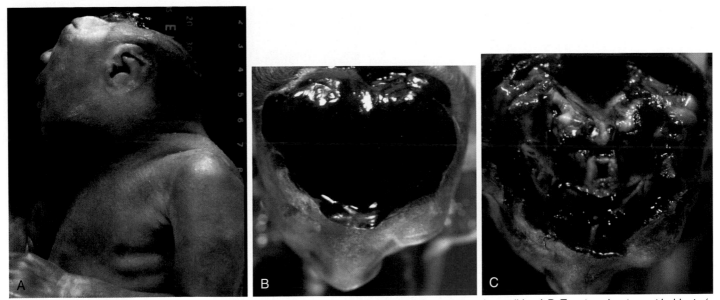

Fig. 10-1. Anencephaly. **A,** Side view of head and neck, showing absent calvarium, exposed cranial contents, and a small head. **B,** Top view, showing residual brain (area cerebrovasculosa) enclosed in hemorrhagic membranes. **C,** Skull base after removal of residual brain. Note small anterior and middle fossae with relatively normal sella and posterior fossa.

DIFFERENT TYPES OF SPINA BIFIDA

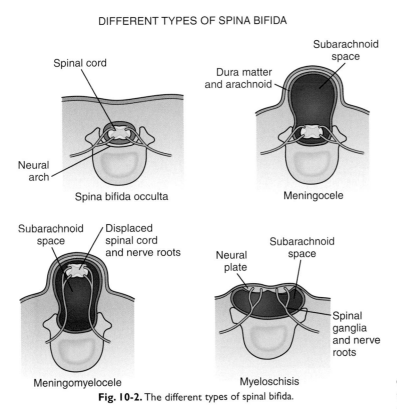

Fig. 10-2. The different types of spinal bifida.

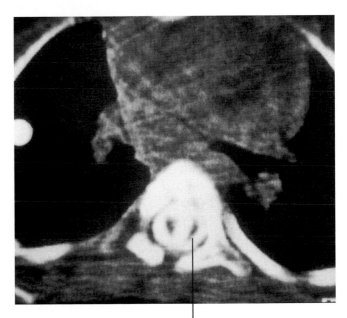

Split spinal cord

Fig. 10-3. Diastematomyelia. CT myelography demonstrating a split cord.

and root elongation. In adults, dermoids are more readily accessible (Fig. 10-8), but removal of lipomas is often incomplete. Neural tube defects are usually detectable in the fetus by finding elevated levels of α-fetoprotein in maternal serum and amniotic fluid. Fetal ultrasonography then localizes the abnormality. Most neural tube defects are preventable by folate supplementation for women of childbearing age. As the defects appear early in embryogenesis, taking folate after confirmation of pregnancy is ineffective.

CHIARI MALFORMATIONS

Chiari malformations are divided into three types. In type I, there is herniation of the cerebellar tonsils through the foramen magnum. The condition is often associated with syringomyelia, but not with hydrocephalus (Fig. 10-9). A number of clinical presentations are described, and the condition may be asymptomatic. Typically, a mixture of cerebellar and pyramidal tract signs is associated with dysfunction of the lower cranial nerves.

A particular type of headache (hindbrain hernia headache) is described, in which a severe, throbbing occipital pain lasting for about a minute is triggered after a few seconds, by coughing, straining, sneezing, or laughing. In most patients, a downbeating nystagmus is conspicuous on downward and outward gaze.

In some cases, the condition is associated with congenital anomalies of the cervical spine (Fig. 10-10). The displaced cerebellar tonsils can be identified by CT myelography, but the investigation of choice is MRI. The position of the tonsils is identified and any associated syringomyelia revealed (Fig. 10-11). Decompression of the cerebellar tonsils, and the underlying brainstem, is achieved by surgery on the foramen magnum (Fig. 10-12).

The type II malformation is associated with downward displacement of both the cerebellar tonsils and the vermis into the spinal canal. As a result of the hindbrain displacement an S- or Z-shaped deformity of the medulla and cord is seen in the upper cervical region (Fig. 10-13). An associated hydrocephalus is usual, accompanied by

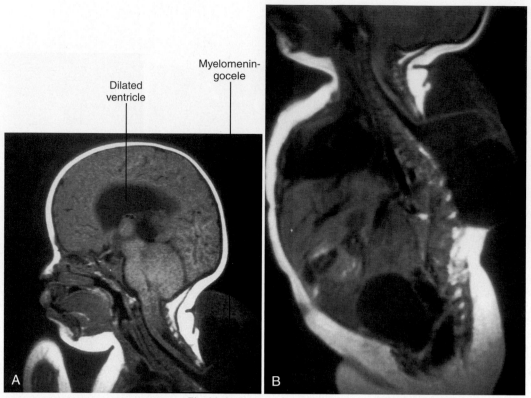

Dilated
ventricle

Myelomenin-
gocele

Fig. 10-4. Myelomeningocele. MRI.

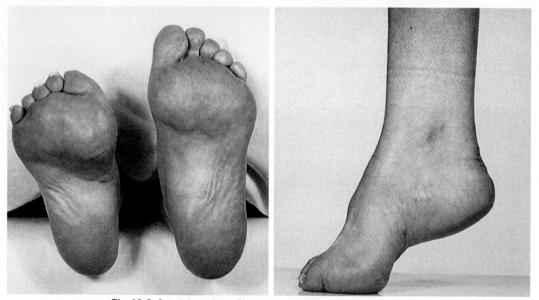

Fig. 10-5. Spinal dysraphism. Shortening of the right foot with pes cavus.

a variety of intracranial structural anomalies (Fig. 10-14). Chiari II malformations are generally associated with lumbosacral meningo-myeloceles with spina bifida cystica (Arnold-Chiari malformation).

The rare type III malformation produces a cerebelloencephalocele through an occipitocervical or high cervical bony defect. The defect is readily visible and palpable (Fig. 10-15). Plain radiographs serve to identify the skull or cervical defect (Fig. 10-16), whereas MRI identifies the herniated brain tissue (Fig. 10-17).

DANDY-WALKER SYNDROME

In the Dandy-Walker syndrome, the cerebellar vermis is hypoplastic or entirely absent, the cerebellum is hypoplastic or flattened, and the fourth ventricle is enlarged. There is an associated hydrocephalus (Fig. 10-18), sometimes with a partial absence of the corpus callosum. The skull is abnormally shaped, with the lateral sinuses and their confluence displaced upward.

The cause of the condition is unknown. It is probably the result of a developmental arrest of the hindbrain in the first trimester. The condition may be an incidental finding, or it may appear with arrested development or, later, as a posterior fossa mass.

The abnormal fourth ventricle and the other features can be identified by MRI (Fig. 10-19). If the intracyst pressure is elevated, shunting is recommended.

LHERMITTE-DUCLOS SYNDROME

Lhermitte-Duclos syndrome is a dysplastic gangliocytoma of the cerebellum and is best regarded as a hamartoma. Histologically, enlarged neurons replace the internal granular cells, and there is distortion of the cerebellar architecture (Fig. 10-20). The condition can lead to ventricular obstruction and secondary hydrocephalus. It may be sporadic or a manifestation of a genetically determined disorder. Cowden's disease, in which there is an autosomal dominant inheritance of a germlike

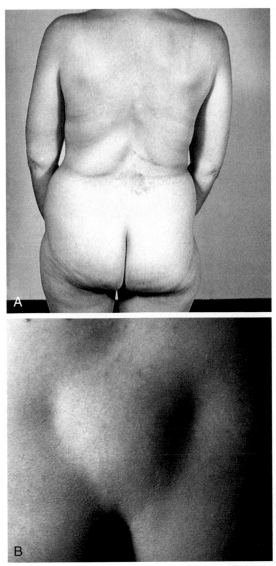

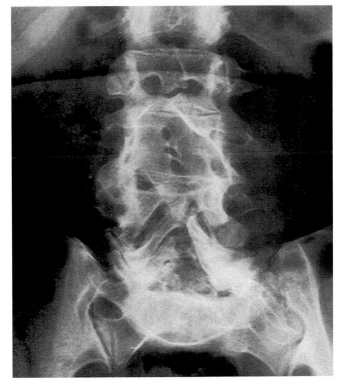

Fig. 10-7. Spinal dysraphism. Lumbar radiograph showing extensive failure of fusion.

Fig. 10-6. Spinal dysraphism. **A,** Nevus over the lumbar region. **B,** Lipoma overlying the lumbosacral junction.

mutation in the *PTEN/MMAC1* gene. Patients with Cowden's disease have abnormalities of the skin, colonic hamartomatous polyps, mucosal fibromas of the mouth, and thyroid neoplasms.

AGENESIS OF THE CORPUS CALLOSUM

Agenesis of the corpus callosum is either partial or complete and may or may not be associated with other malformations. When complete, the lateral ventricles are displaced laterally, and there is upward displacement of the third (Fig. 10-21). The anomaly may be associated with a lipoma of the corpus callosum and with a variety of developmental dyscrasias including absence of the septum pellucidum (Fig. 10-22). Many patients with this disorder are asymptomatic, but in some, subtle defects of interhemispheric transfer of auditory, visual, or sensory information are detectable. Epilepsy is common but in many cases reflects additional CNS pathology, such as neuronal migration disorders with heterotopic gray matter.

ANOMALIES OF THE SEPTUM PELLUCIDUM

Septo-optic dysplasia includes hypoplasia of the optic nerves and chiasm, an absent or rudimentary septum pellucidum, and abnormalities of the corpus callosum and fornix. There may be additional

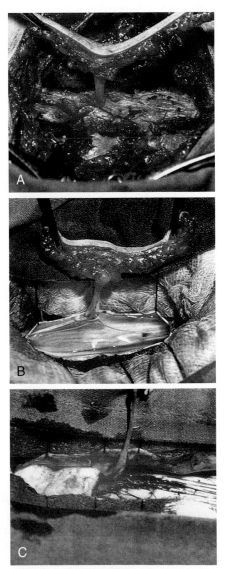

Fig. 10-8. Extension of a track from the skin to a dermoid lying in the conus.

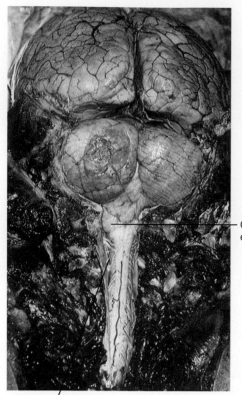

Fig. 10-9. Chiari malformation type I. Tonsillar ectopia associated with an abnormal course of the upper cervical roots.

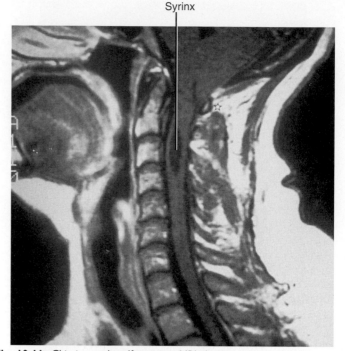

Fig. 10-11. Chiari type I malformation. MRI demonstrating cerebellar ectopia (asterisk) associated with a syrinx in the cervical cord.

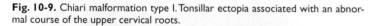
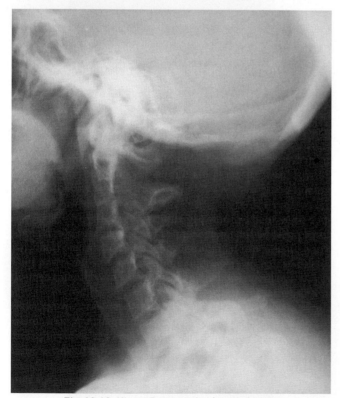

Fig. 10-10. Klippel-Feil anomaly of cervical spine.

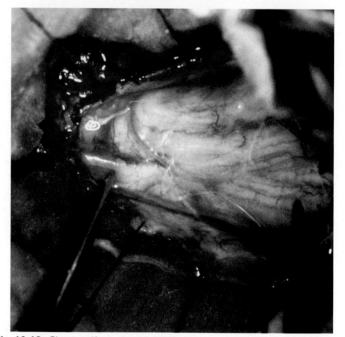

Fig. 10-12. Chiari malformation type I. Operative photograph showing displaced tonsils.

NEURONAL MIGRATION DEFECTS

Agyria and pachygyria represent an absence or reduction in the number of gyri and sulci, coupled with a thickening of the cortical ribbon. The former is not associated with survival beyond infancy (Fig. 10-24).

In polymicrogyria, there are abnormally small gyri separated by small sulci. The abnormality may be focal or may extend to much of the lateral cortical surface. In a rare subtype, cortical architecture is simplified to four layers; the third layer is largely composed of myelinated fibers, and the fourth is a mixture of nerve cells and fibers (Fig. 10-25). Both agyria/pachygyria and polymicrogyria result from abnormal migration of neuronal precursors from the germinal matrix zones to the developing fetal cortex.

anomalies of the hypothalamic–pituitary axis and midline cerebellar structures. The anatomic features are revealed by MRI.

Cavum septum pellucidum and cavum vergae are rostral and caudal cavities bounded above by the corpus callosum and laterally by the septum pellucidum. A cavum septum pellucidum, with or without cavum vergae, is not an uncommon incidental finding on MRI (Fig. 10-23).

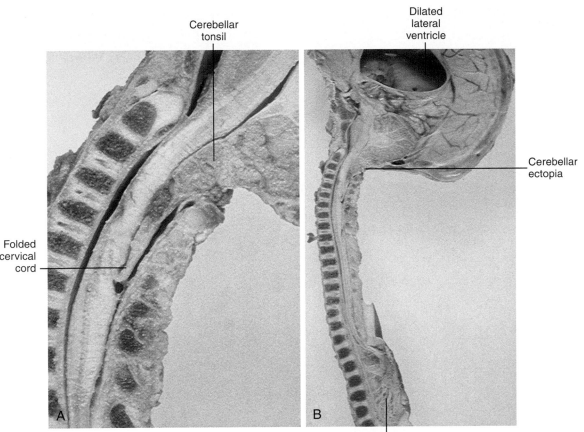

Fig. 10-13. Chiari malformation type II. **A,** Sagittal slice of the brain and vertebral column showing tonsillar and vermian herniation. **B,** An associated myelomeningocele.

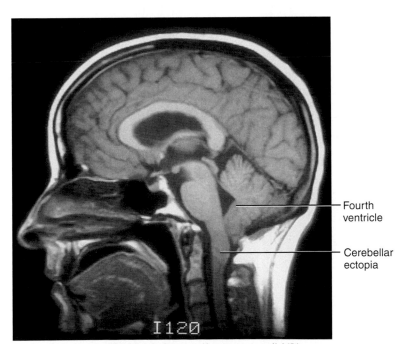

Fig. 10-14. Chiari malformation type II. MRI.

DISORDERS OF DIVERTICULATION

Alobar Holoprosencephaly

Alobar holoprosencephaly consists of a brain with a single midline ventricle with continuity of cerebral cortex across the midline. The basal ganglia and thalami are fused, and there is a rudimentary or absent third ventricle. Callosal agenesis is inevitable. Associated cra-

niofacial and skeletal anomalies include, notably, cleft lip and palate and microcephaly.

Semilobar Holoprosencephaly

In semilobar holoprosencephaly, a partial interhemispheric fissure forms posteriorly, and there are relatively normal occipital lobes but extensively fused frontal and parietal lobes.

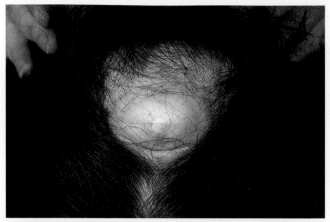

Fig. 10-15. Chiari malformation type III. Clinical appearance.

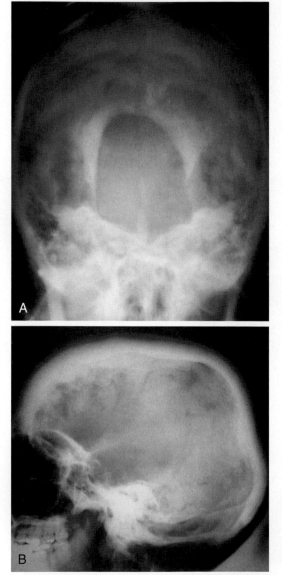

Fig. 10-16. Chiari malformation type III. Skull defect.

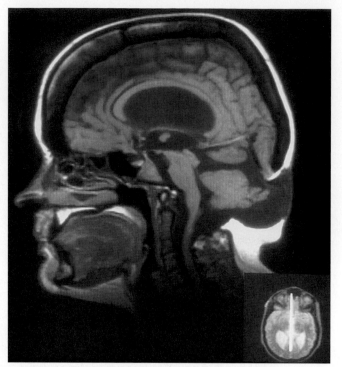

Fig. 10-17. Chiari malformation type III. MRI.

Lobar Prosencephaly

Lobar prosencephaly is the mildest form. Separation of the hemispheres is achieved except for continuity in the region of the frontal poles. There is partial formation of the corpus callosum (Fig. 10-26).

All forms of holoprosencephaly are accompanied by other congenital anomalies of the central nervous system, including olfactory agenesis, and for that reason they are classified as forms of arhinencephaly. Most cases are diagnosed at birth from the various facial abnormalities that result from abnormal fusion. In the few patients who survive the neonatal period, mental retardation, developmental delay, and seizures are the rule. MRI, using T1-weighted coronal sequences, is the best imaging technique for establishing the diagnosis (Fig. 10-27).

NEURONAL HETEROTOPIAS IN CEREBRAL WHITE MATTER

Neuronal heterotopias in cerebral white matter may be diffuse, nodular, or organized into large masses. They appear to be of importance in the genesis of certain types of epilepsy (see Chapter 17).

ARACHNOID CYSTS

Arachnoid cysts are rarely symptomatic. They result from a split in the arachnoid membrane and are most commonly found around the sylvian fissure or over the cerebellum. They may be in communication with the subarachnoid space and, if a valvular mechanism operates at the opening, the cyst can enlarge and become symptomatic (Fig. 10-28). Similar cysts in the leptomeninges are occasionally encountered that have an ependymal lining on a glial base instead of the connective tissue base of the arachnoid cysts; these are glial-ependymal cysts.

PORENCEPHALY

Porencephaly more often represents an acquired than a primary developmental disorder. A cystic space in one or both cerebral hemispheres is lined by ependyma and communicates from the lateral ventricle (Fig. 10-29) to the subarachnoid space. The cysts are often bilateral. The acquired form of porencephaly is the result of cerebral softening secondary to ischemic damage in early life before the time that reactive gliosis can occur. CT or MRI demonstrates the defect (Fig. 10-30).

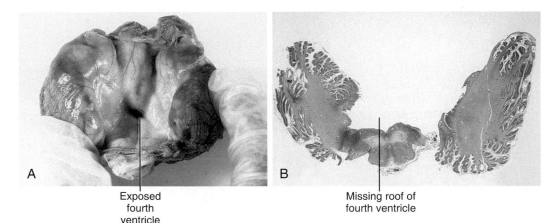

Fig. 10-18. Dandy-Walker syndrome. **A,** Dorsal view of the brainstem and cerebellum, with the midbrain superiorly. The vermis is absent and there is no roof to the fourth ventricle. **B,** Transverse section through the medulla. Normal architecture of the cerebellar hemispheres with an absent vermis and a de-roofed fourth ventricle (Luxol fast blue, H&E).

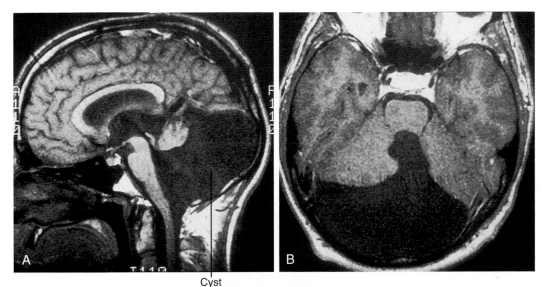

Fig. 10-19. Dandy-Walker syndrome. **A,** Sagittal T1-weighted MRI showing enlarged posterior fossa, a large CSF-containing cyst in communication with the fourth ventricle, and absence of the inferior vermis of the cerebellum. **B,** Axial MRI showing communication of the cyst with the fourth ventricle.

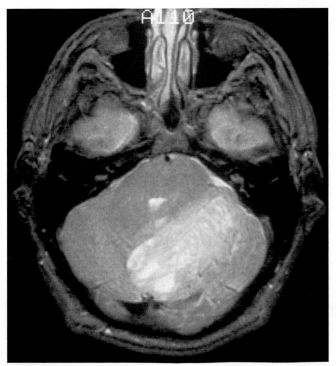

Fig. 10-20. Lhermitte-Duclos syndrome. T2-weighted MRI showing thickened cerebellar folia with displacement of the fourth ventricle.

HYDROCEPHALUS

In hydrocephalus, there is dilatation of the ventricular system, usually in association with raised intraventricular pressure. Communicating and noncommunicating forms can be distinguished because the former are associated with free communication between the ventricular system and the subarachnoid space, whereas the latter result from an obstruction of that communication. Alternative nomenclature has been introduced using the terms *intraventricular* and *extraventricular* obstructive hydrocephalus, depending on whether the obstruction is inside or outside the ventricular system. Ex vacuo hydrocephalus is the result of ventricular dilation secondary to shrinkage of the cerebral hemisphere due to ischemia or atrophy.

Etiology

Only rarely is hydrocephalus the consequence of overproduction of CSF, and then it is a result of a choroid plexus papilloma. Almost all cases result from a failure of resorption or an obstruction of the flow of CSF. In the first few years of life, hydrocephalus is usually the consequence of a developmental abnormality or aqueduct stenosis. In older children, the most common cause is a posterior fossa tumor (Table 10-1). Periodically, in adults, hydrocephalus is found by chance. If there is elevation of intracranial pressure, shunting is recommended. If the hydrocephalus is silent, serial scanning is the most appropriate management.

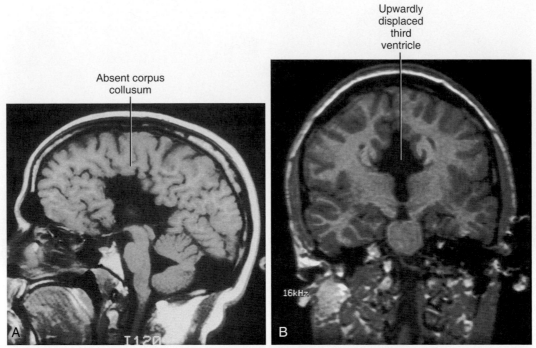

Absent corpus collusum

Upwardly displaced third ventricle

16kHz

Fig. 10-21. Agenesis of the corpus callosum. Sagittal and Coronal T1-weighted MRI.

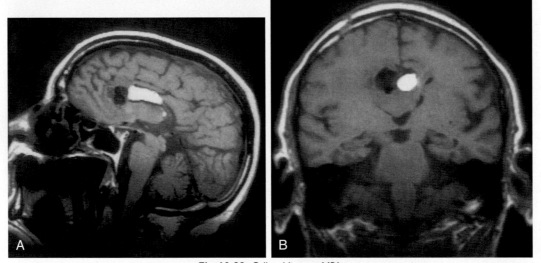

Fig. 10-22. Callosal lipoma. MRI.

Aqueduct Stenosis

Aqueduct stenosis may be sporadic or familial, and when the latter, inheritance is X-linked or autosomal recessive. It is characterized by a vestigial lumen, surrounded by ependyma and without gliosis (Fig. 10-31). In aqueduct atresia, the normal channel is replaced by multiple small canals without associated gliosis, whereas in aqueduct gliosis, the outline of the canal is still visible, with an interrupted ring of ependymal cells and surrounding dense fibrillary gliosis. In all cases, hydrocephalus is the consequence (Fig. 10-32).

Clinical Features

In infants, hydrocephalus results in abnormal skull enlargement. In adults, clinical features include epilepsy, dementia, or CSF rhinorrhea (Fig. 10-33). Less commonly in adults, an acute elevation of intraventricular pressure results in headache with alteration of the conscious state.

Investigation

Cranial ultrasound provides a rapid, accurate, and easily repeated assessment of ventricular size in infants and can establish the diagnosis prenatally.

CT provides a measure of the size of the ventricular system and, by its evaluation of the size of the fourth ventricle, evidence as to whether the obstruction is proximal or distal to that site (Fig. 10-34).

MRI provides greater anatomic detail and gives some information regarding CSF volume and whether flow identified as a flow void is maintained through the aqueduct (Fig. 10-35). Periventricular edema, which concentrates around the frontal and occipital horns, is readily detectable and is conspicuous if the hydrocephalus has developed rapidly.

NORMAL PRESSURE HYDROCEPHALUS

Although random CSF pressure measurements obtained by lumbar puncture are normal in patients with normal pressure hydrocephalus (NPH), intracranial pressure monitoring establishes that, in those patients who respond to shunting, abnormal pressure waves (β waves) are found to occupy at least 5% of the day and to recur at a frequency of up to two per minute.

Although some cases of NPH follow subarachnoid hemorrhage, meningitis, or head injury, many are idiopathic. In those cases, a nonspecific reaction is found in the meninges, accompanied in some by morphologic

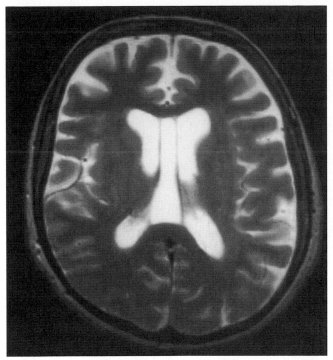

Fig. 10-23. Cavum vergae. MRI.

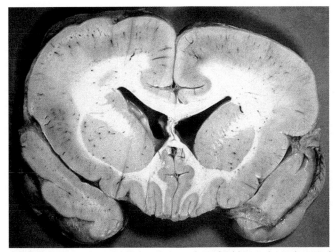

Fig. 10-24. Agyria/pachygyria. Coronal slice of cerebral hemisphere showing lack of gyri and sulci on both frontal convexities. Note the normal gyral pattern on the frontal bases and on the anterior temporal lobes.

changes in the arachnoid granulations. Clearly, the clinical syndrome is not linked to a specific pathology, because some patients at postmortem examination have evidence of either vascular or Alzheimer's disease.

Clinical Features

A typical triad of symptoms is described, incorporating gait disturbance, dementia, and altered urinary control. Shunting is likely to be successful only when the presenting complaint is of a gait disorder. Headache is uncommon.

Gait disturbance is often the most conspicuous part of the syndrome, and usually the earliest. Some patients appear frozen to the spot, unable to initiate locomotion, whereas others show parkinsonian features—a stooped posture and small steps. Patients with multi-infarct dementia and those with Binswanger's encephalopathy have very similar gait patterns.

The initial mentation changes are nonspecific, amounting to a dulling of thought with withdrawal and lack of motivation. The dementia, at least initially, has more subcortical than cortical features. Again, the changes seen in Binswanger's encephalopathy are similar.

Initially there is urinary urgency and frequency, followed by incontinence, which may appear to be of little concern to the patient.

Investigation

In some patients, a substantial, but transient, improvement in gait follows the removal of 25 to 50 mL of CSF, although an absent response to this procedure does not preclude the subsequent possibility of response to shunting. Various CSF infusion tests have been devised to assess whether an inappropriate increase in CSF pressure follows infusion of fluid at a standard rate into the lumbar canal. The procedure is not without hazard and is not widely used. The lumbar or cisternal injection of a radioisotope can sometimes demonstrate striking pooling of the tracer in the lateral ventricles, but the finding fails to correlate with the outcome after shunting.

CT scanning typically demonstrates dilatation of the ventricular system with relatively normal sulci. The size of the sylvian fissures is not important when predicting response to shunting. Periventricular lucencies are detectable on CT but not necessarily distinguishable from those found in Binswanger's disease (Fig. 10-36).

MRI is the preferred imaging technique. Periventricular abnormal signal is detected in T2-weighted images and, in some cases, the pattern of CSF flow through the aqueduct can be identified (Fig. 10-37).

Procedures whose role in diagnosis remain to be established include SPECT, PET, and MR spectroscopy.

Treatment

When the triad of NPH symptoms is complete and a cause has been identified, response to shunting occurs in about two thirds of patients, with a complete response in about half of these. In the idiopathic group, no more than a third are responsive and even fewer if the triad is incomplete. Generally, the incontinence or gait disturbance is more likely to respond than the dementia. There is a surprisingly poor correlation between the degree of reduction of ventricular size after shunting and any clinical response. Shunting complications include infection, epilepsy, and subdural hematoma (Fig. 10-38).

TUBEROUS SCLEROSIS (BOURNEVILLE'S DISEASE)

Tuberous sclerosis is inherited as an autosomal dominant. Its prevalence among children from birth to 5 years of age is 1 in 10,000. Relevant genes (TS1 and TS2), with gene products called tuberin and hamartin, respectively, have been mapped to chromosomes 9q34 and 16p13.3. A mutation in either gene results in the disorder.

Clinical Features

In addition to the CNS, the heart, kidney, skin, and retina are likely to be affected, and other organs less commonly. Skin lesions are the most common manifestation of the condition but are sometimes lacking. Almost inevitable are hypomelanotic macules, frequently accompanied by focal areas of depigmentation in the hair of the scalp, eyelids, or eyebrows. Adenoma sebaceum is a hamartoma found particularly over the cheeks and nasolabial folds (Fig. 10-39). Ungual fibromas are specific for this disease but are found in only about a quarter of the patients. They are more common on the toes than on the fingers and grow either underneath the nail or at the junction of nail and skin (Fig. 10-40). Shagreen patches are found principally over the back; these are roughened areas with a color slightly different from that of the surrounding skin.

Both cysts and angiomyolipomas are found in the kidneys, and either can result in chronic renal failure. Cardiac rhabdomyomas are benign tumors that are symptomatic only if they result in a conduction defect or interfere with the heart's contractile action (Fig. 10-41).

Retinal tumors (hamartomas) are found in about half the patients. Unless the lesions calcify, they are difficult to detect. They are usually asymptomatic.

Pathologic abnormalities found in the CNS include cortical tubers, subependymal nodules, and subependymal giant cell astrocytomas. Cortical tubers appear as slightly pale areas on the surface

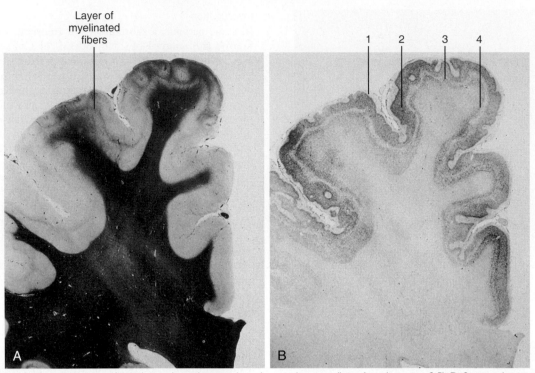

Fig. 10-25. Polymicrogyria. **A,** Coronal section of right hemisphere showing altered cortical pattern (Loyez' myelin stain, ×2.5). **B,** Section showing the four cortical nerve cell layers (thionin, ×2.5).

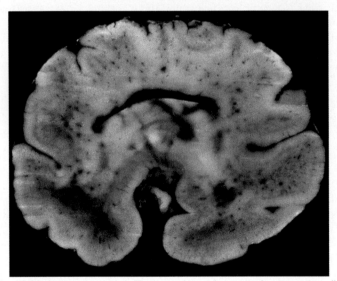

Fig. 10-26. Holoprosencephaly. Thick, simple, gyral pattern, absent corpus callosum, and single hemispheric ventricle.

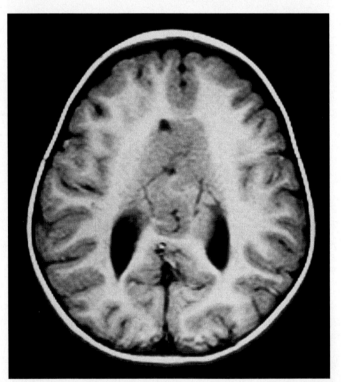

Fig. 10-27. Holoprosencephaly. MRI.

of the brain (Fig. 10-42, *A*), a section of which reveals disruption of the cortical lamination with infiltration by giant cells and astrocytes (Fig. 10-42, *B*). Fibrillary gliosis is present, and calcification is likely. These hamartomatous lesions extend through or beneath the cortex into the white matter. Histologically, they are composed mostly of large cells with mixed astrocytic and neuronal features, usually with large neuronal-type nuclei but with eosinophilic cell bodies more like reactive astrocytes.

Subependymal nodules, derived from similar cells with both neuronal and astrocytic features, are found in the walls of the lateral or third ventricles, whereas subependymal giant cell astrocytomas contain giant cells also derived either from astrocytes or neurons (Fig. 10-43).

Investigation

Calcification in the subependymal nodules is detected by CT scanning (Fig. 10-44). MRI is more valuable for detecting cortical tubers and any associated white matter change (Fig. 10-45).

NEUROFIBROMATOSIS (VON RECKLINGHAUSEN'S DISEASE)

Neurofibromatosis is inherited as an autosomal dominant. The NF1 gene is located on chromosome 17q11. Its prevalence is around 1 in 3000. About half the cases represent new mutations. The NF1 gene product, neurofibromin, influences cell proliferation and differentiation. The NF2 gene is located on chromosome 22q12. Its prevalence is around 1 in 40,000 and, again, some half the cases are new mutations. The gene product is merlin (or schwannomin).

Criteria have been devised to facilitate the diagnosis of NF1 and NF2 (Boxes 10-2 and 10-3). Clinically detectable markers of NF1

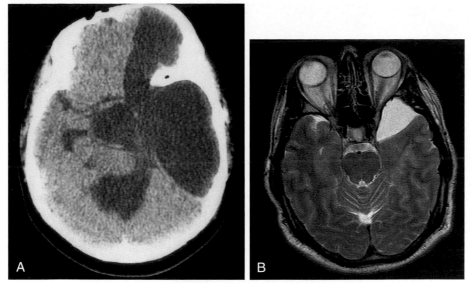

Fig. 10-28. Arachnoid cyst. **A** CT. **B,** Axial T2-weighted MRI appearance.

Large defect

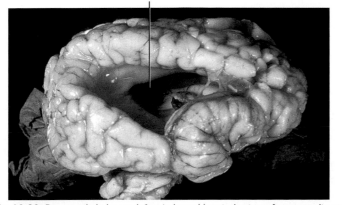

Fig. 10-29. Porencephaly. Large defect in lateral hemispheric surface extending to the lateral ventricle and to the contralateral ventricle and hemisphere.

TABLE 10-1. CAUSES OF HYDROCEPHALUS

Lateral ventricular obstruction	Intraventricular tumor or hemorrhage
Obstruction of foramen of Monro	Suprasellar mass Tuberous sclerosis
Obstruction of third ventricle	Colloid cyst Suprasellar mass Chiasmatic glioma
Obstruction of aqueduct	Aqueductal stenosis Pineal tumor Arteriovenous malformation
Obstruction of fourth ventricle or outflow foramina	Cerebellar tumor Dandy-Walker syndrome Meningitis
Obstruction of subarachnoid space	Meningitis Subarachnoid hemorrhage Chiari malformation

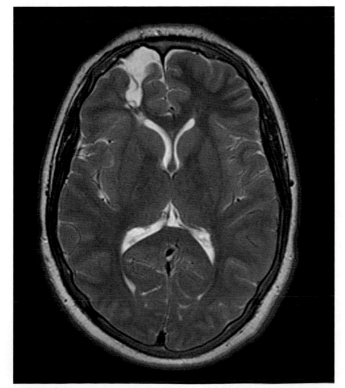

Fig. 10-30. Porencephaly. Axial T2-weighted MRI. There is right frontal porencephaly.

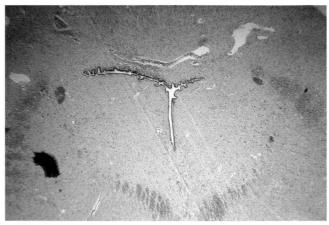

Fig. 10-31. Congenital aqueduct stenosis. Section through aqueduct (Luxol fast blue, H&E, ×6).

include café-au-lait spots, neurofibromas or plexiform neurofibromas, and iris hamartomas (Lisch nodules) (Fig. 10-46).

Intracranial tumors associated with NF1 include optic nerve gliomas, meningiomas, and schwannomas. Pseudoarthroses, principally affecting the tibia or radius, are encountered in patients with NF1. Absence of the greater wing of the sphenoid leads to pulsating exophthalmos (Fig. 10-47).

NF2 is characterized principally by the presence of bilateral eighth-nerve tumors.

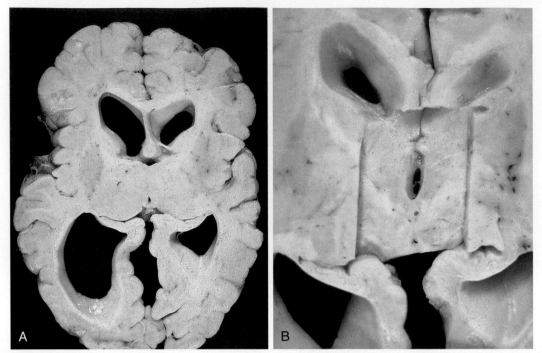

Fig. 10-32. Congenital aqueduct stenosis. **A,** Axial slice indicating hydrocephalus and the small bottom of the third ventricle. **B,** The anterior third ventricle is visible, together with a narrowed aqueduct.

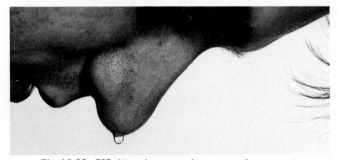

Fig. 10-33. CSF rhinorrhea secondary to aqueduct stenosis.

FAMILIAL DISORDERS AFFECTING THE CEREBELLUM

Ataxia Telangiectasia

Ataxia telangiectasia is caused by mutations in a single gene *(AT-mutated [ATM])*, concerned in various aspects of cell cycle control and DNA damage appraisal. In about 80% to 90% of patients, the ATM protein is totally inactivated, and in the other 10% to 20%, partial inactivation produces a less severe clinical phenotype. The condition is inherited as an autosomal recessive.

In addition to the ataxia, the child is likely to display dysarthria and involuntary movements of a choreoathetoid type as a result of cerebellar degeneration (Fig. 10-48). An associated peripheral neuropathy may be evident clinically or detectable electrophysiologically. The telangiectases, which are found on both the skin and the conjunctivae, develop at a later stage (Fig. 10-49).

The condition is associated with deficiencies of both humoral and cell-mediated immunity. Consequently, recurrent respiratory tract infection in childhood is the rule. Serum levels of IgA and IgG are depressed, and there is a lymphopenia. A proportion of the patients develop malignancy, principally of the lymphoid system or breast. Progressive clinical deterioration is the rule, with most patients dying in early adult life.

Abetalipoproteinemia

Abetalipoproteinemia is inherited as a recessive. Malabsorption of the fat-soluble vitamins A, D, E, and K is accompanied by severely depressed levels of serum lipids, particularly cholesterol. Acantho-cytes (spiky red blood cells) are a characteristic finding in the peripheral blood, detectable either on simple wet films or using scanning electron microscopy (Fig. 10-50). Clinical features include abnormal retinal pigmentation, ataxia, areflexia, and joint position sense loss. The neurologic deficit appears to be secondary to vitamin E deficiency, and it responds, at least in part, to its replacement. Hypobetalipoproteinemia is inherited as a dominant. Lipid levels are less severely depressed, and many cases are asymptomatic. Some patients, however, present in adult life with cerebellar ataxia associated with pyramidal signs. A neuropathy may be seen (see Chapter 2).

Friedreich's Ataxia

Clinical criteria for the diagnosis of Friedreich's ataxia include limb and gait ataxia, areflexia in the lower limbs, and electrophysiologic evidence of a neuropathy. Patients usually present before the age of 15, though later-onset cases are recognized. The relevant gene (the condition is an autosomal recessive) has been mapped to the centromeric region of chromosome 9q. The relevant protein product is frataxin, and its reduction or loss leads to iron accumulation with subsequent neuronal oxidative stress. In most cases, there is an expansion of a GAA triplet repeat of the gene. The fewer the repeats, the later is the onset of disease.

Most patients present in the early part of the second decade, and the condition is the commonest of the familial ataxias presenting in this age group. Progression to a wheelchair existence is the norm, with death, on average, by the mid thirties.

Additional clinical features include pyramidal signs (extensor plantar responses are almost inevitable), dysarthria, nystagmus, and optic atrophy. Scoliosis is usual (Fig. 10-51), and about 50% of patients have pes cavus (Fig. 10-52). Besides areflexia, the neuropathy results in some cases in distal wasting and commonly in impairment of posterior column function.

Evidence of cardiomyopathy, which is not necessarily symptomatic, is common, and some two thirds of patients have an abnormal electrocardiogram. Changes include widespread T-wave inversion, together with evidence of ventricular hypertrophy (Fig. 10-53). There is an association between Friedreich's ataxia and diabetes mellitus.

The spinal cord is atrophic, and there is degeneration of the posterior columns (particularly the gracile fasciculi) and the pyramidal and spinocerebellar tracts. There is severe cell loss in the dentate nuclei of the cerebellum, with atrophy of the superior cerebellar peduncles

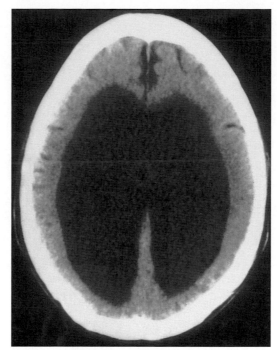

Fig. 10-34. Aqueduct stenosis. CT.

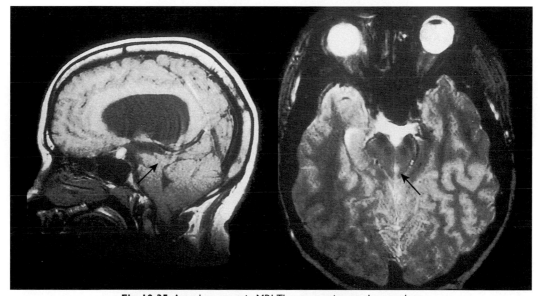

Fig. 10-35. Aqueduct stenosis. MRI. The *arrow* points to the aqueduct.

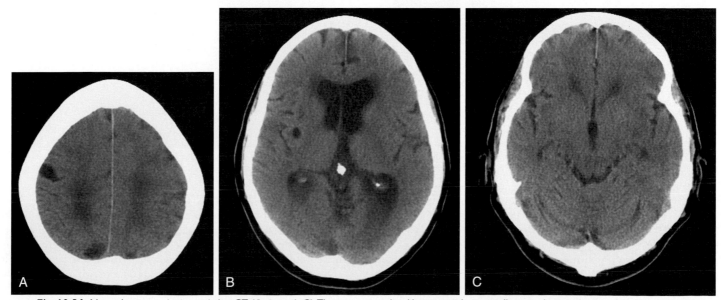

Fig. 10-36. Normal pressure hydrocephalus, CT (**A** through **C**). There is ventricular dilatation with essentially normal cortical sulci and sylvian fissures.

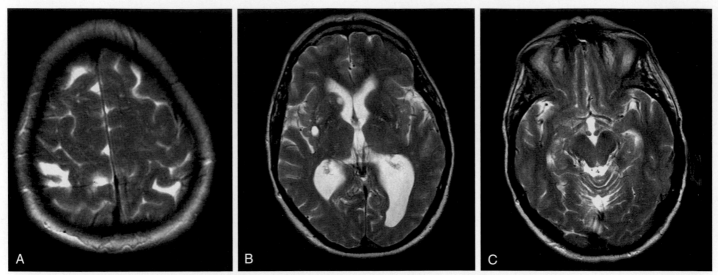

Fig. 10-37. Normal pressure hydrocephalus. MRI at three levels showing the same features.

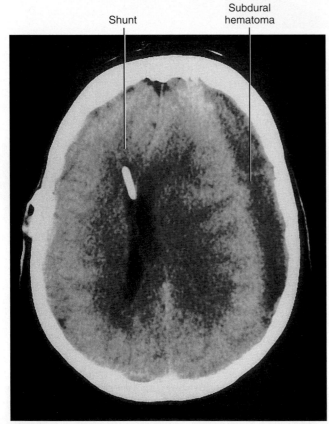

Fig. 10-38. Normal pressure hydrocephalus. Subdural hematoma complicating previous shunting.

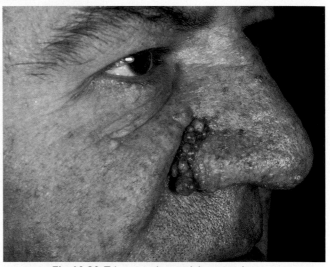

Fig. 10-39. Tuberous sclerosis. Adenoma sebaceum.

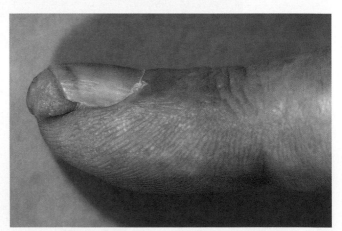

Fig. 10-40. Tuberous sclerosis. Subungual fibroma.

(Fig. 10-54). There is a fallout of large myelinated fibers in the peripheral nerves.

A number of other early-onset familial ataxic syndromes has been described, including one (early-onset cerebellar ataxia with retained reflexes) with features superficially resembling Friedreich's ataxia but with retained reflexes and an absence of cardiomyopathy or skeletal deformity. Genetically, some such cases are phenotypic variants of Friedreich's ataxia, but others are not linked to chromosome 9.

Cerebellar Ataxia Resulting from Isolated Vitamin E Deficiency
Cerebellar ataxia resulting from isolated vitamin E deficiency is a rare autosomal recessive disorder with close similarities to Friedreich's ataxia. The age of onset varies, but most patients present before the age of 20. The condition is caused by mutations of the gene encoding

α-tocopherol transfer protein. Progressive ataxia is the norm, leading to wheelchair confinement at a rather later age than is seen with Friedreich's ataxia. Cardiomyopathy is seen in about 20% of patients. Pathologically, there is posterior column degeneration with lipofuscin accumulation in neurons, including the dorsal root ganglion cells.

Diagnosis is established by showing absent or severely reduced levels of vitamin E, and the effects of the condition can be ameliorated, to some extent, by large doses of vitamin E.

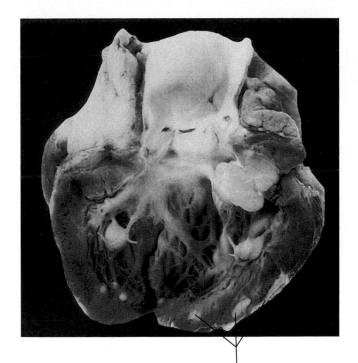

Nodules

Fig. 10-41. Tuberous sclerosis. Cardiac lesions.

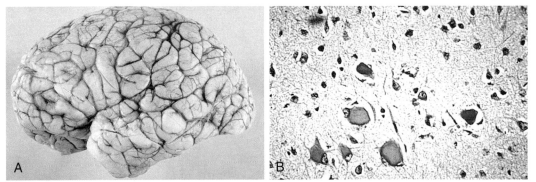

A   B

Fig. 10-42. Tuberous sclerosis. **A,** Lateral surface of the brain showing a typical tuber. **B,** Histology of cortical tuber.

Tuber

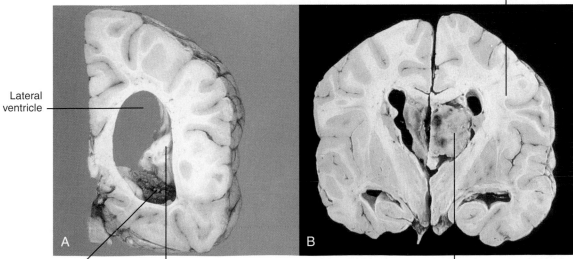

Lateral
ventricle

A   B

Choroid Ependymal nodule   Glioma
plexus

Fig. 10-43. Tuberous sclerosis. **A,** Coronal brain slice showing subependymal nodule. **B,** Coronal brain section showing subependymal nodules with glioma.

Autosomal Dominant Cerebellar Ataxia

The autosomal dominant cerebellar ataxias are principally represented by the spinocerebellar atrophies (types 1 through 17, but not 9) and dentatorubro-pallidoluysian atrophy (DRPLA). The genetic origin of the spinocerebellar ataxias (SCAs) has been defined, and there are multiple chromosomal contributors. The gene products have been identified in some of these—for example, ataxin 1, 2, and 3 for SCAs 1, 2, and 3, respectively. A variety of associated neurologic findings are recognized according to the particular type of SCA.

DRPLA is inherited as an autosomal dominant, the relevant gene being located on chromosome 12p coding for atrophin-1.

Clinical features besides ataxia include movement disorders, myoclonic epilepsy, and dementia. At times, the condition can mimic Huntington's disease.

Sporadic Idiopathic Cerebellar Degeneration

Most cases of degenerative adult-onset cerebellar ataxias are sporadic, and most are caused by olivopontocerebellar degeneration. There is atrophy of the cerebellum, middle cerebellar peduncles, and the pons (Figs. 10-55 and 10-56).

Other forms include cerebello-olivary atrophy and cortical cerebellar atrophy. In the former, the cerebellar degeneration predominates in the vermis, and a mainly midline cerebellar syndrome emerges in which gait ataxia is far more prominent than any limb involvement (Fig. 10-57). Olivary atrophy accompanies the cerebellar pathology. Cortical cerebellar atrophy has a tremor in association with ataxia, either resting or postural.

Neuroacanthocytosis

Both autosomal dominant and recessive inheritances have been proposed for neuroacanthocytosis, which is heterogeneous. It bears some similarity to Huntington's disease, combining evidence of a movement disorder with intellectual impairment and altered personality. Onset is usually in early adult life.

Chorea is the usual movement disorder, but other movements seen include tics, dystonia, and repetitive vocalizations. Depression or loss of the tendon reflexes is common, accompanied by evidence of an axonal neuropathy. There is cerebral and caudate atrophy resembling that seen in Huntington's disease (Fig. 10-58). MRI may detect abnormal signal from the caudate or lentiform nuclei.

Light microscopy or scanning electron microscopy detects acanthocytes (red cells with spiny projections), usually accompanied by echinocytes (red cells with rounded projections) (Fig. 10-59).

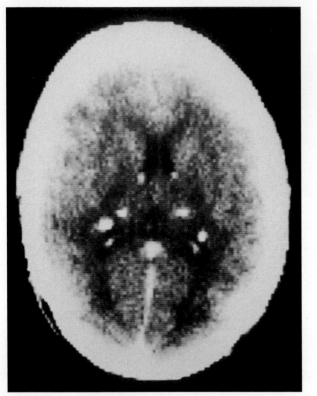

Fig. 10-44. Tuberous sclerosis. CT scan demonstrating calcified subependymal nodules.

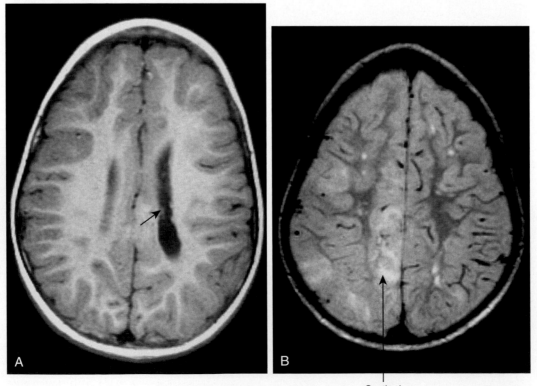

Cortical tuber

Fig. 10-45. Tuberous sclerosis. MRI demonstrating subependymal nodule *(arrow, left)* and cortical tubers *(arrow, right)*.

BOX 10-2	CRITERIA FOR THE DIAGNOSIS OF NEUROFIBROMA 1 (NF1)

Two of the following eight criteria:
• Six café-au-lait spots greater than 15 mm in diameter (adults)
• Multiple axillary or inguinal freckles
• One plexiform neurofibroma, or two or more neurofibromas of other types
• Optic nerve or chiasmatic glioma
• Lisch iris nodules (two or more)
• Thinning of the cortex of long bones
• Sphenoid dysplasia
• A first-degree relative with NF1

BOX 10-3	CRITERIA FOR THE DIAGNOSIS OF NEUROFIBROMA 2 (NF2)

Any one of the first three criteria:
• Bilateral eighth-nerve tumors (as determined by CT or MRI)
• Unilateral eighth-nerve tumor and a first-degree relative with NF2
• Any two of the following, plus a first-degree relative with NF2:
  • Plexiform neurofibroma
  • Neurofibroma of another type
  • Meningioma
  • Glioma
  • Schwannoma
  • Presenile posterior cataract

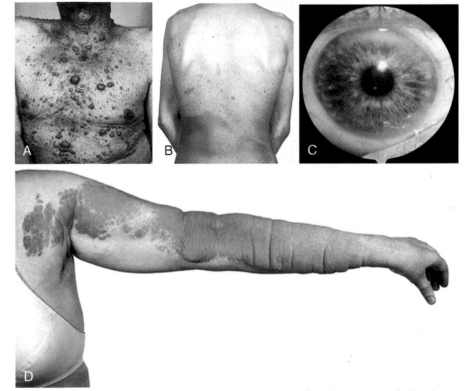

Fig. 10-46. NF1. **A,** Multiple cutaneous neurofibromas. **B,** Café-au-lait patches. **C,** Lisch iris nodules. **D,** Plexiform neurofibroma.

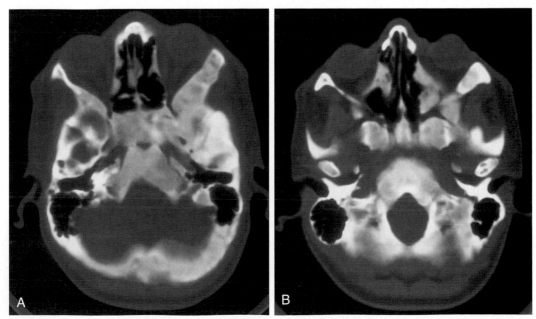

Fig. 10-47. Multiple areas of fibrous dysplasia of skull bones in NF1. CT.

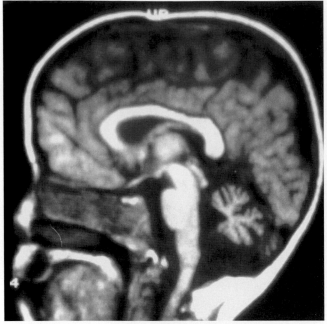

Fig. 10-48. Ataxia telangiectasia. MRI showing cerebellar atrophy.

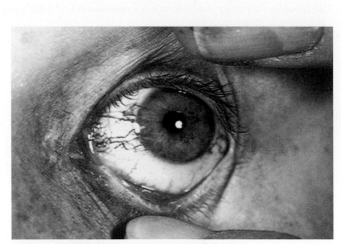

Fig. 10-49. Ataxia telangiectasia. Scleral appearance.

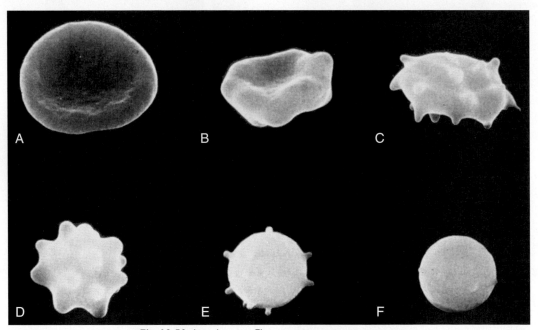

Fig. 10-50. Acanthocytes. Electron microscopy appearance.

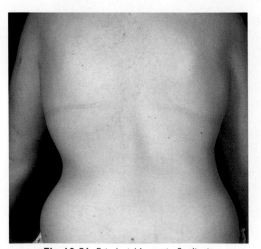

Fig. 10-51. Friedreich's ataxia. Scoliosis.

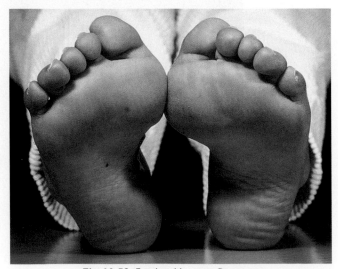

Fig. 10-52. Friedreich's ataxia. Pes cavus.

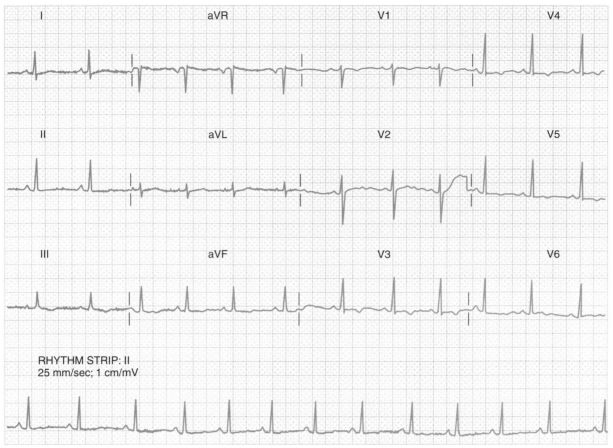

Fig. 10-53. Friedreich's ataxia. Electrocardiogram.

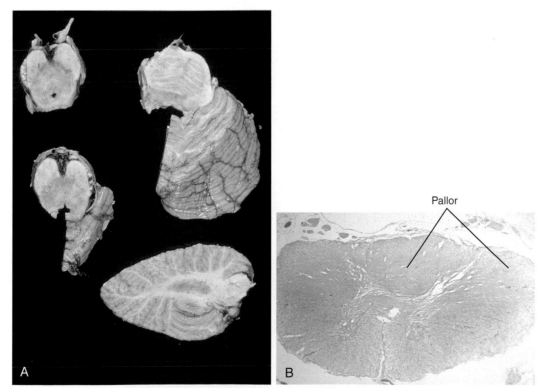

Fig. 10-54. Friedreich's ataxia. **A,** Transverse sections of midbrain and pons, and parasagittal slice of left cerebellar hemisphere. The superior cerebellar peduncles are abnormally small, and the dentate nucleus is small and atrophic. **B,** Cross-section of spinal cord. Loss of myelinated fibers from posterior and lateral columns (Luxol fast blue, H&E).

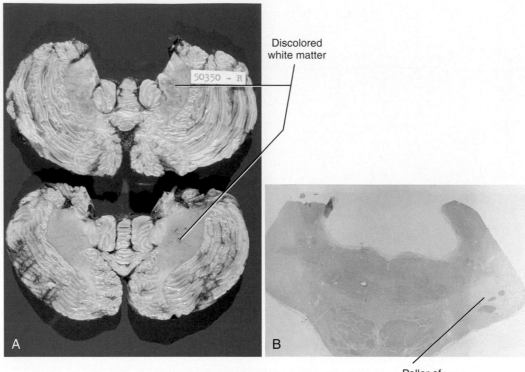

Discolored
white matter

Pallor of
middle
cerebellar
peduncle

Fig. 10-55. Olivopontocerebellar degeneration. **A,** Loss of deep cerebellar white matter, which, particularly around the dentate nuclei, is shrunken and discolored. **B,** Whole mount of pons. Ratio of base to tegmentum reduced from 2:1 to 1:1. Loss of myelinated fibers in middle cerebellar peduncle (Luxol fast blue, periodic acid–Schiff).

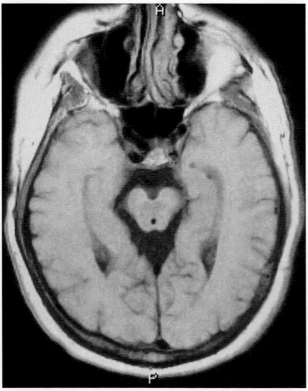

Fig. 10-56. Olivopontocerebellar atrophy. Pontine atrophy. MRI.

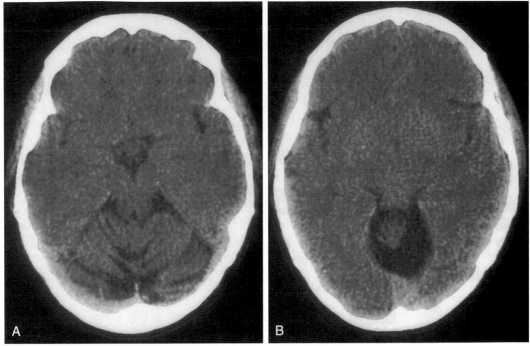

Fig. 10-57. Sporadic late-onset cerebellar ataxia. CT.

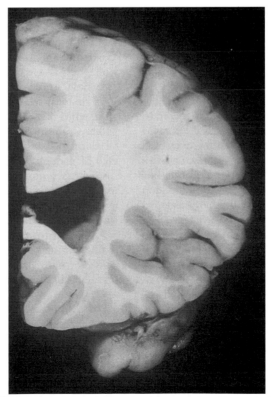

Fig. 10-58. Neuroacanthocytosis. There is caudate atrophy with ventricular dilation.

BOX 11-1   CLASSIFICATION OF HEADACHES AND CRANIAL NEURALGIAS*

Primary Headaches
- Migraine
- Tension-type headache
- Cluster headache and other trigeminal autonomic cephalalgias (TACs)
- Other primary headaches

Secondary Headaches
- Head and/or neck trauma
- Cranial or cervical vascular disorders
- Nonvascular intracranial disorders
- Drugs or toxins, or their withdrawal
- Infections
- Disorders of homeostasis
- Disease or disorders of cranial structures
- Psychiatric disorders
- Facial pain and cranial neuralgias
- Other headaches and cranial pain not classified elsewhere

*Based on International Headache Classification, 2004.

BOX 11-2   TRIGEMINAL AUTONOMIC CEPHALALGIAS

Cluster Headache (CH)
- Episodic CH
- Chronic CH

Paroxysmal Hemicrania (PH)
- Episodic PH
- Chronic PH

Hemicrania continua
SUNA
SUNCT

SUNA, short-lasting unilateral neuralgiform headaches with cranial autonomic symptoms; SUNCT, short-lasting unilateral neuralgiform headache attacks with conjunctival injection and tearing.

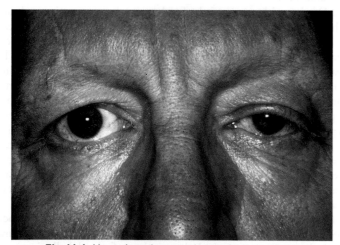

Fig. 11-1. Horner's syndrome in chronic cluster headache.

BOX 11-3   OTHER PRIMARY HEADACHES

Primary Thunderclap Headache
Exertional Cephalalgias
- Exercise-triggered migraine†
- Benign exertion headache
- Cough headache
  - Primary
  - Secondary

Reflex Cephalalgias
- 'Ice-cream headache'
- 'Bath-related headache', etc.

Hypnic Headache (Exploding Head Syndrome)*
Stabbing Headaches

†Migraine triggered by exercise but not occurring spontaneously or under other circumstances.

*Perhaps a parasomnia rather than part of the primary headache spectrum.

TABLE 11-1.   IHC2* CODES FOR MIGRAINE SUBTYPES

IHC2 CODE	SUBTYPE
1.1	Migraine without aura
1.2	Migraine with aura
1.2.3	Typical aura without headache
1.2.4	Familial hemiplegic migraine
1.2.5	Sporadic hemiplegic migraine
1.2.6	Basilar type migraine
1.3	Childhood migraine syndromes
1.4	Retinal migraine
13.17	Ophthalmoplegic migraine

*International Headache Classification, 2004.

---

shown to result from mutations in a neural voltage-gated calcium channel gene *(CACN1A)*. Affected individuals have severe attacks of migraine with aura, often with altered consciousness and vomiting, and many evolve to a progressive cerebellar ataxia. Indeed, FHM1 appears to be allelic with episodic ataxia type 2 and spinocerebellar ataxia type 6. Another form, FHM2, results from mutations in *ATP1A2*, a neuronal Na/K-ATPase gene, whereas FHM3 results from mutations in *SCN1A*, which codes for a neuronal voltage-gated sodium channel. The FHM-associated genes so far identified are involved in the regulation of intercellular levels of K$^+$ and glutamate by neurons and astrocytes—key factors in the genesis of spreading depression, the likely neural basis of migraine. Mutations in these genes are very rarely found in patients with sporadic hemiplegic migraine, but a number of other genes have been linked to more common forms of migraine. Other genetic associations will no doubt be discovered.

BASILAR-TYPE MIGRAINE. Basilar-type migraine is diagnosed when symptoms indicate that aura is generated in the brainstem, or that it involves both posterior hemispheres. The aura may include dysarthria, vertigo, tinnitus, decreased hearing, double vision, ataxia, decreased level of consciousness, simultaneous bilateral visual hallucinations in the temporal and nasal fields of both eyes, total blindness, and simultaneous bilateral paresthesias.

CHILDHOOD MIGRAINE SYNDROMES. It is now well recognized that migraine may present atypically in infancy and childhood with recurrent stereotypic symptoms not necessarily associated with headache. Syndromes include benign paroxysmal torticollis of infancy, cyclical vomiting, recurrent abdominal pain (abdominal migraine, often misdiagnosed as "grumbling appendix"), and benign paroxysmal vertigo of childhood. Such syndromes are often the precursor to more typical migraine attacks in later life. Occasionally, these childhood presentations are also encountered in adults.

These are referred to as acephalalgic attacks. In addition, a wide variety of other commonly encountered episodic, stereotypic neurologic symptoms are probably migraine auras or complications of migraine. These include recurrent vertigo (migrainous vertigo is the most common cause of recurrent vertigo in the absence of definable vestibular pathology), syncope, some instances of seizures, transient global amnesia, and young-onset stroke, particularly in the posterior circulation.

HEMIPLEGIC MIGRAINE. Although patients experiencing hemisensory aura may describe the sensation as "weakness," true hemiplegic migraine is rare. It can occur in familial and sporadic forms. The common form of familial hemiplegic migraine (FHM1) has been

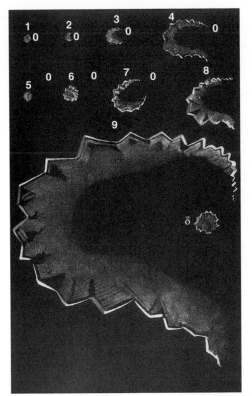

Fig. 11-2. Visual aura. Dr. Hubert Airy's drawing of his own "sinistral teichopsia" was first published in 1870 and shows the temporal evolution of a typical paracentral scotoma that gradually expands into the left hemifield. The advancing edge is jagged and partly colored.

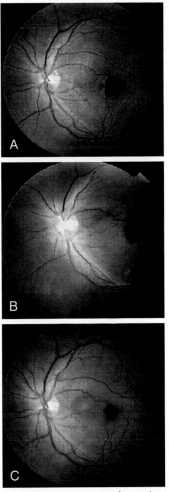

Fig. 11-3. Retinal artery vasospasm in a case of retinal migraine. **A,** Left fundus photographed at routine optometrist appointment 1 month before presenting episode. Normal appearance of disc, vessels, and macula. **B,** During the period of visual loss, constriction of both arteries and veins is seen, with macular pallor, a central cherry red spot, and slight disc pallor. **C,** At 10 minutes after the previous picture, when the patient reported that vision had returned to normal, some pallor remains in the macula (with a central cherry-red spot), but the disc and vasculature have returned to normal.

RETINAL MIGRAINE. Many patients experiencing visual aura say that the symptoms are confined to one eye or the other, but careful analysis during attacks usually demonstrates that the hallucinations are homonymous. Rarely, however, cases are encountered of true monocular aura followed by migraine headache—"retinal migraine." Monocular aura implies dysfunction anterior to the optic chiasm, and retinal artery vasospasm has been observed during episodes (Fig. 11-3). The basis for this is unclear, because the branches of the central retinal artery lack adrenergic innervation. Cases of permanent monocular blindness have been recorded after prolonged attacks.

OPHTHALMOPLEGIC MIGRAINE. Ophthalmoplegic migraine (OM) is a very rare condition characterized by recurrent attacks of migrainous headache associated with reversible paresis of one or more ocular cranial nerves. The third nerve is involved in more than 95% of cases (Fig. 11-4, *A* and *B*). Painful ophthalmoplegia has a wide differential diagnosis. Parasellar, orbital fissure, and posterior fossa lesions must always be excluded by appropriate investigations.

OM is more common in children than adults. The ophthalmoplegia follows the headache, typically within 1 to 4 days. If the third nerve is involved, the pupil is usually spared early in the attack but is often affected later, and recurrent attacks can result in persistent ophthalmoplegia involving the pupil (see Fig. 11-4, *B*).

According to the IHC2, OM has been reclassified under "cranial neuralgias and central causes of facial pain" by analogy to immune-mediated demyelinating cranial neuropathies, because enhancement and swelling of the exit zone of the affected cranial nerve on MRI may occur (see Fig. 11-4, *C*). However, this appearance may be a reflection of blood–nerve barrier permeability changes caused by the migraine mechanism itself, rather than by a primary immune pathology.

The Migraine Mechanism. Migraine is an extremely complex pathophysiologic process. It is essentially a function of the normal human brain, and all are potentially susceptible to varying degrees. Fortunately, the majority of the population is affected only rarely.

Our present understanding is far from complete, but in broad terms, migraine aura and headache result from activation of neuronal networks in the brainstem or the cerebral cortex, or both. It may be possible to identify specific attack triggers. These may be internal (e.g., stress, hormonal changes in women, sleep deprivation, starvation) and external (e.g., certain foods and drinks, head trauma, exercise).

The neural process underlying the migraine mechanism is almost certainly spreading depression. This comprises an advancing wave of excitation that spreads through the neural networks followed by a protracted period of neuronal depression. Cortical spreading depression (CSD) is believed to be the basis for "typical" auras. If the process is confined to the cortex, aura without headache may occur (acephalalgic migraine attack). The headache phase is probably initiated independently in the brainstem. Activation of nociceptive pathways and elements of the trigeminal sensory and autonomic reflex pathways account for the semiology, while activation of anti-nociceptive pathways eventually terminates the attack. Failure of the switch off mechanism results in 'chronic migraine'.

A migraine attack comprises up to four (arguably five) phases, although individual attacks often feature only one or two components. The phases are as follows:

Premonitory symptoms (prodrome)
Aura

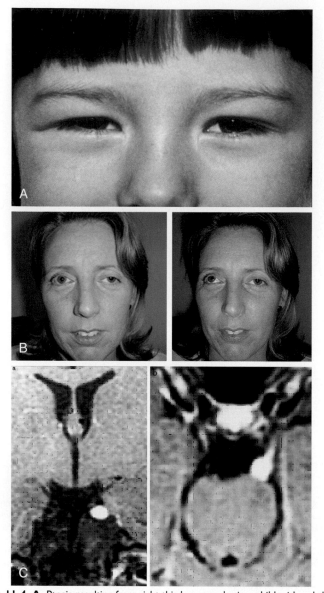

Fig. 11-4. A, Ptosis resulting from right third-nerve palsy in a child with ophthalmoplegic migraine. **B,** Persistent left third-nerve palsy in an adult after repeated ophthalmoplegic migraine attacks over 20 years. *Left:* Primary gaze. Left-sided ptosis and pupillary dilation. *Right:* The patient is attempting to look upward and to the right. **C,** MRI of brain, showing typical enlargement and marked contrast enhancement of the cisternal portion of the left third cranial nerve during an attack of ophthalmoplegic migraine.

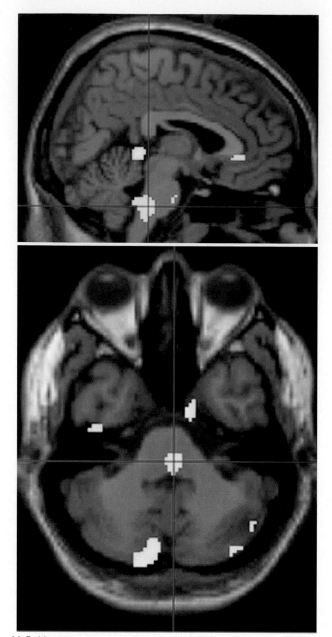

Fig. 11-5. Migraine generator site in the brainstem. Images from a PET study of an attack of migraine without aura, triggered by glyceryl trinitrate. Dorsal pontine activation ipsilateral to the headache is specific to the migraine attack. Nonspecific activation is also seen in the cerebellum and anterior cingulate.

Headache phase—activation of the trigeminocervical complex, the trigeminovascular system, and the trigeminal autonomic reflex

Resolution and postdrome (the postdrome may be considered a fifth phase)

PREMONITORY SYMPTOMS (PRODROME). A minority of patients experience premonitory symptoms, such as a change in mood, heightened sensory awareness, and increased thirst. It is thought that such symptoms stem from the hypothalamus and involve dopaminergic mechanisms.

Aura and Headache

SPREADING DEPRESSION. Migraine without aura is associated with activation of migraine generator nuclei in the brainstem, which have been imaged during attacks by both functional MRI and PET (Fig. 11-5). Migraine 'generators' have been located variously in the periaqueductal gray matter, the basal ganglia, and the dorsal pons in different studies, and it seems likely that the brainstem generator site may vary. In cases of unilateral migraine headache, the generator is ipsilateral to the headache. Cluster headache (see later) is seen to be initiated in the

hypothalamus using similar techniques, whereas the rare syndrome of hemicrania continua (see p. 294) may show activation of both hypothalamic and brainstem sites.

Migraine aura is initiated in the cortex (Fig. 11-6). As noted earlier, CSD comprises an initial brief excitatory phase, corresponding to the "positive" component of the aura (e.g., "flashing lights," the jagged edge of the teichopsia, paresthesias), followed by a protracted neural inhibitory phase causing "negative" symptoms (e.g., scotoma, numbness). CSD proceeds as a wave across the cortex without regard to vascular boundaries, with a velocity of around 3 to 5 mm/min. The rate of propagation presumably determines the duration of aura, and the function of the cortical areas involved determines the symptoms.

NEUROGENIC INFLAMMATION. Blood vessels in the meninges and the circle of Willis are invested with a meshwork of nerve fibers derived from the ophthalmic branch of the trigeminal nerve. These fibers are characterized by varicosities on the terminal axons containing many neuropeptides and transmitters, including nitric oxide, histamine,

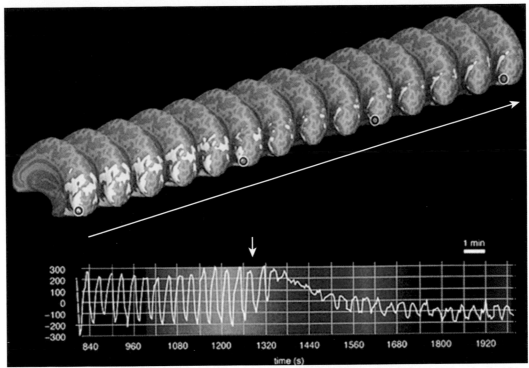

Fig. 11-6. Visual aura results from cortical spreading depression (CSD). Functional blood oxygen level–dependent (BOLD) MRI study of teichopsic aura. The background signal oscillations over the affected occipital cortex give way to an initial signal increase *(arrow)*, indicating hyperemia caused by the excitatory phase of CSD. This lasts 3 to 4.5 minutes and is followed by progressive hypoperfusion, resulting from neuronal suppression, lasting 1 to 2 hours.

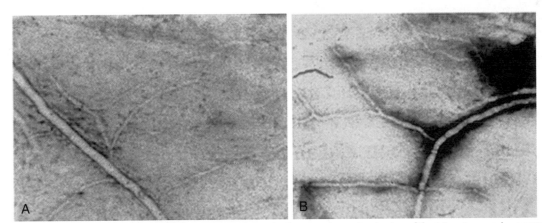

Fig. 11-7. Vasodilation and plasma protein extravasation (PPE) from meningeal vessels after experimental activation of the trigeminovascular system in the rat. **A,** Control. **B,** Stimulated. Triptans abolish PPE in this model.

serotonin, calcitonin gene–related peptide, and substance P. Depolarization of these fibers (by CSD or antidromically from the brainstem) results in the release of these various effectors into the vessel walls. This results in swelling of the vessel walls and local plasma extravasation (i.e., neurogenic inflammation) (Fig. 11-7). Nociceptive information is relayed orthodromically to the brainstem by these sensitized trigeminal nerve fibers.

ALLODYNIA AND THE TRIGEMINAL AUTONOMIC REFLEX. Brainstem activation generated ab initio, or by nociceptive input from the trigeminovascular system, results in activation of second-order neurons in the trigeminocervical complex (TCC). This comprises the trigeminal nucleus caudalis and the contiguous dorsal horn of the upper cervical segments. Nociceptive information from the TCC is modulated by other brainstem nuclei and relayed to the thalamus and sensory cortex.

Cranial afferent sensitization (particularly the first division of the trigeminal nerve) and activation of the TCC are thought to underlie the allodynia commonly experienced during a migraine attack.

This may be confined to the cranial territory but may extend more widely—for example, to the neck, back, and limbs.

Brainstem activation may also stimulate the trigeminal autonomic reflex, resulting in ipsilateral parasympathetic symptoms and signs that vary in magnitude in different primary headache syndromes. As noted earlier, this is a cardinal feature of the TACs, but it can also occasionally occur in migraine.

The term *red migraine* was used in the past to denote cases with prominent facial flushing resulting from the skin vasodilation caused by the reflex. The red ear syndrome is another manifestation. However, facial pallor (white migraine) during migraine attacks is much more common and presumably results from the general sympathetic stress response.

RESOLUTION AND POSTDROME. The mechanisms by which migraine symptoms are maintained and terminated are not known. The pathways of the migraine mechanism extend to the vomiting center and chemoreceptor trigger zone (area postrema). Nausea is a cardinal feature of most attacks, and vomiting can sometimes be severe and prolonged (Fig. 11-8), although some sufferers note that vomiting signals the end of an attack. Sleep and avoidance of sensory input may also help.

After resolution of the headache phase, some migraine sufferers experience a postdrome of symptoms reminiscent of their premonitory syndrome. Polyuria may be a feature.

Complications of Migraine.
As noted earlier, there is increasing evidence that many cases of vertigo, syncope, and transient global amnesia are manifestations of migraine. Very rarely, status migrainosus, in which severe and refractory symptoms persist for more than 72 hours without respite, can occur. Aura symptoms can also sometimes be protracted and even permanent, referred to as persistent aura without infarction.

Serious complications related to migraine are rare, but there is extensive literature relating migraine to the following:

Cerebral infarction, particularly in the posterior circulation, mainly in young adults. The risk of stroke in migraineurs is markedly increased by smoking and the use of combined oral contraceptives (Fig. 11-9).

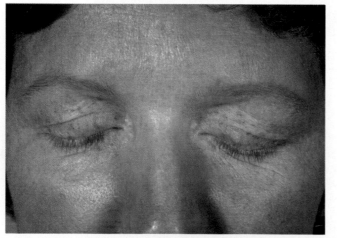

Fig. 11-8. Petechial hemorrhages on the upper eyelids after severe vomiting during a migraine attack.

Epilepsy, including migraine-triggered seizures, epilepsy evolving from migraine, the childhood syndrome of benign occipital epilepsy with intercalated migraine, and migralepsy.

Coma, a feature of certain types of familial hemiplegic migraine and basilar type migraine, particularly in childhood.

CLUSTER HEADACHE AND OTHER FORMS OF TACs. Cluster headache is so called because of the curious tendency of attacks to occur at a similar time on consecutive days for weeks or months on end, followed by protracted intervals free of attacks. The symptomatic intervals are termed cluster periods. Nocturnal attacks are particularly characteristic, and attacks may be provoked by alcohol during the cluster period.

The pain typically wakes the patient at about 2 to 3 AM, and rather than lie still in the quiet as a typical migraine sufferer would do, the cluster headache patient is usually restless and may well even hit the affected area in an attempt to gain relief. The attacks are much more severe than typical migraine but generally last less than an hour. The headache is unilateral, almost always in the territory of the first division of the trigeminal nerve, and it is almost always accompanied by symptoms and signs of ipsilateral parasympathetic autonomic reflex activity and sometimes sympathetic paresis of the pupil, as noted earlier. Usually, only one or perhaps two attacks occur in a single day.

Chronic cluster headache is defined by cluster periods of more than a year, or with less than 1 month of remission between cluster periods. Chronic cluster may be primary or may evolve from episodic cluster headache.

Other forms of TAC are very rare but easily confused with chronic cluster headache (Table 11-2). Paroxysmal hemicrania resembles cluster headache closely, except that the attacks are generally of shorter duration (each lasting only a few minutes) and more frequent (usually at least five daily, and often more). The chronic form is more common than the episodic. Hemicrania continua is essentially an amalgam of chronic cluster headache and paroxysmal hemicrania but with unremitting symptoms. Both of these syndromes usually respond rapidly to treatment with indomethacin.

SUNA/SUNCT (see Table 11-2) is very difficult to treat but may respond to intravenous lidocaine and to Na^+ channel blockers, such as lamotrigine.

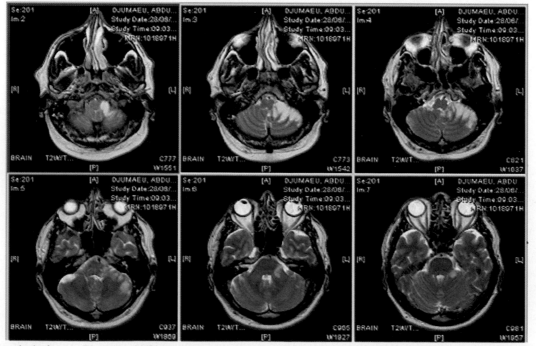

Fig. 11-9. Migrainous cerebral infarction. T2-weighted MRI showing infarction in the distribution of the left anterior cerebellar artery (*arrow*). The patient's initial symptoms included left-sided sensorineural deafness and vertigo resulting from occlusion of the internal auditory artery, and they were followed by a headache identical to the patient's habitual migraine attacks.

TABLE 11-2.   FEATURES OF CHRONIC CLUSTER HEADACHE COMPARED WITH OTHER FORMS OF TAC

	CHRONIC CLUSTER HEADACHE	CHRONIC PAROXYSMAL HEMICRANIA	HEMICRANIA CONTINUA	SUNA OR SUNCT
Time course	<1 month's remission per year	<1 month's remission per year	Unremitting	Episodic or chronic
Pain duration	15-180 min	2-30 min	20 min to days	2 sec to 10 min
Attack frequency	1-8 per day	5-40 per day	Persistent	3-200 per day
Trigeminal autonomic symptoms	Yes	Yes	Yes	Yes
Indomethacin responsive	No	Yes	Yes	No

SUNA, short-lasting unilateral neuralgiform headache with cranial autonomic symptoms; SUNCT, short-lasting unilateral neuralgiform headache attacks with conjunctival injection and tearing; TAC, trigeminal autonomic cephalalgia.

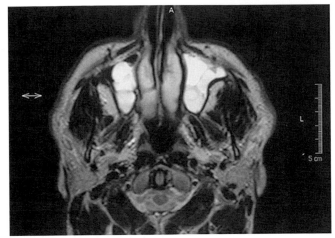

Fig. 11-10. Sinusitis. There is opacification of the maxillary sinuses.

SYMPTOMATIC MIGRAINE.   Headaches with migrainous characteristics can occur as a result of a variety of systemic diseases and intracranial and extracranial pathologies. Such instances probably result from activation of the migraine mechanism. For example, migraine can be provoked by platelet disorders and has been linked to patent foramen ovale. Cases of migraine caused by pathology in regions contiguous with or connected to the anatomic structures involved in the migraine mechanism (e.g., brainstem strokes, cerebral tumors, vascular malformations) have also been reported, and "migraine" can be a feature of some genetic disorders such as MELAS (see Chapter 3) and CADASIL (see Chapter 4).

SECONDARY HEADACHES

Headache is a feature of many systemic diseases and pathologies that affect the pain-sensitive cranial structures, including the scalp, skull bones, meninges, and cerebral vasculature. The cause of secondary headache in some of the conditions listed in Box 11-1 is self-evident. Head and neck injury is discussed later, and other disorders of the neck, intracranial and extracranial vascular disorders, and infections are dealt with elsewhere in this book. It is exceedingly uncommon for headache to be the presenting or exclusive manifestation of an intracranial neoplasm.

As noted earlier, chronic and recurrent headaches are often attributed incorrectly to eye strain and sinus, but true secondary headaches can indeed arise from both. However, chronic sinusitis (Fig. 11-10) is not validated as a cause of headache unless it relapses to an acute infective stage. Headache resulting from refractive errors is localized to the frontal and periorbital regions, aggravated by prolonged visual tasks, and disappears within 7 days of correction of the refractive error.

Giant Cell Arteritis.   Giant cell arteritis is a patchy inflammatory process that affects large and medium-sized vessels that possess an internal elastic lamina, which is characteristically disrupted. Involved vessels may become swollen and even completely occluded. The inflammatory reaction usually includes noncaseating, multinucleated giant cells (Fig. 11-11).

Commonly used alternative names for this disease—temporal arteritis and cranial arteritis—are misnomers, because the pathology often involves vessels throughout the cerebral circulation and even more widely, including the coronary arteries, the vascular supply to the gut, and the vasa nervorum.

Patients rarely present with giant cell arteritis at an age younger than 50. Headache is the most common manifestation and is usually severe, unremitting, and boring in quality. It is often focal but sometimes more widespread, and it is worsened by cold exposure. The extracranial circulation is usually involved, and the scalp is typically tender. The superficial temporal artery, in particular, is frequently swollen and nonpulsatile (Fig. 11-12). Additional diagnostic clues include pain and jaw fatigue on chewing (jaw claudication) and throat and tongue pain. In many cases, there are the additional features of polymyalgia rheumatica, with weight loss, general malaise, and, in particular, pain and stiffness in the limbs on waking.

The most important complication is visual failure, caused by anterior ischemic optic neuropathy. This usually appears with acute, painless, unilateral blindness, but the onset may be much more insidious and may be bilateral. The optic disc becomes swollen and then pale (Fig. 11-13). It is vital to make the diagnosis and initiate treatment before this occurs, as the visual impairment is irreversible. Other neurologic complications can include stroke and transient ischemic attacks, and rarely sixth-nerve and pupillary sparing third-nerve palsies caused by nerve infarction.

The ESR is nearly always increased, and usually substantially so. It is wise to obtain an emergency temporal artery biopsy to confirm the diagnosis before initiating treatment with high-dose steroids. It is essential that multiple fine sections of a long segment of vessel be examined, as the process is patchy. The response to high-dose steroids is usually dramatic and gratifying, and it nearly always prevents the visual complications. Treatment usually has to be continued for at least 2 years.

Idiopathic Intracranial Hypertension (IIH).   Sometimes referred to as pseudotumour cerebri, or less appropriately, benign intracranial hypertension is a condition of unknown cause that affects obese women of reproductive age. Menstrual irregularities are a common feature, and the condition has been linked to polycystic ovary syndrome. When a male patient presents with this syndrome, it is likely to reflect some underlying disorder, such as occult cerebral venous sinus thrombosis, or stenosis of a transverse sinus (Fig. 11-14). It may also be a complication of collagen vascular disease and procoagulant states. An identical syndrome can be precipitated by a variety of drugs, notably tetracyclines, naladixic acid, retinoic acid, and vitamin A, and by rapid withdrawal of steroids.

There is some evidence that the idiopathic condition results from impaired bulk flow of CSF through the arachnoid granulations that line the venous sinuses, as a consequence of local thrombophilia-hypofibrinolysis. There is no cerebral edema, and the rate of CSF production equals the absorption rate, but a higher intracranial pressure is then required to achieve this.

The headache is nonspecific and typically holocranial, unremitting, and worsened by coughing and stooping. Rarely, there may be nausea and vomiting, pulsatile tinnitus, and diplopia resulting from a false-localizing sixth-nerve paresis. The sole major morbidity is

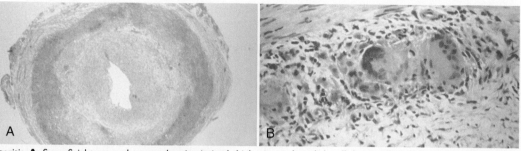

Fig. 11-11. Giant cell arteritis. **A,** Superficial temporal artery showing intimal thickening and medial wall damage. **B,** Inflammatory infiltrate in the internal elastic lamina, including noncaseating giant cells.

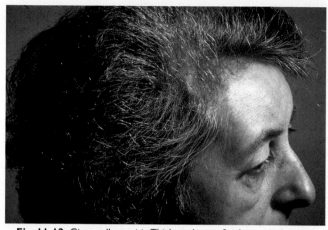

Fig. 11-12. Giant cell arteritis. Thickened superficial temporal artery.

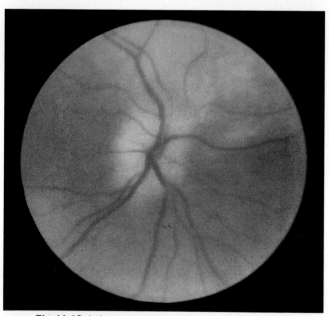

Fig. 11-13. Ischemic optic neuropathy in giant cell arteritis.

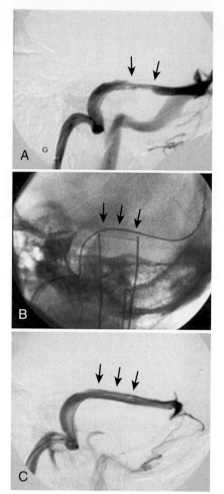

Fig. 11-14. Intracranial hypertension secondary to stenosis of lateral venous sinus **A,** Oblique lateral subtracted venogram of the lateral sinuses. Guide catheter (G) is in the left internal jugular vein. A smaller catheter enters the left sigmoid sinus and crosses the stenosis *(arrows)* in the left transverse sinus. The right transverse sinus is hidden from view but the right sigmoid sinus and right internal jugular vein are seen. **B,** Similar view (unsubtracted) showing guidewire passing through the stent *(arrows)*, deployed at the level of the stenosis. **C,** Subtracted venogram (same view as **B**) showing the site of the stenosis *(arrows)* dilated by the stent, with good flow through the left lateral sinus.

progressive, or even sudden, visual failure caused by decompensation of papilledema. Early visual symptoms can include transient visual obscurations with changes in posture. Acuity and color vision are unaffected.

Papilledema is present in nearly all cases, and it is often very marked (Fig. 11-15). It is usually possible to confirm enlarged blind spots and sometimes inferonasal visual field defects by confrontation testing, but formal perimetry is helpful for serial observations (Fig. 11-16).

Neuroimaging is mandatory to exclude an intracranial mass. The ventricles may appear slit-like, but this is certainly not invariable. CT can exclude drusen in the optic nerve head (Fig. 11-17), and MR venography can identify venous sinus thrombosis and stenosis. Fluorescein retinal angiography can be helpful to confirm papilledema

in equivocal cases (Fig. 11-18), but measurement of CSF opening pressure at lumbar puncture is essential to confirm the diagnosis. This may also relieve the symptoms immediately and can be repeated therapeutically and to monitor progress during treatment.

A vigorous weight loss program is a key element of treatment, together with acetazolamide, a carbonic anhydrase inhibitor that reduces CSF production. A short course of high-dose steroids may be given to patients with severe visual symptoms. Venous sinus stenting may be undertaken in appropriate cases (see earlier). Refractory cases may require lumboperitoneal shunting, although recently good results have been claimed for ventricular shunting using a stereotactic frame. Incipient visual failure may require optic nerve sheath fenestration (Fig. 11-19).

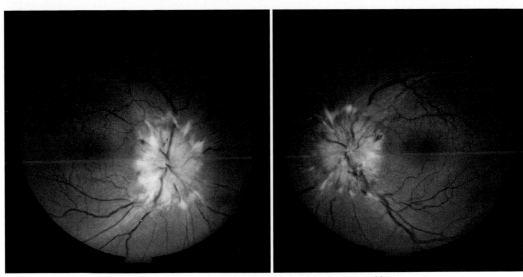

Fig. 11-15. Severe bilateral papilloedema in idiopathic intracranial hypertension.

VISUAL FIELDS IN BENIGN INTRACRANIAL HYPERTENSION

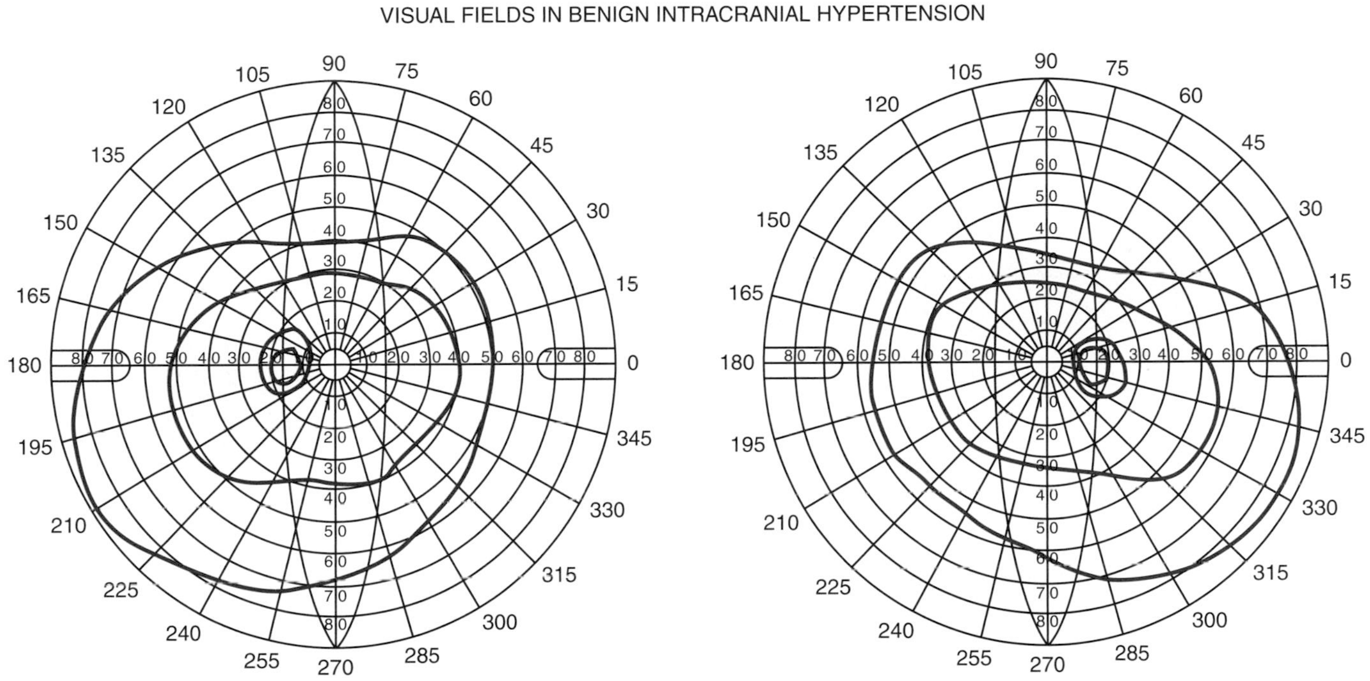

Fig. 11-16. Idiopathic intracranial hypertension. Enlarged blind spots on perimetry.

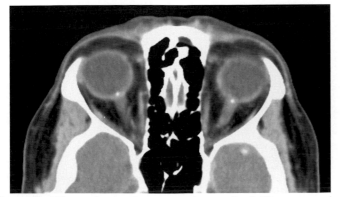

Fig. 11-17. CT scan showing drusen at optic nerve heads. These can produce changes at the optic disc that can mimic papilledema.

Intracranial Hypotension. The headache of intracranial hypotension is strikingly postural, being precipitated within 15 minutes by sitting or standing and largely relieved by lying down. It is typically holocranial, it is exacerbated by Valsalva maneuvers, and it may be associated with nausea, vomiting, neck stiffness, and photophobia.

The condition can arise in a number of ways. By far the most common is after lumbar puncture, but it may occur spontaneously, or be precipitated by coughing or straining, and it may appear as a thunderclap headache (see earlier). In such instances, the condition usually results from a persistent CSF leak from the dura around the spinal cord, commonly in the cervical or thoracic region. Occasionally, leaks are multiple.

The diagnosis is usually made by brain MRI. This typically shows diffuse "thickening" of the meninges, with dural enhancement with gadolinium (Fig. 11-20). This appearance seems to be the result of dilation of meningeal vessels, particularly veins, to maintain the total intracranial volume despite CSF leakage. There may also be descent of the cerebellar tonsils. Rarely, subdural hematomas develop. The CSF pressure at lumbar puncture is typically less than 6 cm H_2O.

The site of a leak can sometimes be identified by MRI, CT myelography, or radioisotope cisternography. The syndrome usually resolves spontaneously with bed rest and fluids. Otherwise, empirical use of theophylline or caffeine may help headache after lumbar puncture, as may steroids. In refractory cases, epidural blood patching, epidural saline infusion, and fibrin glue injection have been advocated. Rarely, direct surgical repair of the defect may be required.

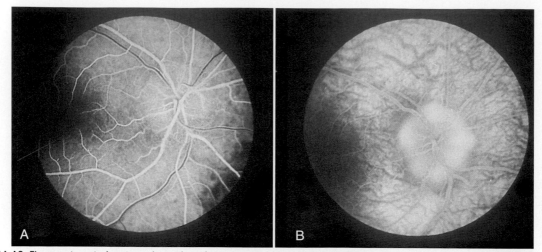

Fig. 11-18. Fluorescein retinal angiography in idiopathic intracranial hypertension. **A,** Increased vascularity of the disc. **B,** Leakage of dye.

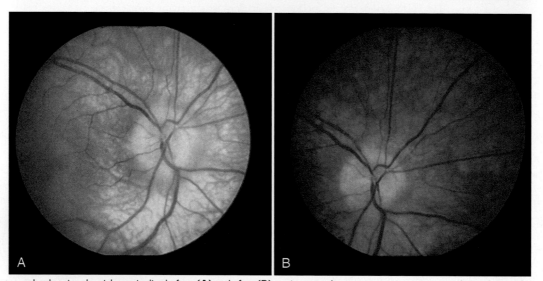

Fig. 11-19. Fundal photographs showing the right optic disc before **(A)** and after **(B)** optic nerve decompression in a patient with rapid visual failure caused by idiopathic intracranial hypertension.

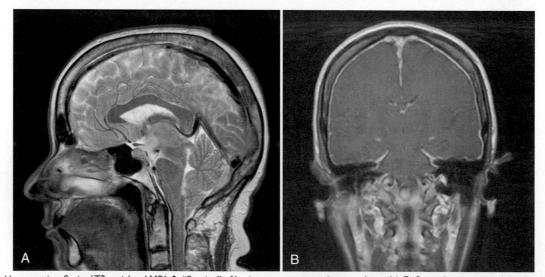

Fig. 11-20. Intracranial hypotension. Sagittal T2-weighted MRI. **A,** "Sagging" of brainstem structures (pons and tonsils). **B,** Smooth symmetrical dural enhancement over vertex.

NEURALGIAS

CRANIAL NEURALGIAS

Trigeminal Neuralgia

Trigeminal neuralgia comprises paroxysmal attacks of very severe, unilateral facial pain, usually in the distribution of the second or third division of one trigeminal nerve; the first division is affected in less than 5% of cases (compare Cluster Headache, earlier). Rarely, the pain affects two or even all three divisions. During an attack period, the pain always occurs on the same side, and in the extremely rare instance of bilateral attacks, both sides are never affected simultaneously. The syndrome is more common in women than in men, and it usually occurs in individuals older than 50 years. In younger patients, pathology affecting the trigeminal nerve or its brainstem

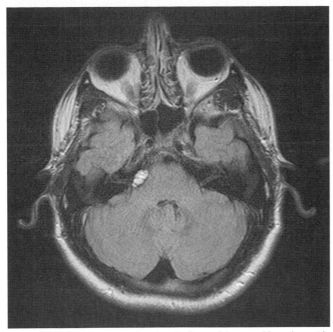

Fig. 11-21. Symptomatic right trigeminal neuralgia caused by a dermoid.

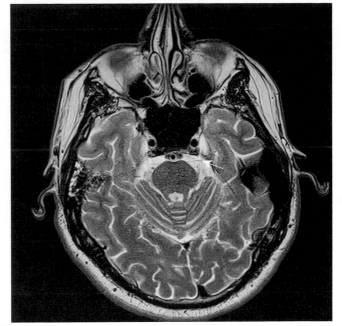

Fig. 11-23. Vascular cross-compression of the left trigeminal nerve in a patient with trigeminal neuralgia. Note the vessel crossing the left trigeminal nerve.

TRIGGER ZONES

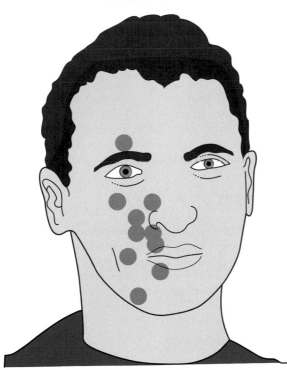

Fig. 11-22. Trigger zones in trigeminal neuralgia.

connections, such as a plaque of multiple sclerosis or nerve tumor, should be suspected (Fig. 11-21).

The pain is classically lancinating and may be described as like an electric shock or red-hot needle. The attacks often occur many times a day, and sometimes a more protracted, dull aching pain persists between paroxysms. An important characteristic is that the pain can usually be triggered by tactile stimuli in certain areas (trigger zones [Fig. 11-22]) and also, for example, by chewing, cleaning the teeth, or a cold wind. After a paroxysm, there is a refractory period during which an attack cannot be triggered. This distinguishes trigeminal neuralgia from TACs, in which there is no refractory period. After a period of weeks, the attacks often remit, only to return weeks or months later. Sometimes, the pain is so severe that it evokes reflex

spasm of the facial muscles (tic doloreux, once thought to be a form of focal epilepsy 'neuralgia epileptiforme').

The condition is often misdiagnosed as being caused by dental or sinus disease, sometimes leading to inappropriate interventions.

Examination is normal in idiopathic cases but neuroimaging may identify vascular cross-compression of the symptomatic nerve at the root entry zone, typically by the superior cerebellar artery (Fig. 11-23). Ephaptic discharges from the irritated sensory nerve fibers are thought to produce secondary excitation of the trigeminal nucleus, leading to pain. Vascular cross-compression can certainly be found in normal, asymptomatic individuals, but persistent pulsatile irritation by an arteriosclerotic vessel is thought to injure the nerve. This might explain the higher prevalence of the condition in older people.

Anticonvulsants, such as carbamazepine, may suppress the symptoms, and selective destruction of pain fibers in the trigeminal ganglion by thermocoagulation, cryothermy, glycerol injection, or vascular decompression of the nerve via a posterior fossa approach (Jannetta procedure) may cure the condition. Stereotactic radiosurgery has its advocates, but, rarely, a total trigeminal sensory rhizotomy may be the only recourse, with the resulting risk of anesthesia dolorosa.

Vascular cross-compression has been implicated in several other paroxysmal cranial nerve disorders. Evidence is reasonably convincing for hemifacial spasm (seventh nerve) and glossopharyngeal neuralgia (ninth nerve), but much less so for vertigo, motion intolerance, and tinnitus (eighth nerve), torticollis (eleventh nerve), and essential hypertension (left retro-olivary sulcus).

Glossopharyngeal Neuralgia

Glossopharyngeal neuralgia is an extremely rare syndrome characterized by intense, shocklike paroxysmal pain in the region of the tonsillar fossa or the ear, at the base of the tongue, or beneath the angle of the jaw on one side. The pain is therefore felt in the distribution of the auricular and pharyngeal branches of the vagus nerve as well as the glossopharyngeal nerve. Swallowing, coughing, and sometimes talking and chewing can trigger attacks. Between paroxysms, there may be a constant background pain in the throat and ear region. The threat of pain may prevent the patient from eating or drinking. The condition shows a pattern of exacerbations and remissions that is similar to that of trigeminal neuralgia, and, as noted, vascular cross-compression is generally considered to be the cause. The management is as for trigeminal neuralgia.

TABLE 11-3. RARE CRANIAL NEURALGIAS

SYNDROME	NERVE	SITE OF PAIN AND ADDITIONAL FEATURES
Nervus intermedius neuralgia	VII (nervus intermedius branch)	Auditory canal Altered taste, salivation, lacrimation
Superior laryngeal neuralgia	X (superior laryngeal branch)	Lateral throat, under jaw, and ear Precipitated by swallowing, shouting Trigger point in hypothyroid membrane
Nasociliary neuralgia	V (nasociliary branch)	Nostril, radiating to forehead Triggered by touching lateral aspect of nostril
Supraorbital neuralgia	V (supraorbital nerve)	Supraorbital notch, forehead Focal tenderness in supraorbital notch
Occipital neuralgia	C2 (greater or lesser occipital nerves)	Occipital region Affected area may become numb

Other Cranial Neuralgias

A number of other idiopathic paroxysmal cranial neuralgias have been described (Table 11-3). All are rare. Local anesthesia of the suspect nerve can be diagnostic, and nerve ablation may be curative.

Neck–tongue syndrome comprises unilateral pain, lasting seconds or minutes, in the occipital region or upper neck, associated with an abnormal sensation in the tongue on that side. This may involve numbness, paresthesias, or a sensation of involuntary movement (lingual pseudoathetosis). Head turning typically precipitates the symptoms. It appears to be caused by irritation of the C2 sensory root, typically by a protuberant atlantoaxial joint. Proprioceptive fibers in the lingual nerve connect to the hypoglossal nerve in the tongue, which in turn connects to the C2 nerve root. Surgical decompression of the root relieves the symptoms.

POSTHERPETIC NEURALGIA

It has been estimated that some 50% of individuals reaching the age of 80 will have had at least one attack of shingles, a condition that results from reactivation of dormant herpes (varicella) zoster in the dorsal root ganglia of the spinal cord or the sensory roots of the cranial nerves. Attacks of shingles usually occur spontaneously, but reactivation may follow intercurrent illness, particularly hematologic malignancies, lymphomas, and immunosuppressive disorders; zoster occurs in about 10% of patients with lymphoma and 25% of patients with Hodgkin's disease. It may also follow trauma to the involved nerves or dermatomes.

The clinical syndrome comprises burning, and tingling pain with occasional stabbing components, followed in less than a week by small cutaneous blisters that follow the distribution of one or more dermatomes. In rare instances, the rash may not be evident (zoster sine herpete). The thoracic dermatomes are most often involved, but no region is immune. The trigeminal distribution is affected in 10% to 15% of patients, with the ophthalmic division being singled out in some 80% of such cases. Shingles may also involve the geniculate ganglion and thus its sensory component, the nervus intermedius, causing a facial palsy and a zoster eruption over the anterior external auditory meatus, soft palate, and pinna (Ramsay Hunt syndrome) (see Chapter 15, Fig. 15-58). Nervus intermedius neuralgia may also be a feature.

Involvement of the ganglia of Corti and Scarpa may cause additional otic symptoms such as vertigo, tinnitus, and deafness. Rarely, other ipsilateral cranial nerve palsies—causing unilateral external ophthalmoplegia, for example—can also occur in this context (Garcin's syndrome).

The pain of acute shingles resolves within a month in 90% of cases. Some 10% of patients, almost always older than 50, develop postherpetic neuralgia, and the incidence of this complication increases with age. A burning discomfort persists for 3 or more months after the initial shingles attack, and the involved dermatomes

exhibit hypesthesia, hyperalgesia, or allodynia. Although this may resolve within a year, up to 40% of patients suffer protracted discomfort that is often refractory to treatment. There is some evidence that treatment with acyclovir within 3 days of onset of shingles reduces the risk of postherpetic neuralgia.

CAUSALGIA AND REFLEX SYMPATHETIC DYSTROPHY

Causalgia and *reflex sympathetic dystrophy* (sometimes referred to as algodystrophy and Sudeck's atrophy) are poorly understood phenomena that are part of the spectrum of the complex regional pain syndrome (CRPS). Reflex sympathetic dystrophy (type 1 CRPS) is thought to result from reflex sympathetic responses to minor injury. Similar symptoms and signs following more severe nerve trunk injury are usually referred to as causalgia (type 2 CRPS). Opinion is divided as to whether these entities are part of a continuum.

The hands are most often involved, but the lower limbs can also be affected. The trigger is usually accidental trauma, such as a Colles' fracture, or a needlestick injury to the sciatic nerve. The trigger may be surgery, such as median nerve decompression or release of Dupuytren's contracture.

The syndrome has three components:

Pain that is typically burning, throbbing, shooting, or aching, together with hyperalgesia, hyperpathia, and allodynia.
Trophic changes, such as loss of hair and atrophy of the skin and nails in the affected dermatomes. There is atrophy of the underlying soft tissues, with stiffness and contractures leading to loss of function and localized bone demineralization (Sudeck's atrophy).
Autonomic dysfunction in those dermatomes, commonly including excess sweating (less often anhidrosis), local edema, heat and cold insensitivity, and vasomotor abnormalities (typically redness or cyanosis).

In the acute stage, there may be pain, swelling, and warmth distal to the injury, sometimes associated with features of denervation; trophic changes follow, then muscle wasting and contractures (Fig. 11-24). Plain radiographs of the affected part reveal localized osteopenia with preservation of joint spaces.

HEAD INJURY

Head injury and its chronic complications pose a considerable burden for medical services and the community. Road traffic accidents, falls, and intoxication-associated assaults are the most common causes in adults and tend to result in more severe head injuries. Sporting head injuries are generally milder and more common in children and young adolescents.

SEVERITY OF HEAD INJURY

The Glasgow Coma Scale (GCS) (Table 11-4) is generally accepted as the best clinical descriptor of head injury severity. The total score is based on the patient's highest responses. It may be falsely low in the presence of shock or hypothermia, after a seizure, and in cases of intoxication or sedative drug administration. The GCS can also be difficult to score if the patient is agitated, dysphasic, or intubated or has significant facial injury or spinal cord dysfunction. Critically, it takes no account of eye movement abnormalities as demonstrated by the doll's head maneuver.

A score of less than 8 denotes severe head injury, and the patient will be comatose or have severe depression of the conscious level. A score of 8 to 12 denotes moderate head injury, and 13 to 15, mild head injury. However, it is now recognized that even "mild" head injury, which constitutes some 80% of cases admitted to the hospital, can cause brain damage with serious long-term complications if there is any impairment of consciousness, amnesia, or alteration in mental state at the time of injury or subsequently.

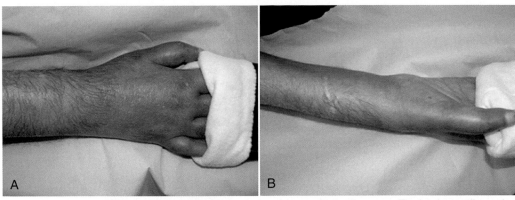

Fig. 11-24. Reflex sympathetic dystrophy. **A** and **B,** Two views of the right hand after injury to the median nerve. The hand is swollen and severely allodynic. There is hyperhidrosis and atrophy of the thenar eminence.

TABLE 11-4.   GLASGOW COMA SCALE

ITEM	SCORE	OBSERVATION
Eye opening	4	Spontaneous
	3	To verbal command
	2	To pain
	1	No response
Best verbal response	5	Oriented
	4	Confused
	3	Inappropriate words
	2	Incomprehensible sounds
	1	None
Best motor response	6	Obeys commands
	5	Localizes to pain
	4	Withdraws to pain
	3	Flexion to pain
	2	Extension to pain
	1	No response to pain
Maximum total score	15	—

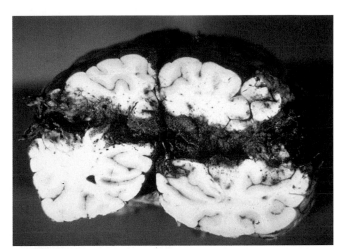

Fig. 11-25. Through-and-through missile injury. The bullet entered the brain on the right.

Head injury associated with impairment of consciousness (concussion) results in some loss of memory for events before the event (retrograde amnesia) and after it (anterograde amnesia—in this context referred to as posttraumatic amnesia). Very often, a mixed amnesic picture is evident, but posttraumatic amnesia is always more severe and protracted than the retrograde amnesia, and its duration is correlated with the severity of head injury. Concussion does not cause loss of autobiographical memory; apparent impairment in this context indicates malingering or hysteria.

MECHANISMS OF BRAIN INJURY

Head injuries may be penetrating, such as those caused by missiles and stab wounds, or closed (or blunt), as typically sustained in road traffic accidents and brawls.

Penetrating injuries (Figs. 11-25 and 11-26) have a high mortality rate because of direct damage to vital structures, and from cerebral edema, hemorrhage, and infection. Individuals who survive such injury often have neurologic and cognitive deficits, and there is a high incidence of posttraumatic epilepsy.

In closed head injuries, the force of impact may be transmitted linearly (translational force) or may result in rotational or angular forces centered on the midbrain and thalamus. These forces can produce focal and diffuse injuries (Table 11-5).

Loss of consciousness results from disruption of neuronal function in the reticular activating system, which is situated at the impact fulcrum point in the midbrain and diencephalon. It is difficult to produce concussion experimentally if the neck is restrained, which emphasizes the importance of head restraints and seat belts in vehicles. These forces can also produce cranial nerve lesions even in the absence of parenchymal brain injury on imaging. Olfactory nerve damage is particularly common and often missed on initial examination. If persistent for more than 6 months after injury, olfactory nerve damage is permanent.

Focal Injuries

Skull Fractures and Imaging in Head Injury.   Brain damage resulting from head injury can occur in the absence of skull fracture, but the presence of a fracture makes such damage much more likely. CT brain scanning is the investigation of choice in head injury cases and is indicated in any patient with skull fracture (suspected or proven by radiography) (Fig. 11-27, 11-29), depressed consciousness, or neurologic deficit.

The role of imaging in the investigation of mild head injury is more controversial. Less than 10% of patients with simple concussion have intracranial bleeding, and less than 2% require neurosurgical treatment. The frequency of surgically significant intracranial hematoma in adults without neurologic deficit, skull fracture, or postconcussive symptoms, except mild headache, is less than 1%. In such cases, all that is required is a period of observation. However, CT is recommended routinely for all head-injured children less than 16 years old, for patients who cannot be observed after discharge, for intoxicated patients, and for those with bleeding diatheses or on anticoagulants.

Frontal and orbital fractures often produce periorbital hematomas ("raccoon eyes") (Fig. 11-28), and, if the dura in the region of the paranasal sinuses is breached, there may be CSF rhinorrhea. Fractures of the squamous temporal and parietal bones (Fig. 11-29) can injure the middle meningeal artery, resulting in extradural hematoma (see p. 302), and base-of-skull fractures can injure the facial and auditory nerves, causing deafness, vertigo, and facial palsy. Extension of the fracture to the auditory canal can result in bleeding from the external canal and CSF otorrhea. Such fractures can also be associated with bleeding behind the mastoid (Battle's sign) (Fig. 11-30).

Intracranial Hemorrhages. After head injury, brain hemorrhage may occur at a number of sites depending on the site and force of impact. Cerebral contusions, which are found in some 90% of fatal head injury cases, generally occur in parts of the brain that are in contact with uneven bony surfaces of the skull deep to the site of impact, such as the crests of the frontal and temporal lobe gyri (Fig. 11-31). Contrecoup contusions on the side of the brain opposite the point of impact are thought to be caused by negative pressures that develop as the brain moves relative to the skull (Fig. 11-32).

Extradural hematoma (EDH) is a particular risk in young people who suffer head injury during sport—for example, being hit on the head by a cricket ball. EDH is found in some 10% of severe head injury cases. Classically, the patient is concussed but recovers consciousness and may seem relatively normal for some time (the lucid interval) but subsequently lapses into coma, preceded by headache, focal symptoms, and sometimes seizures. A more protracted course may occur when the bleeding is primarily venous. A skull fracture across the path of the middle meningeal artery is found in about 90% of cases. CT is virtually diagnostic, as the hematoma has a very characteristic lens-shaped appearance, with shift of midbrain structures (Fig. 11-33). If this condition is not diagnosed and treated promptly by surgical removal of the clot (Fig. 11-34), the resulting pressure cone leads to death (Fig. 11-35).

Acute subdural hematoma (acute SDH) results from rupture of parasagittal bridging veins in the subdural space. Hemorrhage tends to be more extensive than in EDH, as the extravasated blood can spread more freely in this compartment. A lucid interval may occur after injury, but more often there is persistent impairment of consciousness from the outset. Associated cerebral contusion is common.

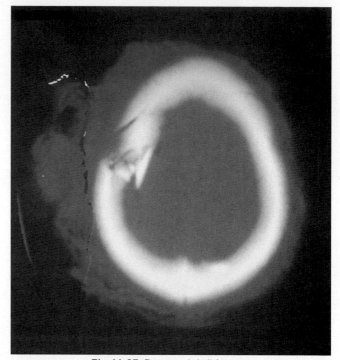

Fig. 11-27. Depressed skull fracture.

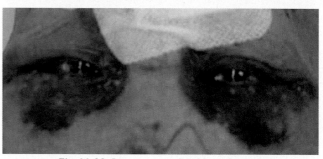

Fig. 11-28. Raccoon eyes after frontal fracture.

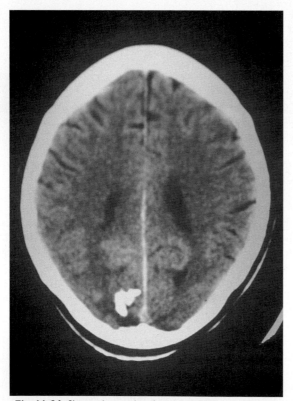

Fig. 11-26. Shrapnel wound in the occipital lobe on CT scan.

TABLE 11-5. PATHOLOGIC CONSEQUENCES OF CLOSED HEAD INJURY

FOCAL INJURIES	DIFFUSE INJURIES
Scalp lacerations	Diffuse axonal injury
Skull fractures	Brain swelling
Intracranial hemorrhages	Global ischemia
Contusions	
Extradural hematoma	
Subdural hematoma	
Subarachnoid hemorrhage	
Midbrain hemorrhage	
Intraventricular hemorrhage	
Lesions resulting from raised intracranial pressure	

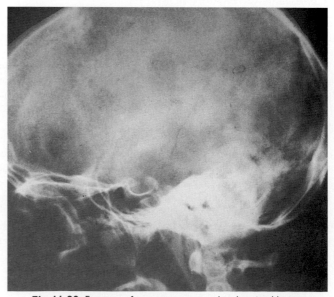

Fig. 11-29. Fracture of squamous temporal and parietal bones.

On CT, the high-density lesion differs in shape from that of an EDH (Fig. 11-36), but it may also be associated with shift of midline structures unless bilateral hematomas are present. These clots may not require surgical removal if modest in size, and they often resolve spontaneously (Fig. 11-37). As the clot matures, its intensity on CT decreases and at a critical point it becomes isodense, its presence marked only by any space-occupying effects on surrounding structures. T1-weighted MRI will demonstrate the lesion, however (Fig. 11-38).

Chronic subdural hematomas can be difficult to diagnose clinically. There is often no clear history of head injury, and they may be an incidental finding on imaging. When symptoms arise, they tend to be nonlocalizing, such as fluctuating consciousness levels, cognitive decline, apathy, and diffuse headache. There may be hyperreflexia and primitive reflexes. The hematoma is usually readily identified on CT or MRI imaging (Fig. 11-39).

Subarachnoid, Midbrain, and Intraventricular Hemorrhage. Hemorrhages of the subarachnoid, midbrain, and intraventricular type are associated with severe head injury and a poorer prognosis (Fig. 11-40). Hemorrhage in the midbrain can result from the effects of the impact itself but can also be secondary to raised intracranial pressure and herniation. When an intracerebral hematoma is in continuity with an acute subdural, the term *burst lobe* is used.

Diffuse Injury

Diffuse Axonal Injury. It is likely that nearly all head injuries, and certainly those of sufficient severity to cause impairment of consciousness, result in axonal injury as a result of shear stresses on axons

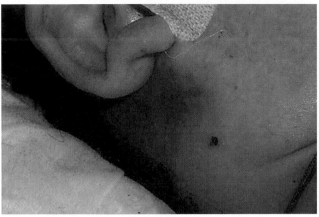

Fig. 11-30. Battle's sign in base-of-skull fracture.

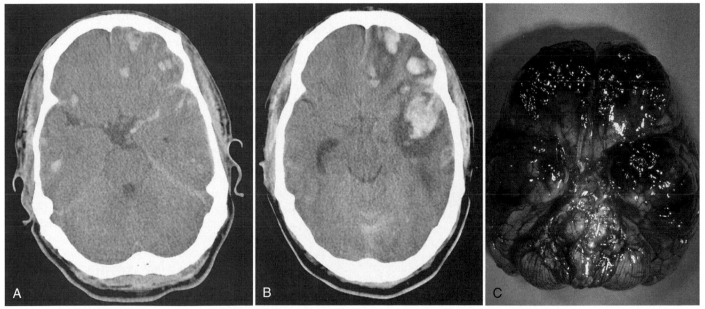

Fig. 11-31. CT brain scan showing contusions in left frontal and temporal lobes. **A,** Scan at presentation. **B,** Scan 24 hours later. Note dramatic worsening of the contusions. **C,** Postmortem specimen showing contusions in the frontal and temporal lobes.

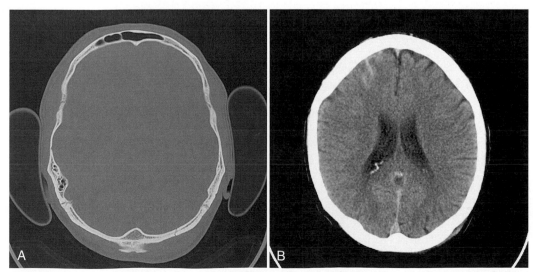

Fig. 11-32. CT brain scans showing contrecoup hemorrhages. Bone **(A)** and soft tissue **(B)** window showing left occipital fracture and soft tissue swelling and right frontal (contrecoup) contusion.

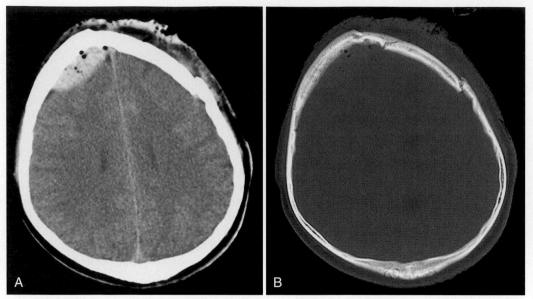

Fig. 11-33. CT scans. **A,** Right frontal extradural hematoma. **B,** Bony window demonstrating skull fracture.

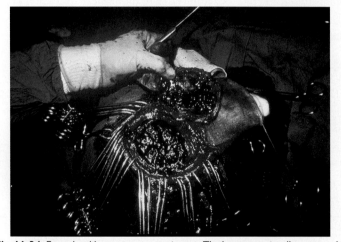

Fig. 11-34. Extradural hematoma at craniotomy. The hematoma is adherent to the bone flap and dura.

and dendritic connections. This axonal damage results in white matter lesions in the cerebrum and brainstem that may be focal or diffuse (Fig. 11-41). Some axons are damaged at the time of impact (primary axotomy), but it is now established that brain trauma establishes a chronic process of axonal degeneration (secondary axotomy) (Fig. 11-42). Acute axonal injury in the reticular activating system is probably the basis of loss of consciousness in concussion. When extensive, diffuse axonal injury may result in severe brain swelling and irreversible coma.

Brain Swelling. Any significant intracranial clot formation will be associated with raised intracranial pressure. Depending on the severity and location, this may lead to lateral (subfalcine) or transtentorial herniation, which in turn can be associated with additional midbrain hemorrhage. Even in the absence of frank hemorrhage on the CT scan, there is almost always acute cerebral edema from the effects of ischemia and diffuse axonal injury. This may be associated with effacement of the brain sulci and slit-like ventricles on the CT scan, but it may be inconspicuous. Intracranial pressure monitoring may be required to manage this complication. Subsequent MRI can reveal the true extent of damage from diffuse axonal injury (Fig. 11-43).

Global Ischemia. Cerebral hypoperfusion is usually secondary to systemic hypotension after multiple injuries or as a result of raised intracranial pressure.

CHRONIC COMPLICATIONS OF HEAD INJURY

The Glasgow Outcome Scale defines four states after head injury: (1) death or vegetative state, (2) severe disability, (3) moderate disability, and (4) good recovery. However, the incidence of moderate and severe disability in young people after mild head injury is actually similar to that of survivors of moderate and severe head injury, suggesting that cognitive and motor dysfunction can continue to progress long after apparent recovery.

Postconcussion Syndrome

The most common chronic neurologic complication of head injury is postconcussion syndrome, which is found in 90% of concussed patients at 1 month, and in 25% a year or more after injury. This syndrome comprises a number of sometimes disabling symptoms, particularly headache, dizziness, and cognitive difficulties (Box 11-4). There is controversy as to the extent that this syndrome has an organic basis. Presumed emotional and psychological symptoms are prominent, and unresolved litigation issues may confound the situation. Countries where such litigation is infrequent have a low incidence of postconcussion disability, and it is rare in children. However, formal neuropsychometric tests can show significant abnormalities months after concussion and, as noted, some degree of diffuse axonal injury is probably universal.

Posttraumatic Headache

Headache is the single most common chronic symptom after head injury. It may be part of postconcussion syndrome or an isolated complaint. The symptoms are most often compatible with tension type headache but can have migrainous qualities or even resemble cluster headache.

The mechanism of posttraumatic headache is unclear, but it is probably heterogeneous. Most cases probably stem from activation of the migraine mechanism of primary headache (see earlier). This can also involve cervical inputs when there was an associated whiplash injury (see later). Migraineurs are particularly likely to experience exacerbation of migraine after head injury. Acute posttraumatic headache usually settles after about 3 months and is said to be less common after severe than after mild head injury. Psychosocial factors may play a part in chronic cases.

Dementia Pugilistica and Alzheimer's Disease

Although there is controversy over the extent of brain damage after a single episode of concussion, there is clear evidence of cumulative damage, both on neuropsychological testing and from pathologic

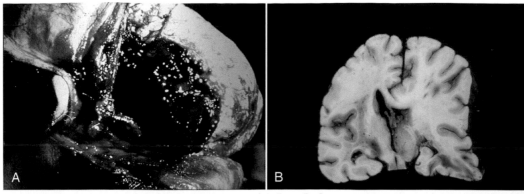

Fig. 11-35. Extradural hematoma at postmortem examination. **A,** After removal of skull cap. **B,** Coronal section of brain showing marked cerebral compression and shift of midline structures caused by the clot.

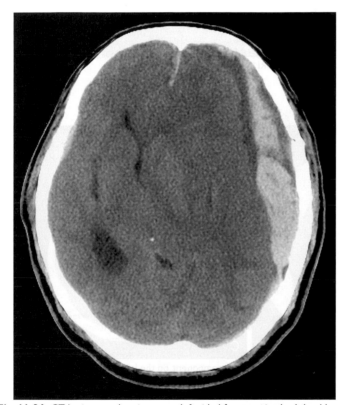

Fig. 11-36. CT brain scan showing acute left-sided frontoparietal subdural hematoma with midline shift.

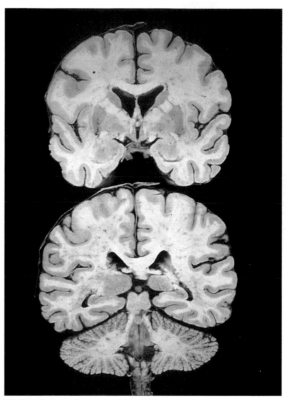

Fig. 11-37. Resolution of acute subdural hematoma at postmortem examination. This patient had had a traumatic subdural hematoma diagnosed on MRI, 3 months before he died of a myocardial infarction.

studies, in individuals such as boxers who sustain repeated head injuries. In dementia pugilistica, there is memory impairment, slowness of thinking and movement, dysarthria, and gait ataxia, often with features of parkinsonism. Neuroimaging and pathologic features can include cortical atrophy, ventricular dilation, cavum septum pellucidum, and evidence of diffuse microhemorrhages (Fig. 11-44).

There is epidemiologic evidence of an association between previous head injury and the subsequent development of Alzheimer's disease. This is particularly strong for patients with previous severe head injury who lack the ApoE-ε4 allele, a known risk factor for Alzheimer's disease. Pathologic changes similar to those in Alzheimer's disease, such as prominent amyloid deposition, selective damage to cholinergic structures, and chronic neuroinflammation, may be found in the postmortem examination.

Psychiatric Disorders
As noted, psychological and psychiatric disorders, such as depression, are common in postconcussion syndrome, but head injury of any severity can also be associated with affective disorders, including schizophrenia (Fig. 11-45).

SPINAL INJURY

Spinal trauma can result in (1) injury confined to the vertebral column without involvement of the spinal cord or nerve roots and (2) damage to the cord or nerve roots without evidence of spinal fracture or dislocation; or a combination of both.

INJURY TO BOTH BONY AND NEUROLOGIC STRUCTURES

The anatomic level and extent of spinal injury are assessed by clinical examination supplemented by neuroimaging, often a combination of (1) plain radiographs and CT scanning, looking for fractures, dislocations, and instability, and (2) MRI to examine damage to neurologic structures.

Vertebral Injury
Vertebral injury in isolation is by far the most common form of spinal trauma. Whiplash injuries of the cervical and lumbar spine are a very common consequence of road traffic accidents. Spinal trauma resulting from forces transmitted in the axial plane, such as falling

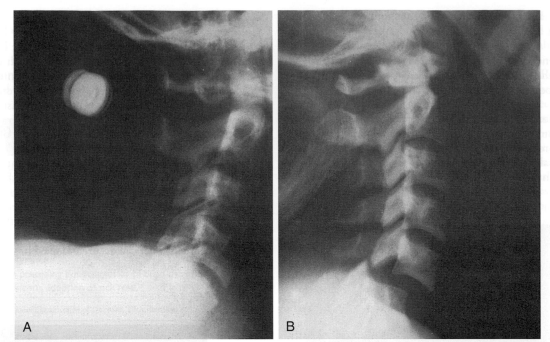

Fig. 11-50. Lateral cervical spine radiograph fails to reveal a dislocation at C5-C6 **(A)** until the shoulders have been depressed **(B)**.

TABLE 11-6.	ASIA CLASSIFICATION OF SPINAL CORD INJURY SEVERITY
ASIA IMPAIRMENT SCALE	**EXTENT OF IMPAIRMENT**
A = Complete	No motor or sensory function below level of lesion, including S4–S5.
B = Incomplete	Sensory but not motor function is preserved below the neurologic level, including S4-S5.
C = Incomplete	Motor function is preserved below the neurologic level, but more than half the key muscles are MRC grade <3.
D = Incomplete	As C, but more than half the key muscles are MRC grade >3.
E = Normal	Normal motor and sensory function.

ASIA, American Spinal Injuries Association; MRC, Medical Research Council.

Spinal cord injuries are classified as complete or incomplete with reference to the eventual motor or sensory neuroanatomic level below which neurologic function is lost. However, there are paradoxical situations in *apparently* complete injuries, where function is partly preserved below this level. The American Spinal Injuries Association impairment scale has been widely adopted to classify the extent of impairment (Table 11-6).

SPINAL CORD SYNDROMES

Incomplete traumatic cord lesions may result in a defined spinal cord syndrome. These syndromes can of course also be encountered with a wide range of other pathologies.

Central Cord Syndrome

Hyperflexion and hyperextension cord injury, particularly in the cervical region, may result in traumatic hematomyelia or posttraumatic syringomyelia, with necrosis and cavitation of central areas of the cord over several segments (Fig. 11-51). When symptomatic, such lesions typically result in the clinical features of syringomyelia (see Chapter 14), but traumatic lesions often cause severe neck and cape or half-cape distribution pain that is burning in quality and associated with allodynia.

Brown-Séquard Syndrome

The Brown-Séquard syndrome results from damage to one half of the spinal cord in the sagittal plane. This results in loss of ipsilateral motor function and impaired dorsal column sensory modalities

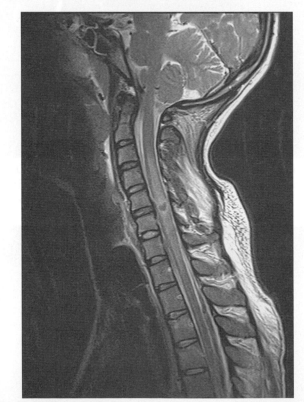

Fig. 11-51. T2-weighted MRI of cervicothoracic cord showing high signal resulting from a posttraumatic syrinx.

below the lesion, together with contralateral loss of pain and temperature sensation beginning one to two segments below this level but with preservation of dorsal column function on that side. Partial Brown-Séquard lesions are more often encountered than the complete syndrome.

Anterior Cord Syndrome

Anterior cord syndrome is more commonly encountered as a result of spinal cord infarction than as a direct result of trauma It is described in detail in Chapter 14.

Conus and Cauda Equina Syndromes

The conus medullaris is the terminal expansion of the lower extremity of the spinal cord. The cauda equina comprises nerve roots L3 to S5, which exit from the conus.

Conus lesions typically result in a mixed and symmetrical upper and lower motor neuron pattern of weakness and reflex changes in the legs, with impaired bladder and bowel sphincter dysfunction as an early feature. Sensory impairment is usually confined to the perianal area. Cauda equina syndrome is a purely lower motor neuron disorder that is typically asymmetrical, with sacral and perineal sensory impairment. Impotence is common, and bladder dysfunction tends to occur late, along with urinary retention.

Infections of the central nervous system can be divided into those that primarily involve the coverings of the brain or spinal cord (i.e., meningitis) and those that involve the CNS parenchyma (i.e., cerebritis, encephalitis, or myelitis). Focal circumscribed parenchymal or meningeal infections present as abscesses or, in the subdural space, as empyema. There can be combinations of any of these (e.g., meningoencephalitis, encephalomyelitis).

The etiologic agents of these diseases include viruses, conventional bacteria, acid-fast bacilli, spirochetes, a variety of fungi, and several kinds of protozoal or metazoal parasites. The most important of these diseases are described by site and etiology.

THE MENINGITIDES

VIRAL MENINGITIS

Viral meningitis is most commonly identified in younger individuals, and it tends to cluster in the summer and autumn months. It produces an acute illness with fever and signs of meningeal irritation. Alteration of the level of consciousness is uncommon. Additional features, which are partly dependent on the causative agent, include a rash, arthralgia, muscle pain, sore throat, and vomiting or diarrhea.

The CSF protein concentration is normal or slightly raised. There is a lymphocytic pleocytosis with counts reaching 1000/mm³. Rarely, the pleocytosis is initially polymorphonuclear before becoming lymphocytic. (This depends on the rapidity with which CSF is sampled after the onset of the infection, and not on the particular virus responsible.) The CSF glucose concentration is usually normal, but exceptionally (e.g., in mumps, herpes zoster, herpes simplex type 2, and lymphocytic choriomeningitis) it is moderately depressed. Attempts to identify the responsible agent, either by its isolation or by demonstrating a significant rise in CSF antibody titers, meet with limited success. Newer techniques for viral detection include immunofluorescence, enzyme immunoassay, and polymerase chain reaction (PCR). An apparently viral meningitis that recurs (a rare occurrence with true viral meningitis) raises the possibility of Lyme disease, syphilis, collagen vascular disease, or an infective process bordering the meninges. Treatment is symptomatic.

BACTERIAL MENINGITIS

Haemophilus influenzae, Neisseria meningitidis, and *Streptococcus pneumoniae* historically accounted for about three quarters of those cases of community-acquired bacterial meningitis in which the responsible agent was isolated. The incidence of *H. influenzae* infection has declined substantially since the introduction of conjugated *H. influenzae* type B vaccine. Nosocomial meningitis (typically occurring in hospitalized patients as a result of recent neurosurgery or head injury) is usually caused by gram-negative organisms, staphylococci, or streptococci. In most cases, the agent reaches the meninges via the bloodstream, at least for community-acquired cases, probably through the choroid plexus. CNS damage is at least in part a result of release of cytokines such as interleukin-1 and tumor necrosis factor. The cytokines stimulate leukocyte adhesion to endothelial cells with resultant

breaching of the cell wall and exudation of albumin. Substantial brain edema is the norm. Other agents released by leukocytes and thought to be the mediators of the pathophysiologic changes observed during bacterial meningitis include reactive oxygen species and nitric oxide. In those patients who succumb, postmortem examination reveals clouding of the meninges with opalescent streaks surrounding the cortical veins over the hemisphere convexities (Fig. 12-1, *A*). In deaths occurring slightly later in the disease process, the calvarial surfaces are often covered by dense subarachnoid pus, with relative sparing (grossly) of the inferior and basal surfaces (Fig. 12-1, *B*). The pus extends deeply into the sulci (Fig. 12-1, *C*).

Microscopy reveals polymorphonuclear and mononuclear cells (the relative proportions depend on how rapidly death has ensued after onset of the infection) with hemorrhages lying between the pia and arachnoid. A fibrinous exudate appears and extends into the sulci and Virchow-Robin spaces (Fig. 12-2). Vasculitis follows in the superficial cortical vessels and over the base of the brain. Brain infarction occurs in up to 20% of cases. The cranial nerves are often engulfed in the fibrinous exudate.

Clinical features include fever, headache, signs of meningeal irritation, and clouding of consciousness. Those patients admitted in coma have a poor prognosis, as do very young and elderly patients. The finding of focal neurologic signs is likely to reflect a complicating vasculitis. Signs of meningeal irritation are sometimes lacking in the neonate, in elderly patients, and in deeply comatose patients. A petechial rash occurs in about 50% of cases of meningococcal meningitis but is seen in meningitis caused by other organisms (e.g., *Escherichia coli*).

Lumbar puncture for evaluation of the CSF remains the mainstay of diagnosis, although the procedure is potentially hazardous if there is acute brain swelling, a finding particularly associated with *H. influenzae* infection. The CSF pressure is usually elevated. The protein concentration is raised in most patients, although seldom to greater than 5 g/L. The cell count, predominantly polymorphonuclear, may reach 100,000/mm³. In rare cases, the cell count is barely raised, or even normal. Glucose concentrations of less than 2.2 mmol/L are found in about half the cases. When comparison is made between the glucose concentration in the CSF and that in the plasma, the delay before the plasma glucose concentration is reflected in the CSF should be considered. Gram staining is positive in up to three quarters of cases. Failure to identify the organism by either Gram staining or culture is encountered in up to a quarter of cases.

Counterimmunoelectrophoresis and latex agglutination are available for most bacterial pathogens, but the sensitivity of these measures varies considerably. PCR permits detection of nuclear material.

Radiologic investigation is seldom warranted in the acute stages of the illness, except in the unlikely event of the patient's being found to have papilledema. CT scanning at this stage often reveals gyral enhancement. Later scanning reveals communicating hydrocephalus in a small proportion of cases. Repeated CSF examination serves little useful purpose in management unless the clinical response to treatment is unsatisfactory. The development of seizures or focal neurologic signs, or a late deterioration in the patient's clinical condition, merits imaging. In patients with recurrent meningitis, a search for an anatomic defect that has allowed access of organisms to the CNS is

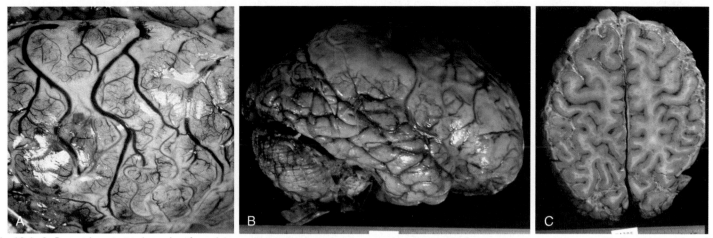

Fig. 12-1. A, Bacterial meningitis. Lateral surface of the cerebral hemisphere showing a purulent exudate. **B,** *Streptococcus pneumoniae* meningitis. Predilection of purulent exudate for the convexities with relative sparing of the inferior part of the convexity and the base. **C,** Deep sulcal infiltration by pus, as shown in an axial slice.

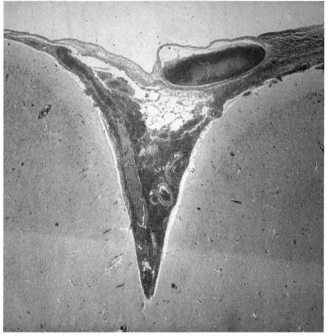

Fig. 12-2. Bacterial meningitis. Section showing exudate in the subarachnoid space of a cerebral sulcus (H&E, ×8.)

mandatory. Abnormalities underlying recurrent meningitis include fistulas in the frontal or ethmoid sinuses or defects of the cribriform plate (Fig. 12-3).

Sporadic bacterial meningitides are usually caused by *S. pneumoniae, E. coli,* other gram-negative bacilli, or staphylococci. Epidemic meningitis, a serious public health concern, is largely caused by *N. meningitidis.* This infection can spread rapidly in schools or military barracks. *Listeria monocytogenes* is the causative agent of a subacute meningitis that can be subtle in its early stages and then progress through a fatal course if not recognized and properly treated. Typically, it leads to a rhomboencephalitis, with brainstem and cerebellar signs in addition to the features of a meningitis.

TUBERCULOUS MENINGITIS

After tuberculous bacteremia, small tuberculous foci (Rich's foci) may become established in the brain, spinal cord, or meninges. Expansion of the focus produces a granulomatous mass lesion (tuberculoma), and its rupture into the subarachnoid space or ventricular system results in meningitis.

A number of different pathologic processes are identified in tuberculous meningitis and are partly determined by the host's tuberculin

sensitivity. Rupture of the focus into the subarachnoid space produces a gelatinous exudate that concentrates in the basal cisterns (Fig. 12-4). Microscopic examination reveals an inflammatory reaction containing lymphocytes, plasma cells, and, prominently, epithelioid histiocytes. Tubercle bacilli may be sparse or plentiful (Fig. 12-5). There is an accompanying vasculitis (Fig. 12-6). Later, a fibrotic reaction appears and hydrocephalus is common.

The initial clinical manifestations of the disease are nonspecific, with malaise, fever, headache, and muscle pain. Signs of meningeal irritation appear insidiously over 1 to 3 weeks, with headache, neck stiffness, and dulling of the consciousness state. As the exudate organizes and a secondary vasculitis emerges, infection appears in the infarcted brain tissue. Focal neurologic deficits appear, including cranial nerve signs, seizures, and hemiplegia or paraplegia (Fig. 12-7). In one series of adults, independent predictors of tuberculous meningitis were age less than 36 years, a length of history exceeding 6 days, a white blood cell count exceeding 15,000/mm^3, a total CSF cell count exceeding 900/mm^3, and a neutrophil percentage exceeding 75.

An abnormal chest radiograph is found in about half the cases, but tuberculin skin tests are often negative. CSF examination is essential. The cell count is usually 100 to 400/mm^3. Rarely, in patients with impaired tuberculin sensitivity, the cell count is normal. In a small group of patients, the illness begins abruptly, the clinical features resemble bacterial meningitis, and the cell count often exceeds 1000/mm^3 with a predominance of polymorphonuclear leukocytes. The protein concentration usually measures 1 to 5 g/L. Sometimes, the glucose concentration is normal but most typically it is moderately depressed, lying between 1.7 and 2.5 mmol/L in about half the cases. A failure to demonstrate the organism on Ziehl-Neelsen staining is common but is less likely if serial CSF specimens are examined. CSF adenosine deaminase activity is raised, but it is also elevated in pyogenic meningitis. PCR and related methods achieve a sensitivity that has been reported to range between 20% and 100%. False positives can occur. Mycobacterial DNA remains detectable in the CSF for up to 1 month after starting therapy.

CT may demonstrate enhancing basal exudates, low-density areas in the basal ganglia, and hydrocephalus. MRI is probably a more sensitive technique for detecting the various pathologies (Fig. 12-8).

The general recommendation regarding therapy is that all patients should be started on isoniazid, rifampicin, and pyrazinamide. A fourth drug is added, usually either streptomycin or ethambutol. After a short intensive phase of treatment, continuation therapy is given, usually in the form of isoniazid and rifampicin, with or without pyrazinamide. Drug resistance is common. Treatment is continued for at least 6 months. The role of adjunct steroid therapy is controversial.

Tuberculoma once accounted for a third of intracerebral tumors occurring in the United States and the United Kingdom, and it is still

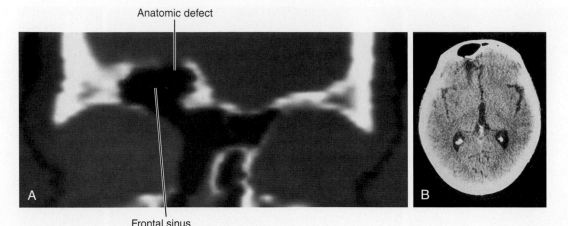

Anatomic defect

Frontal sinus

Fig. 12-3. Recurrent pneumococcal meningitis. CT scan showing a defect in the posterior wall of the frontal sinus. **A,** Coronal section. **B,** Axial section.

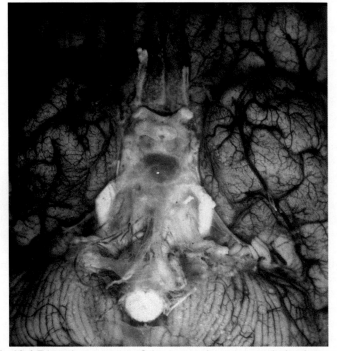

Fig. 12-4. Tuberculous meningitis. Gelatinous exudate occupying the basal cisterns.

common in third-world countries. Many cases in the United Kingdom occur in the Asian community. The tumors are usually infratentorial in children and supratentorial in adults (Fig. 12-9). They are multiple in up to a third of cases. Many, but not all, tuberculomas are superficial and involve the leptomeninges; some are entirely intraparenchymal.

Histologically, there is a central caseating core surrounded by a collagen capsule containing epithelioid histiocytes, lymphocytes, and multinucleate giant cells (also histiocytic) (Fig. 12-10). Organisms are found on microscopy in about 70% of cases. Some 30% to 50% of patients have evidence of extracranial tuberculosis, and a similar percentage have a history of previous infection. The chest radiograph is abnormal in about half. Typically, the patient presents with signs of raised intracranial pressure. Seizures occur in at least 50% of cases, but fever is uncommon, and only a third have hemiparesis. The most common CSF abnormality is a raised protein concentration. Skin testing is often negative, and the erythrocyte sedimentation rate is usually normal. CT identifies low- or high-density areas, often with marked edema. Enhancement may occur either diffusely or in a ring form (Fig. 12-11). The lesions are usually isointense on T1-weighted MR images but have more variable signal characteristics with T2 weighting. Typically, an irregular enhancing rim is seen with gadolinium. The lesions can be parenchymal or dural, and single or multiple

(Fig. 12-12). The condition is managed medically. Only seldom is surgery required. Extensive edema is treated with corticosteroids.

CRYPTOCOCCAL MENINGITIS

Cryptococcus neoformans is a yeast, 2 to 15 μm in greatest diameter, surrounded by a polysaccharide capsule (Fig. 12-13). In cryptococcal meningitis, the organism, found in the soil near bird colonies, gains access to the body via the respiratory tract, leading to a pulmonary infection that may be silent. After hematogenous dissemination, infiltration of the leptomeninges occurs, with meningeal thickening and proliferation of the organisms around penetrative vessels in the Virchow-Robin space (Fig. 12-14). Granulomatous masses may appear in the cerebral substance or spinal cord (Fig. 12-15, *A*) but are usually limited to the leptomeninges in immunocompetent patients. The chest radiograph is abnormal in about 25% of cases. The CSF pressure is usually raised with a lymphocytic pleocytosis, a mildly elevated protein concentration, and a depressed glucose level. Staining the CSF with India ink or nigrosin identifies the encapsulated budding cells in up to 90% of cases. CSF culture is performed. Alternative routes to the diagnosis consist of detection of cryptococcal antigen by latex agglutination or enzyme-linked immunosorbent assay (ELISA).

In immunosuppressed patients, most notably those with AIDS, cryptococcal CNS infection evokes a minimal inflammatory reaction, both in terms of the CSF and the histologic appearance of the brain at autopsy in fatal cases, when there are myriads of organisms but almost no inflammatory cells. In addition to the meningeal and subarachnoid proliferation, which gives the brain surfaces an oily, slippery texture, the organisms proliferate deep into the brain perivascular spaces, commonly in the basal ganglia. The latter lesions expand the perivascular spaces without invasion of the brain and without any reaction, producing a spongy appearance in cut surfaces of the brain at autopsy (Fig. 12-15, *B*).

Imaging reveals nonspecific changes including edema and hydrocephalus. Traditionally, treatment has been with amphotericin B, with or without 5-fluorocytosine.

PARENCHYMAL INFECTIONS: CEREBRITIS, ENCEPHALITIS, ABSCESS, SUBDURAL EMPYEMA

FUNGAL ENCEPHALITIS

Aspergillosis

Aspergillosis is usually confined to immunocompromised individuals or to patients with uncontrolled diabetes mellitus. The organism gains access to the CNS via the respiratory tract. A meningeal syndrome is unusual. Typically, the organism invades small or large

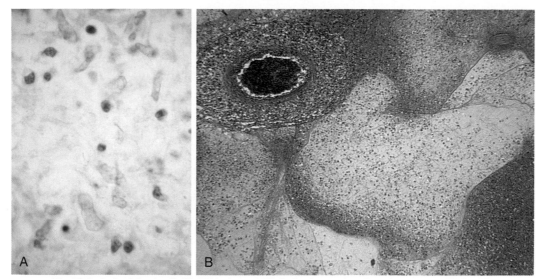

Fig. 12-5. A, Acid-fast bacilli (Ziehl-Neelsen, ×950). **B,** Exudate in the subarachnoid space (H&E, ×60).

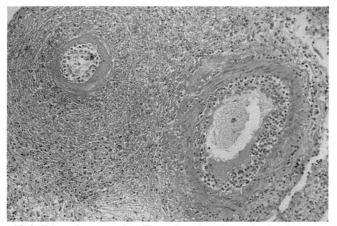

Fig. 12-6. Tuberculous vasculitis. Two subarachnoid vessels showing extensive fibrinoid necrosis (H&E, ×62.5).

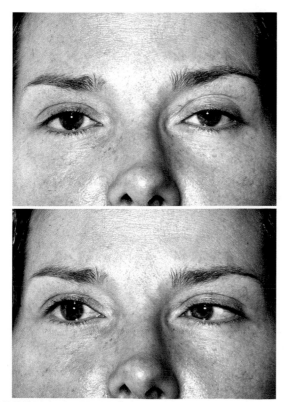

Fig. 12-7. Tuberculous meningitis. Right VI nerve palsy. **A,** Forward gaze. **B,** Right lateral gaze.

blood vessels, with secondary thrombus formation leading to vessel occlusion and focal infarction (Fig. 12-16). Mycotic aneurysms can occur, resulting in subarachnoid and intraparenchymal hemorrhage. In some cases, a focal mass lesion appears (Fig. 12-17, *A*). The diagnosis is usually established by tissue biopsy. Lesions are usually full of organisms, shown by appropriate stains to be septate hyphal forms that frequently branch at a 45-degree angle (Fig. 12-17, *B*). Treatment is normally a combination of surgery with amphotericin B and 5-fluorocytosine.

Mucormycosis

Mucormycosis encompasses infections (zygomycosis, chromomycosis) with a variety of similar fungi, all of which have large broad hyphae and are clinically aggressive. These infections are virtually confined to individuals with a predisposing illness (e.g., diabetes mellitus). The clinical picture is similar to that seen with aspergillosis, although the organism gains access to the nervous system via the paranasal sinuses. Consequently, facial and ocular pain is common, followed by proptosis, ophthalmoplegia, and evidence of arterial or retro-orbital venous occlusion. Carotid occlusion may follow. Imaging demonstrates bone destruction and soft tissue mass formation (Fig. 12-18). The condition is often fatal. Treatment combines removal of invaded bone with the use of amphotericin B.

Coccidioidomycosis

Coccidioides is a soil-based fungus found in Central and South America and parts of the United States (Fig. 12-19). The disease initially affects the lung (Fig. 12-20), with later spread to the CNS. There, a granulomatous reaction occurs in the meninges and sometimes in the parenchyma. The granuloma contains giant cells, lymphocytes, plasma, and epithelioid cells and bears a close resemblance to the granuloma found in tuberculous meningitis (Fig. 12-21).

The usual picture is of a slowly evolving meningitic syndrome, with headache, malaise, and signs of systemic illness, sometimes progressing over several months. The CSF changes include an elevated protein concentration and cell count, and a depressed glucose level. In some cases, the organism can be identified. Alternatively, antibody can be detected by various techniques. Treatment is with amphotericin B.

Candida

Disseminated candidal infection is almost confined to individuals who have some systemic illness, including AIDS, and particularly to those individuals who have been treated with antibiotics, steroids, or both. It usually manifests as a meningitis or focal encephalitis. Treatment is with amphotericin B, and sometimes with 5-fluorocytosine.

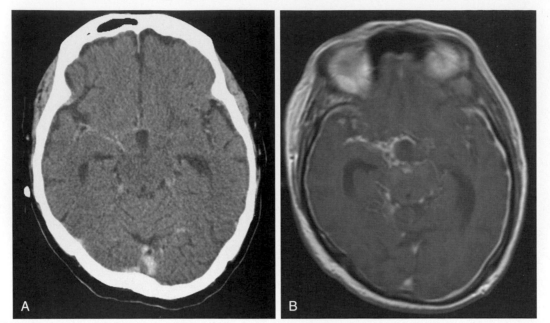

Fig. 12-8. Tuberculous meningitis. **A,** Postcontrast CT. **B,** MRI. The basal and dural convexity meningeal enhancement is better appreciated with MRI.

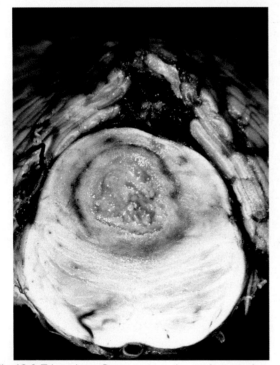

Fig. 12-9. Tuberculoma. Gross specimen showing lesion in the pons.

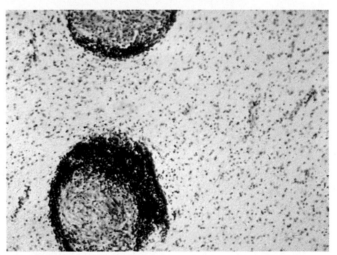

Fig. 12-10. Tuberculoma. Two foci with an intense surrounding inflammatory reaction.

Histoplasmosis

Histoplasmosis infection by *Histoplasma capsulatum* is endemic in the central and eastern states of the United States (particularly in the Ohio River Valley). The lung usually bears the brunt of the disease, but disseminated infection can occur with CNS involvement, including a meningitis or disseminated parenchymal granuloma.

PARASITIC INFECTION

Hydatid Disease

Hydatid disease is caused by infestation with the cystic stage of *Taenia echinococcus* (echinococcus granulosus). The cyst is unilocular, with a double wall, from the inner layer of which capsules are budded. The heads of the worms are produced from the inner walls of the

capsules (Fig. 12-22). The cyst is most commonly found in the liver and lungs. Involvement of the brain may be asymptomatic or result in epilepsy (Fig. 12-23).

Cysticercosis

Cysticercosis is the encysted stage of the pork tapeworm, *Taenia solium*. Proglottids released from the gut of carriers of the tapeworm contain ova, which can enter food through fecal contamination. Ingestion of contaminated food allows the ova to penetrate the gut and develop into the cystic stage of the disease. Muscle involvement leads to enlargement simulating hypertrophy, sometimes with weakness and, eventually, calcified deposits (Fig. 12-24).

The CNS is infested in 60% to 90% of patients with cysticercosis. Cysts form in the brain parenchyma associated with varying degrees of inflammatory reaction and edema (Fig. 12-25, *A*). Later, a fibrous wall resembling that of an abscess with calcification may develop. When removed, these mature fibrous-walled cysts may contain a visible organism (Fig. 12-25, *B*), although in many cases the larva has died and degenerated. The larva in a cyst has a characteristic structure, although when degenerated, this may be lost. The outer wall is acellular chitin, beneath which is a thin layer of basal epithelial cells. Deep to these, various internal

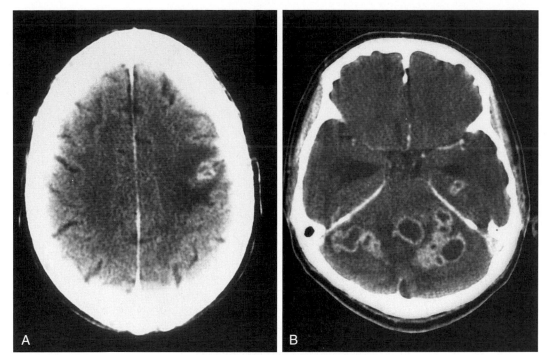

Fig. 12-11. Tuberculoma. CT scan. **A,** Single enhancing lesion in left hemisphere. **B,** Multiple, predominantly ring-enhancing lesions, principally in the cerebellum.

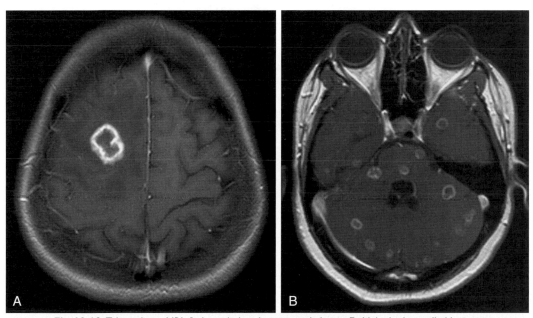

Fig. 12-12. Tuberculoma. MRI. **A,** Irregularly enhancing single lesion. **B,** Multiple thin-walled lesions.

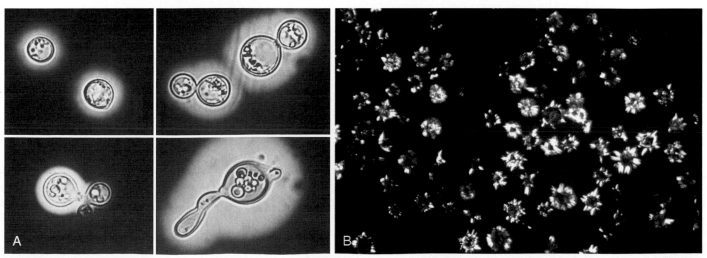

Fig. 12-13. Cryptococcal meningitis. *Cryptococcus neoformans.* **A,** Nigrosin preparation (×120). **B,** Buffered cresyl violet under polarized light (×110).

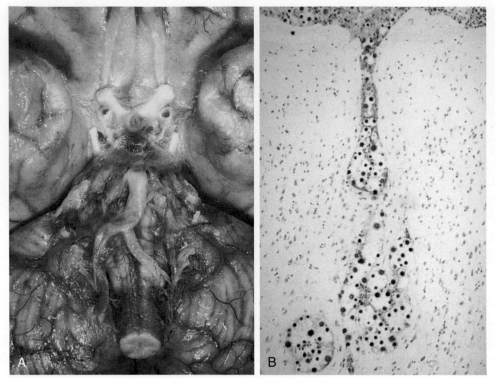

Fig. 12-14. Cryptococcal meningitis. **A,** Opacity of the basal leptomeninges. **B,** Cryptococci distending the perivascular space of a cortical blood vessel (Nissl, ×40).

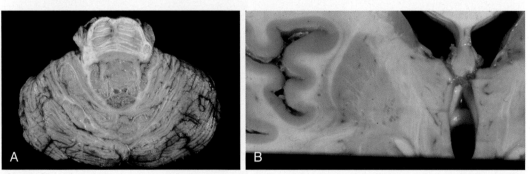

Fig. 12-15. A, Cryptococcoma. Slice of cerebellum and pons. A large cryptococcoma replaces a major part of the ventral cerebellar vermis, obliterating the fourth ventricle. **B,** Cryptococcal meningitis in a patient with AIDS. Typical spongiform appearance of the basal ganglia.

structures, mostly the gut, are apparent (Fig. 12-25, *C*). The scolices are not usually apparent in tissue sections. Many patients remain asymptomatic and have a normal neurologic examination. Epilepsy occurs in about half the cases. Arachnoiditis, secondary to invasion of the arachnoid by the cysticerci, leads to meningeal fibrosis and obstructive hydrocephalus. If the inflammatory reaction is particularly florid, a vasculitic syndrome ensues, with multiple infarcts.

Diagnosis is based on imaging and serologic testing, but it sometimes awaits histologic examination of single lesions mistaken as tumors. CT or MRI may demonstrate multiple cysts with or without calcification (Fig. 12-26), areas of infarction secondary to vasculitis, obstructive hydrocephalus, or foci of edema associated with contrast enhancement. If the disease is active, an inflammatory reaction, sometimes with eosinophils, is found in the CSF.

Most cysticercus lesions are parenchymal and abscess-like, but when organisms encyst in the subarachnoid space or in a ventricle, they may form multiple thin-walled cysts (racemose form) (Fig. 12-27, *A*). In some locations, these can lead to obstructive hydrocephalus (Fig. 12-27, *B* to *D*).

Immunoblot is the serologic investigation of choice. In individuals with multiple active lesions, it is 98% sensitive and 100% specific. Assays using unfractionated antigens are less specific, but they are more reliable if used on CSF rather than serum.

Albendazole is the drug of choice for treating cerebral cysticercosis. An alternative is a single-day course of praziquantel coupled with steroids. Transient worsening of symptoms after a few days of initiating therapy is common, so therapy is usually combined with corticosteroids. The use of antiparasitic agents has to be critically examined in patients with diffuse disease or with hydrocephalus, as it is thought that maximal inflammation and associated edema occur as the encysted organisms are killed.

BACTERIAL CEREBRITIS

Invasive infection of the cerebral parenchyma by conventional bacteria is conventionally termed cerebritis, but the term *encephalitis* would be equally appropriate. The organisms reach the brain mostly by hematogenous means; cerebritis from a precursor meningitis is uncommon. Organisms proliferate and invade outward from an initial focus, which may be a microinfarct secondary to the originating septic embolus. The initial focus is filled with polymorphonuclear leukocytes, and is surrounded by spreading edema along with the organisms. Host defenses attempt to wall off the infection, producing an abscess, but until or unless the fibrous capsule of the abscess is formed, the infection will continue to invade the brain tissue, with associated mass effect from the edema. Vasculitic involvement of parenchymal vessels leads to associated infarcts.

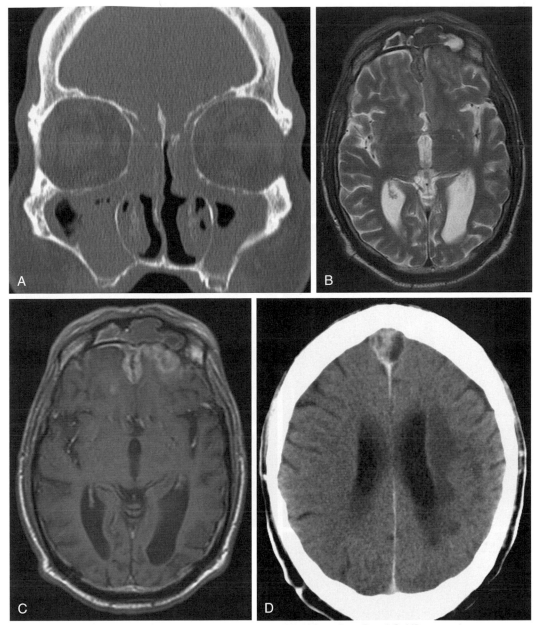

Fig. 12-16. Aspergillosis. **A,** Extensive sinus disease with bone destruction of anterior cranial fossa floor. **B** and **C,** MR images showing intracranial spread along dura. **D,** Two weeks later, there is increasing dural spread with an infarct of the middle cerebral artery CT.

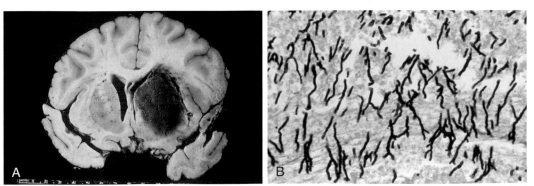

Fig. 12-17. Aspergillosis. **A,** An aspergilloma with hemorrhage and necrosis involving the basal ganglia. **B,** Organisms revealed as septate hyphal forms with frequent branches at 45-degree angles.

CEREBRAL BACTERIAL ABSCESS

Intracerebral abscess most commonly occurs secondary to an infective source in the paranasal sinuses or the middle ear. Pulmonary infection provides a hematogenous source of infection. Septic emboli (as from bacterial endocarditis) result in small infarcts, which then become the site of bacterial growth. Cerebral abscess is a recognized hazard in patients with congenital cyanotic heart disease, those with pulmonary arteriovenous malformation, and those using IV drugs. Oral or dental bacterial disease is another potential source of transient bacteremia that can seed in the CNS. Some of the abscesses in that situation contain unusual filamentous organisms, such as *Nocardia*. In up to 20% of cases, the source of the infection is not apparent.

alongside the falx as well as over the convexities. The condition is frequently complicated by cortical venous thrombosis.

Patients may present with signs of sinus infection or severe focal, then generalized, headache. Signs of sepsis are usual. Later, focal neurologic deficit appears and is associated with a decline in the consciousness state and epilepsy, which often proves intractable. CT scanning is sometimes negative in subsequently proven cases. The collection of pus may be quite thin, although there is often a zone of enhancement between the inner surface of the collection and the adjacent cortex (Fig. 12-33). MRI is the preferred imaging procedure (Fig. 12-34).

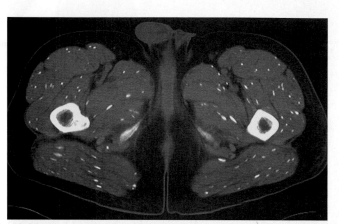

Fig. 12-24. Cysticercosis. Multiple cysts in the thighs. Some cysts show calcification, and they are characteristically arranged along the planes of the muscle fibers.

ENCEPHALITIS

VIRAL ENCEPHALITIS

Although viral encephalitis is a worldwide phenomenon, the usual infective agent varies from one part of the globe to the other. In the United Kingdom and United States, sporadic viral encephalitis is most commonly caused by herpes simplex; in the United States, western equine, St. Louis, and eastern equine viruses are encountered in warm-weather months as epidemic encephalitis. Increasingly recognized forms of the disease include West Nile encephalitis and Nipah virus encephalitis.

In some patients, prodromal symptoms occur, and in others there is an abrupt onset of fever, depression of the conscious state, and headache. Either focal or generalized seizures are common. A wide variety of physical signs are seen and do not allow a confident prediction of the underlying agent. Indeed, the condition can sometimes be difficult to distinguish from a metabolic encephalopathy. Various arthropod-borne viruses (arboviruses) transmitted to humans by either the mosquito or the tick produce epidemic encephalitis in the United States and other countries where these vectors and viruses exist.

About 90% of cases of herpes simplex encephalitis (HSE) are caused by HSV-1, the remainder being caused by HSV-2. HSE can occur as a primary infection, by reinfection by a second virus type, or as the result of reactivation of latent virus. HSV-2 is the usual agent in immunocompromised individuals. HSE has a predilection for the temporal and basal frontal lobes (Fig. 12-35). The lesions are often hemorrhagic. Microscopy reveals a necrotizing vasculitis with

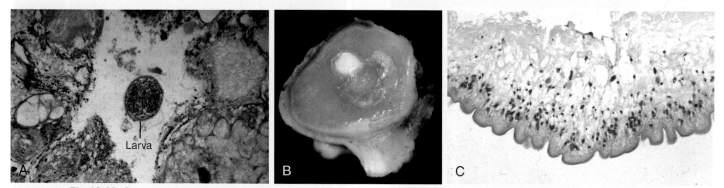

Fig. 12-25. Cysticercosis. **A,** A larva can be seen in the center of the section. **B,** Cyst containing a visible organism. **C,** Larval structure.

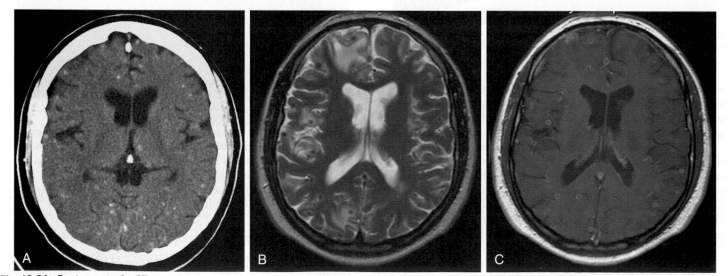

Fig. 12-26. Cysticercosis. **A,** CT scan showing multiple calcific foci. **B,** T2-weighted MRI showing hypointense foci. **C,** Thin-walled ring enhancement after contrast administration.

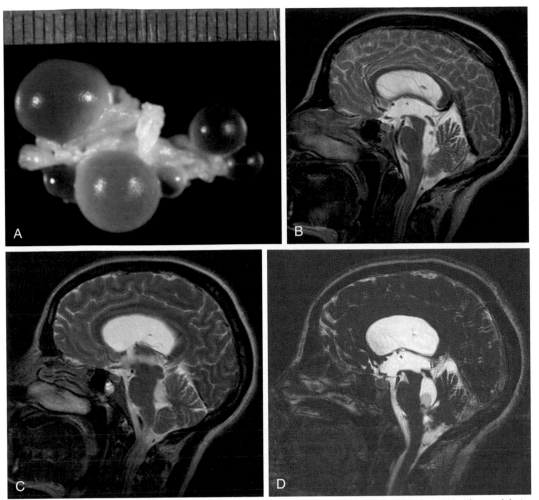

Fig. 12-27. Cysticercosis. Racemose form (**A**). Sagittal T2-weighted MRI on day 1 (**B** and **C**) and day 2 (**D**). Initially, the cyst with a nodule is at the top of the fourth ventricle. The following day, it is at the bottom.

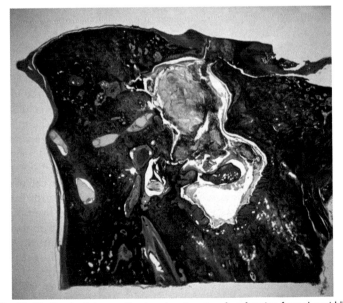

Fig. 12-28. Cerebral abscess. Section showing site of perforation from the middle ear to the middle cranial fossa and adherent temporal lobe (hematoxylin and Van Gieson, ×3).

(in some sections) intranuclear (Cowdry type A) inclusions in both glial cells and neurons (Fig. 12-36). Immunochemical techniques can more easily identify the viral antigen (because diagnostic inclusions are usually quite rare), and viral particles can be detected by electron microscopy. Although the early inflammatory reaction contains polymorphonuclear leukocytes, a chronic reaction with macrophages

and lymphocytes soon appears, followed by an intense gliosis (Fig. 12-37). Focal atrophy may be conspicuous in those surviving the acute illness (Fig. 12-38).

Investigation. The CSF is rarely normal in biopsy-proven cases of acute viral encephalitis (perhaps 5% of herpes cases). Lumbar puncture is potentially hazardous if there is significant cerebral edema. Typically, there is a lymphocytic pleocytosis of around 10 to 200 cells/mm³ and an elevated protein concentration of around 0.5 to 5 g/L. There is quite often a hemorrhagic component, and xanthochromia may be present. In cases caused by herpes simplex, the CSF glucose concentration is normal. CSF PCR has greatly aided diagnosis. Within the first week of HSE, PCR for HSV DNA is positive in up to 95% of cases. PCR can also be used for other agents—for example, cytomegalovirus (CMV). False-negative studies in HSE are most commonly found in the first 24 to 48 hours, and then again beyond 10 days of the illness. Specificity is over 95%.

The EEG is abnormal and in herpes simplex cases may reveal periodic lateralized epileptic discharges (Fig. 12-39).

Investigation is usually initiated by CT scanning or MRI. In patients with HSE, CT demonstrates attenuation in one or both temporal lobes, sometimes with mass effect, hemorrhage, and areas of enhancement (Fig. 12-40). Rarely, the CT scan is normal. MRI, in the early stages, reveals edema of the cortex with an abnormal signal, which, at least initially, is confined to the gray matter with sparing of the underlying white matter (Fig. 12-41). The areas affected are typically the temporal lobes, as well as the insular cortex and angular gyrus.

Brain biopsy is seldom required for diagnosis of HSE. The virus particles can be seen by EM in the nuclei of infected cells, and viral antigen can be detected by immunochemistry for up to 3 weeks after

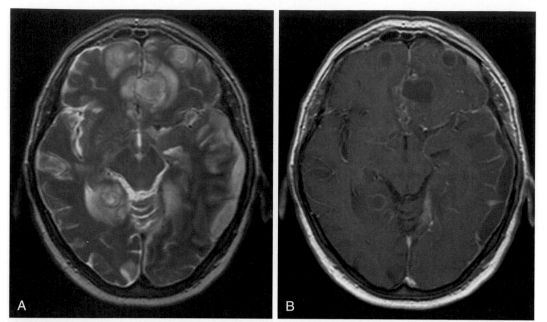

Fig. 12-32. Cerebral abscess. Axial T2-weighted MRI **(A)** and postcontrast T1-weighted MRI **(B)** showing multiple abscesses and subdural Right.

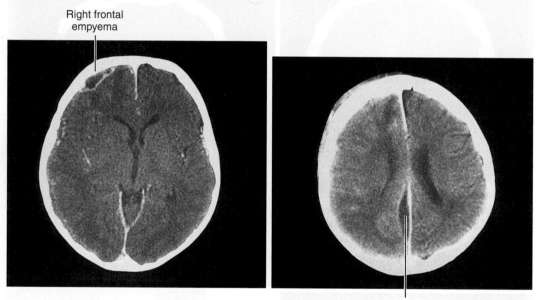

Right frontal
empyema

Hemispheric
collection

Fig. 12-33. Subdural empyema. CT scan showing right frontal **(A)** and interhemispheric **(B)** collections.

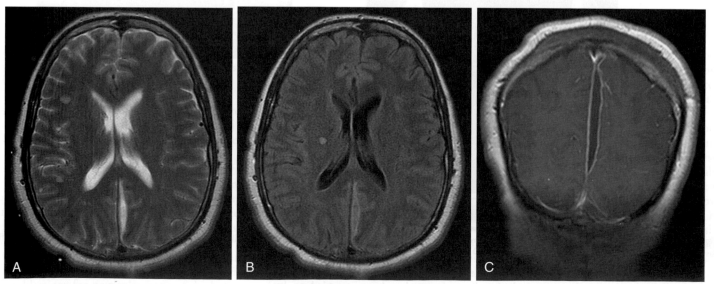

Fig. 12-34. Subdural empyema. MRI.

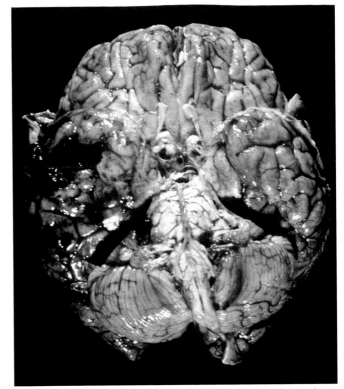

Fig. 12-35. Herpes simplex encephalitis. Basal view showing hemorrhage and necrosis in the right temporal lobe. There is brain swelling.

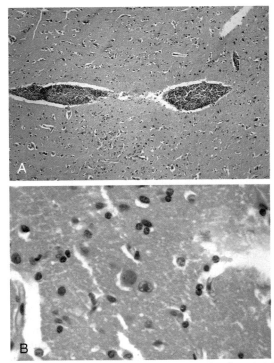

Fig. 12-36. Herpes simplex encephalitis. **A,** Perivascular lymphocytic inflammation (H&E, ×25). **B,** Large eosinophilic inclusion, Cowdry type A (H&E, ×400).

cases, the inflammatory process mostly affects spinal and cerebral gray matter, and includes mainly mononuclear cells and microglia. Other viruses, notably Coxsackie, are thought, rarely, to cause a similar syndrome.

Subacute Sclerosing Panencephalitis

Subacute sclerosing panencephalitis (SSPE), an inclusion-body encephalitis, follows measles infection after a mean period of about 5 years; however, the range is considerable. The exact way in which the virus evokes this reaction is unclear, but the responsible viruses are genetically distinct from other strains of measles virus that do not

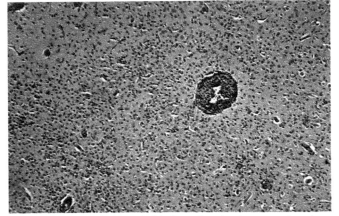

Fig. 12-37. Herpes simplex encephalitis. Several weeks after onset, there is severe inflammation containing lymphocytes, microglia, and astrocytes (H&E, ×25).

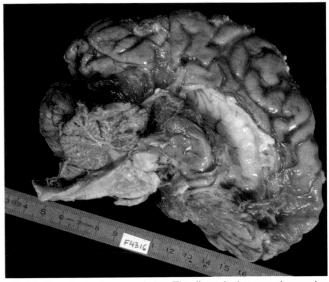

Fig. 12-38. Herpes simplex encephalitis. The illness had occurred several years before. There is severe atrophy of the temporal and medial frontal lobes, together with a portion of the temporo-occipital gyrus but relative preservation of the posterior frontal and parietal cortices.

cause SSPE. There is no relationship between SSPE and postmeasles acute encephalomyelitis or the subacute measles encephalitis that sometimes occurs in immunocompromised individuals. The condition is confined to children and adults less than 25 years old. It is more likely if the initial exposure occurs before the age of 18 months. Vaccination reduces the risk by 10 to 20 times.

Patients present with a behavioral disturbance followed by dementia, myoclonus, and incoordination. Eventually, the patient becomes mute and decorticate, but survival exceeding 10 years has been recorded. The EEG shows a characteristic slow-wave discharge alternating with periods of relative electrical silence. The CSF contains oligoclonal IgG measles antibody. Low-density areas in the subcortex and periventricular white matter are found on imaging. Pathologic examination reveals neuronal loss, astrocytic proliferation, microglial reaction, and loss of myelinated fibers (Fig. 12-45). The nerve cells contain homogeneous rounded inclusion bodies. There is perivascular cuffing (Fig. 12-46).

There is no specific treatment.

Rabies Encephalitis

Retrograde axoplasmic transport is the means by which the virus gains access to the CNS from the peripheral nerve. Transmission is usually through the bite of an infected animal. After local pain, the condition rapidly evolves, with agitation and reflex muscle spasms triggered by minor stimulation. Paralytic rabies evolves a little more slowly. Rapidly progressive weakness appears, affecting limbs and pharyngeal,

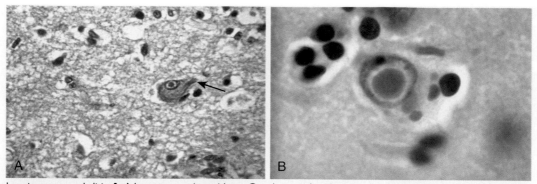

Fig. 12-46. Subacute sclerosing panencephalitis. **A,** A large neuron *(arrow)* has a Cowdry type A inclusion in its nucleus, and a neurofibrillary tangle in its cytoplasm (GFAP immunostain/hematoxylin). **B,** Inclusion body, high-power view (Lendrum's phloxine tartrazine, ×1500).

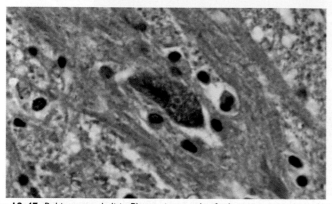

Fig. 12-47. Rabies encephalitis. Photomicrograph of a brainstem pigmented neuron containing a Negri body, an eosinophilic cytoplasmic inclusion.

of multiple enhancing lesions described here is insufficient to ensure a diagnosis of *Toxoplasma* encephalitis or to exclude lymphoma. The lesions are usually sensitive to a combination of pyrimethamine and sulfadiazine. A therapeutic trial is given with serial scanning over a period of 1 to 2 weeks to confirm that the lesions are resolving (Fig. 12-59, C and D). Treatment is continued indefinitely.

Amebic Encephalitis. Two types of free-living amebas infect the CNS. One, a group that includes *Acanthamoeba* species and *Balamuthia* species, produces a focal or multifocal necrotizing and hemorrhagic encephalitis that has been described principally in patients with AIDS, in whom it is fulminant (Fig. 12-60). The other type, which has no described predilection for immunosuppressed patients, is *Naegleria fowleri,* an inhabitant of polluted warm freshwater lakes and streams, described particularly in the southern regions of the United States. *Naegleria* enters the body through the nasopharynx when individuals swim, dive, or water-ski in infected waterways, and then it penetrates through the skull base to the brain where it produces a diffuse, fulminant, and nearly 100% fatal encephalitis.

CEREBRAL LYMPHOMA IN AIDS

Besides toxoplasmosis, cerebral lymphoma is an important cause of a focal brain lesion in patients with AIDS, occurring in up to 5% of these patients. The tumor is a B-cell non-Hodgkin's lymphoma, and it contains the Epstein-Barr (EB) viral genome and expresses some EB proteins. The lesions may be single or multiple, are often periventricular, and occur in the form of a steroid-sensitive focal mass or as a diffuse infiltrating process. Homogeneous or patchy enhancement is the usual CT finding (Fig. 12-61). MRI identifies the same process. In patients with AIDS, the enhancement is more usually ring shaped than diffuse (Fig. 12-62). The vitreous of the eye and the CSF are involved in one quarter of patients, but systemic deposits are rare. Aggressive chemotherapeutic regimes are employed, and many therapists prefer to delay the use of radiotherapy.

CNS DISEASES CAUSED BY SPIROCHETES

SYPHILIS

Syphilis is caused by the spirochete *Treponema pallidum,* which can reach the nervous system early in the course of the disease, even during the primary stage. In the secondary stage of syphilis, meningeal involvement, as determined by the presence of a CSF pleocytosis, is present in the majority of patients, but most remain asymptomatic. The initial pathologic event in the nervous system is a meningitis, which in some cases is so acute as to be indistinguishable from viral meningitis. In most patients, however, this stage of the infection is occult, to be succeeded, months or years later, by the tertiary stage of the disease, a reflection then of both parenchymal and meningitic pathology.

Meningovascular Syphilis
In meningovascular syphilis, an endarteritis of cerebral or spinal vessels occurs, with infiltration of the media and adventitia by inflammatory cells. Intimal hyperplasia accompanied, in larger vessels, by fibrosis and inflammatory cell infiltration can result in vessel occlusion (Heubner's endarteritis) (Fig. 12-63). The meninges thicken and become infiltrated by lymphocytes and plasma cells, the clinical features reflecting the relative balance of these varying pathologic processes. Larger-vessel occlusion leads to cerebral or spinal infarction. Basal meningeal infiltration and thickening result in cranial nerve palsies and hydrocephalus. Thickening of the spinal meninges and dura (pachymeningitis) results in root pain and focal radicular signs, followed by evidence of cord compression (Fig. 12-64).

The CSF is inevitably abnormal, with a lymphocytic pleocytosis, a moderately elevated protein concentration, and positive serology in greater than 80% of patients. Vascular imaging demonstrates concentric narrowing of large vessels, with focal dilation and constriction of smaller vessels. Unless focal infarction has occurred, response to penicillin is usually impressive and reflected by CSF improvement.

Tabes Dorsalis
About 70% of cases of tabes dorsalis appear 5 to 20 years after the primary infection. The condition mostly affects men between the ages of 30 and 50. Pathologically, there is atrophy of the dorsal roots associated with posterior column degeneration and thickening of the overlying meninges, which are infiltrated by mononuclear cells (Fig. 12-65). Some authorities believe this is a dorsal spinal cord manifestation of meningovascular syphilis.

Typically, the condition develops insidiously with root pain, radicular sensory loss associated with ataxia, and areflexia. Severe brief sharp pains (lightning pains) can occur in the legs or trunk. Bladder dysfunction appears. The pupils are usually abnormal, and there is frequent involvement of other cranial nerves. Optic atrophy is common, secondary to an inflammatory reaction in the pia of the optic nerves and chiasm. Autonomic dysfunction with hyperactivity can lead to a variety of crises affecting the gut, the bladder,

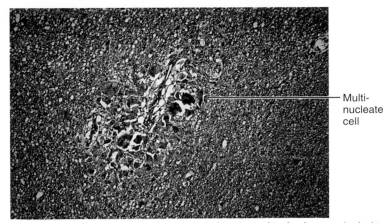

Fig. 12-48. AIDS encephalopathy. Central area of inflammation and myelin loss around a blood vessel in the deep cerebral white matter. There are several multinucleated cells (Luxol fast blue, H&E, ×25).

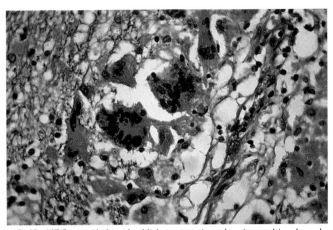

Fig. 12-49. AIDS encephalopathy. High-power view showing multinucleated cells with horseshoe orientation of the nuclei (Luxol fast blue, H&E, ×100).

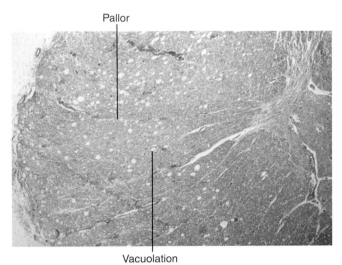

Fig. 12-51. AIDS vacuolar myelopathy. Lateral portion of cord showing vacuolation and pallor of lateral column compared with more normal white matter adjacent to the ventral horn (Luxol fast blue, PAS, ×31).

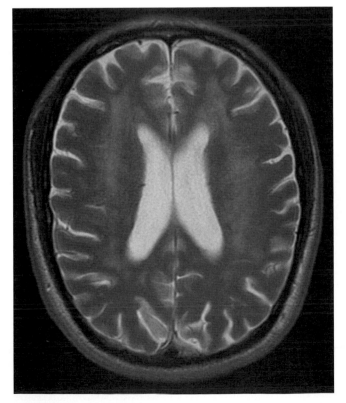

Fig. 12-50. AIDS encephalopathy. The patient was a 45-year-old HIV-positive man MRI showing atrophy and diffuse white matter change.

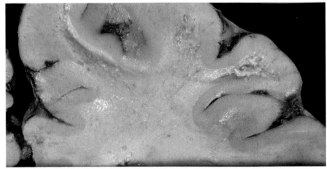

Fig. 12-52. Progressive multifocal leukoencephalopathy. Upper half of right hemisphere, coronal section. Discoloration, granularity, and collapse of white matter.

or the larynx. Loss of pain sensitivity is associated with perforating ulcers and profound joint dysfunction (Charcot's joints) (Figs. 12-66 and 12-67).

About half the patients have an elevated cell count or protein concentration in the CSF. Positive serology, in the CSF, occurs in about three quarters.

General Paresis

General paresis, now rare, was once common. It accounted for 1539 deaths in England and Wales in 1925. It is more frequent in women and presents most commonly 5 to 20 years after the primary infection. Pathologically, there is meningeal thickening accompanied by cortical atrophy, which primarily affects the frontal and parietal lobes (Fig. 12-68). Spirochetes invade the brain, resulting in neuronal death, gliosis, and patchy subcortical demyelination (Fig. 12-69). There is a striking infiltration of the infected brain parenchyma by activated microglia.

The condition produces alteration of judgment, sometimes leading to the development of grandiose ideas. Intellectual function deteriorates, followed by a number of specific neurologic symptoms and signs including dysarthria, tremor, and seizures. About 50% of cases have small, irregular pupils, which eventually become fixed to light (Argyll Robertson pupils) (Fig. 12-70). Later, pyramidal signs emerge, and the patient becomes incontinent.

The CSF is inevitably abnormal, with syphilis serology virtually always positive.

Congenital Syphilis

About 50% of babies born to mothers with syphilis are symptomatic. Neurologic features include an infantile meningitis, strokes during the first decade of life, and paretic syndromes emerging during the second and third decades. Various stigmata have been identified, including interstitial keratitis (Fig. 12-71) and dental abnormalities—Hutchinson's teeth—centrally notched and peg-shaped incisors (Fig. 12-72).

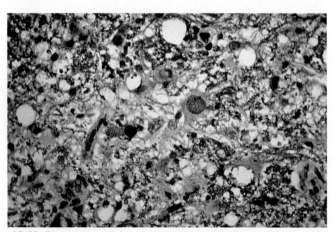

Fig. 12-53. Progressive multifocal leukoencephalopathy. Section at edge of lesion. Central infected oligodendrocytes surrounded by reactive astrocytes (Luxol fast blue, H&E, ×100).

LYME DISEASE

Lyme disease is caused by the tick-borne spirochete *Borrelia burgdorferi*. Deer are the only natural hosts for the adult ticks, but the immature ticks are found on other species (Fig. 12-73). The main animal reservoir for the spirochetes may be mice; immature ticks pick up the infection from mice and later transmit it to deer, humans, or other large vertebrates (including dogs). Having entered the body, the organism invades a multitude of tissues and can be cultured from the brain, the CSF, the blood, and the skin. Pathologic reactions found in peripheral nerve, root, or plexus include meningeal inflammation, perivascular inflammatory cell formation, and focal demyelination.

The disease follows a three-stage course. Initially, there is a skin reaction, erythema chronicum migrans (Fig. 12-74), associated with systemic symptoms including muscle pain, malaise, fever, and headache. About 10% to 15% of patients then develop neurologic sequelae, including cranial nerve damage (particularly fifth and seventh nerves), and radicular signs associated with meningitic and encephalitic features.

Finally, some patients (more so in the United States than in Europe) develop an arthritis, which may be confined to a single joint or be more widely distributed. Typically, this comes and goes over months or years.

At the stage of meningitic symptoms, there is a CSF lymphocytosis associated with an elevated protein concentration and, in some patients, an elevated IgG concentration together with oligoclonal IgG. The encephalitic picture includes drowsiness, personality change, impairment of memory, movement disorders, and seizures. Although virtually any cranial nerve can be affected, the facial nerve is particularly susceptible. Radicular features include pain, sensory loss, weakness, and reflex abnormalities. Occasionally, mononeuritis multiplex or plexopathy appears. In a small number of cases, a late remitting and relapsing neurologic syndrome emerges with some resemblance to multiple sclerosis. The diagnosis can be confirmed by finding elevated serum antibody levels to *B. burgdorferi*. The presence of intrathecal antibody synthesis is the only laboratory test for diagnosing active CNS infection.

Patients with substantial neurologic involvement require intravenous ceftriaxone or cefotaxime. A vaccine for the disease is available.

LEPTOSPIROSIS

Leptospirosis is caused by the spirochete *Leptospira interrogans*. In addition to the hepatic and renal manifestations of the disease, both meningitic and encephalitic syndromes are recognized.

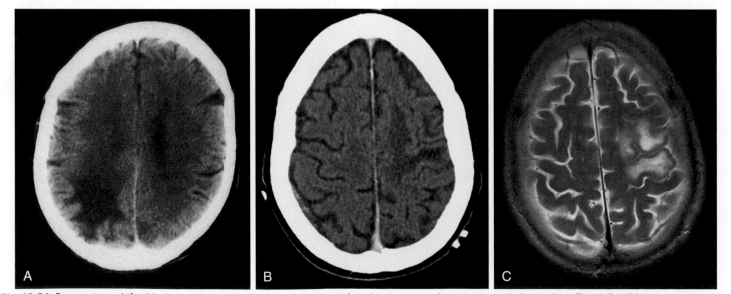

Fig. 12-54. Progressive multifocal leukoencephalopathy. **A,** CT scan showing a low-density area in the posterior right hemisphere. **B** and **C,** MRI demonstrating signal change in the left hemisphere.

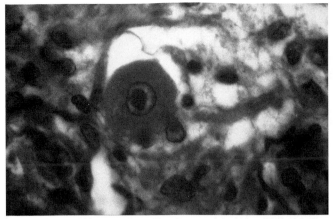

Fig. 12-55. Trigeminal herpes zoster. Cowdry type A inclusions in the nucleus of a ganglion cell and a satellite cell (H&E, ×1300).

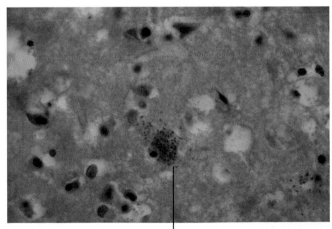

Fig. 12-56. Toxoplasmosis. Macroscopic appearance. The white matter is granular and cavitated.

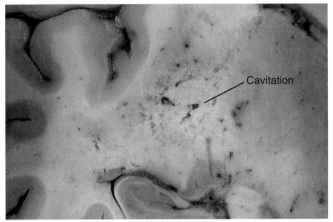

Free forms

Fig. 12-57. Toxoplasmosis. Encysted and free forms of the organism can be seen.

Aseptic meningitis may be the presenting feature of the disease, although it may remain asymptomatic. The CSF cell count is elevated, and there is an elevated protein concentration and, occasionally, a depressed glucose concentration. The organism can sometimes be isolated from the CSF or its presence inferred by abnormal serologic findings. Encephalitis or myelitic complications occur in a small proportion of cases. Virtually any combination of neurologic signs and symptoms can be seen, including manifestations of subarachnoid or intracerebral hemorrhage. The peripheral nervous system can be affected in a way similar to that seen in Lyme disease. Various antibiotics are used, including doxycycline and penicillin.

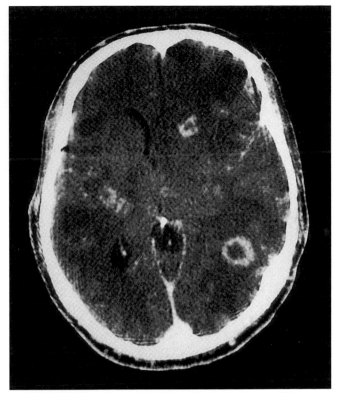

Fig. 12-58. Toxoplasmosis. Multiple enhancing lesions on CT scan.

PRION DISEASE

The prion diseases (transmissible spongiform encephalopathies) are characterized by the presence of PrP^{Sc}, an abnormal form of the normal cellular protein, PrP^{c}. The conditions are sometimes familial, sometime acquired, and sometimes sporadic; iatrogenic transmission is well described.

The function of the normal prion protein, encoded by the prion gene on chromosome 20, is unknown. The disease-associated form, PrP^{Sc}, is relatively insoluble and protease resistant, and it accumulates in tissues, producing amyloid structures. At codon 129 of the prion protein gene *(PRNP)*, an individual can encode for methionine (M) or valine (V). Approximately 80% of the sporadic cases of Creutzfeldt-Jakob disease (CJD) in the United Kingdom, and, to date, all cases of variant CJD, are MM. Prion diseases occurring in animals include scrapie, transmissible mink encephalopathy, chronic wasting disease of deer and elk in the United States, and bovine spongiform encephalopathy. Those described in humans include kuru, CJD, Gerstmann-Sträussler-Scheinker syndrome, and fatal familial insomnia.

The spongiform encephalopathies are characterized by the pathologic appearance of vacuolation in the neuropil of gray matter, principally in the frontal and occipital cortices, but also in the basal ganglia or cerebellum (Fig. 12-75). All the conditions are associated with the accumulation of an amyloid protein, sometimes in the form of amyloid plaques (Fig. 12-76).

CREUTZFELDT-JAKOB DISEASE

Most cases of CJD are sporadic, with an annual incidence of 1 in 1,000,000. The condition peaks, in terms of presentation, in the seventh decade. Case-to-case transmission has occurred through the use of corneal or dura mater grafts and by the use of human growth hormone derived from pituitary glands removed at autopsy. In adults, a small number of cases are familial, displaying autosomal dominant inheritance.

Typically, the disease presents quite rapidly with personality change, seizures, focal neurologic deficit, and dementia. Myoclonus, with sensitivity to sound, light, or touch, soon emerges in the majority, often in the form of rhythmically repetitive contractions.

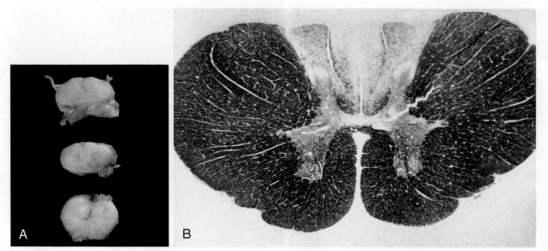

Fig. 12-65. Tabes dorsalis. **A,** Three spinal cord sections showing shrinkage and discoloration of the dorsal cord and thickening of the leptomeninges at the lumbar level. **B,** Section of lumbar cord showing posterior column degeneration.

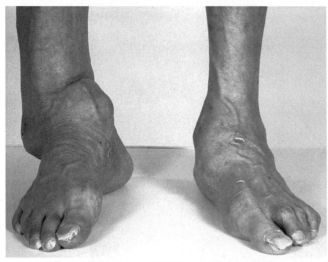

Fig. 12-66. Tabes dorsalis. Charcot joint, right ankle.

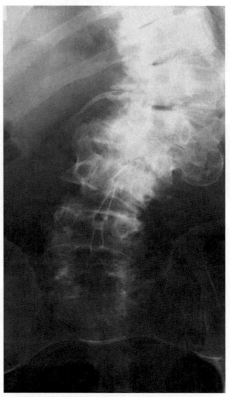

Fig. 12-67. Tabes dorsalis. Charcot spine.

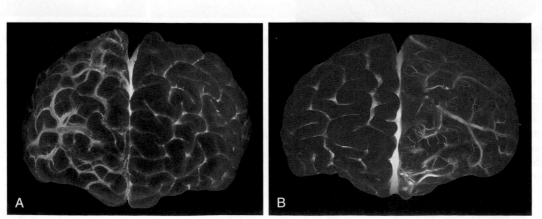

Fig. 12-68. General paresis. **A,** Normal frontal lobes with leptomeninges removed on the right. **B,** General paresis. The leptomeninges have been removed on the left. There is atrophy together with leptomeningeal calcification.

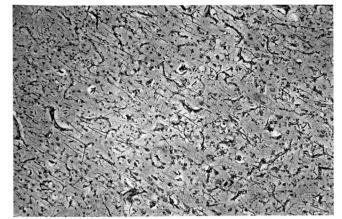

Fig. 12-69. General paresis. Section of cerebral cortex. There is proliferation and infiltration by silver-positive microglia (silver carbonate).

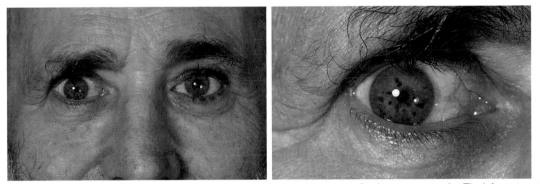

Fig. 12-70. Argyll Robertson pupil. The right pupil is small and slightly irregular and was fixed to a near stimulus. The left eye is artificial.

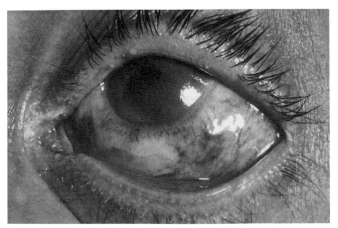

Fig. 12-71. Congenital syphilis. Interstitial keratitis.

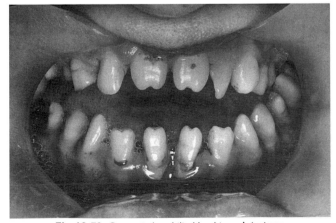

Fig. 12-72. Congenital syphilis. Hutchinson's incisors.

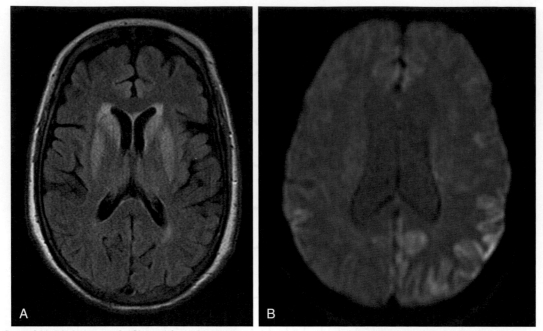

Fig. 12-78. Sporadic Creutzfeldt-Jakob disease. **A,** Classical form demonstrating bilateral caudate and putaminal signal change. **B,** Cortical variant demonstrating patchy cortical high signal best seen with diffusion-weighted imaging.

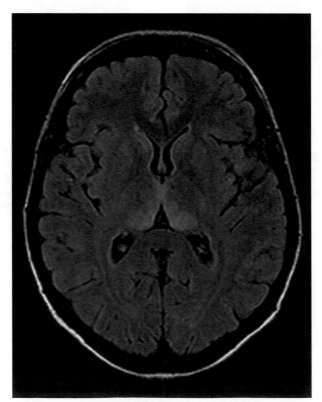

Fig. 12-79. Variant Creutzfeldt-Jakob disease. MRI. Bilateral medial thalamic and putaminal signal change.

MULTIPLE SCLEROSIS AND OTHER DEMYELINATING DISORDERS

MULTIPLE SCLEROSIS

The prevalence of multiple sclerosis (MS) varies from country to country, with relatively high rates for both the United States and the United Kingdom. The figure for every 100,000 of the population rises from about 100 to 150 in England to around 150 to 200 in the Orkneys and Shetland. A similar prevalence shift occurs in North America, with rates of about 20 per 100,000 in the southern United States rising to around 100 per 100,000 in parts of Canada. The prevalence of MS in other parts of the world probably also increases with increasing distance north or south of the equator, although certain exceptions apply, particularly for Japan, which has a low incidence of the disease. The prevalence of the disease in nonwhite populations living in relatively high-risk areas is less than that of whites in the same area, but it is higher than would be anticipated from the prevalence in the country of origin.

Individual predisposition to the disease appears to be acquired by about the age of 15. Hence, adults migrating from high-risk areas to low-risk areas, or vice-versa, have subsequent MS rates compatible with their country of origin, whereas children who migrate acquire the risk of their new residence.

In addition to this geographic influence, a genetic factor operates in MS, with first-degree relatives of sufferers having 10 to 50 times the risk for the disease as normal controls. The concordance rate for monozygotic twins is of the order of 25%. Various associations have been described between human leukocyte antigen status and susceptibility to multiple sclerosis. The most substantial association in the United Kingdom is with DR2. Definite or possible sites of linkage have been described for chromosomes 1, 5, 6, 7, 14, and 17.

PATHOLOGY

The lesions of MS concentrate particularly around the lateral ventricles (Fig. 13-1). Other sites commonly affected include the optic nerves (Fig. 13-2), the regions around the fourth ventricle, the pons, and the spinal cord (Fig. 13-3). Chronic lesions take on a brownish

gray discoloration and can be confused with gray matter at autopsy (Fig. 13-4). In the initial stages, focal areas of myelin destruction are associated with an inflammatory cell infiltrate consisting predominantly of macrophages and T lymphocytes. Areas of ongoing demyelination are characterized by macrophage activation and phagocytosis of myelin protein together with a vigorous gliosis. Digestion of the myelin sheath by macrophages leads to the appearance of lipid material in these cells (Fig. 13-5). The lesions are sharply circumscribed, with an abrupt change from well-myelinated tissues with minimal inflammation and gliosis, to the lesional zones full of inflammatory cells and large reactive astrocytes. In the chronic stages, the lymphocytic infiltration is far less intense, and without evidence of active myelin breakdown. Fibrillary gliosis is prominent and there is a substantial reduction in axon density (Fig. 13-6), but some axons survive in chronic plaques despite a complete absence of myelin. Oligodendrocytes are reduced or absent.

This apparent uniformity of pathologic response is misleading, because it conceals substantial heterogeneity in the underlying demyelinating process. Four patterns have been described, all of which occur in the setting of an inflammatory process consisting predominantly of T lymphocytes and macrophages. Debate continues as to whether these patterns are permanently distinct or whether evolution can take place from one to another.

Patterns I and II
Patterns I and II display perivenular plaques that containing macrophages and T cells. In type II, however, there is evidence of local precipitation of immunoglobulin and active complement in the regions of active myelin breakdown (Fig. 13-7). In both types I and II, demyelinated plaques are centered on small veins and venules, and they have sharply demarcated edges with perivenous extensions.

Pattern III
Pattern III lesions contain an inflammatory infiltrate. Deposition of Ig and complement is missing. The demyelination is not perivenular; indeed, a rim of preserved myelin may be found around the inflamed

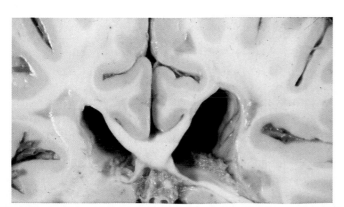

Fig. 13-1. Multiple sclerosis. Coronal brain section showing periventricular plaques.

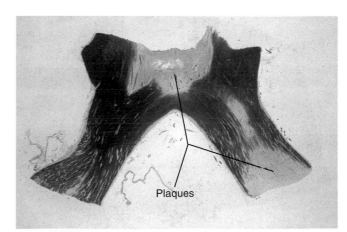

Fig. 13-2. Multiple sclerosis. Plaques of demyelination involving the optic nerves and chiasm (Heidenhain's myelin stain).

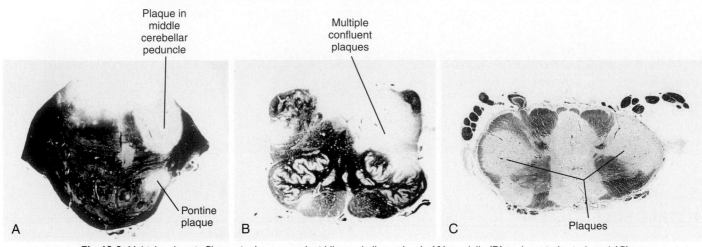

Fig. 13-3. Multiple sclerosis. Plaques in the pons and middle cerebellar peduncle **(A)**, medulla **(B)**, and cervical spinal cord **(C)**.

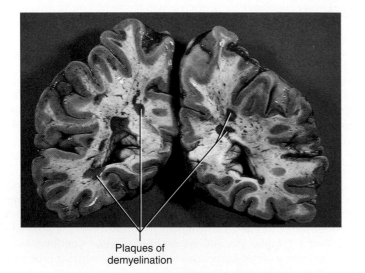

Fig. 13-4. Multiple sclerosis. Coronal brain section showing numerous plaques of demyelination, particularly in the periventricular areas.

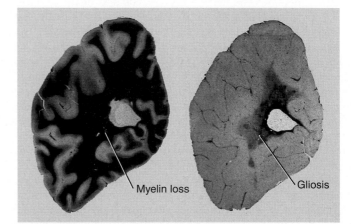

Fig. 13-6. Multiple sclerosis. Plaques in relation to the occipital horn of the lateral ventricle *(left)* (Heidenhain's myelin stain), and the corresponding gliosis *(right)* (Holzer preparation).

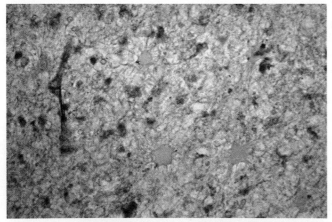

Fig. 13-5. Lipid-containing macrophages in relation to a multiple sclerosis plaque (Luxol fast blue, PAS, ×100).

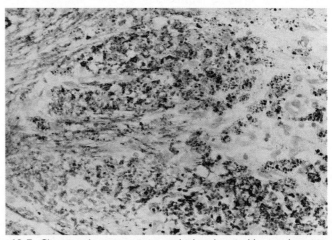

Fig. 13-7. Chronic relapsing remitting multiple sclerosis. Massive deposition of C9neo (a complement antigen) at the actively demyelinating border. C9neo antigen *(red)* is present on myelinated fibers and in macrophages.

vessels in the plaque. Typically, there is preferential loss of myelin-associated glycoprotein, with relative sparing of other myelin protein (e.g., proteolipoprotein and myelin basic protein) (Fig. 13-8). This appearance suggests a substantial reduction of oligodendrocytes at the active plaque border.

Pattern IV

In pattern IV, inflammatory infiltration is again present but without deposition of Ig and complement C9neo (a complement antigen). An almost complete loss of oligodendrocytes is found in active as well as inactive lesions. This pattern appears to be confined to patients with primary progressive MS.

Histopathologic studies of MS brains have demonstrated axonal injury in lesions undergoing inflammatory demyelination, possibly as a result of inflammatory substances produced by activated immune and glial cells. It is possible that this axonal loss during the remitting and relapsing phase of the disease remains subclinical because of a variety of CNS compensatory mechanisms. As disease duration increases, a substantial reduction in axonal density can be demonstrated using techniques employing a measure of axonal function (Fig. 13-9). In

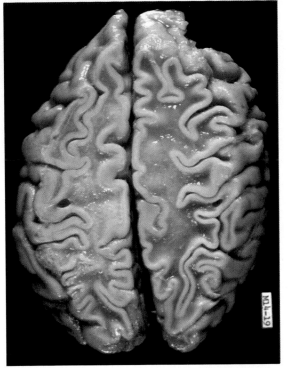

Fig. 13-51. Adrenoleukodystrophy. Extensive white matter changes throughout both hemispheres.

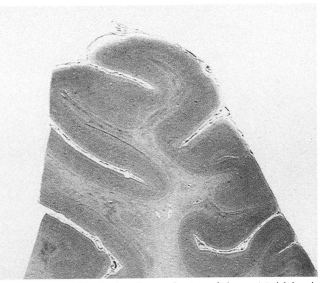

Fig. 13-52. Pelizaeus-Merzbacher disease. Section of the occipital lobe showing extensive loss of myelin with some perivascular sparing, producing a tigroid appearance.

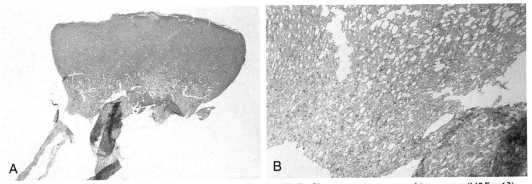

Fig. 13-53. Canavan's disease. **A,** Spongy vacuolation (H&E, ×10). **B,** Characteristic spongy white matter (H&E, ×63).

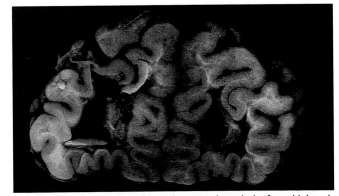

Fig. 13-54. Alexander's disease. Coronal section through the frontal lobes showing demyelination with cystic degeneration of deep white matter.

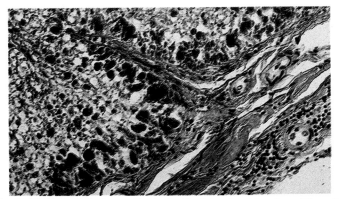

Fig. 13-55. Alexander's disease. Hyaline bodies lining the pial surface of the spinal cord and surrounding a penetrating blood vessel (hematoxylin, van Gieson, ×400).

DEGENERATIVE DISEASE OF THE SPINE

Structural changes in the intervertebral disc are an inevitable consequence of aging, although in many the changes remain asymptomatic. With increasing age, the water content of the nucleus pulposus falls, and splits appear in the surrounding annulus fibrosus. If the split is radial rather than circumferential, and it is located posteriorly, elements of the nucleus pulposus can herniate through the split into the spinal canal, or elements of the annulus can protrude beyond their normal boundaries. These disc protrusions are common even in middle age, and although they may appear to narrow the spinal canal, they are asymptomatic in the vast majority of patients. A congenital weakness of the annulus may predispose to these changes. Shrinkage of the nucleus produces prolapse or folding of the annulus, which, in turn, by traction on the adjacent vertebral body, leads to osteophyte formation. At the same time, degenerative changes, including appearance of osteophytes, develop on the apophyseal joints.

The symptoms associated with degenerative disease of the spine are therefore the consequence either of protrusion of the annulus or disc, or of narrowing of an intervertebral foramen or the spinal canal by osteophyte formation, combined, in some cases, with buckling of the ligamentum flavum. The ligamentum may also thicken and become abnormally stiff because of chondroid or osseous metaplasia. Because intervertebral joints are complex true joints, synovial irritation from mechanical stresses may cause synovial hypertrophy and lead to the formation of synovial cysts, which may also compress the spinal cord or nerve roots. A congenitally narrow canal or congenitally short pedicules predispose to some of these effects. Posterior protrusion of the annulus fibrosus or a herniated nucleus pulposus results in cord compression at the cervical level, or, in the lumbar region, compression of nerve roots at the level of the cauda equina. Posterolateral protrusion of the annulus or a noncalcified (soft) disc, or osteophytosis in relation to the apophyseal joint or vertebral body, can all produce compression of the nerve root in the intervertebral foramen, more commonly in the cervical than in the lumbar region.

Myelopathy is more likely to develop in a narrow canal subject to a higher range of motion. The role of the dentate ligaments in determining the pattern of cord damage in myelopathy is uncertain. Typically, in the cord, the lateral columns are most affected, with demyelination and gliosis of the white matter and loss of nerve cells and gliosis of gray matter.

Differences between the cervical and lumbar spines exist in the relationship between the emerging nerve roots and the adjacent vertebral body. In the cervical spine, for example at the C4-5 level, the C5 nerve roots exit above the pedicle of C5 (in the inferior aspect of the C4-5 neural foramen) and are liable to compression by a disc protrusion between C4 and C5 (Fig. 14-1). The L5 nerve root, however, emerges from the theca opposite the L4 vertebral body and then passes over the posterolateral aspect of the L4-5 disc before coursing along the L5 vertebral body to emerge beneath the L5 pedicle at the next intervertebral foramen. Consequently, a disc protrusion at L4-5 usually affects the L5 root and involves the L4 root only if it extends sufficiently laterally or distally.

CERVICAL DISC DISEASE

Cervical Spondylosis
Degenerative disease in the cervical spine occurs most often at the C5-6 and C6-7 levels.

Cervical Radiculopathy
Typically, patients give a history of neck pain accompanied, if there is root involvement, by pain radiating to the medial aspect of the scapula, the shoulder, or the arm itself. Pain secondary to root compression follows a myotomal or, perhaps, sclerotomal distribution. Sensory symptoms, whether paresthesias or numbness, serve to localize the affected root (Fig. 14-2). Clinical examination reveals restricted neck movement, sometimes with an altered neck posture. Neck movements often trigger a stereotypical pain. The distribution of muscle weakness follows the pattern of innervation of the affected root (Fig. 14-3). Eventually, wasting may appear (Fig. 14-4).

Localization of the root involved is aided by examination of the reflexes. Depression or absence of the biceps and supinator reflexes accompanies a C5 or C6 lesion, with inversion of these reflexes if there is an added spinal cord compression at that level. Depression of the triceps reflex is encountered in C7 root lesions, and sometimes in C6 root lesions. Areas of cutaneous sensory loss reflect the distribution of the affected root.

Cervical Myelopathy
Cord compression resulting from spondylitic disease is most often the result of disease at the C5-6 or C6-7 disc space, although multiple-level compression is common, particularly if there is a contribution from a congenitally narrow canal or ankylosing spondylitis. Root sensory symptoms are uncommon, as the majority of patients insidiously develop signs and symptoms of cord compression. The clinical features depend on the level of compression. Five patterns have been described (Table 14-1).

INVESTIGATION

Plain Radiography
Degenerative changes in the cervical spine are common in older persons. Some evidence of spondylitic disease can be seen on the radiographs of 95% of men and 70% of women older than 65 years. A diagnosis of cervical radiculopathy is certainly supported if prominent foraminal narrowing is confined to the clinically affected root. Oblique views of the cervical spine assist identification of zygapophyseal or neurocentral osteophyte protrusion into the intervertebral foramen (Fig. 14-5).

Electrophysiology
Electrophysiology can provide confirmatory evidence of cord or root involvement. Segmental denervation suggests a diagnosis of radiculopathy, as can measurements of the H reflex from the relevant upper arm muscle. Somatosensory evoked responses have proved of limited value in the evaluation of a root or cord syndrome.

RELATIONSHIPS OF A NERVE ROOT

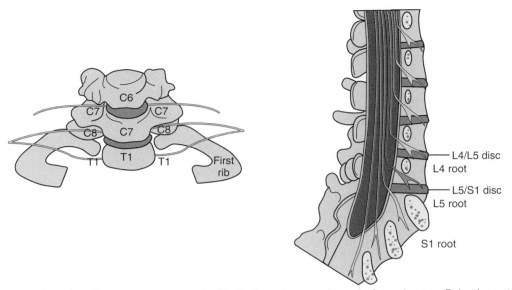

Fig. 14-1. Relationship of nerve roots to the vertebral body, disc, and articular facets. **A,** Cervical regions. **B,** Lumbar regions.

CERVICAL ROOT SYMPTOMS

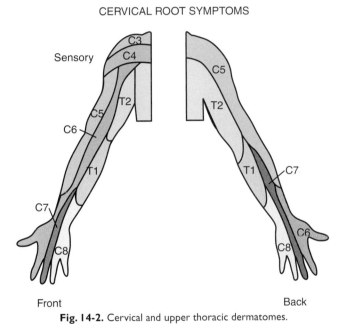

Fig. 14-2. Cervical and upper thoracic dermatomes.

MOTOR AND REFLEX CHANGES

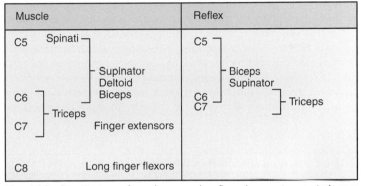

Muscle		Reflex	
C5 Spinati	Supinator Deltoid Biceps	C5	Biceps Supinator
C6 C7	Triceps Finger extensors	C6 C7	Triceps
C8	Long finger flexors		

Fig. 14-3. Distribution of weakness and reflex changes in cervical root compression.

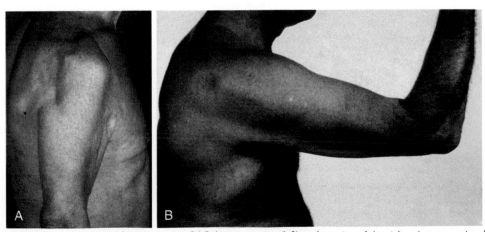

Fig. 14-4. Wasting of right deltoid, supraspinatus, and infraspinatus in a C4-5 disc protrusion *(left)*, and wasting of the right triceps associated with a C5-6 disc protrusion *(right)*.

Computed Tomographic Myelography
CT myelography is now performed only if the patient is intolerant of MRI, or if MRI is contraindicated (Fig. 14-6).

Magnetic Resonance Imaging
MRI is the imaging method of choice for both cervical radiculopathy and myelopathy. Using thin-section, high-resolution techniques, the nerve roots can be traced into the foramina, and compression can be identified (Fig. 14-7). Also, imaging identifies the site and degree of cord compression (Fig. 14-8). In some 15% of cases of cord compression, high signal intensity is seen on T2-weighted images. In general, the presence of signal change correlates with a more severe myelopathy, but its resolution after surgery correlates with a better outcome (Fig. 14-9).

MANAGEMENT

Cervical Radiculopathy
Most patients with cervical spondylitic radiculopathy recover spontaneously. Analgesia suffices for most patients. Benefit from immobilization of the neck in a collar is unproved, as are the numerous physical treatments that are undertaken. Surgery for referred pain secondary to a soft disc prolapse is successful, but intervention for symptoms related to osteophyte formation is seldom justified.

Cervical Myelopathy
After an initial phase of deterioration, many patients with spondylitic cervical myelopathy are stable for years. Furthermore, no adequately controlled surgical trial has ever been performed in this field. Cervical laminectomy has a limited role. Increasing age, loss of the normal cervical lordosis, and the presence of high signal change in the cord on MRI reduce the possibility of postoperative improvement. An anterior cervical decompression is more commonly performed, with or without an interbody graft (Fig. 14-10). Imaging appearance is better with grafting but there is no evidence that this improves clinical outcome.

THORACIC DISC DISEASE

Symptomatic thoracic disc disease is rare, and because of its effects, it is often confused with benign tumors. It predominates in men and principally affects the lower thoracic region. It can present as a slowly evolving spastic paraparesis, but many patients complain of exercise-induced symptoms, whether sensory, motor, or mixed. Disc calcification is found in about half the cases. The disc protrusion and calcification are identifiable using CT myelography or MRI (Fig. 14-11). Treatment is surgical, but the complication rate is relatively high.

LUMBOSACRAL DISC DISEASE

Degenerative disease of the lumbar spine involves the lower two levels in greater than 90% of cases. Posterolateral, lateral, and central patterns of protrusion are described (Fig. 14-12). Pain is a prominent feature in posterolateral disc protrusion.

Posterolateral Disc Protrusion
Pain is a prominent feature in lumbar disc disease and can be referred to the buttock and upper thigh in the absence of root involvement. Areas commonly affected by pain include the lower lumbar spine, in or around the midline, together with the region of the sacroiliac joint and the medial aspect of the buttock. There may be local tenderness in these areas. Although a history of antecedent spinal injury is common, in many patients the trauma was relatively trivial. Radicular pain may coincide with back pain or appear in isolation. Diagnosis of the affected root is complicated by the anatomic pathway pursued by the roots and is also frustrated by the variability in the segmental innervation of the lower limb muscles. Typically, radicular pain is exacerbated by straining. Pain extending from the back to the anterior thigh suggests involvement of an upper lumbar root. Identifying posterior thigh or buttock pain is of limited value in distinguishing an L5 from an S1 root lesion. Lateral calf pain is more likely with the latter and medial calf pain with the former. Sensory symptoms are common and generally segmental.

The lateral recess is defined as the area between the thecal sac and the pedicle. The pain arising from compression of the root at this level is similar to that caused by a posterolateral disc protrusion, although it is often exacerbated by exercise.

Examination aspects include assessment of the spine, performance of various stretch tests, and evaluation of any focal signs, which

TABLE 14-1.   PATTERNS OF CERVICAL MYELOPATHY

PATTERN	FEATURES
1. Transverse lesion	Long-tract involvement below, and segmental lower motor neuron (LMN) findings at, the level of lesion
2. Motor syndrome	Mixed LMN and upper motor neuron findings, with little or no sensory involvement
3. Central cord syndrome	Fixed deficits principally involving the upper limbs
4. Brown-Séquard syndrome	
5. Myelopathy and root pain	

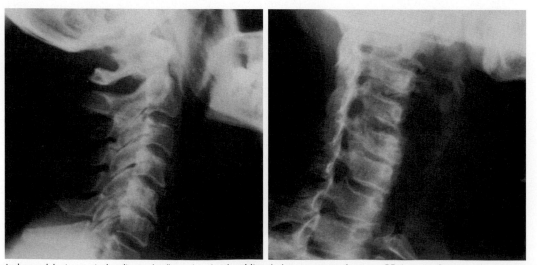

Fig. 14-5. Cervical spondylosis: cervical radiographs (lateral and right oblique) showing osteophytes at C5-6 protruding into the intervertebral foramen.

depend on the distribution of the affected nerve root (Fig. 14-13). With L4 compression, there is weakness of quadriceps and tibialis anterior, with sensory change over the medial aspect of the skin and depression of the knee jerk (Fig. 14-14). L5 root compression may manifest solely as weakness of extensor hallucis longus. Any sensory change is found over the medial aspect of the dorsum of the foot and the lateral shin. In an S1 root syndrome, weakness can occur in the buttock, the hamstrings, or the calf. The ankle reflex is likely to be depressed or absent. Sensory change predominates over the lateral aspect of the foot and calf.

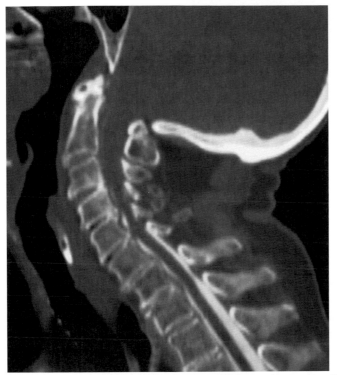

Fig. 14-6. CT myelography. Cervical myelopathy at C5-6 caused by anterior disc bulge and posterior flaval buckling.

Central Disc Protrusion

After a central disc protrusion, which can occur without antecedent back pain, cauda equina compression occurs, often abruptly. Severe pain results, with paravertebral localization or with radiation into both lower limbs. Typically, there is severe distal lower limb weakness (Fig. 14-15) with footdrop, together with depression of the ankle reflexes and impaired sphincter function. Saddle anesthesia is common.

INVESTIGATION OF LUMBOSACRAL DISC DISEASE

Plain Radiography

Plain radiographs are of very limited value in the investigation of a lumbar radiculopathy. Flexion–extension views are used to assess for slip, and oblique views can be useful to confirm pars interarticularis defects (Fig. 14-16).

Computed Tomographic Myelography

CT myelography is relevant only when the patient is intolerant of MRI or when MRI is contraindicated.

Magnetic Resonance Imaging

MRI is the imaging technique of choice for the accurate definition of suspected lumbar disc herniation. It is indicated in a patient with assumed nerve root compression when initial conservative management has failed and there are supportive signs on physical examination. Conservative management is supported by evidence that disc herniations, as assessed by imaging, can spontaneously diminish in size. Interpretation of any abnormality has to take account of the findings in the normal population. In asymptomatic individuals, particularly those older than 60, disc herniations are found in up to a third and spinal stenosis in up to a fifth.

An early sign of disc deterioration is the appearance of fluid-filled cracks, which manifest as high signal areas on T2-weighted images. Accompanying changes include altered signal in the adjacent endplates (Fig. 14-17). Tears in the annulus fibrosus are visible. Simple disc bulges consist of a diffuse extension of the disc beyond the margin of the vertebral endplates. A localized displacement of disc material beyond the intervertebral space is defined as a herniation. Herniations can be subdivided into protrusions, extrusions, and free

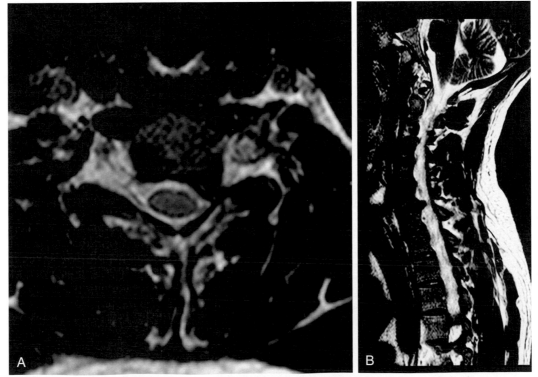

Fig. 14-7. Cervical radiculopathy. MRI showing left-sided discal prolapse. **A,** Sagittal. **B,** Axial.

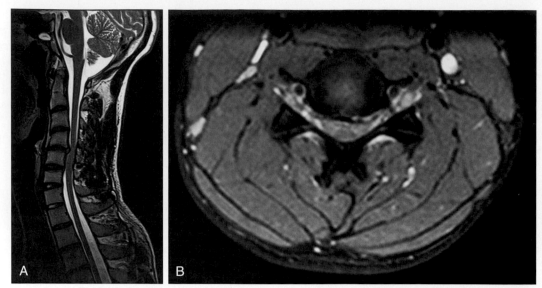

Fig. 14-8. Cervical myelopathy. MRI showing early cord compression. **A,** Sagittal. **B,** Axial.

fragments, according to the size of the herniation and its area of contact with the parent disc (Fig. 14-18).

Other Techniques

Electrophysiologic techniques and, in particular, sampling for evidence of denervation are sometimes employed if uncertainty exists regarding the segmental level affected by a lumbar disc prolapse, although variability of segmental innervation of the lower limb muscles is common. The accuracy of the procedure is enhanced by inclusion of the paravertebral muscles. Preoperative nerve root blocks may aid identification of the affected root.

SPINAL STENOSIS

Although in many patients spinal stenosis is congenital, in others it is secondary to hypertrophy of the bony elements of the lumbar canal, ligamental hypertrophy, or disc degeneration. The stenosis may principally affect the central canal, the lateral recess, or the intervertebral foramen and nerve root canal (Fig. 14-19).

Canal stenosis usually affects middle-aged men. Typically, paroxysmal numbness or paresthesias, rather than pain, appear in the lower limbs on walking and sometimes when standing. The symptoms often spread, usually from the distal parts of the extremities to the proximal, and then resolve after resting or lying flat for a few minutes. Physical examination tends to be unrewarding. Stenosis of the lateral recess results in leg pain and paresthesias.

The boundaries of the lateral recess are formed by the posterior aspect of the vertebral body and disc, the pedicle, and the superior articular facet. Root impingement in the recess is often caused by bony hypertrophy of the superior facet and can mimic the effect of disc herniation.

MRI is the investigation of choice. Findings include a congenitally narrow canal, facet joint degeneration, hypertrophy of the ligamentum flavum, and degenerative disc disease (Fig. 14-20). A variety of other disorders can cause spinal stenosis, including achondroplasia and Paget's disease (Fig. 14-21). Rarely, a clinical syndrome suggesting neurogenic claudication is encountered in patients with severe stenosis of the terminal aorta (Fig. 14-22).

Spinal or foraminal stenosis is managed surgically or with epidural injection if the symptoms are disabling. Central lumbar disc prolapse is managed by immediate surgery. Posterolateral disc prolapse is initially managed conservatively, or with nerve root injection if there is severe pain (Fig. 14-23) but by surgery if symptoms fail to resolve with rest or recur at frequent intervals. If a focal root syndrome is identified clinically and confirmed by investigation, relief of limb pain by surgery is excellent.

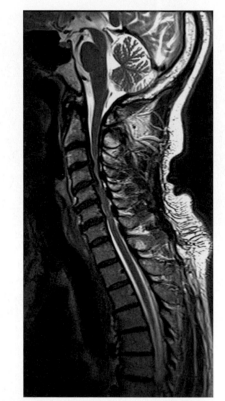

Fig. 14-9. Cervical myelopathy. Multilevel degenerative change with cord compression and abnormal cord signal at the site of compression.

PAGET'S DISEASE OF THE SPINE

Spinal involvement from Paget's disease most commonly results in bony overgrowth of part or all of one or more thoracic or lumbar vertebrae (Fig. 14-24). An increasing bony mass, or a complicating fracture, can result in spinal cord or nerve root damage, or in the syndrome of neurogenic claudication. Pain is common. The skull is affected in up to two thirds of cases. A variety of changes are described on plain skull radiographs, including "cotton wool" skull and platybasia with basilar invagination. CT demonstrates the spectrum of bony change (Fig. 14-25). On MRI (T1 weighted), the hyperintensity of the yellow marrow is usually maintained. Later, marrow signal lessens and finally becomes hypointense (Fig. 14-26). Involvement of the skull base can result in cranial nerve compression or basilar impression with secondary hydrocephalus.

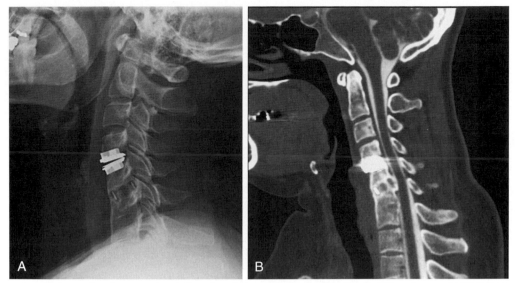

Fig. 14-10. Cloward's procedure. Postoperative changes and evolution of surgical procedures. **A,** Plain film. **B,** CT myelogram. At C6-7 (first operation), fusion is noted (Cloward's procedure). At C5-6 (second operation), there is a spacer device in the disc space (to prevent exit foramen narrowing) and fusion. At C4-5 (third operation), there is a spacer device that allows some degree of movement.

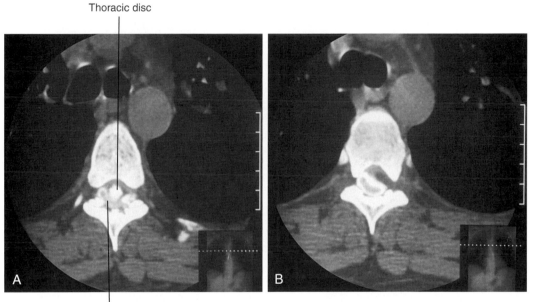

Fig. 14-11. Thoracic disc disease. CT myelography at two levels showing severe cord compression.

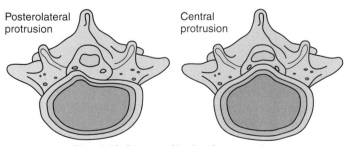

Fig. 14-12. Patterns of lumbar disc protrusion.

RHEUMATOID ARTHRITIS AND THE SPINE

The cervical spine is not uncommonly affected in rheumatoid arthritis. Subluxation at the atlantoaxial or the lower intervertebral joints is the characteristic finding. Significant subluxation at the atlantoaxial joint is defined as a separation of at least 3 cm in men and 2.5 cm in women. Other changes found in the cervical spine include osteoporosis with reduction of disc space but relatively little osteophyte formation, and erosion of the vertebral endplates (Fig. 14-27).

Although some or all of these changes can by asymptomatic, lancinating pain is usually a prominent feature and is frequently referred to the occipital region of the skull via branches of the occipital nerve (C3)—"occipital neuralgia." Physical examination of the neck can sometimes identify a prominent C2 spinous process.

Neurologic consequences of subluxation include a spastic tetraparesis, which is usually managed by a posterior fusion of atlas, axis, and occiput. Plain CT is preferable to radiography when evaluating the odontoid peg. MRI is preferable to CT, because it allows delineation of the whole spine, the extent of any pannus formation, and the degree of spinal cord compression. Pannus formation is suggested by the absence of the odontoid fat pad on T1-weighted images.

MOTOR, REFLEX AND SENSORY CHANGES

Muscle		Reflex	
L4 L5	Tibialis anterior Extensor hallucis longus	L4	Knee (+L2, 3)
		L5	No reflex
S1	Gastrocnemius, soleus	S1	Ankle

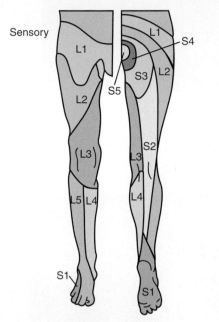

Fig. 14-13. Motor, sensory, and reflex changes in lumbosacral root disorders.

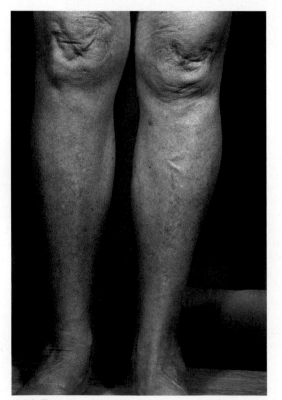

Fig. 14-14. Flattening of right tibialis anterior in an L4 root syndrome.

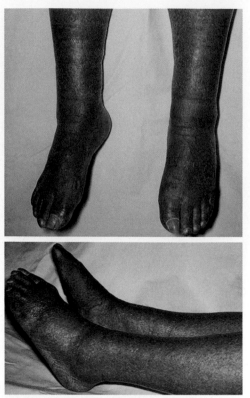

Fig. 14-15. Central disc prolapse. Bilateral footdrop.

INFECTION

SPINAL EPIDURAL ABSCESS

Hematogenous spread of infection is the usual source of an epidural abscess, but in some cases the condition is triggered by a spinal procedure, which can include epidural injection as well as open surgery. Typically, the infective process, usually caused by *Staphylococcus aureus,* begins in the vertebral body before spreading to the epidural space. The abscess most often occurs in the lumbosacral region. Secondary involvement of the spinal vessels is common. Triggering factors, found in about half the cases, include diabetes, intravenous drug abuse, alcoholism, and renal failure.

Back pain is almost invariable at the outset, with evidence of a febrile illness in the majority of patients. Neurologic findings include root or cord sensory loss, limb weakness, and sphincter disturbance. The length of history tends to be bimodal, lasting over days or several weeks. An elevated erythrocyte sedimentation rate and C-reactive protein are usual, but the white cell count is sometimes normal. Unless the abscess has ruptured through the theca, the CSF findings reflect the presence of a parameningeal focus of infection, with an elevated white cell count (polymorphonuclear leukocytes or lymphocytes) and protein concentration but with a normal glucose level. Identification of the causative agent is achieved, in descending order of frequency, from operative tissue, blood culture, and CSF culture.

Investigation

Postcontrast CT is capable of demonstrating any paraspinal soft-tissue mass but the diagnostic imaging of choice is MRI (Fig. 14-28). The abscess appears hyperintense on T2-weighted and hypointense on T1-weighted images. The dura may be visible as a thin line between the abscess and the CSF. With contrast, diffuse or peripheral enhancement is seen (Fig. 14-29). Additional abnormalities that may be seen include vertebral osteomyelitis or discitis and paravertebral abscess formation. Antibiotic therapy is the mainstay of treatment, the duration of which is unsettled, but morbidity remains considerable. Surgery is generally to be avoided if possible. In general, abscesses identified early and treated promptly allow preserved motor

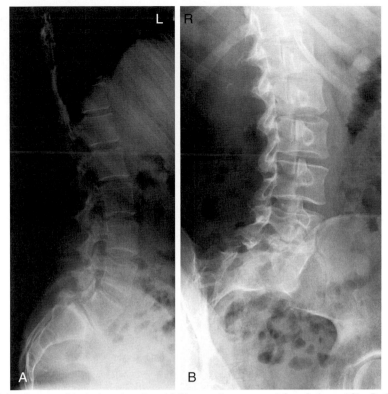

Fig. 14-16. Lumbar spondylosis. Anterior slip at L5-S1 secondary to pars defect. **A,** Lateral film. **B,** Oblique film.

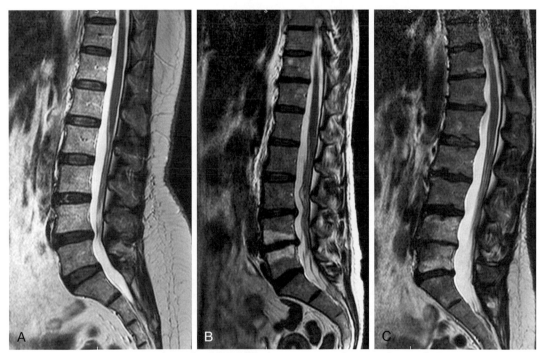

Fig. 14-17. Lumbar spondylosis. Degenerative changes in disc and endplate. MRIs showing increasingly severe changes. **A,** Dehydrated disc. **B,** Disc dehydration, adjacent endplate changes, and slight loss of disc height. **C,** Complete loss of disc height and extensive vertebral body signal change.

and sensory function and retained sphincter control, but presentation with plegia and incontinence implies a poor prognosis.

TUBERCULOUS DISEASE OF THE SPINE

Tuberculous disease of the spine concentrates in the thoracolumbar region. Involvement of multiple vertebrae is the rule. The disease usually commences in the vertebral body adjacent to the cartilage plate and then extends to adjacent levels. The vertebral interspace is relatively spared but becomes involved when the disease is extensive. Primary involvement of the posterior vertebral elements is less common. Eventually, passage through or around the anterior or posterior

longitudinal ligament leads to paraspinal abscess formation (Fig. 14-30). Anterior spread from the thoracolumbar site leads to tracking along the psoas sheath. Posterior spread results in cord compression. Vertebral collapse with kyphosis is an additional mechanism sometimes responsible for spinal cord damage (Fig. 14-31).

In that the disease originates from hematogenous spread in almost all cases, initial features of the illness include fever, malaise, and weight loss. Subsequently, pain emerges, associated with focal tenderness. A radicular element to the pain is often prominent. Tracking of the abscess in the cervical region can lead to a neck swelling, whereas, from the thoracolumbar region, tracking along the psoas sheath results eventually in a mass in the iliac fossa, pelvis, or groin

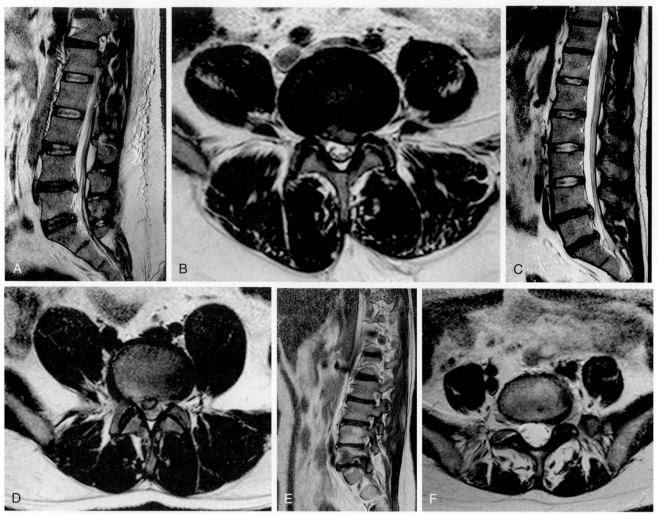

Fig. 14-18. Lumbar disc herniation with root entrapment. Three pairs of MRIs showing paracentral disc bulge (**A** and **B**), sequestrated paracentral fragment (**C** and **D**), and disc bulge in exit foramen (**E** and **F**).

(Fig. 14-32). The neurologic deficit that follows in a proportion of cases is typically a spastic paraparesis (Fig. 14-33).

Investigation

Blood tests are of limited value in the diagnosis of tuberculous disease of the spine. Plain radiographs are usually, but not inevitably, abnormal. Typically, there is erosion of the vertebral bodies with disc space narrowing and, in the later stages, shadowing secondary to paravertebral abscess formation (Fig. 14-34). Later, more frank bone destruction with vertebral collapse or deformity becomes evident (Fig. 14-35). The MRI characteristics of tuberculous spondylitis differ from those encountered with pyogenic infection. Although an increased signal from the disc on T2-weighted images is the rule in pyogenic infection, it is likely to be absent with tuberculous disease. Involvement of multiple vertebrae is the rule, with relative preservation of the intervening discs, a picture liable to cause confusion with metastatic disease (Fig. 14-36). Involvement of the posterior vertebral elements is often more prominent than appreciated from other imaging techniques.

Treatment is with standard antituberculous therapy, combined, where there is neurologic deficit, with surgery. Laminectomy is required if the disease is affecting the posterior neural arch. For anterior paravertebral masses, an anterior approach is usually undertaken.

BRUCELLOSIS

Human brucellosis is caused by one of four species of *Brucella*. Animal contact with inhalation of organisms it the most frequent cause of infection. The clinical features of the condition are nonspecific. Bone involvement is commonly in the form of spondylitis, the pro-

cess beginning in the superior endplate. Lumbar involvement is most common.

Brucella myelitis can occur in isolation or as part of a meningo-encephalitic syndrome. In addition, cord involvement may follow primary vertebral disease, with or without extradural granuloma formation. Most patients have evidence of systemic brucellosis. Back pain is common, associated with a spastic paraparesis or quadriparesis, with sphincter involvement in some. The sensory deficit is less conspicuous. Plain radiographs of the spine are often normal, and MRI is required.

The manifestations of *Brucella* meningoencephalitis are protean. The CSF pressure is usually elevated, with an increased protein concentration and a lymphocytic pleocytosis. There may be oligoclonal bands.

The polymerase chain reaction is highly specific and sensitive for the detection of *Brucella* agglutinins, usually using antigens prepared from *Brucella abortus,* which cross-react with most other, although not all, *Brucella* species.

SCHISTOSOMIASIS

Spinal cord disease in patients with schistosomiasis is usually caused by infection by *Schistosoma mansoni*. Granuloma formation both inside and outside the cord has been described (Fig. 14-37). The cauda equina can also be affected. Typically, a transverse myelitis appears, sometimes acutely. The CSF shows an increased protein concentration, a lymphocytic pleocytosis, and elevated antibody levels. CT myelography or MRI detects a diffuse swelling of the lower cord, sometimes with cyst formation (Fig. 14-38).

The treatment of choice is praziquantel. It is unsettled as to whether the addition of steroid therapy confers additional benefit.

HTLV-1–ASSOCIATED MYELOPATHY

HTLV-1–associated myelopathy (tropical spastic paraparesis) is caused by human T-cell lymphotropic virus type 1. It is endemic in the Caribbean, Central and South America, the Middle East, Southern Japan, equatorial regions of Africa, and Melanesia.

The virus is transmitted by whole-blood transfusion, by use of contaminated needles, via breast milk, and through sexual intercourse. Most infected individuals are asymptomatic. Clinically, the condition embraces optic atrophy, spastic paraparesis, ataxia, and neuropathy.

There may be a mild inflammatory reaction in the CSF, with a slightly elevated protein concentration.

ARACHNOID CYSTS

Most arachnoid cysts are congenital and either extradural or intradural. Extradural cysts consist of a saclike protrusion of the arachnoid through the dura mater. They are single and appear posteriorly, most often in the thoracic region. In about half the cases, the communication with the subarachnoid space remains patent. Many of these cysts are asymptomatic, but some, perhaps by a ball-valve mechanism, increase in size and become symptomatic. Clinical features include local pain, radicular sensory symptoms, and manifestations of cord compression. Symptoms can be exacerbated by any procedure that raises intrathecal pressure. Intradural arachnoid cysts, like their extradural counterparts, may be enclosed or in communication with the subarachnoid space. They are usually multiple and often incidental findings discovered during investigation of unrelated neurologic symptoms.

Plain radiography changes, including erosion of the vertebral pedicles, widening of the intervertebral foramen, and widening of the spinal canal, can occur with extradural cysts. MRI readily demonstrates these cysts. A third type of arachnoid cyst, found in the sacral region, is believed to arise from the nerve root sheath. Apparent compression of the ganglion or nerve root may result but generally without clinical sequelae (Fig. 14-39).

ARACHNOIDITIS

Spinal arachnoiditis can arise de novo or alongside other pathologic processes. It can be triggered by operative procedures on the spine or by infection, and historically it was associated with the performance of myelography using oil-containing media. After an inflammatory reaction in the arachnoid, a fibrotic process ensues, leading to thickening of the membranes, obliteration of the subarachnoid space, cyst formation, and vessel occlusion. Any part of the spine can be affected. Pain is usually the earliest and often the most prominent symptom. Additional features include limb numbness, paresthesias, and weakness. The condition is usually slowly progressive. Sometimes there is a mixture of upper and lower motor neuron signs.

MRI is the investigation of choice. T1-weighted images demonstrate an indistinct cord outline, but the features are best revealed on

THE LUMBAR CANAL

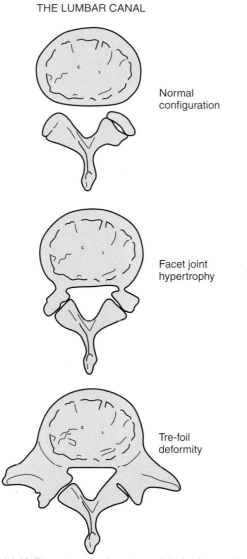

Normal configuration

Facet joint hypertrophy

Tre-foil deformity

Fig. 14-19. The various configurations of the lumbar canal.

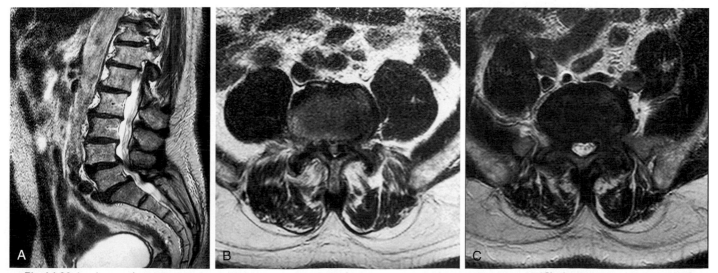

Fig. 14-20. Lumbar canal stenosis. MRI. Sagittal **(A)** and axial **(B)** images through L4-5, and axial images through L5-S1 **(C)**, showing spinal stenosis at L4-5.

T2-weighted images. These demonstrate CSF loculation and obliteration of the subarachnoid space. At the level of the cauda equina, the nerve roots show clumping (Fig. 14-40). Contrast enhancement is variable and shows different patterns. Linear, nodular, and diffuse thick enhancement has been described. There is no specific treatment.

VASCULAR ABNORMALITIES OF THE SPINE AND CORD

SPINAL (PIAL) ARTERIOVENOUS MALFORMATIONS

Spinal arteriovenous malformations (AVMs) are much less common than intracranial AVMs. They are histologically identical but, because of their location, spinal AVMs tend to cause a greater degree of neurologic deficit when they bleed. Treatment options are similar to those used intracranially, but they carry a greater risk. The nidus lies within the cord, it is usual to have multiple feeding vessels, and transit time is rapid. In some instances, there are associated arterial or venous aneurysms (Fig. 14-41). Venous drainage is both rostral and caudal. They may present with a slowly evolving mixed motor and

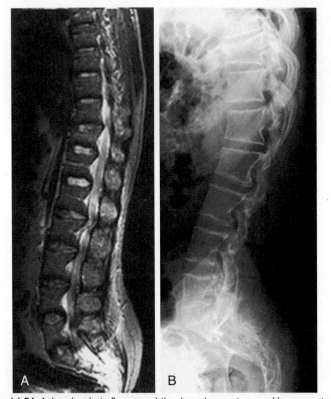

Fig. 14-21. Achondroplasia. Severe multilevel canal stenosis caused by congenitally short pedicles and superadded degenerative change. **A,** MRI. **B,** Plain radiographic film. Note posterior vertebral body scalloping, which is a feature of achondroplasia.

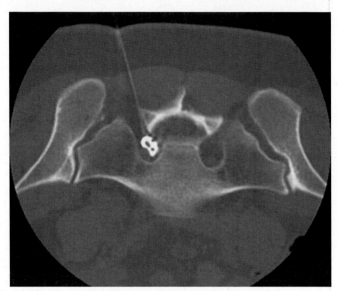

Fig. 14-23. CT-guided left S1 nerve root injection for pain relief. Contrast agent is injected first to confirm the position.

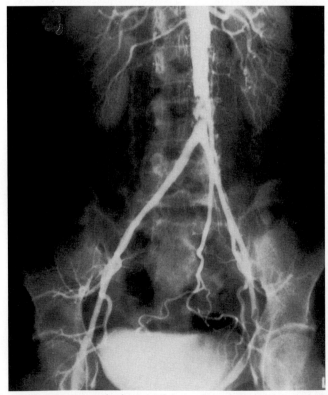

Fig. 14-22. Intermittent claudication of the cauda equina secondary to a severe distal stenosis of the terminal aorta.

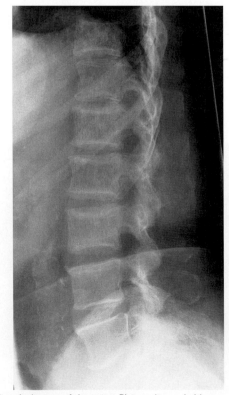

Fig. 14-24. Paget's disease of the spine. Plain radiograph. Note coarsening of the trabecular pattern.

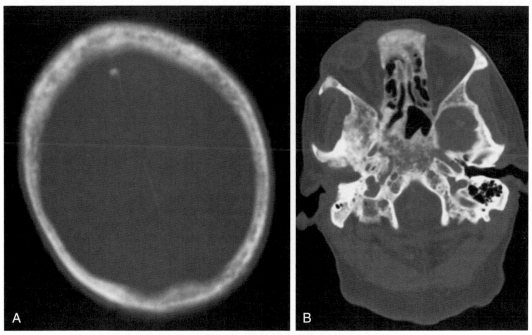

Fig. 14-25. Paget's disease of the skull. CT. **A,** Skull vault. **B,** Patchy skull base involvement.

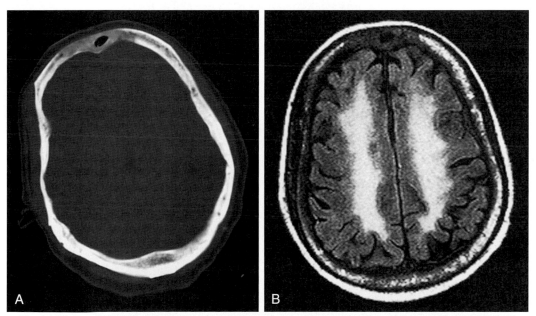

Fig. 14-26. Paget's disease of the skull. Anterior pagetoid patch with altered marrow signal on MRI. **A,** CT. **B,** MRI.

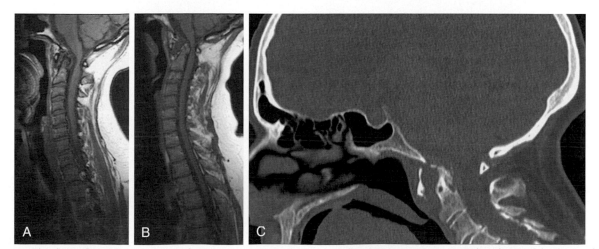

Fig. 14-27. Rheumatoid arthritis. **A** and **B,** MRI of cervical spine in same patient 6 years apart showing increasing pannus with widening of the distance between the peg and the anterior arch of C1, with a corresponding decrease in the diameter of the vertebral canal. **C,** CT showing erosion of the peg.

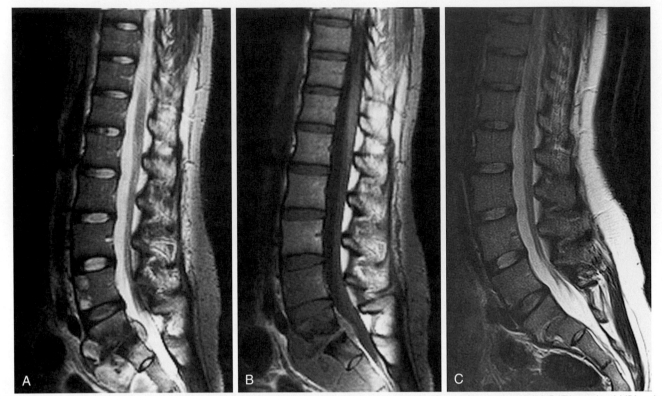

Fig. 14-28. Anterior spinal epidural abscess with disc involvement and anterior subligamentous spread. **A,** Sagittal T2-weighted MRI. **B,** T1-weighted MRI with contrast enhancement. **C,** Three-year follow-up. Note fusion at disc space.

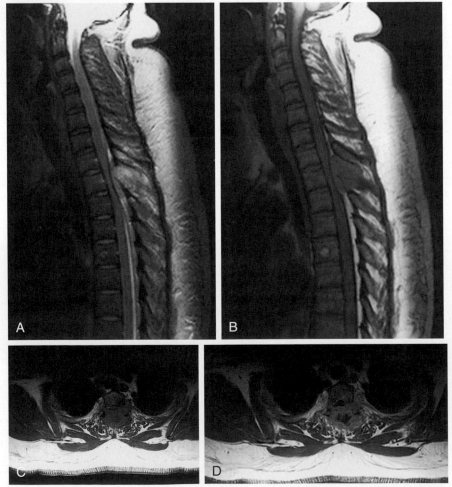

Fig. 14-29. Spinal epidural abscess MRI. Sagittal T2 **(A)** and T1 **(B)** and axial pre and post contrast T1 **(C, D)** showing epidural abscess with posterior spread.

sensory syndrome, but pain is more common than with spinal dural arteriovenous fistulas (AVFs). Most, however, present with sudden deterioration secondary to subarachnoid hemorrhage. They are distributed more evenly along the spinal axis than are spinal dural AVFs.

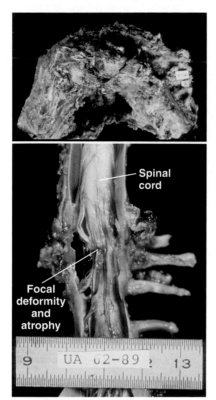

Fig. 14-30. Spinal tuberculosis. **A,** Severe kyphosis. **B,** Marked focal atrophy of the cord at the site of compression.

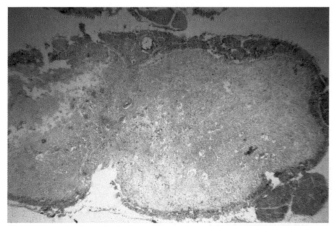

Fig. 14-31. Spinal tuberculosis. Low-power view of the spinal cord showing almost complete myelin loss (Luxol fast blue, H&E).

SPINAL DURAL ARTERIOVENOUS FISTULAS

Spinal dural arteriovenous fistulas are most common in the thoracolumbar region, and tend to appear with a gradually evolving, mixed motor, sensory, and sphincteric syndrome in which the symptoms are frequently exacerbated by exercise. They are more common than AVMs and tend to occur in late middle-aged men. Typically, the motor deficit, which is principally in the lower limbs, combines upper with lower motor neuron components, a pattern described as the necrotizing myelopathy of Foix and Alajouanine. There is typically a single fistulous point on the dural sleeve of an exiting nerve root. Arterial blood is therefore diverted into the pial venous network that surrounds and drains the cord, decreasing the perfusion pressure in the cord (the difference between arterial and venous pressures), with consequent ischemia. The pathologic basis of the paresis or plegia is ischemic necrosis of the affected levels of the spinal cord. Subarachnoid hemorrhage as a presenting feature is rare.

The dilated tortuous veins draining these malformations are more likely to be found on the dorsal than on the ventral surface of the cord (Fig. 14-42).

MRI demonstrates, in dural fistulas, serpiginous low-signal-intensity lesions over the dorsal surface of the cord on T2-weighted images, together with high-signal areas in the cord on both T1- and T2-weighted images, with evidence of cord expansion (Fig. 14-43).

Different treatment options have been advocated, including direct microneurosurgery and endovascular occlusion, the choice partly determined by the size of the shunt (Fig. 14-44).

CAVERNOUS HEMANGIOMA (CAVERNOMA)

Cavernomas (cavernous hemangiomas) are found in the spinal cord as well as intracranially. They consist of sinusoidal vascular spaces lined by a single layer of endothelial cells. As in cerebral cavernomas, the vessel walls in most of the lesions are in close contact, creating a back-to-back histologic appearance. Some connective tissue lies between the spaces, but there is no true capsule. Recurrent hemorrhage occurs in the lesions, as do foci of thrombosis and calcification. On T2-weighted MRI, cavernomas appears as a hyperintense nidus, often of heterogeneous appearance, with a surrounding hypointense zone resulting from hemosiderin. The imaging appearance is identical to that of intracranial cavernomas.

VERTEBRAL BODY HEMANGIOMAS

Hemangiomas are commonly seen in vertebral bodies and are usually of no clinical significance. Occasionally, they spread extraosseously into the vertebral canal, and patients present with either backache or a spastic paraparesis resulting from cord compression. Diagnosis is made with CT or MRI and treatment is usually surgical, often after embolization to decrease perioperative blood loss and vertebroplasty to help support the vertebral body (Fig. 14-45).

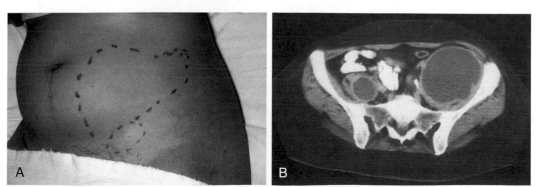

Fig. 14-32. A, Spinal tuberculosis, an abdominal mass. **B,** Contrast-enhanced CT scan showing bilateral psoas abscesses.

SUBACUTE COMBINED DEGENERATION OF THE SPINAL CORD

Subacute combined degeneration of the spinal cord (SACD) is secondary to vitamin B$_{12}$ deficiency, although, rarely, similar cases have been attributed to pure folate deficiency. In the United Kingdom and United States, B$_{12}$ deficiency is rare and SACD is uncommon. Vitamin B$_{12}$ deficiency leads to inadequate methyltransferase activity, resulting in high serum folate concentrations and the incorporation of uridyl residues into DNA. The resulting DNA is abnormally fragile. In addition, elevated levels of methylmalonic acid, the consequence of adenosylcobalamin deficiency, may be toxic to myelin.

Myelin degeneration commences in the posterior columns, later involving the lateral and anterior columns, predominantly in the cervicothoracic region (Fig. 14-46). Subsequently, axonal degeneration appears. The changes are associated with a spongy degeneration of the supportive glia (Fig. 14-47). Similar lesions are found in the optic nerves and occasionally in the cerebral white matter. Degenerative changes can extend to the peripheral nervous system, and some patients present with neuropathy without obvious myelopathy.

Sensory symptoms are prominent from the beginning with peripheral paresthesias affecting the legs more than the hands. Subsequently, weakness and stiffness of the legs appear, and there may be changes in mood and behavior. Lhermitte's sign is found in about 20% of patients. The clinical progression may be rapid or gradual. Findings include predominant posterior column sensory loss and paraplegia, although often with depressed or absent ankle reflexes.

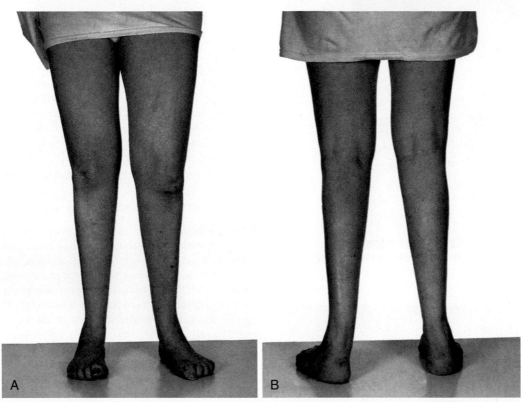

Fig. 14-33. Front **(A)** and back **(B)** views of wasting of the lower limbs secondary to previous tuberculosis of the spine.

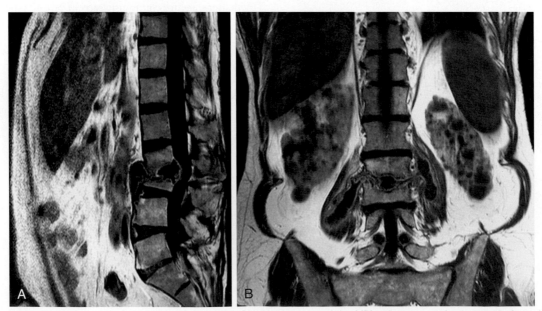

Fig. 14-34. Spinal tuberculosis in a patient with polycystic kidneys. Note spread into both psoas muscles. MRI with contrast enhancement. **A,** Sagittal view. **B,** Coronal view.

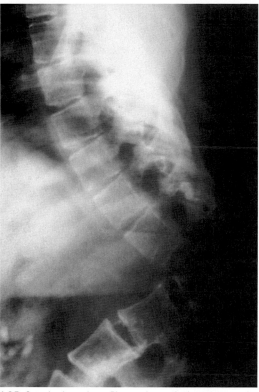

Fig. 14-35. Spinal tuberculosis. Plain radiograph showing gross kyphosis.

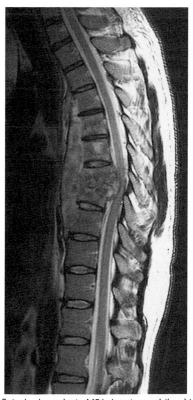

Fig. 14-36. Spinal tuberculosis. MRI showing multilevel involvement.

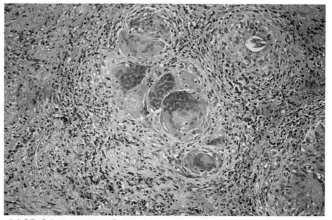

Fig. 14-37. Schistosomiasis. Section demonstrating a granulomatous process with aggregates of multinucleated giant histiocytes (H&E, x25).

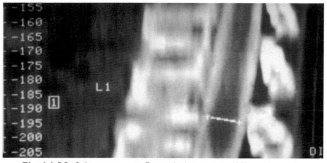

Fig. 14-38. Schistosomiasis. Expanded conus on CT myelography.

When the anemia is substantial, the patient has a yellow-lemon color. The hair is likely to be prematurely gray. About half the patients have an atrophic tongue (Fig. 14-48). Abnormal skin pigmentation occurs, including patches of vitiligo (Fig. 14-49). Anemia is sometimes absent and macrocytosis, although usual, is not inevitable. The neutrophils tend to be hypersegmented, and sometimes there is a pancytopenia. The bone marrow is megaloblastic but, rarely, can appear normoblastic. The vitamin B_{12} concentration is usually less than 100 ng/L. Levels of methylmalonic acid and homocysteine are elevated.

A number of autoantibodies are found. Abnormal electophysiologic findings include altered peripheral nerve conduction and central delay in conduction velocities as determined by somatosensory evoked potentials. MRI may show dorsal column high-signal change (Fig. 14-50). If diagnosed early, the condition responds briskly to substitution therapy, which is continued permanently.

RADIATION MYELOPATHY

The incidence of radiation myelopathy after spinal cord irradiation has been reported to be between 0.6% and 17.5%. A transient form, typically associated with Lhermitte's phenomenon, occurs within a few months of irradiation and appears to resolve spontaneously. In addition, a chronic progressive myelopathy, whose occurrence is related to cumulative dosages exceeding 4000 cGy, appears around a year, but sometimes as long as 5 years, after irradiation. Concomitant chemotherapy may increase the risk. Sensory signs insidiously emerge, sometimes in a Brown-Séquard distribution, followed by paralysis and sphincter disturbance. A variant form has been described in which the brunt of the damage is borne by the anterior horn cells.

Pathologic changes include gray and white matter necrosis together with a prominent vasculopathy consisting of arteriolar fibrosis, fibrinoid necrosis, and vessel occlusion. The disease is preventable by limiting the exposure of the spinal cord.

SYRINGOMYELIA

In syringomyelia, cystic cavitation of the spinal cord occurs, most prominently in the cervical region, sometimes associated with similar cavitation of the brainstem (syringobulbia) (Fig. 14-51). The condition is closely associated with a number of developmental abnormalities close to the cervicocranial junction, including abnormal fusion of the cervical vertebrae (Fig. 14-52) and Chiari's malformation type I (Fig. 14-53).

Syringomyelia may also appear in relationship to an intramedullary tumor (Fig. 14-54) and as a posttraumatic phenomenon.

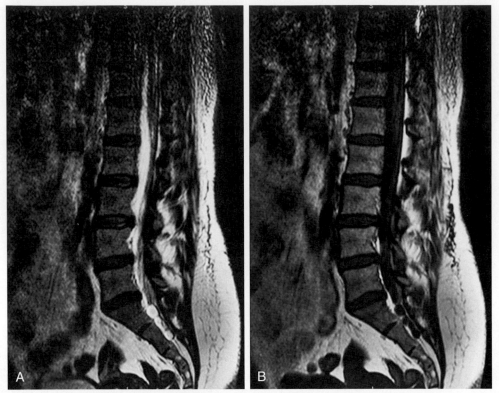

Fig. 14-39. A and **B,** Two MR images of spinal arachnoid cyst at S2.

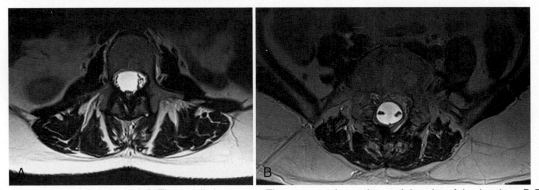

Fig. 14-40. Arachnoiditis. Two patterns are recognized. **A,** The so-called empty sac: The roots are plastered around the edge of the thecal sac. **B,** The roots are clumped and adherent to each other.

Distinction of syringomyelia from hydromyelia has been made: The former is believed to be distinct from the central canal, and hydromyelia is defined as a dialatation of the canal itself. Because of its position, the syrinx interrupts decussating spinothalamic fibers in the anterior commissure. Subsequent expansion of the cavity leads to disruption of the anterior and posterior horns, and finally of the lateral and posterior columns.

Descriptions of the natural history of this condition are somewhat redundant. Early diagnosis and surgical drainage of the cyst along with correction of a Chiari abnormality, if present, prevent progression (in most cases) to the classic picture of the disease. By then, there is prominent dissociated anesthesia in the cervical dermatomes, often leading to repeated trauma to the hands (Fig. 14-55). Later, involvement of touch and proprioceptive function is likely. Paradoxically, pain can be a prominent symptom. The motor involvement includes weakness and then wasting in upper limb muscles (Fig. 14-56) and a spastic paraparesis. The upper limb reflexes become depressed, and the lower limb reflexes exaggerated. Autonomic dysfunction occurs, including Horner's syndrome (Fig. 14-57), altered sweating over the arms and face, and sphincter disturbances. At a later stage, the shoulder joint may be affected by a Charcot arthropathy. Kyphoscoliosis is sometimes found. These late features are now rare. Early

syringomyelia is detected either because of greater awareness of the condition or because of investigation for a suspected Chiari malformation.

Investigation

MRI is the investigation of choice (Fig. 14-58). When MRI is contraindicated, CT permits identification of the cerebellar ectopia and the expanded cord. CT myelography can demonstrate delayed opacification of the syringomyelic cavity (Fig. 14-59). If a Chiari malformation is identified, foramen magnum decompression is usually performed.

SPINAL CORD INFARCTION

The spinal cord is supplied by separate anterior and posterior arterial systems. The anterior two thirds or more of the cord is supplied by the anterior spinal artery. At the cervical level, this is fed by branches of the vertebral arteries; at all thoracic levels, by paired radicular arteries; and, in addition, at the lower thoracic and lumbar levels, by a particular radicular artery, the artery of Adamkiewicz. The overlapping arrangement results in border-zone (watershed) areas, notably in the thoracic cord, which become vulnerable to ischemia if there is a

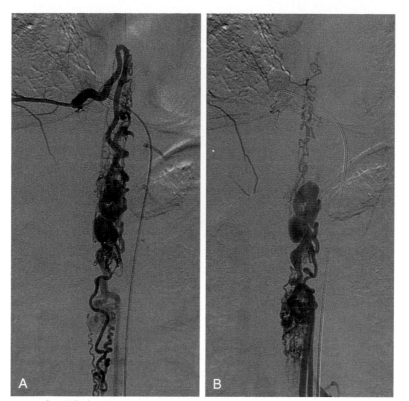

Fig. 14-41. Spinal arteriovenous malformation. **A** and **B,** Sequential angiographic images showing a diffuse nidus, venous dilatation, and caudal and rostral venous drainage.

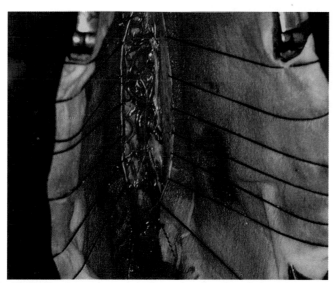

Fig. 14-42. Spinal arteriovenous malformation. Operative findings demonstrating the tortuous draining veins.

hypoperfusion state (Fig. 14-60). The posterior aspect of the cord is supplied by the posterior spinal arteries, supplemented by posterior radicular vessels.

Although transient ischemic events can occur in the cord—for example, as a steal phenomenon associated with coarctation—a vascular event is typically of rapid onset resulting in a mixture of motor, sensory, and sphincteric symptoms. Involvement of the anterior spinal artery, typically directly by atheroma or indirectly by loss of flow in radicular arteries after aortic dissection, produces a flaccid weakness with lower motor neuron features in some cases. Infarction of the posterior cord is less common and produces a predominant sensory deficit. Venous infarcts occur but are seldom diagnosed in life.

Investigation is of limited value, although MRI may reveal evidence of cord swelling with or without altered signal at the relevant level (Fig. 14-61). There is no specific treatment.

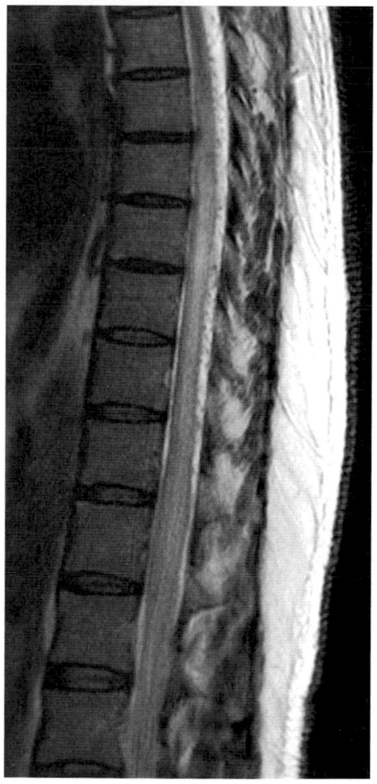

Fig. 14-43. Spinal dural arteriovenous fistula. MRI showing high signal intensity in a swollen cord with vessels on the dorsal surface.

SPINAL EXTRADURAL HEMATOMA

Spinal extradural hematoma is a rare condition. It can occur spontaneously, as a result of trauma, in association with a bleeding diathesis, or with thrombocytopenia in cancer patients. Any spinal level can be affected. The condition usually commences abruptly with severe local pain, exacerbated by spinal movement. Subsequently, focal neu-

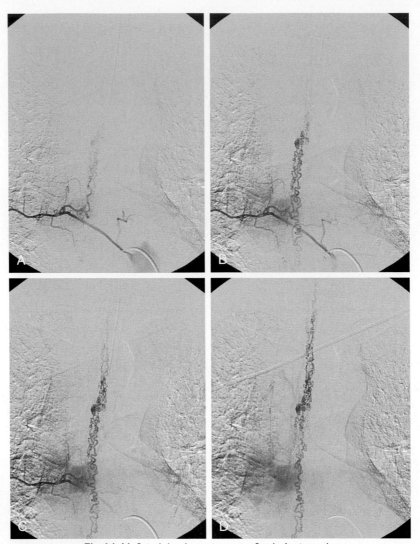

Fig. 14-44. Spinal dural arteriovenous fistula. Angiography.

rologic deficit emerges, determined by the level of the hematoma. MRI allows localization of the hematoma to the extradural space, and defines its complete extent and age and the degree of cord or cauda equina compression (Fig. 14-62). Urgent surgical intervention is required.

AMYLOIDOSIS

In patients on long-term hemodialysis, deposition of amyloid occurs in joints, bone, and the carpal tunnel. Rarely, the amyloid is deposited in the extradural tissues of the spinal canal, leading to cord compression. The amyloid in these instances is derived from β_2-microglobulin.

The cord and its vessels are subject to accumulation of β-amyloid, just as cerebral vessels are in patients with Alzheimer's disease and amyloid angiopathy. Rarely, this results in intramedullary hemorrhage or ischemia.

ANTERIOR HERNIATION OF THE CORD

This increasingly recognized condition appears with a slowly progressive cord syndrome, often a Brown-Séquard syndrome, but less often as paresis or sphincter dysfunction. There is usually an anterolateral dural defect through which the cord herniates. Treatment is by surgical repair, which prevents further deterioration, although the degree of recovery is unpredictable. The MRI images are characteristic (Fig. 14-63).

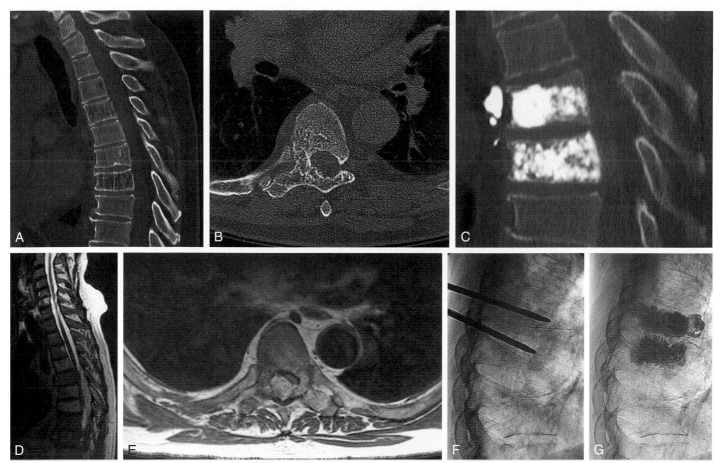

Fig. 14-45. Extraosseous hemangioma. CT **(A, B, C)**, MR **(D, E)**, and before **(F)** and after **(G)** vertebroplasty. The cord is displaced and compressed anterolaterally **(D, E)** by hemangioma that involves multiple vertebral bodies and posterior elements **(A, B)**. Characteristic vertical striation is seen on CT **(A)**.

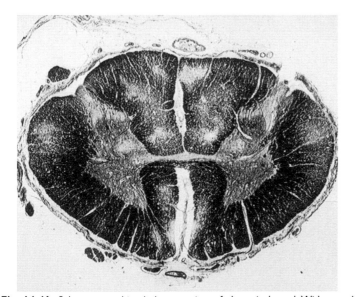

Fig. 14-46. Subacute combined degeneration of the spinal cord. Widespread myelin loss (Weigert-Pal, ×6).

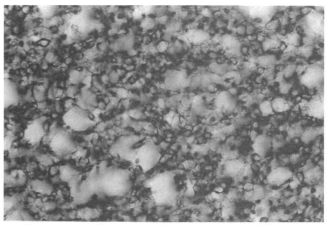

Fig. 14-47. Subacute combined degeneration of the spinal cord. Vacuolation in the myelin sheaths in the posterior columns (Luxol fast blue, cresyl violet).

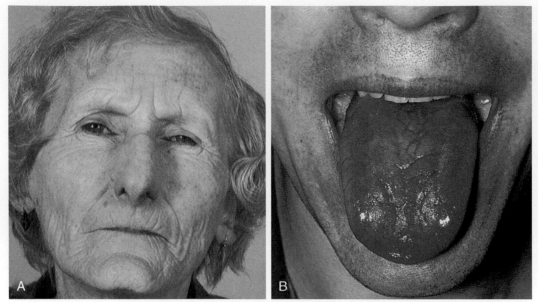

Fig. 14-48. Subacute combined degeneration of the spinal cord. **A,** Facial appearance. **B,** Tongue appearance.

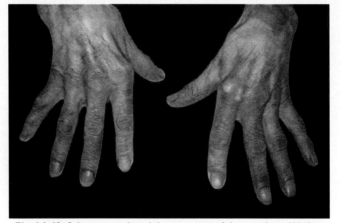

Fig. 14-49. Subacute combined degeneration of the spinal cord. Vitiligo.

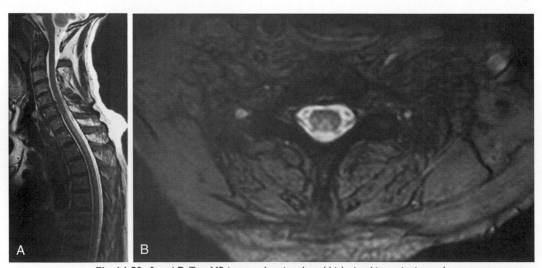

Fig. 14-50. A and **B,** Two MR images showing dorsal high signal intensity in cord.

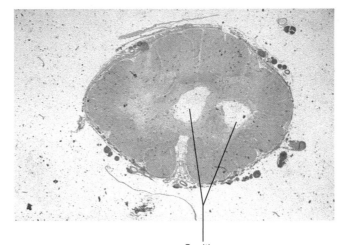

Cavities

Fig. 14-51. Syringomyelia. Cervical cord showing two cavities.

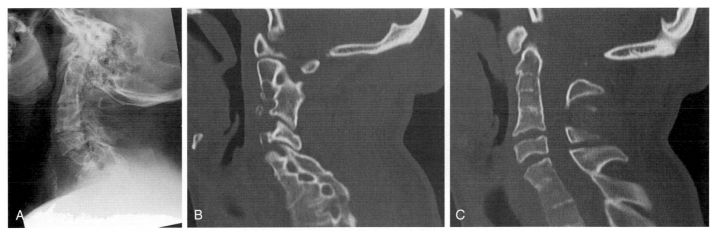

Fig. 14-52. Klippel-Feil syndrome. Plain film **(A)** and CT **(B, C)** showing fusion of vertebral bodies and posterior elements.

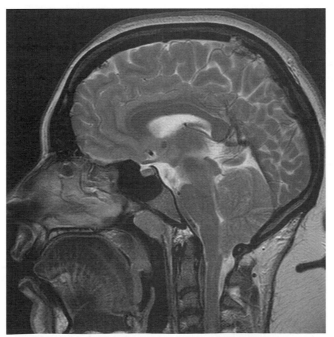

Fig. 14-53. Chiari type I malformation. MRI showing tonsillar descent to just below C1.

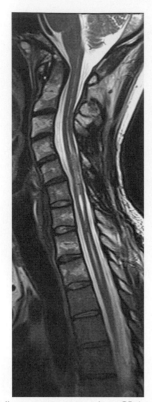

Fig. 14-54. Intramedullary tumor centered at C5-6 with caudal and rostral syrinxes.

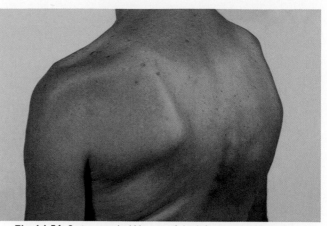

Fig. 14-56. Syringomyelia. Wasting of the left periscapular muscles.

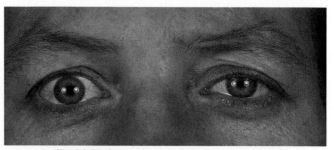

Fig. 14-57. Syringomyelia. Left Horner's syndrome.

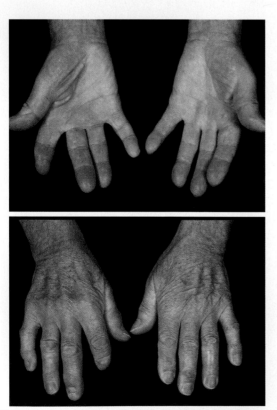

Fig. 14-55. Syringomyelia. Wasting of the small muscles of the hands and loss of the terminal phalanx of the right index finger.

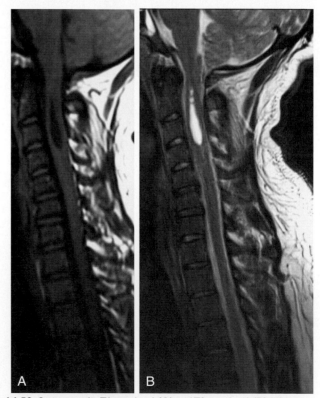

Fig. 14-58. Syringomyelia. T1-weighted **(A)** and T2-weighted **(B)** MRI.

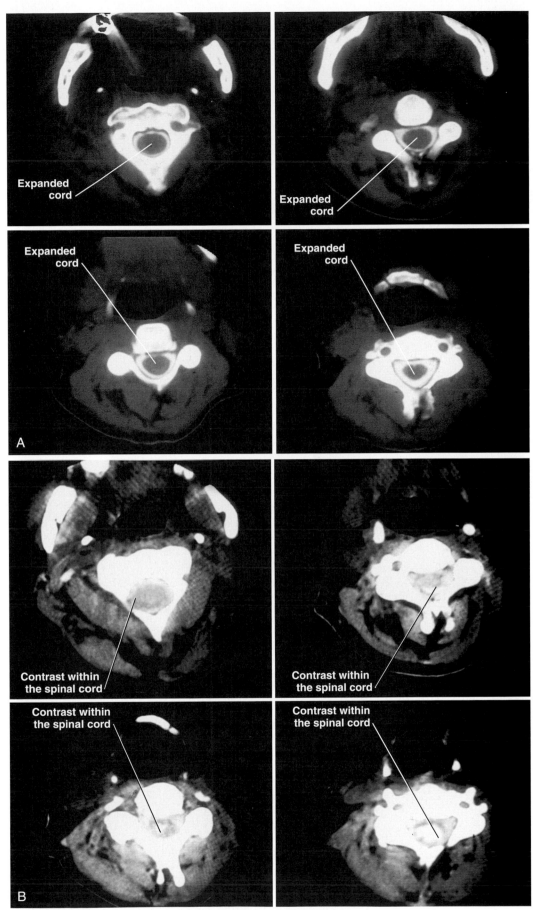

Fig. 14-59. Syringomyelia. CT myelography. **A,** Expanded cord. **B,** Delayed uptake of contrast into the syringomyelic cavity.

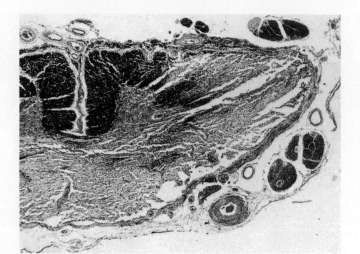

Fig. 14-60. Spinal cord infarction. Section through part of the upper thoracic cord in a patient with severe atheroma and infarction of the cord in the posterior spinal artery territory. There is sparing of the anterior columns and most of the gray matter (solochrome cyanin).

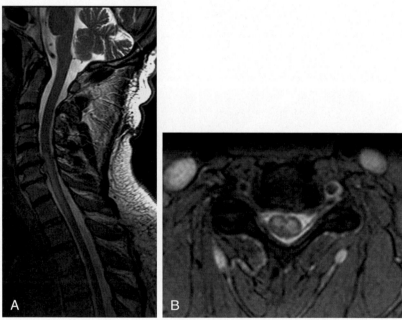

Fig. 14-61. Spinal cord infarction. MRI. Sagittal **(A)** and axial **(B)** T2-weighted images. Note that the anterior cord is more vulnerable than the dorsal cord, and gray matter is affected more than white matter.

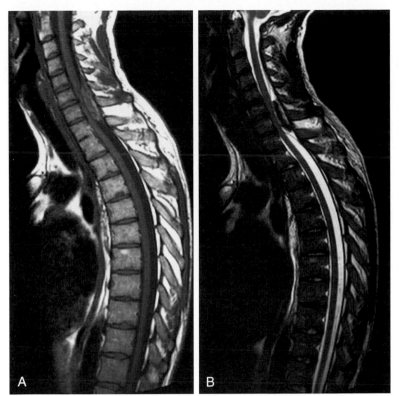

Fig. 14-62. Thoracic spinal extradural hematoma. Sagittal MRI. **A,** T1-weighted. **B,** T2-weighted. Note profound hypointensity on T2-weighted MRI and heterogeneous signal on T1-weighted MRI.

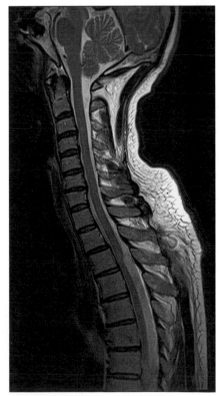

Fig. 14-63. Anterior herniation of the cord at T3. There is some intramedullary signal change. Note anterior kink, with no mass behind the cord.

THE FIRST CRANIAL NERVE (OLFACTORY)

Disturbances of olfaction are uncommon in neurologic practice. Alteration of taste and smell are recognized complications of head injury and can follow an apparently trivial upper respiratory tract infection. Rarely, unilateral or bilateral anosmia is the presenting feature of a subfrontal meningioma. Dulling of olfaction occurs in elderly patients, accompanies Parkinson's disease, and is a relatively early feature of Alzheimer's disease.

THE SECOND CRANIAL NERVE (OPTIC)

A wide variety of pathologic processes affect the optic nerve and its central pathway. In general, optic nerve compression produces insidious visual failure, with a marked impairment of color vision, an afferent pupillary defect, and a central scotoma, later breaking out into the periphery and, yet later, optic atrophy.

ORBITAL TUMORS

Meningiomas
Meningiomas of the optic nerve sheath lead to gradual visual failure associated with mild proptosis (Fig. 15-1). Meningiomas in the optic canal have usually extended into the canal from the orbit or from the region of the anterior clinoid process. The lesions are easily missed clinically but are identified by neuroimaging as an expansion in the region of the optic nerve sheath (Fig. 15-2).

Optic Nerve Gliomas
Optic nerve gliomas in childhood are essentially benign, slow-growing tumors with histologic characteristics of the pilocytic astrocytomas (Fig. 15-3). There is a recognized association of optic nerve and chiasmatic gliomas with neurofibromatosis-1 (NF1). As many as 15% of individuals with NF1 are reported to have optic nerve or chiasmatic enlargement on imaging. The underlying pathologic substrate of that swelling is mixed.

Malignant gliomas of the optic nerve or chiasm occur rarely in adult life. There is often rapid visual failure with ocular pain and early involvement of the other eye. The tumor behaves like an anaplastic astrocytoma. On MRI, the benign childhood glioma appears as a diffuse enlargement of the optic nerve or chiasm, which appears relatively bright on T2-weighted images (Fig. 15-4).

Other Disorders of the Optic Nerve
Optic neuritis is one of the most common presenting features of multiple sclerosis (MS). The condition is usually unilateral. Pain is common, followed by visual failure. Recovery of vision occurs in the majority of patients. Scanning sometimes detects an abnormality in the nerve, either in the form of an enlargement or as an area of increased signal on T2-weighted images (Fig. 15-5).

Many toxic and deficiency disorders affect the optic nerve. They, and the various familial optic atrophies, are characterized by symmetry, with the appearance of bilateral, symmetrical, central, or centrocecal scotomas (Fig. 15-6).

Vascular disease of the optic nerve is common in older patients, more often secondary to atheromatous disease of the posterior ciliary arteries than to an arteritis. Typically, an altitudinal or arcuate field defect appears, with disc swelling followed by optic atrophy (Fig. 15-7).

Sarcoidosis can affect the optic nerve in a variety of ways. Most common is an optic nerve granuloma, which can occupy either the optic nerve head or its retrolaminar portion. Optic atrophy eventually appears (Fig. 15-8).

Papilledema is often asymptomatic initially, although some patients complain of transient visual obscurations typically triggered by head movement. Visual field changes at this stage are confined to enlargement of the blind spots. With prolonged papilledema, the optic nerve sheath expands (Fig. 15-9), and nerve fiber atrophy appears, which leads to various visual field changes including arcuate defects and peripheral constriction.

Disorders of the Chiasm
Chiasmatic compression is usually secondary to pituitary tumor, craniopharyngioma, meningioma, or aneurysm (Fig. 15-10). The relationship of the chiasm to the pituitary gland is variable, so there is no single pattern of visual loss associated with pituitary expansion. The field loss is typically asymmetrical but follows, at least eventually, a bitemporal pattern. Compression of the chiasm from below produces a superior bitemporal hemianopia (Fig. 15-11).

Retrochiasmatic Lesions
Retrochiasmatic lesions of the visual pathway produce increasingly congruous homonymous defects as the occipital cortex is approached. Lesions of the tract and lateral geniculate body are less common than those of the radiation or cortex. Involvement of the optic radiation in the temporal lobe produces a homonymous defect that predominates in the superior quadrants (Fig. 15-12). Parietal lobe lesions produce a defect that is usually complete. Lesions of the occipital lobe typically produce highly congruous defects, which may be scotomatous, quadrantic, or complete.

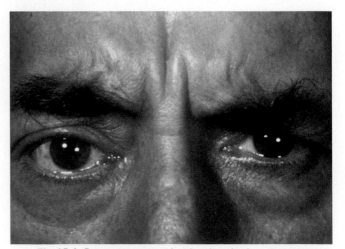

Fig. 15-1. Proptosis associated with right orbital meningioma.

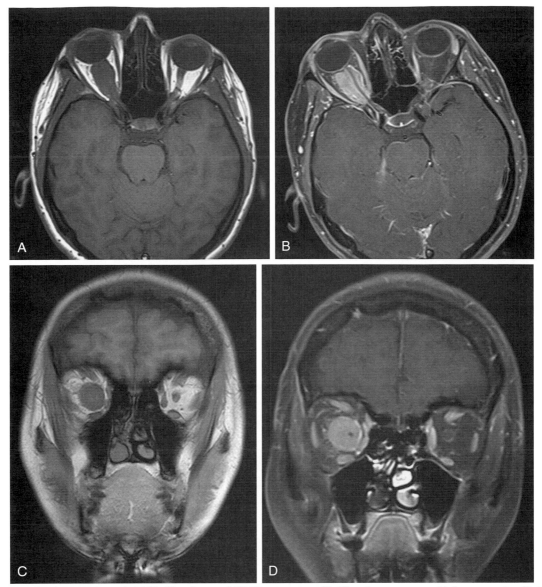

Fig. 15-2. MRI. Optic nerve sheath meningioma. Axial **(A, B)** and coronal **(C, D)** precontrast **(A, C)** and postcontrast with fat suppression **(B, D)** T1-weighted images showing the optic nerve surrounded by an enhancing meningioma.

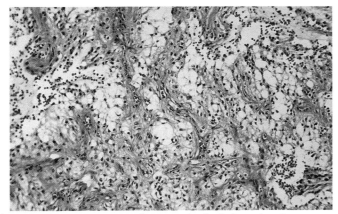

Fig. 15-3. Pilocytic astrocytoma demonstrating fascicular and cystic patterns.

PUPILLARY SYNDROMES

Horner's Syndrome

The sympathetic fibers destined for the eye pursue a tortuous but uncrossed pathway. Fibers innervating the sweat glands of the face pass with branches of the external carotid artery, except for those destined for a small area of the forehead, which accompany the internal carotid. Interruption of the sympathetic fibers to the eye leads to a combination of ptosis and miosis. Enophthalmos, which is apparent rather than real, is suggested by a narrowed palpebral fissure, the consequence of depression of the upper and elevation of the lower lids (upside-down ptosis). The miosis is relatively slight but can be accentuated by taking the patient into a darkened room. In the acute stages of a complete Horner's syndrome, the face is warm and the conjunctival vessels are dilated (Fig. 15-13).

Various pharmacologic agents have been used to localize the site of the lesion. As a screening test, 4% cocaine eye drops are instilled into both eyes. The normal pupil dilates, but the Horner's pupil fails to do so, irrespective of whether the lesion is preganglionic or postganglionic (Figs. 15-14 and 15-15). A 1% solution of hydroxyamphetamine releases noradrenaline at postganglionic nerve endings. Where these stores are depleted, as in a postganglionic sympathetic lesion, the pupil fails to dilate, but it will do so in preganglionic lesions, which have no effect on the stores (Fig. 15-16). Demonstration of pupillary supersensitivity in postganglionic lesions to dilute sympathomimetic agents is better achieved with 1% phenylephrine than with 1:1000 adrenaline.

If a Horner's syndrome is the sole clinical finding, there is little justification for investigation beyond performing a chest radiograph. Accompanying signs are likely if the syndrome is secondary to lateral medullary infarction, trauma, or tumors of the neck, or tumors of the lung apex.

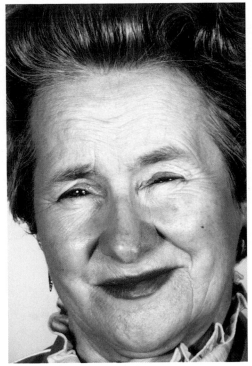

Fig. 15-61. Left hemifacial spasm.

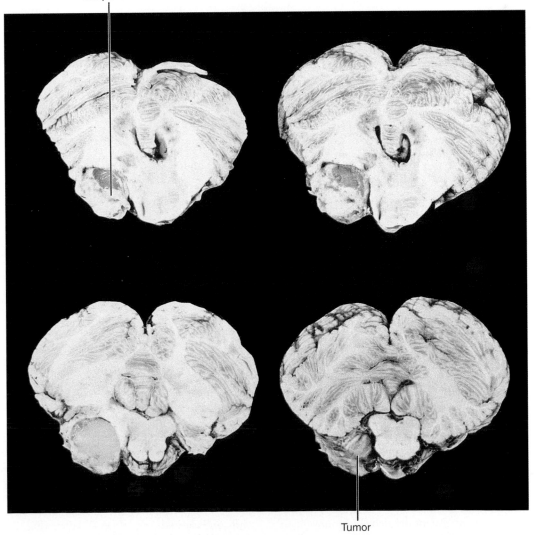

Fig. 15-62. Vestibular schwannoma. Sections at four levels between the medulla and the midbrain.

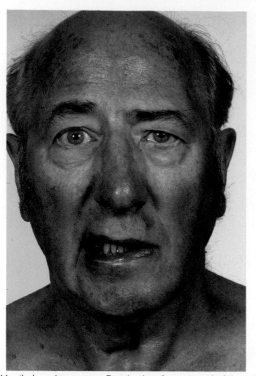

Fig. 15-63. Vestibular schwannoma. Facial palsy after removal of the schwannoma.

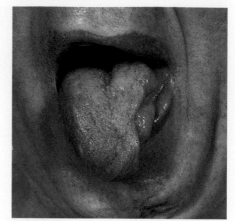

Fig. 15-64. Vestibular schwannoma. Atrophy of the left side of the tongue after a faciohypoglossal anastomosis.

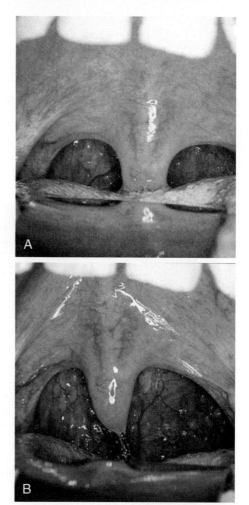

Fig. 15-65. Left tenth-nerve palsy. **A,** The left side of the soft palate is slightly depressed. **B,** The palate deviates to the right during phonation.

THE NINTH, TENTH, ELEVENTH, AND TWELFTH CRANIAL NERVES

The Ninth Cranial Nerve (Glossopharyngeal)

The glossopharyngeal nerve is predominantly sensory. Its function is best tested by applying a painful stimulus to the tonsillar fossa. Isolated lesions of the nerve are rare. In glossopharyngeal neuralgia, paroxysms of pain (analogous to the facial pains of trigeminal neuralgia) occur in the tongue or throat.

The Tenth Cranial Nerve

The tenth nerve is (or at least some of its components) are more readily assessed. It is responsible for the efferent component of the gag reflex. In a unilateral tenth-nerve palsy, the soft palate lies lower on the affected side and, along with the posterior pharyngeal wall, deviates to the intact side during phonation (Fig. 15-65). The vocal cord on the affected side lies fixed in a position midway between abduction and adduction, resulting in a slightly hoarse voice.

The Eleventh Cranial Nerve (Accessory)

The spinal component of the eleventh cranial nerve arises from the C1 to C4 segments and supplies sternomastoid and the upper fibers of the trapezius.

Lesions of the nerve outside the jugular foramen cause paralysis of the sternomastoid and the upper fibers of the trapezius, the lower half being spared because of its innervation by spinal segments C3 and C4 (Fig. 15-66).

The Twelfth Cranial Nerve (Hypoglossal)

A lesion of the hypoglossal nerve produces ipsilateral wasting and fasciculation of the tongue (Fig. 15-67). There is little effect on phonation or swallowing. Bilateral involvement of the tongue at the lower motor neuron level produces severe immobility. The problem is usually part of a bulbar palsy, with attendant deficiencies of movement in the palate, pharynx, and larynx, the consequence most commonly of motor neuron disease.

COMBINED CRANIAL NERVE PALSIES

The jugular foramen syndrome of Vernet is characterized by signs of damage to cranial nerves nine, ten, and eleven. One cause is the glomus jugulare tumor (paraganglioma of the glomus jugulare) arising from chemoreceptor cells found in the adventitia of the jugular vein, but also from the region of the middle ear, the tympanic branch of the glossopharyngeal nerve, and the postauricular branch of the vagus (Fig. 15-68). In the middle ear, the tumors produce deafness, often with vertigo and tinnitus together with facial weakness. With tumors in the region of the jugular foramen, palsies of the ninth, tenth, and eleventh cranial nerves ensue (Fig. 15-69). The proximity of such tumors to the twelfth nerve as it emerges from the anterior condylar canal explains the frequently coexisting hypoglossal palsy

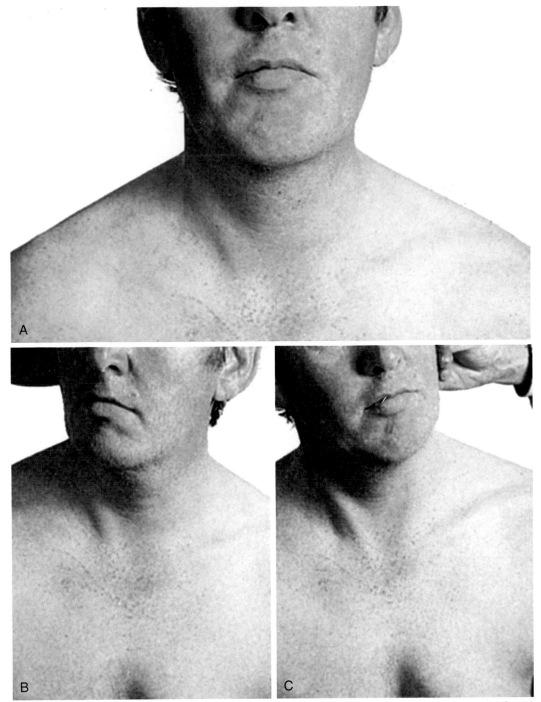

Fig. 15-66. Eleventh cranial nerve palsy. **A,** Wasting of the left sternomastoid. **B** and **C,** Failure to contract during neck rotation.

(Fig. 15-70). Positive staining of the tumors for chromogranin confirms their neurosecretory status.

Prominent vascular channels are a feature of these tumors and can be visualized by angiography. CT demonstrates the tumor and any associated bone erosion (Fig. 15-71). MRI demonstrates the tumor, which tends to display a mixture of hypointense and hyperintense signal on T2-weighted images (Fig. 15-72). Carcinomatous or lymphomatous meningitis commonly affects multiple cranial nerves. Those particularly involved include the optic, oculomotor, and seventh cranial nerves (Fig. 15-73). Multiple cranial nerve palsies in cancer patients may also reflect skull-base metastases or the result of direct invasion by nasopharyngeal carcinoma. CT scanning in carcinomatous meningitis demonstrates effacement of the basal cisterns and sulci, with their enhancement after contrast injection. Rarely, inflammatory or viral illnesses may produce a picture of acute multiple cranial neuropathies.

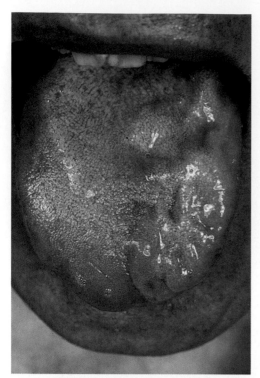

Fig. 15-67. Left twelfth-nerve palsy.

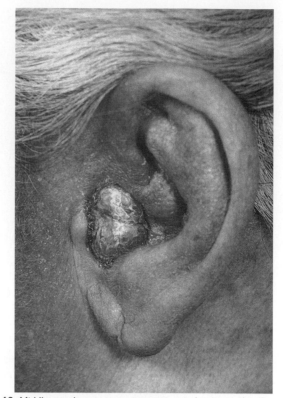

Fig. 15-68. Middle ear glomus tumor presenting at the external auditory meatus.

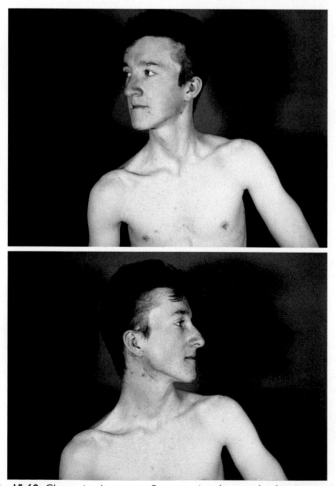

Fig. 15-69. Glomus jugulare tumor. Postoperative photographs showing wasting of the right sternomastoid.

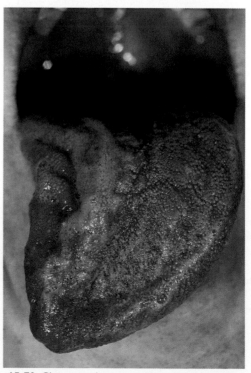

Fig. 15-70. Glomus jugulare tumor. Hypoglossal nerve paresis.

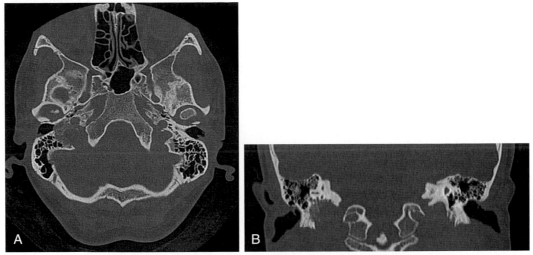

Fig. 15-71. Glomus jugulare tumor. Axial **(A)** and coronal **(B)** CT images. Note loss of cortex in right jugular fossa.

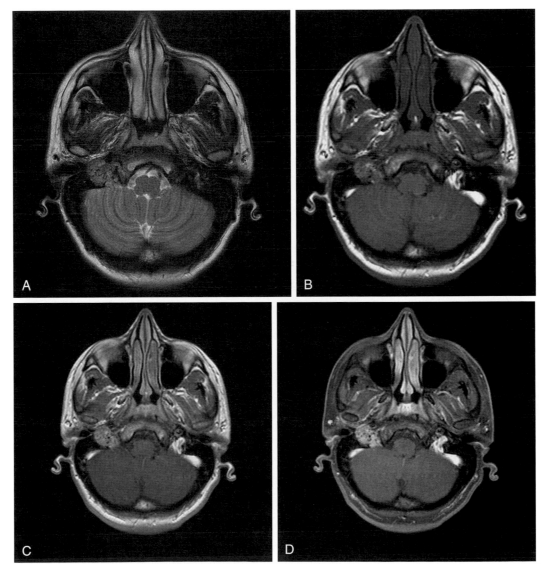

Fig. 15-72. Glomus jugulare tumor in the patient seen in Fig. 15-71. MRI. Axial T2-weighted **(A)**, T1-weighted **(B)**, postcontrast T1-weighted **(C)**, and postcontrast T1-weighted with fat suppression **(D)**. Note enhancing mass in the right jugular fossa with flow voids.

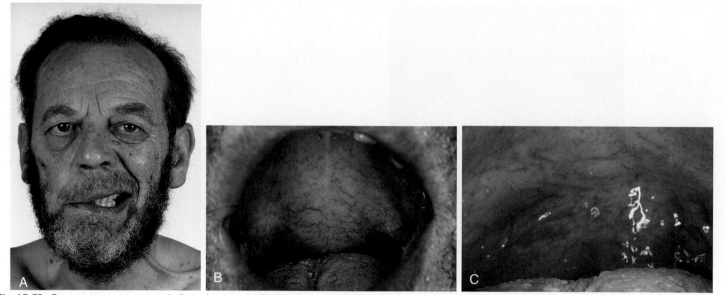

Fig. 15-73. Carcinomatous meningitis. **A,** Right facial paresis. **B,** The position of the palate at rest. **C,** The position of the palate during phonation. There is a right palatal palsy.

NEUROLOGIC ASPECTS OF SYSTEMIC DISEASE

RADIATION DAMAGE

Irradiation damage to the brain parenchyma occurs as an acute, early delayed, or late phenomenon. The acute reaction is more likely when large masses have been treated, using large dosages. It is managed by dexamethasone, best given prophylactically.

An early delayed syndrome appears a few months after completing treatment and manifests on imaging as worsening edema with increased mass effect. Inevitably, it is difficult to distinguish from tumor recurrence. The problem resolves spontaneously whether or not corticosteroid therapy is used, but resection of the affected tissues may be necessary to avoid herniation and alleviate other neurologic sequelae of the mass effect. Resected tissues are edematous, often with infiltrating tumor cells if a glioma was the target of the radiation therapy, and some vessels may show fibrinoid degeneration and thrombosis.

Delayed focal necrosis appears usually within 2 to 3 years of therapy with conventional dosages of external beam radiation therapy, and more rapidly after stereotactic radiosurgery or brachytherapy. The incidence rises to some 10% of patients with malignant gliomas who survive for a year or more and have received standard fractionated radiotherapy. The white matter is principally affected. Blood vessels are particularly targeted, with vascular wall thickening with hyalinosis, focal fibrinoid degeneration of vascular walls with thrombosis, and microhemorrhage plus a reactive vascular proliferation. The vascular damage results in secondary infarction, and a direct effect on glial tissue culminates in demyelination of the white matter (Fig. 16-1).

The problem presents as a slowly evolving mass lesion. The area is associated with edema and may be difficult to distinguish on imaging from a primary neoplasm. With both CT and MRI, the changes are nonspecific, with mass effect, edema, and patchy enhancement (Fig. 16-2). On MR images, the lesions may show a sharp cutoff at the boundary of the irradiated area. Corticosteroids are sometimes helpful in relieving symptoms related to the edema, but in many cases surgical excision is necessary both for diagnosis and for symptom relief. Other imaging techniques, including fluorodeoxyglucose PET, SPECT, and MR spectroscopy, have been used to attempt the distinction from recurrent tumor, but none of these has been definitive when compared with diagnosis based on resected tissue. When the radiation has been given for a high-grade glioma, resected tissue shows a mixture of the radiation effect and progressive or recurrent tumor in almost all instances. When the radiation has been given for metastatic carcinoma or melanoma, recurrent tumor is found less often.

Besides focal necrosis, diffuse cerebral injury can result from irradiation, leading to diffuse atrophy associated with white matter signal change on MRI (Fig. 16-3). Few patients survive long enough for this pattern to emerge. The changes are likely to be accompanied by evidence of cognitive decline. Child and infant brains are more sensitive to the effects of radiotherapy than adult brains.

RADIATION DAMAGE TO EXTRACRANIAL VESSELS

Radiation-induced occlusive disease of the carotid and vertebral arteries in the neck has been reported in patients treated with radiotherapy for a variety of carcinomas or lymphomas affecting the neck

area. Typically, there are multiple sites of arterial narrowing or occlusion, with a distribution different from that seen with atheromatous disease (Fig. 16-4).

The patients present with a variety of cerebrovascular syndromes after a median period of 15 to 20 years. Damage to intracranial vessels can also occur, typically involving the supraclinoid portion of the internal carotid artery or the proximal middle cerebral artery. In some cases, the affected vessels become ectatic and tortuous.

ALCOHOL AND THE NERVOUS SYSTEM

Quite apart from the effects of acute intoxication, various central and peripheral nervous system disorders are associated with chronic alcohol abuse. Scanning of some alcoholics reveals ventricular dilation and enlargement of the cortical sulci, changes that may be at least partly reversible after a period of abstinence (Fig. 16-5). Better defined, both clinically and pathologically, is a cerebellar syndrome in which there is depletion of Purkinje cells, predominantly in the anterior and superior vermis (Fig. 16-6). Scanning demonstrates the distribution of the atrophic process (Fig. 16-7). Typically, the patient presents with gait ataxia and relatively normal upper limb coordination. Nystagmus is not conspicuous.

The Wernicke-Korsakoff syndrome is particularly associated with alcoholism, although the same disorder can result from a deficiency of thiamine induced, for example, by prolonged vomiting. In the acute stages, the lesions, sometimes hemorrhagic, are distributed in the mammillary bodies, the periaqueductal gray matter of the midbrain, the floor of the fourth ventricle, and the periventricular parts of the thalamus and hypothalamus (Fig. 16-8). The maximal changes are found in the mammillary bodies, which later become atrophic (Fig. 16-9, *A*), accompanied by atrophy of the periaqueductal gray matter and other structures (see Fig. 16-9, *B*). Microscopic features include patchy cell necrosis, but with some sparing of neuronal cell bodies, astrocytic and microglial proliferation, hemorrhages, and, in some cases, vascular proliferation (Fig. 16-10).

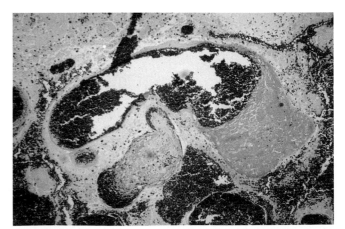

Fig. 16-1. Radionecrosis. Necrotic vessel with extensive fibrinoid degeneration of its wall (H&E, ×25).

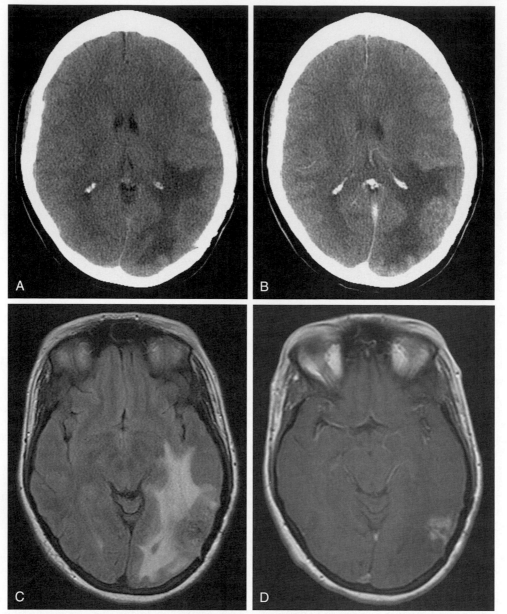

Fig. 16-2. Radionecrosis: edema and irregular enhancement. CT scans before **(A)** and after **(B)** contrast enhancement. **C**, FLAIR MRI. **D**, T1-weighted MRI after contrast enhancement.

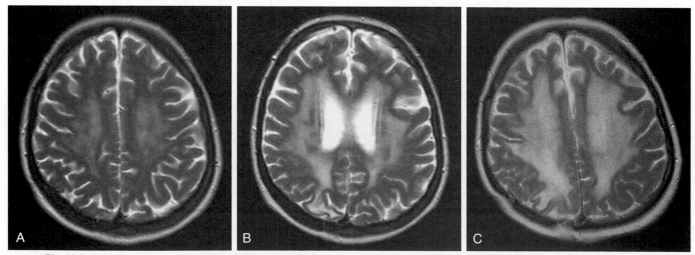

Fig. 16-3. Radionecrosis. Axial T2-weighted MRI showing effects of radiotherapy on white matter at 1 year **(A)**, 4 years **(B)**, and 7 years **(C)**.

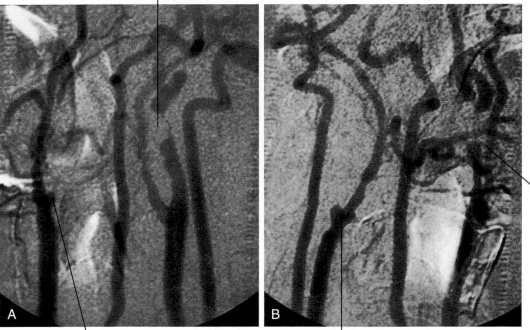

Left internal
carotid stenosis

Left internal
carotid stenosis

A

B

Right carotid
occlusion

Right carotid
occlusion

Fig. 16-4. Irradiation damage of the neck vessels after therapy for carcinoma of the thyroid. **A,** the right internal carotid is occluded soon after its origin. **B,** The left internal carotid has a distal stenotic segment.

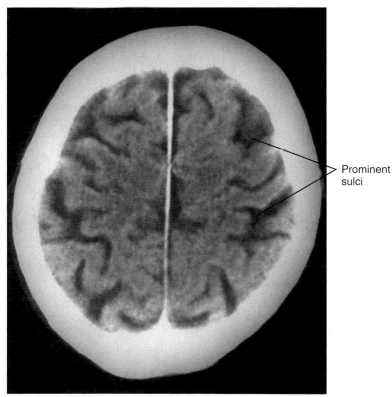

Prominent
sulci

Fig. 16-5. Chronic alcoholism. CT demonstrating cortical sulcal enlargement.

Typically, the condition comprises ophthalmoplegia, ataxia, and a disturbance of orientation. The ophthalmoplegia consists of lateral rectus or horizontal gaze palsies, combined with nystagmus in both the horizontal and vertical planes (Fig. 16-11). The ataxia predominantly affects gait and reflects a pathologic process that, like the isolated alcoholic cerebellar syndrome, principally affects the superior cerebellar vermis. In fact, some patients have concomitant alcoholic cerebellar degeneration, and some authors consider the cerebellar pathology as part of the Wernicke's disease spectrum. Typically, the patient is drowsy, confused, and amnesic. With recovery, an amnestic syndrome emerges with impairment of recent memory but relatively intact intellectual function. A confabulatory element has been over-emphasized. Early, vigorous treatment with thiamine is particularly successful in reversing the ophthalmoplegia but less so in returning memory to normal. Scanning identifies the hemorrhagic lesions in some cases (Fig. 16-12).

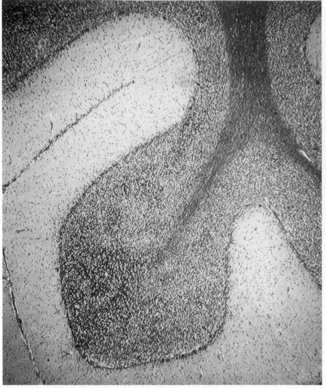

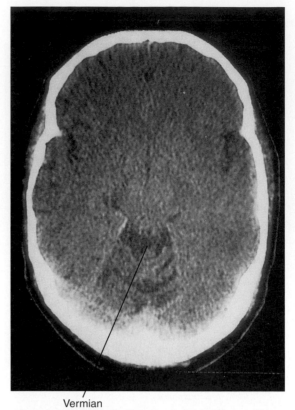

Fig. 16-6. Alcoholic cerebellar degeneration. Reduction of granule and Purkinje cells with replacement gliosis (Luxol fast blue, H&E, ×40).

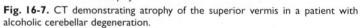

Vermian atrophy

Fig. 16-7. CT demonstrating atrophy of the superior vermis in a patient with alcoholic cerebellar degeneration.

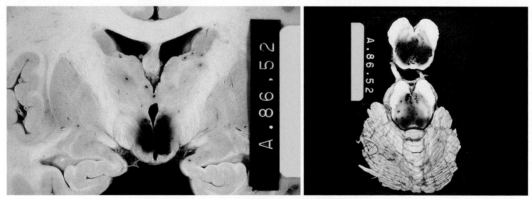

Fig. 16-8. Wernicke-Korsakoff syndrome. **A,** Coronal section of brain through mammillary bodies showing hemorrhages extending up from the mammillary bodies along the sides of the third ventricle. **B,** Hemorrhages extending through the midbrain.

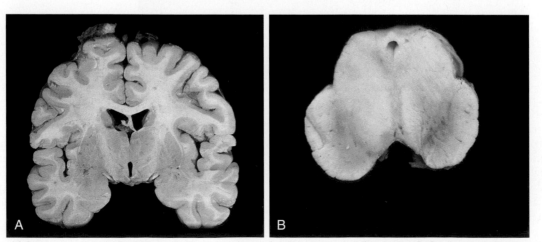

Fig. 16-9. Wernicke-Korsakoff syndrome. **A,** Small, shrunken, and slightly dark mammillary bodies. **B,** Small periaqueductal cavity.

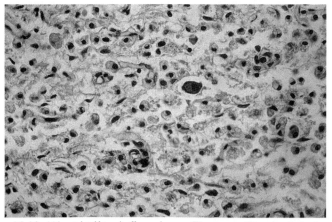

Fig. 16-10. Wernicke-Korsakoff syndrome. The mammillary body is largely replaced by a sheet of macrophages, mixed with proliferating capillaries but containing a surviving normal neuron (Luxol fast blue, H&E).

CENTRAL PONTINE MYELINOLYSIS

Central pontine myelinolysis occurs in a number of conditions, although in the early reports, the condition was confined to alcoholics. Important, though not inevitable in the pathogenesis of the condition, is a hyponatremic state that has been corrected overrapidly. Postmortem examination demonstrates discoloration of the basis pontis (Fig. 16-13), microscopy of which reveals demyelination with relative axonal sparing and an absence of any inflammatory reaction (Fig. 16-14).

The condition occurs both in alcoholics and in individuals with serious medical disorders or substantial malnourishment. After initial recovery, as hyponatremia is reversed, secondary deterioration occurs, with quadriparesis combined with dysphagia and dysarthria. Tegmental pontine involvement results in various defects of horizontal eye movement. Survival may lead to a locked-in state.

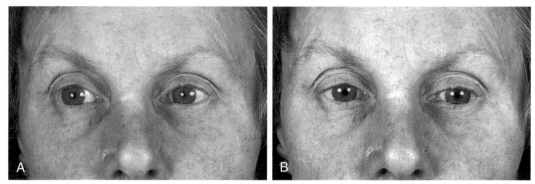

Fig. 16-11. Wernicke-Korsakoff syndrome. Partial horizontal gaze paresis, more marked to the left. **A,** Gaze to the right. **B,** Gaze to the left.

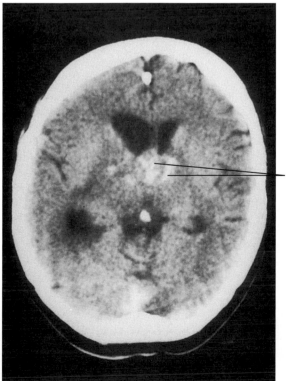

Fig. 16-12. Wernicke-Korsakoff syndrome. CT demonstrating thalamichemorrhages.

Thalamic hemorrhages

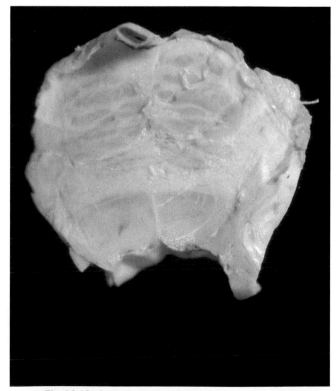

Fig. 16-13. Central pontine myelinolysis. Gross specimen.

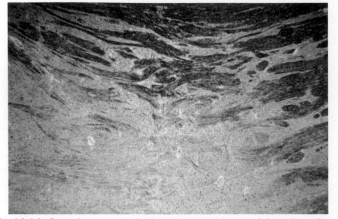

Fig. 16-14. Central pontine myelinolysis, showing the central demyelinated zone (Luxol fast blue, H&E, ×6).

Extrapontine myelinolysis accompanies these features, in some cases with lesions at various sites including the cerebellum, lateral geniculate body, external capsule, and hippocampus. The clinical picture in such cases is correspondingly complex and includes a variety of movement disorders.

Imaging with MRI reveals hyperintense lesions on T2-weighted and hypointense lesions on T1-weighted images (Fig. 16-15).

Prognosis is generally poor, although some patients make a complete recovery. There is no firm evidence that an effective therapy exists for this condition.

MARCHIAFAVA-BIGNAMI DISEASE

Marchiafava-Bignami disease is virtually confined to alcoholics. Pathologically, there is extensive demyelination and axonal damage to the corpus callosum, along with the central white matter of the cerebral hemispheres together with the optic chiasm and the middle cerebellar peduncles. No specific clinical picture corresponds to the pathologic changes, although frontal lobe features are often prominent. Imaging displays the extensive white matter changes (Fig. 16-16).

The peripheral nerve and muscle disorders associated with alcoholism have been described elsewhere.

THE NEUROLOGY OF ENDOCRINE DISEASE

PITUITARY DISORDERS

The visual symptoms and signs associated with pituitary tumors have been discussed elsewhere. Patients with acromegaly eventually develop muscle weakness and wasting, although muscle biopsy changes are often not conspicuous. The creatine kinase activity may be mildly elevated. Carpal tunnel syndrome is a recognized complication of acromegaly. Infrequently, a diffuse hypertrophic demyelinating neuropathy is encountered.

ADRENAL DISORDERS

The myopathy associated with Cushing's disease (or corticosteroid therapy) is considered in Chapter 3. At least 50% of patients with Cushing's syndrome have muscle weakness. In patients who have had bilateral adrenalectomy for Cushing's syndrome, a marked elevation of serum adrenocorticotropic hormone levels may follow, associated with hyperpigmentation and proximal muscle weakness—Nelson's syndrome (Fig. 16-17).

In Cushing's syndrome itself, the myopathy is of gradual onset in the majority, although a variant with acute onset and muscle pain is recognized. Typically, the pelvic girdle muscles are those principally affected (Fig. 16-18). Although muscle weakness is a prominent symptom of Addison's disease, a specific myopathy has not been described.

THYROID DISORDERS

Thyrotoxicosis is associated with muscle weakness in about three quarters of the patients. Light microscopy changes on muscle biopsy are often inconspicuous, and the more evident changes on EMG are nonspecific. Serum creatine kinase levels are usually normal. Many patients with hypothyroidism complain of muscle cramps or weakness. A true myopathy is rare and is reversed along with the facial changes of the condition by treatment of the thyroid deficiency (Fig. 16-19).

Hoffman's syndrome consists of muscle hypertrophy, pain, and slowness of movement in adults with hypothyroidism. The muscles dimple excessively on percussion in a manner resembling myotonia.

A diffuse neuropathy had been described rarely in thyrotoxicosis but more frequently in hypothyroidism, then taking the form of a predominant sensory syndrome with peripheral nerve demyelination and slowed conduction velocities. Hypothyroidism is also associated with the carpal tunnel and tarsal tunnel syndromes.

Dysthyroid eye disease is said to be the commonest cause of diplopia in middle-aged individuals. The patient has evidence of lid retraction or lid lag, or both (Fig. 16-20). Typically, there appears to be a defect of elevation, suggesting a superior rectus palsy (Fig. 16-21). Further assessment reveals that the apparent palsy is caused by tethering of the inferior rectus in the orbit. Less commonly, other orbital muscles are involved in the fibrotic reaction. Tests of thyroid function frequently reveal a euthyroid state. Thyroid-stimulating immunoglobulins are present in most patients. The abnormally expanded muscle is readily demonstrated by CT scanning or MRI of the orbits (Fig. 16-22). More recently, a steroid-responsive encephalitis associated with autoimmune thyroid disease has been described.

PARATHYROID DISORDERS AND ABNORMALITIES OF CALCIUM METABOLISM

Muscle pain and stiffness occur in primary hyperparathyroidism, but actual weakness is very uncommon. Patients with osteomalacic myopathy have muscle and skeletal pains, proximal muscle weakness, and bony tenderness. The alkaline phosphatase level is markedly elevated, with a normal or depressed calcium concentration. Muscle biopsy may reveal type II fiber atrophy. Radiographs may reveal looser zones (Fig. 16-23).

PAGET'S DISEASE

In Paget's disease, abnormal osteoclastic activity leads to both increased bone resorption and, secondarily, increased new bone formation. Neurologic complications follow bone fracture or result from direct compression of neural tissue by either abnormal bone or bone that has undergone malignant transformation. The skull is affected in about half the cases, the changes being earlier and more readily detectable by CT than by conventional radiology (Fig. 16-24). Bone scintigraphy demonstrates the extent of the bone lesions and can be used to monitor the effects of treatment (Fig. 16-25).

Cranial nerve palsies result from compression in the skull exit foramina and particularly affect the eighth nerve. Deformity of the skull base, with softening, leads to invagination of the odontoid process and secondary compression of the brainstem and cerebellum. Hydrocephalus follows in some cases. Spinal involvement is usually multifocal (see Chapter 14).

PANCREATIC DISEASE

Insulinomas are rare, with an incidence around 1 in 1,000,000 of the population. Symptoms are likely to appear when plasma glucose concentrations fall below 2.5 mmol/L. Neurologic symptoms,

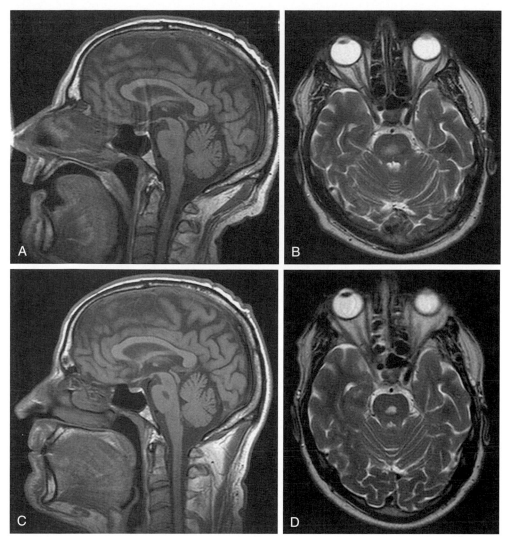

Fig. 16-15. Central pontine myelinolysis. Sagittal T1-weighted MRI **(A, C)** and axial T2-weighted MRI **(B, D)** at presentation **(A, B)** and after 1 month **(C, D)** showing initial ill-defined central pontine edema resolving to a well-defined lesion.

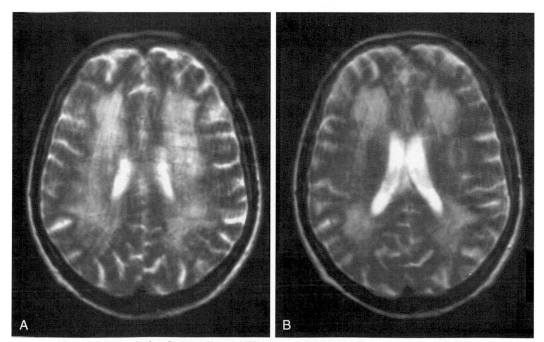

Fig. 16-16. Marchiafava-Bignami disease. MRI demonstrating extensive white matter signal change.

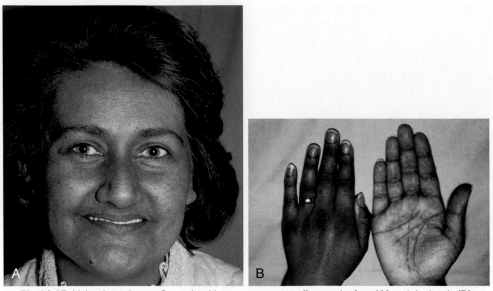

Fig. 16-17. Nelson's syndrome. Generalized hyperpigmentation affecting the face **(A)** and the hands **(B)**.

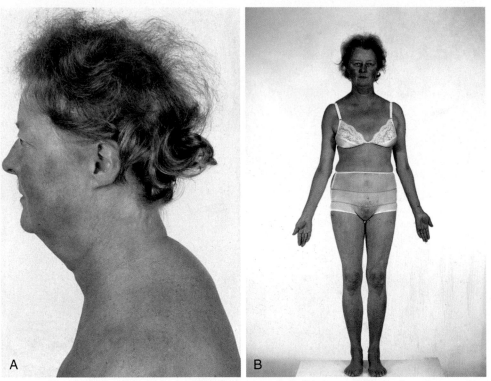

Fig. 16-18. Cushing's syndrome, clinical appearance. **A,** Buffalo hump. **B,** Proximal wasting.

which are typically episodic, include drowsiness, altered behavior, brainstem manifestations, seizures, and focal deficits, suggesting a cerebrovascular event. Many patients develop symptoms during a 24-hour fast, and virtually all become symptomatic during a 72-hour fast.

The hypoglycemia is accompanied by inappropriate hyperinsulinemia (proinsulinemia and C-peptidemia). Localization of the tumor, at operation, is aided by the use of intraoperative ultrasound. Imaging techniques tend to be unreliable. Distal pancreatectomy is performed if the tumor is in the tail of the gland (Fig. 16-26).

NEUROLOGIC FEATURES OF VASCULITIS

In vasculitic disorders, there is evidence of inflammation and necrosis of blood vessels, including both arteries and veins. Both the peripheral and central nervous system can be affected. Some of the vasculitic

syndromes are associated with granuloma formation. Some of the conditions under this umbrella are summarized in Box 16-1.

SYSTEMIC NECROTIZING VASCULITIS

This group includes polyarteritis nodosa (PAN), allergic angiitis with granulomatosis (Churg-Strauss syndrome), and an intermediate form. In PAN, there is inflammation with lymphocytes and macrophages or histiocytes of small and medium-sized arteries in many different organs. Histologic features include a chronic inflammatory cell infiltration, internal elastic lamina proliferation, and fibrinoid necrosis of the vessel wall. Neurologic complications occur in at least 50% of patients with PAN and include mononeuritis multiplex, sensorimotor neuropathy, radiculopathy, and brachial plexopathy. Some of these reflect occlusion of the vasa nervorum. CNS involvement takes the form of infarction of the brain or spinal cord, or an encephalopathic syndrome embracing altered cognition with seizures. Involvement of

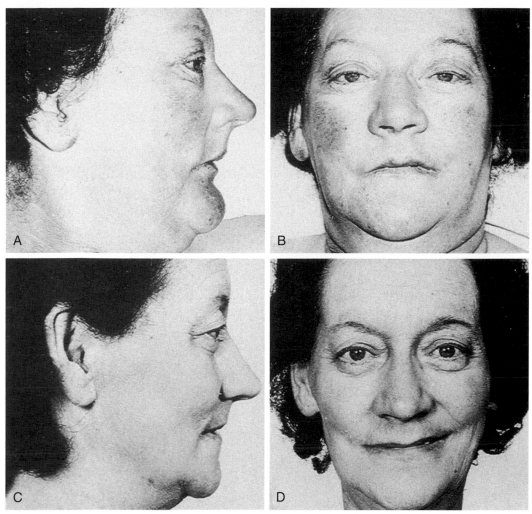

Fig. 16-19. Myxedema. Facial appearance before **(A, B)** and after **(C, D)** replacement therapy.

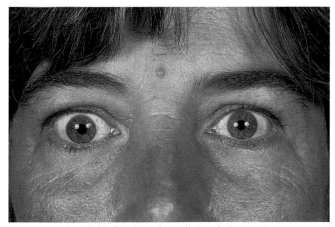

Fig. 16-20. Dysthyroid eye disease. Lid retraction.

the visual pathway by the ischemic process is common. The neurologic features of Churg-Strauss syndrome are similar: pathologically, there is a prominent component of eosinophils among the inflammatory cells. Leukocytoclastic vasculitides have a number of triggers and are characterized by acute inflammation with polymorphonuclear leukocytes involving both small arteries and veins.

HYPERSENSITIVITY VASCULITIDES

In hypersensitivity vasculitides, there is polymorphonuclear leukocyte infiltration of the walls of small vessels and postcapillary venules, particularly in the skin. As a consequence, fibrinoid necrosis,

microinfarction, and hemorrhages appear. Drug reactions are included in this category.

Types I, II, and III cryoglobulinemia are defined on the basis of whether the circulating cryoglobulin is of IgM or IgG type, mixed, or with activity against polyclonal IgG. A hyperviscosity state with secondary vascular wall damage results in various ischemic manifestations of the central and peripheral nervous systems.

SYSTEMIC GRANULOMATOUS VASCULITIDES

The prime example of systemic granulomatous vasculitides is Wegener's granulomatosis. The initial lesion in Wegener's is a focus of granular necrosis with fibrinoid degeneration, accompanied by polymorphonuclear leukocytes, histiocytes, and giant cells. The upper respiratory tract and the kidneys are particularly targeted. Segmental fibrinoid necrosis follows (Fig. 16-27).

The condition typically begins in the upper respiratory tract with a nonspecific granulomatous rhinitis or sinusitis. The condition progresses to bony destruction of the nasal bones, sinuses, and sometimes the orbits. Focal extension of these masses into the orbit or the middle or posterior cranial fossae account for many of the neurologic complications. Saddle-nose deformity is common (Fig. 16-28) and is associated with abnormalities on bone scanning (Fig. 16-29). At this stage of the disease, granulomatous masses are often visible on chest radiograph.

Neurologic complications appear in up to half the patients. In addition to the effect of direct invasion by granulomatous tissue, remote granuloma may appear in individual cranial nerves or in the cerebrum. Vasculitis accounts for the other neurologic complications, including cerebral infarction, intracerebral or subarachnoid hemorrhage, and

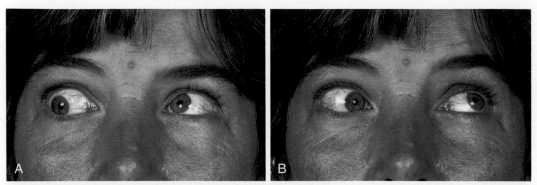

Fig. 16-21. Dysthyroid eye disease. **A,** Impaired dexro-elevation of right eye and **B,** Depressed Laevo-elevation of the right eye associated with bilateral lid retraction.

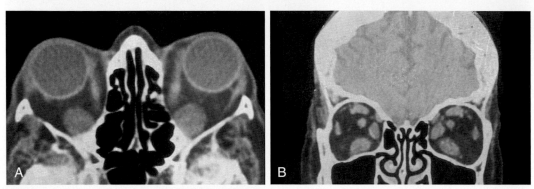

Fig. 16-22. Dysthyroid eye disease. CT of the orbit. **A,** Axial view. **B,** Coronal view. The principal muscles affected are the medial and inferior recti.

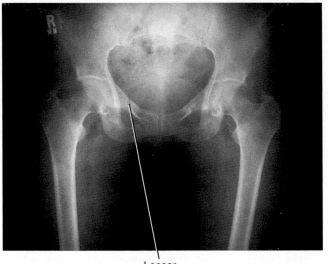

Looser
zone

Fig. 16-23. Osteomalacia. Looser zone on a pelvic radiograph.

ischemic optic neuropathy. Typically, the peripheral nervous system is affected in the form of mononeuritis multiplex, polyneuritis, or radiculitis. Antiproteinase-3 antibodies are almost invariably present in untreated active Wegener's granulomatosis.

Granulomatous Angiitis
Granulomatous angiitis is a rare disorder sometimes triggered by zoster infection and characterized by an inflammatory reaction confined to vessels of the CNS. Leptomeningeal arterioles and venules are particularly affected by an often patchy inflammatory process containing lymphocytes, plasma cells, and granulomas associated with multinucleate giant cells (Fig. 16-30). In some cases, zoster viral particles have been demonstrated in the lesions by immunohistochemistry or electron microscopy. Larger cerebral vessels can be affected, and this may produce classic infarcts in specific arterial territories. Clinical features

include headache, intellectual change, and focal signs. The erythrocyte sedimentation rate is sometimes elevated, and a CSF pleocytosis with an elevated protein concentration is almost inevitable. Besides an association with zoster infection, the condition has been described in association with lymphoma, sarcoidosis, and HIV infection. Angiography may demonstrate focal areas of narrowing and dilatation of the intracranial vessels. The condition is treated with steroids, sometimes with the addition of cyclophosphamide, and, when zoster is the cause, with high dosages of acyclovir or ganciclovir.

CONNECTIVE TISSUE DISORDERS

SYSTEMIC LUPUS ERYTHEMATOSUS

Vasculitis with disruption of the vessel wall is rare in systemic lupus erythematosus (SLE). When present, it consists of a fibrinoid necrosis of small arteries, arterioles, and capillaries. Nonvasculitic vasculopathy is likely to be caused by circulating antiphospholipid antibodies (IgG and IgM) that possess procoagulant activity. Anticardiolipin antibodies are present in more than 50% of patients, and high titers increase the risk of occlusive cerebrovascular disease (Fig. 16-31).

Other neurologic features include headache, psychiatric disorders, seizures, cranial or peripheral nerve disorders, spinal cord syndromes, and movement disorders (Fig. 16-32). The movement disorders described include a parkinsonian-like state, hemiballismus, and chorea. The peripheral nerve syndromes are similar to those seen in PAN, although, in addition, a Guillain-Barré syndrome has been described (Fig. 16-33) in patients with neurologic disease. CSF abnormalities include an elevated cell count and protein concentration, abnormal IgG indices, oligoclonal IgG, and decreased C4 levels.

SCLERODERMA

In scleroderma, there is extensive microvasculopathy, with tissue fibrosis affecting a variety of organs, including the skin, gut, lungs, and heart (Fig. 16-34). Neurologic manifestations include headache, encephalopathy, and seizures. Limited cutaneous systemic sclerosis,

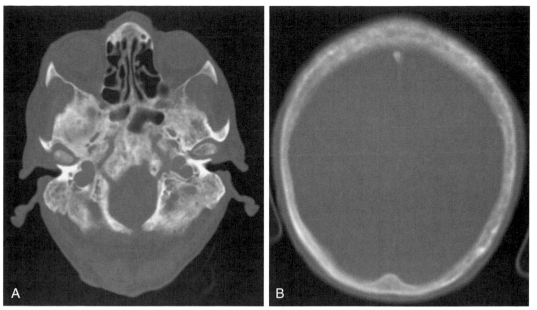

Fig. 16-24. Paget's disease of the skull. CT appearances of skull base **(A)** and vault **(B)**.

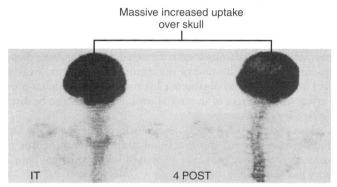

Massive increased uptake over skull

IT   4 POST

Fig. 16-25. Paget's disease. Abnormal isotope bone scan.

or the CREST syndrome (*c*alcinosis cutis, *R*aynaud's phenomenon, *e*sophageal dysfunction, *s*clerodactyly, and *t*elangiectasia) (Fig. 16-35).

A systemic necrotizing arteritis occurs rarely in scleroderma or CREST syndrome and can lead to stroke (Fig. 16-36). Anticentromere and antitopoisomerase or anti-RNA polymerase III antibodies are present in most patients with scleroderma.

SJÖGREN'S SYNDROME

Sjögren's syndrome is characterized by a mononuclear infiltrative process affecting the lacrimal and salivary glands and resulting in xerophthalmia and xerostomia. Other organs affected include the thyroid, lung, and kidney. Most reports of neurologic involvement have stressed peripheral nerve damage, but the CNS is not immune. In some cases, CNS manifestations are the first declaration of the disease. Both cerebral and spinal involvement occur. Clinical features include hemiparesis, focal seizures, cerebellar signs, and internuclear ophthalmoplegia. A diffuse meningoencephalitic syndrome occurs, associated with a CSF pleocytosis in which polymorphonuclear leukocytes predominate. Imaging demonstrates focal infarction in those with cerebral involvement. Damage to the nervous system probably results principally from a vasculitis syndrome. Typically, antibodies are found against the cellular ribonucleoprotein antigens Ro and La. The former are found more frequently, but the latter are more specific.

Peripheral nerve complications have been more fully documented than central ones and include trigeminal sensory neuropathy, mononeuritis multiplex, and a sensory polyneuropathy. The last can result in a profound sensory disorder analogous to that encountered as a paraneoplastic syndrome. An autonomic neuropathy (including

Adie's pupils), which may be silent, accompanies the sensory disorder in up to half the cases. The CSF is usually normal. Examination of dorsal root ganglia reveals infiltration by mononuclear cells accompanied by a varying degree of neuronal loss. Peripheral nerves show loss of large myelinated fibers. As with the CNS complications, some patients with this type of peripheral nervous system damage may have, at the time of presentation, little evidence of a sicca syndrome. The course of the disease and the speed of its development are very variable, and the response to treatment is uncertain.

BEHÇET'S DISEASE

Behçet's disease is diagnosed on the basis of recurrent orogenital ulceration occurring in association with evidence of ocular inflammation. Other features include thrombophlebitis, gastroenteritis, and cutaneous vasculitis. Pathologically there is leukocytoclastic vasculitis with or without fibrinoid necrosis, together with perivascular lymphocytic infiltration.

Neurologic complications occur in up to a quarter of patients. Although isolated headache is seen in a higher proportion, virtually all patients with neurologic involvement have evidence of an aseptic meningitis accompanied by a CSF pleocytosis and an elevated protein concentration. Focal neurologic features include seizures, motor and cerebellar signs, paraplegia, cerebral venous thrombosis, and ocular palsies. The brainstem is the site most often affected by focal disease (Fig. 16-37).

Imaging is virtually always abnormal in patients with neurologic disease. Findings include focal lesions, cortical and cerebellar atrophy, and evidence of sagittal sinus thrombosis. Patchy or homogeneous enhancement of the focal lesions is usual in the active stages of the disease. The imaging abnormalities tend to resolve as the symptoms subside (Fig. 16-38).

VASCULITIS ASSOCIATED WITH INFECTION

In herpes zoster ophthalmicus, a delayed contralateral hemiparesis may occur as a result of a granulomatous vasculitis ipsilateral to the skin eruption. Other infective agents associated with vasculitis include *Treponema pallidum* and *Borrelia burgdorferi*.

SARCOIDOSIS

Neurologic complications occur in about 5% of patients with sarcoidosis. Rarely, the disease is confined to the nervous system. Pathologically, there are nonnecrotizing granulomas, containing epithelioid

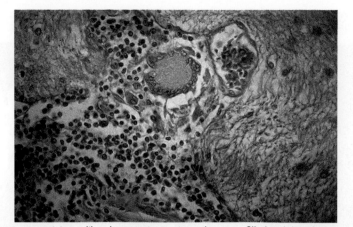

Fig. 16-30. Granulomatous angiitis. White matter containing a dilated serpentine perivascular space filled with lymphocytes and a multinucleated giant cell (H&E, ×100).

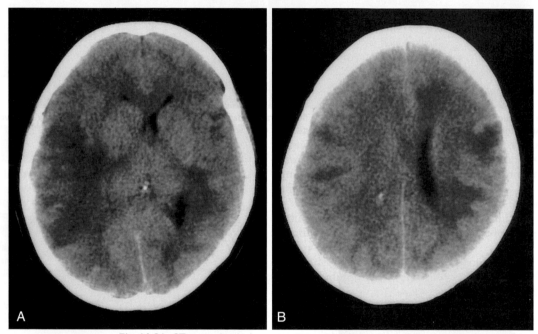

Fig. 16-31. CT at two levels demonstrating multiple infarction in SLE.

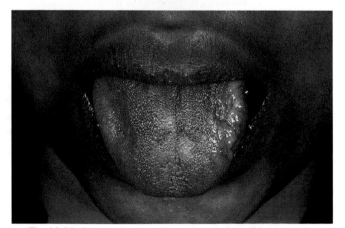

Fig. 16-32. Systemic lupus erythematosus. Left twelfth-nerve palsy.

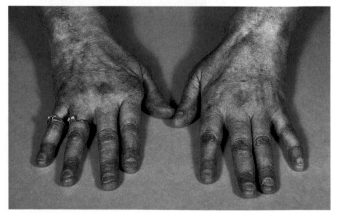

Fig. 16-33. Systemic lupus erythematosus. Wasting of the small hand muscles.

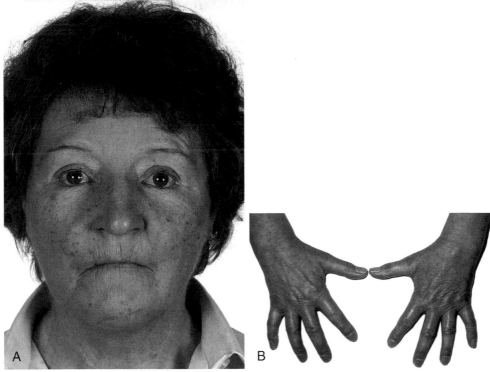

Fig. 16-34. Scleroderma. Facial and hand appearance.

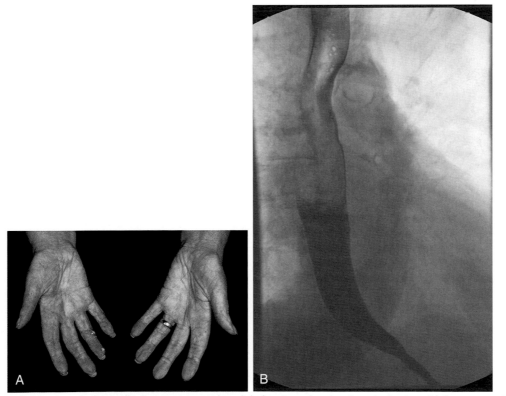

Fig. 16-35. CREST syndrome (calcinosis cutis, *Raynaud's* phenomenon, esophageal dysfunction, sclerodactyly, and telangiectasia). Appearance of the hands **A,** and of the esophagus on barium swallow **B,** Note smooth dilatation with residue of food in lumen due to dysmotility.

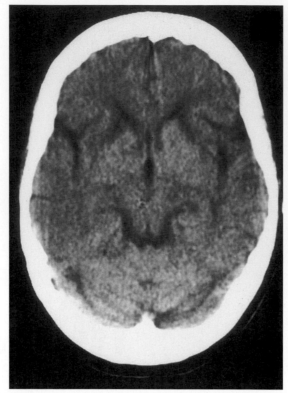

Fig. 16-36. CREST syndrome (*calcinosis* cutis, *Raynaud's* phenomenon, *esophageal* dysfunction, *sclerodactyly*, and *telangiectasia*). CT demonstrating bilateral caudate infarcts.

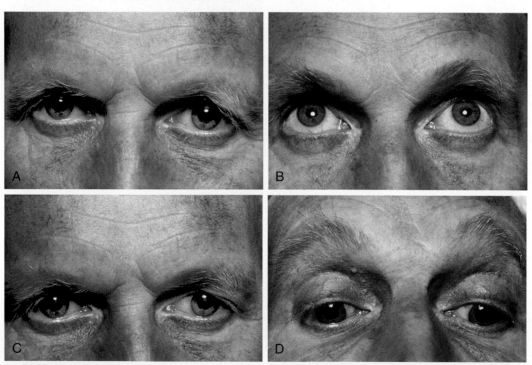

Fig. 16-37. Neuro-Behçet's disease. There is a bilateral horizontal gaze paresis **(A, C)** with preserved vertical gaze **(B, D)**.

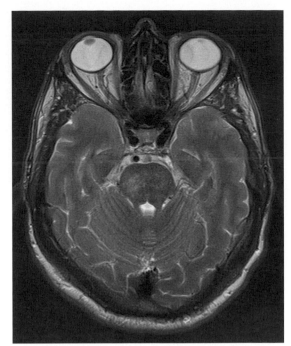

Fig. 16-38. Neuro-Behçet's disease. MRI demonstrating brainstem lesions.

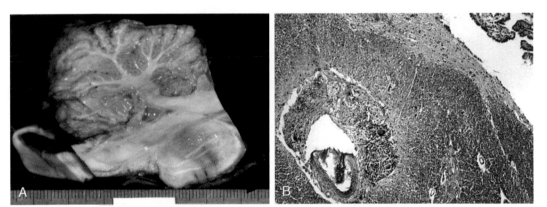

Fig. 16-39. Neurosarcoidosis. **A,** Granulomatous mass blocking the lower fourth ventricle. **B,** Granuloma in the roof of the temporal horn (Luxol fast blue, H&E, ×100).

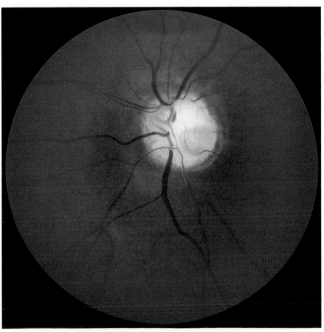

Fig. 16-40. Sarcoidosis. Optic atrophy.

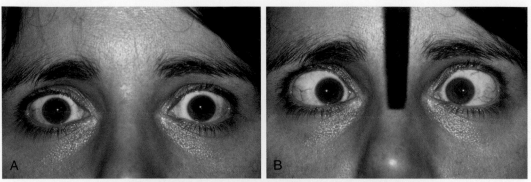

Fig. 16-41. Sarcoidosis. Partial right iridoplegia. **A,** Dilated pupil. **B,** Incomplete near response.

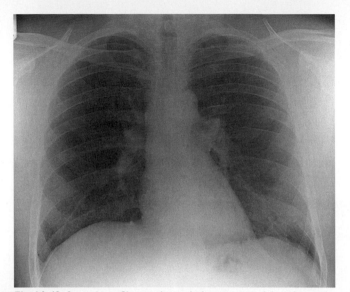

Fig. 16-42. Sarcoidosis. Chest radiograph demonstrating hilar adenopathy.

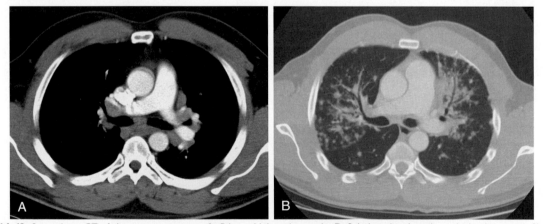

Fig. 16-43. Sarcoidosis. CT of chest in two patients. **A,** Bilateral hilar adenopathy. **B,** Subpleural and peribronchial pulmonary infiltrates.

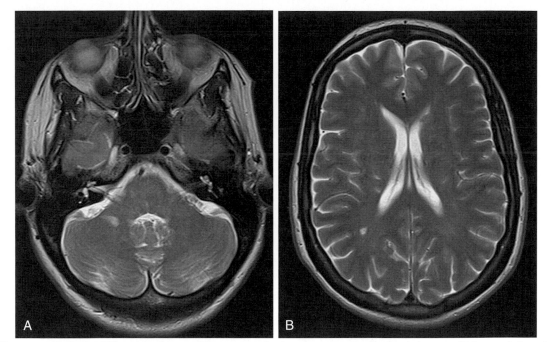

Fig. 16-44. Neurosarcoidosis. Axial T2-weighted images. There are predominantly periventricular signal changes, which can mimic multiple sclerosis.

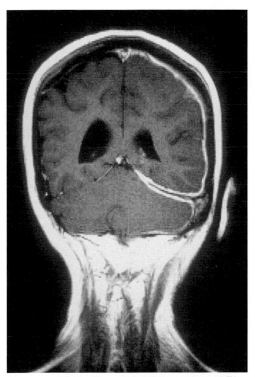

Fig. 16-45. Neurosarcoidosis. Coronal gadolinium-enhanced T1-weighted MRI. Bright meningeal enhancement over left hemisphere and tentorium cerebelli.

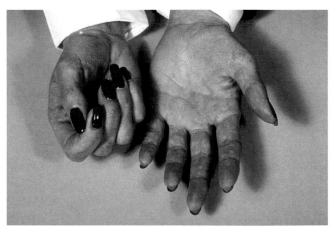

Fig. 16-46. Conversion syndrome. Fixed posture of the fingers of the right hand.

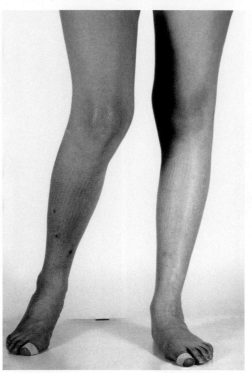

Fig. 16-47. Conversion syndrome. The right knee is flexed and the right ankle plantar flexed.

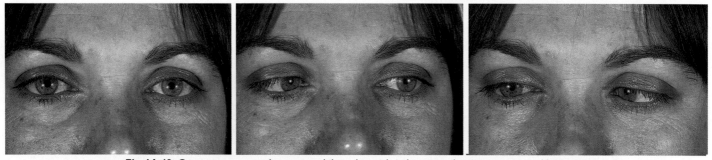

Fig. 16-48. Convergence spasm. An apparent bilateral partial sixth-nerve palsy was accompanied by miosis.

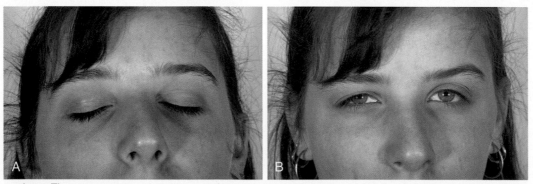

Fig. 16-49. Conversion syndrome. The apparent ptosis was at times complete or incomplete and unilateral **(A)**, and then showed evidence of contraction of the ipsilateral orbicularis oculi, causing a narrowing of the palpebral fissure and depression of the eyebrow **(B)**.

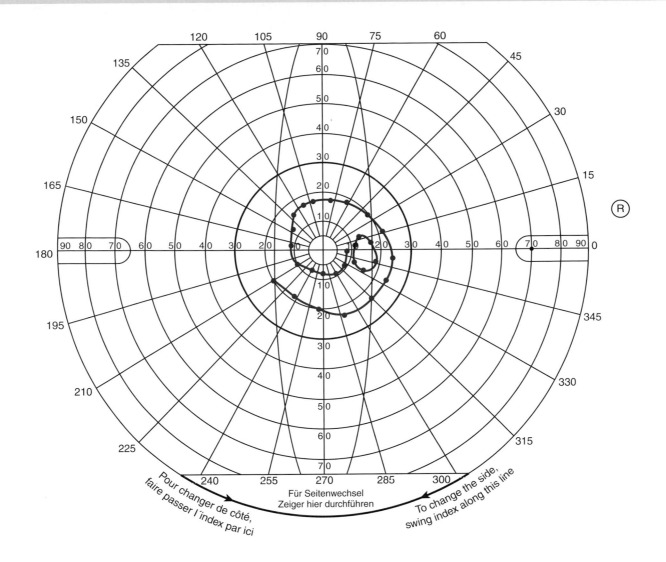

Fig. 16-50. Spiraling visual defect as part of a conversion syndrome.

Epilepsy is defined as recurrent (two or more) epileptic seizures, unprovoked by any immediate identifiable cause. Febrile seizures and neonatal seizures are classified separately. The seizures, the result of an abnormal discharge of a group of brain neurons, may include alteration of consciousness, and motor, sensory, autonomic, or psychic events perceived by the individual or observed by others.

The idiopathic epilepsies are partial or generalized disorders with characteristic clinical and electrophysiologic features associated with a genetic predisposition. Cryptogenic epilepsy refers to those cases in which no etiologic agent has been identified. Symptomatic seizures are those where a risk factor has been defined by clinical characteristics, age of onset, and electrophysiologic findings.

The incidence of epilepsy lies between 40 and 70 per 100,000, although higher figures apply in developing countries.

Epileptic seizures are thought to arise at cortical sites. Partial seizures begin focally, whereas generalized seizures imply initial widespread bilateral cortical discharges. Classification of epilepsy divides seizures into focal, generalized, and unclassifiable forms (Box 17-1).

PARTIAL SEIZURES

Any part of the body can be affected by a focal motor seizure, which may then remain localized to that part or spread (march) along the motor cortex producing successional jerking of adjacent body areas (Jacksonian seizures). The hands and face are the most common sites for this activity. Seizures emanating from the sensory cortex produce paresthesias or numbness. The march may be analogous to that of a motor seizure. In occipital lobe seizures, visual symptoms predominate, while frontal lobe seizures are commonly nocturnal and frequently associated with body turning, pelvic thrusting, and vocalization.

The distinction between simple and complex partial seizures is based on the presence of altered consciousness in the latter. Disturbances of smell and taste, often of a disagreeable nature, are characteristic and may be accompanied by vertigo, abdominal sensations, and psychic symptoms. There may be a sense of intense familiarity (déjà vu) or unfamiliarity (jamais vu). When consciousness is altered, there may be automatisms, sometimes of a semi-elaborate nature.

GENERALIZED SEIZURES

The tonic phase of a tonic–clonic seizure is associated with contraction of axial then limb muscles. If upright, the patient falls, often with injury. Tongue biting is secondary to jaw contraction. Subsequently, clonic movements appear, followed by flaccidity, which may be accompanied by urinary or fecal incontinence. A period of sleep commonly follows. On waking, confusion and disorientation are usual and headache and limb pains common. In some seizures, vertebral compression is sufficiently severe to produce fractures (Fig. 17-1).

Absence seizures are largely confined to childhood, although some 50% of patients with this seizure type develop tonic–clonic seizures in adult life. The patient is unaware of the episodes, which last about 10 to 20 seconds. Activity ceases, and there may be slight movement around the eyes and lips. Occasionally, limb movement occurs.

Myoclonic seizures are accompanied by brief, shocklike contractions of muscle, either focally or in a generalized distribution. Atonic seizures lead to a sudden loss of muscle tone, with falls and injury.

CAUSES OF EPILEPSY

The idiopathic generalized epilepsies account for about 20% to 30% of all epilepsies and have a significant genetic component. The most common are childhood absence epilepsy, juvenile absence epilepsy, and epilepsy with generalized tonic–clonic seizures alone. A gene encoding the CLC-2 voltage-gated chloride channel (*CLCN2* gene) located on chromosome 3q26 has been found in association with all these forms of idiopathic generalized epilepsy. Some forms of focal epilepsy have also been found to have a genetic component, including autosomal dominant lateral temporal lobe epilepsy and autosomal dominant nocturnal frontal lobe epilepsy.

Malformations of cortical development account for a significant number of cases of epilepsy, particularly those arising in childhood.

BOX 17-1 EPILEPSY CLASSIFICATION

Partial (Focal, Local) Seizures
- Simple partial seizures (consciousness retained)
  - With motor symptoms
  - With somatosensory or special sensory symptoms
  - Autonomic symptoms
  - With psychic symptoms
- Complex partial seizures (consciousness impaired)
  - Beginning as simple partial seizures and progressing to impairment of consciousness
    - With no other features
    - With features as in simple partial seizures
    - With automatisms
  - With impairment of consciousness at onset
    - With no other features
    - With features as in simple partial seizures
    - With automatisms
- Partial seizures evolving to secondary generalized seizures
  - Simple partial seizures evolving to generalized seizures
  - Complex partial seizures evolving to generalized seizures
  - Simple partial seizures evolving first to complex partial seizures and then to generalized seizures

Generalized Seizures (Convulsive or Nonconvulsive)
- Absence seizures
  - Typical absence seizures
  - Atypical absence seizures
- Myoclonic seizures
- Clonic seizures
- Tonic seizures
- Tonic–clonic seizures
- Atonic seizures (astatic seizures)

Unclassified Epileptic Seizures

In polymicrogyria, the normal gyral pattern is replaced by multiple small gyri separated by shallow sulci (Fig. 17-2). An X-linked pattern of inheritance linked to chromosome Xq28 is recognized, and a recessive pattern is linked to 16q12.2-21. Lissencephaly is characterized by a smooth cerebral surface, with a range from complete gyral absence (agyria) (Fig 17-3) to regional absence (pachygyria).

In periventricular nodular heterotopia, there are subependymal gray matter nodules. The condition is heterogeneous, with both X-linked dominant and autosomal recessive patterns of inheritance described.

The term focal cortical dysplasia is applied to a variety of disorders of cortical anatomy. Various subtypes of focal cortical dysplasia have been proposed, including architectural dysplasia, cytoarchitectural dysplasia (in which, in addition to the characteristics of architectural dysplasia, there are giant neuro-filament-enriched neurons) and Taylor-type cortical dysplasia, with giant dysmorphic neurons and balloon cells in addition to cortical laminar disruption (Fig 17-4). Although MRI is not necessarily abnormal in these sub-groups, the appearance of a distinctive signal change (increased signal intensity in the subcortical white matter on T2-weighted images) is considered suggestive of the Taylor-type cortical dysplasia.

INVESTIGATION

Electroencephalography is of crucial importance in corroborating a clinical diagnosis of epilepsy. It should not be used in isolation but to supplement a meticulous recording of clinical events, provided by the patient or by an observer of the attacks. Interictal epileptiform activity is found in about 50% of routine recordings in adults with epilepsy.

Two awake recordings demonstrate discharges in 85% of patients, and four awake recordings in 90%. A sleep-deprived record produces an abnormal result in about 80% to 85% of cases.

Bilateral synchronous spike–wave discharges characterize idiopathic generalized epilepsy and help to distinguish absence seizures from complex partial seizures (Fig. 17-5). In patients with neocortical epileptogenic foci, confirmed with invasive electrodes, some 40% of ictal recordings produce localizing surface EEG abnormalities. In general, occipital and temporal neocortical seizures are more likely to be localized than frontal or parietal seizures.

In complex partial seizures, the seizures strongly lateralize to the side of the temporal spike discharges. Focal unilateral delta activity also correlates closely with the side of seizure origin (Fig. 17-6). In patients with temporal lobe epilepsy compatible with mesial temporal sclerosis, lateralization of hippocampal atrophy on MR images correlates closely with ictal and interictal EEG lateralizations.

If surface recording and neuroimaging together fail to determine the likely lateralization of temporal discharges, invasive EEG may be required. In nontemporal epilepsy, for example emanating from the inferior or mesial frontal lobe, invasive recording is more commonly needed.

Magnetoencephalography provides a better spatial resolution of signals than does conventional EEG, and it may allow better localization of spike activity—for example, to the temporal tip cortex or the mediobasal temporal lobe.

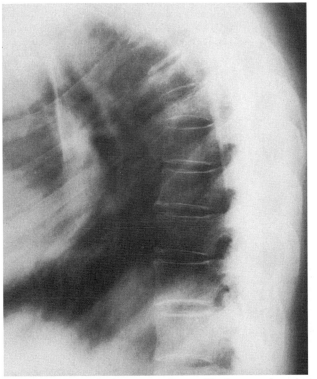

Fig. 17-1. Crush fracture of a thoracic vertebra resulting from a prolonged seizure.

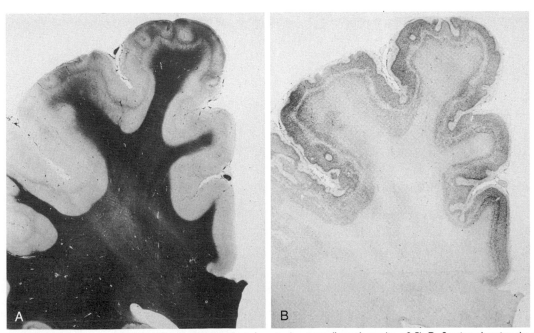

Fig. 17-2. Polymicrogyria. **A,** Coronal section, right hemisphere, showing altered cortical pattern (Loyez's myelin, ×2.5). **B,** Section showing the four cortical nerve cell layers (thionin, ×2.5).

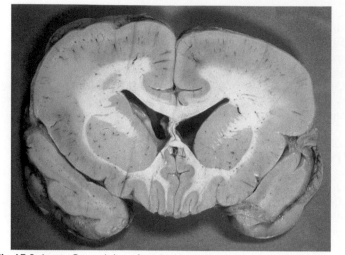

Fig. 17-3. Agyria. Coronal slice of cerebral hemisphere showing lack of gyri except in the hippocampal region.

MAGNETIC RESONANCE IMAGING

To achieve the highest sensitivity and specificity in MRI, specific protocols have been devised for the investigation of particular epilepsy types. Those required include T1-weighted thin-slice volumetric sequences, T2-weighted FLAIR sequences, and high-resolution T2-weighted spin echo sequences. When such specialized imaging is applied, focal lesions can be detected in 85% of patients with intractable epilepsy, even though standard MR images were previously reported as normal (Fig. 17-7). In general, CT should not be used in this context, as its sensitivity is substantially less.

Hippocampal Sclerosis

Initial MRI features of hippocampal sclerosis were reported to be atrophy, demonstrated on T1-weighted coronal images and increased signal intensity on T2-weighted spin echo images (Fig. 17-8). The hippocampal sclerosis so demonstrated is not necessarily diffuse. The finding of ipsilateral hippocampal atrophy is a good prognostic feature for seizure control after anterior temporal

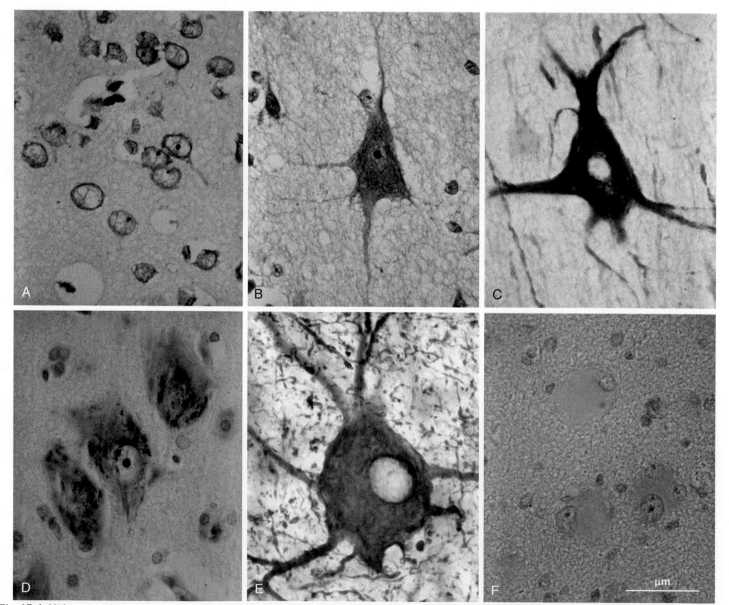

Fig. 17-4. High-power photomicrographs showing cytologic features of different types of focal cortical dysplasia. **A,** Thionin-stained clusters of rounded cells with large nuclei and a thin rim of cytoplasm, interpreted as immature neurons. **B,** Thionin-stained large pyramidal neuron in cytoarchitectural dysplasia. **C,** Large pyramidal neuron showing intense immunostaining for neurofilaments. **D** and **E,** Large dysmorphic neurons as observed by thionin staining (**D**) and neurofilament immunostaining (**E**) in Taylor-type cortical dysplasia. **F,** Thionin-stained balloon cells, frequently observed at the border between gray and white matter in Taylor-type cortical dysplasia. (Bar = 25 μm.)

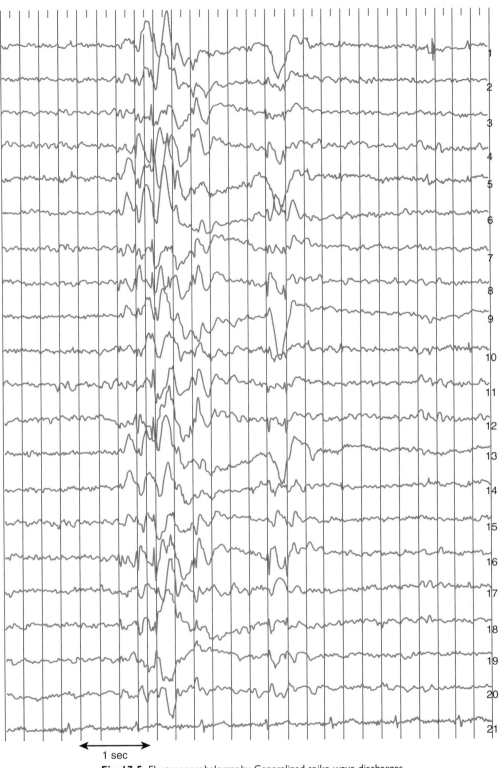

1 sec

Fig. 17-5. Electroencephalography. Generalized spike-wave discharges.

lobectomy. Formal measurement of hippocampal volume improves assessment of hippocampal atrophy, and assessment of increased signal intensity can be improved by measurement of hippocampal T2 relaxation time.

Malformations of Cortical Development

The range of MCDs identified by MRI include schizencephaly, agyria, macrogyria, polymicrogyria, subependymal gray matter heterotopias, tuberous sclerosis, focal cortical dysplasia, and dysembryoplastic neuroepithelial tumors. Although the grosser abnormalities are detectable by CT, more subtle changes are detected only by MRI techniques.

Band heterotopia may be associated with epilepsy, with or without cognitive dysfunction (Fig. 17-9). Subependymal heterotopia predominates in women. The abnormality is usually bilateral and

typically occurs around the occipital horn of the lateral ventricle. The associated seizures tend to be partial rather than generalized (Fig. 17-10). As noted earlier, increased signal intensity in the subcortical white matter on T2-weighted images is thought to be particularly suggestive of Taylor-type cortical dysplasia (Fig. 17-11). By contrast, it is recognized that areas of unequivocal abnormal T2 signal may have no histopathologic equivalent. Furthermore, transient MRI abnormalities are a recognized feature in some patients with epilepsy.

Gangliogliomas

Gangliogliomas and gangliocytomas are comparatively rare benign neuronal tumors. Typically, the lesions show low intensity on T1-weighted and high intensity on T2-weighted images. They may enhance with gadolinium.

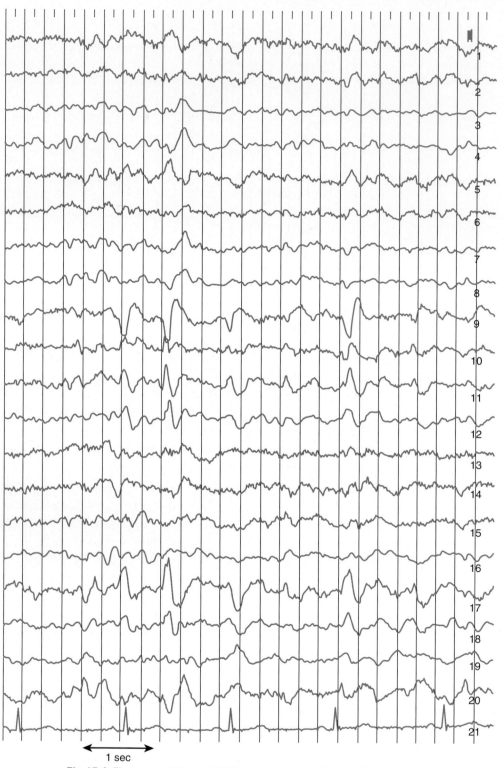

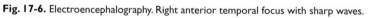

1 sec

Fig. 17-6. Electroencephalography. Right anterior temporal focus with sharp waves.

Dysembryoplastic Neuroepithelial Tumors

Dysembryoplastic neuroepithelial tumors account for about 1 to 2% of CNS neoplasms and predominate in the temporal lobes. They account for a significant proportion of intractable complex partial seizures and have a characteristic MRI appearance (Fig. 17-12). MRI is also of value in the postoperative appraisal of patients who have had surgery. The extent of hippocampal resection can be assessed.

Functional MRI that is sensitive to regional cerebral blood volume and flow allows imaging comparable to that achieved with PET but with greater spatial resolution. The technique is used to localize the motor cortex before resection of adjacent neocortex and to lateralize language function (Fig. 17-13).

In MR spectroscopy, naturally occurring nuclei that resonate (e.g., ^{1}H, ^{31}P) are used to detect compounds in the brain that are of relevance in epilepsy imaging. Although, historically, measures of N-acetylaspartate (NAA) were taken as a measure of neuronal loss, it appears from hippocampal surgical specimens that only about a quarter of the NAA concentration is accounted for by neuronal loss. It appears more likely that NAA is a marker of metabolic dysfunction, so that, for example, abnormalities of NAA may be reversed after seizure control.

MR spectroscopy with ^{1}H has also been used for the analysis of neurotransmitters—for example, gamma-aminobutyric acid (GABA). MR spectroscopy with ^{31}P has been used to investigate the metabolic changes associated with partial seizures. In some such studies, the technique was superior to MRI in determining the lateralization of the seizure focus.

SINGLE-PHOTON EMISSION COMPUTED TOMOGRAPHY

Interictal SPECT has a relatively low sensitivity and specificity in the detection of an epileptogenic area. Better results are achieved with newer radiotracers that have a longer half-life. Ictal SPECT achieves a higher sensitivity and specificity in lateralizing complex partial seizures, and postictal SPECT falls between ictal and interictal. Detection of focal hypoperfusion by subtraction SPECT co-registered to MRI (SISCOM) appears to improve the sensitivity and specificity of postictal SPECT in patients with partial epilepsy.

A postictal switch occurs in the epileptogenic zones as a state of hyperperfusion converts to one of hypoperfusion. The conversion probably occurs within a minute of the end of a complex partial seizure. The switch to a hypoperfusion state may be earlier for extratemporal seizures. Because the switch is so variable, it is recommended that both hypoperfusion and hyperperfusion images be analyzed in postictal SPECT studies (Fig. 17-14).

POSITRON EMISSION TOMOGRAPHY

Positron emission tomography can be used to measure cerebral blood flow, using ^{15}O-labeled water, and regional cerebral glucose metabolism using fluorodeoxyglucose labeled with radioactive fluoride (^{18}F) (FDG). In addition, binding of specific ligands can be mapped—for example, of [^{11}C]flumazenil (FMZ) to the central benzodiazepine–GABA$_A$ receptor complex. More clinically relevant data have emerged from studies in partial as opposed to generalized epilepsy.

In the interictal state, an epileptic focus is characterized by an area of reduced blood flow and glucose metabolism that is somewhat larger than its pathologic substrate. During partial seizures, increased blood flow and glucose metabolism occur in the relevant area. In complex partial seizures, the degree of temporal lobe hypometabolism correlates closely with outcome after temporal lobectomy. The area of hypometabolism in complex partial seizures may extend beyond the boundaries of the temporal lobe, to

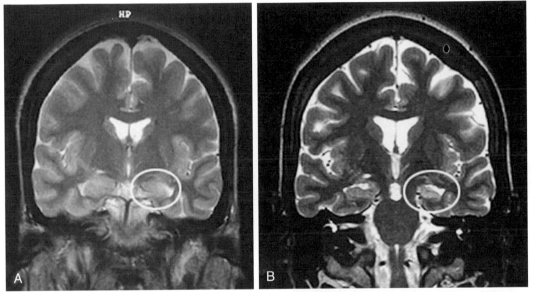

Fig. 17-7. T2-weighted standard MRI. **A,** Epilepsy-dedicated MRI. **B,** The standard MRI shows no signal abnormalities or hippocampal atrophy.

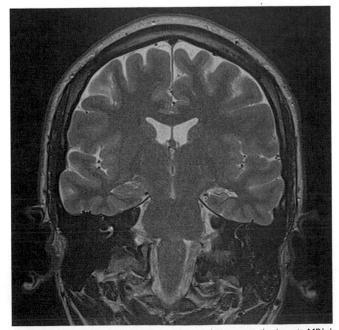

Fig. 17-8. Complex partial seizures secondary to hippocampal sclerosis. MRI demonstrating increased signal and small size of left hippocampal head.

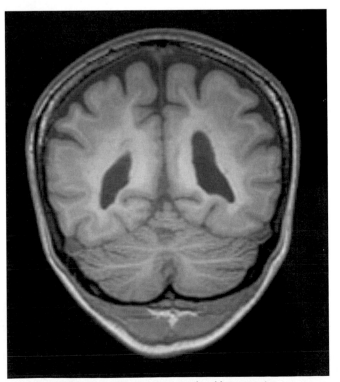

Fig. 17-9. MRI demonstrating band heterotopia.

include the thalamus and the frontal cortex, thereby limiting the potential value of the investigation. In addition, false localization may occur.

Binding of FMZ is reduced by about 30% in epileptogenic foci, apparently correlating with histologic evidence of neuronal loss in those individuals coming to surgery (Fig. 17-15).

Using FMZ-PET analyzed by statistical parametric mapping, hippocampal abnormalities can be detected in a third of patients with refractory epilepsy who have had normal quantitative MRI. In at least some such cases, resection of the relevant anterior temporal lobe appears capable of achieving seizure control. Not only do some subjects show decreased hippocampal binding but others show increased binding in the temporal lobe white matter. It has been suggested that the latter may represent microdysgenesis as a mechanism for epilepsy in those particular patients.

Areas of malformation of cortical development are likely to show adjacent or coinciding areas of single or multiple increases or decreases in FMZ volume of distribution (Fig. 17-16).

In patients with neocortical epilepsy related to the frontal, parietal, or occipital lobes, FMZ-PET images may demonstrate focal abnormalities of FMZ volume of distribution, some with increases, some with decreases, and some with both (Fig. 17-17). In some patients with refractory temporal lobe epilepsy and normal MRI, FMZ binding can demonstrate an abnormality correlating with clinical and EEG data (Fig. 17-18).

THERAPY

A comprehensive account of epilepsy treatment is not relevant to this text, but an outline of the mechanisms of action of antiepileptic drugs is pertinent (Fig. 17-19). The $GABA_A$–receptor complex has at least three subunits (α, β, and δ), which combine as a five-member structure forming an anion-permeable channel. Barbiturates bind to the β subunit to potentiate the action of endogenous GABA transaminase. Vigabatrin irreversibly binds to GABA transaminase, thereby elevating brain GABA levels. GABA-mediated inhibition can also be enhanced by blocking GABA uptake into glia and neurons after its release during synaptic transmission.

Tiagabine blocks uptake of synaptically released GABA into both presynaptic neurons and glial cells, whereas gabapentin acts presynaptically to promote GABA synthesis or release.

Ethosuximide acts by inhibition of one class of voltage-dependent calcium ion currents. Valproate may have a similar effect. Another neurotransmitter system involved in epileptic activity uses glutamate and perhaps aspartate. Targeted receptor sites include α-amino-3-hydroxy-5-methylisoxazole propionic acid (AMPA) and N-methyl-D-aspartate (NMDA). Blockage of the NMDA receptor produces antiepileptic effects.

Phenytoin, carbamazepine, and possibly valproate reduce the rate of recovery from inactivation of depolarized voltage-dependent

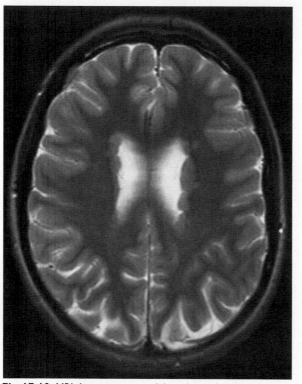

Fig. 17-10. MRI demonstrating nodular subependymal heterotopia.

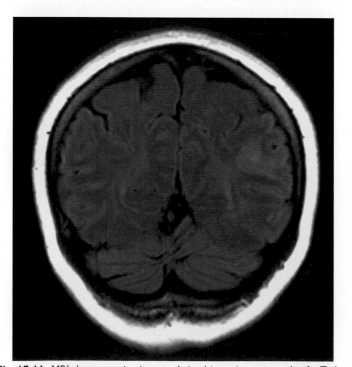

Fig. 17-11. MRI demonstrating increased signal intensity as a result of a Taylor-type cortical dysplasia.

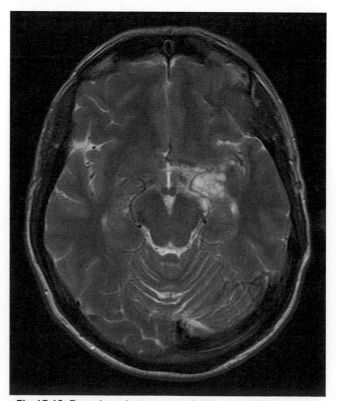

Fig. 17-12. Dysembryoplastic neuroepithelial tumor. MRI appearance.

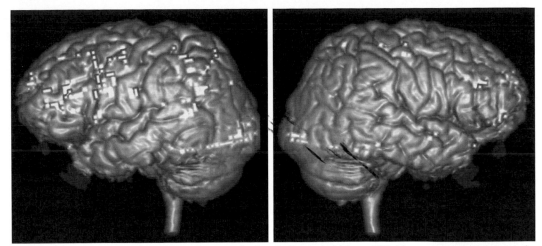

Fig. 17-13. Patient with intractable epilepsy secondary to mesial temporal sclerosis. Presurgical bilateral Wada's test indicated left hemisphere language dominance. Functional MRI activity *(yellow)* showed clear left hemisphere dominance. Note extensive language activity outside classic language areas.

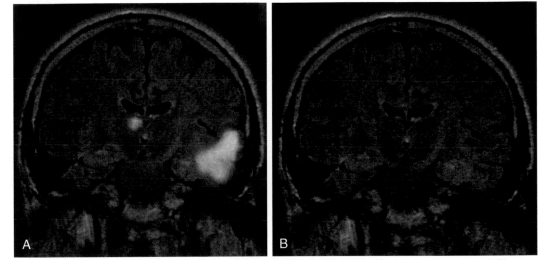

Fig. 17-14. SPECT images in a patient with intractable partial epilepsy performed with tracer injection 12 seconds after an attack. Hyperperfusion SISCOM images **(A)** localized the seizure to the left temporal lobe, whereas hypoperfusion images were nonlocalizing **(B)**.

sodium channels, thereby blocking sustained repetitive firing of action potentials in depolarized neurons. Lamotrigine inhibits glutamate and aspartate release and may have additional effects on calcium channels. Oxcarbazepine may act by reducing glutamate release via a blocking action on presynaptic calcium channels. Topiramate influences sodium channel activity, suggesting a mode of action comparable to that of phenytoin. Felbamate probably acts via its effect on the NMDA receptor.

ADVERSE DRUG EFFECTS

Side effects are common with antiepileptic drugs. Some are common to many of these agents, and others are specific to a particular drug. Sedation, unsteadiness, and nystagmus are common symptoms or signs of intoxication with almost any anticonvulsant. A skin rash can occur with any of the drugs in use, and in some instances can amount to a Stevens-Johnson syndrome (Fig. 17-20). Phenytoin can produce a characteristic facial appearance coupled with gum hypertrophy (Fig. 17-21). Vigabatrin is capable of damaging retinal ganglion cells, leading in some instances to a constricted visual field in which binasal defects predominate (Fig. 17-22).

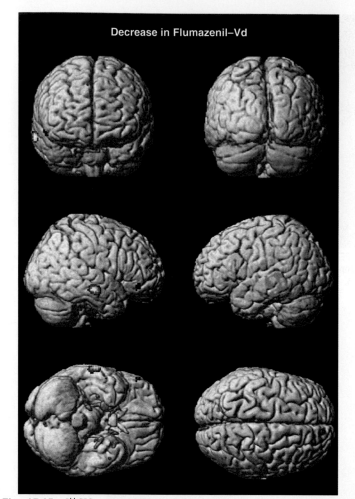

Decrease in Flumazenil–Vd

Fig. 17-15. [¹¹C]flumazenil-PET in MRI-negative complex partial seizures. Pathology of the resected neocortex showed an area of focal cortical dysplasia. The patient did not experience any fits after surgery.

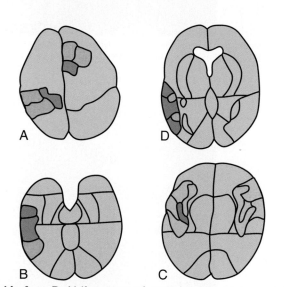

A   D

B   C

Fig. 17-16. A to **D,** Malformations of cortical development, associated with epilepsy. Malformations *(gray)* (from MRI data), increases in [¹¹C]flumazenil binding *(red),* and decreases in *blue.*

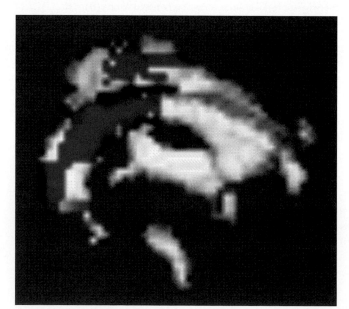

Fig. 17-17. Frontal lobe epilepsy. Increased [¹¹C]flumazenil volume of distribution around the posterolateral ventricles bilaterally.

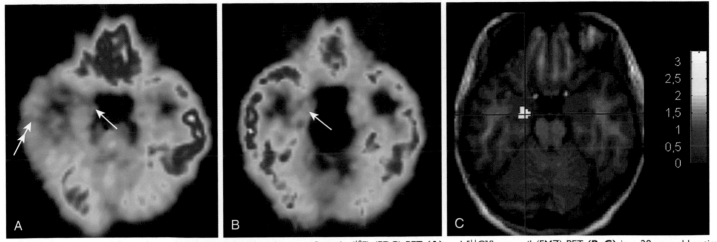

Fig. 17-18. Comparison of fluorodeoxyglucose labeled with radioactive fluoride (^{18}F) (FDG)-PET **(A)** and [^{11}C]flumazenil (FMZ)-PET **(B, C)** in a 28-year-old patient with complex partial seizures, interictal left temporal epileptiform discharges, and left temporal seizures on video telemetry. MRI (including T1- and T2-weighted images, FLAIR, and quantitative hippocampal volumetry and T2 mapping) was normal. FDG-PET **A,** Extensive hypometabolism in the left temporal lobe, affecting both the medial temporal cortex *(arrow)* and the inferior and lateral *(double arrow)* temporal neocortex. **B,** FMZ-PET shows a circumscribed decrease of FMZ volume of distribution (Vd) in the left temporal lobe *(arrow)*. **C,** Statistical parametric mapping localizes a significant decrease of FMZ-Vd in the left anterior hippocampus, compared with 21 controls.

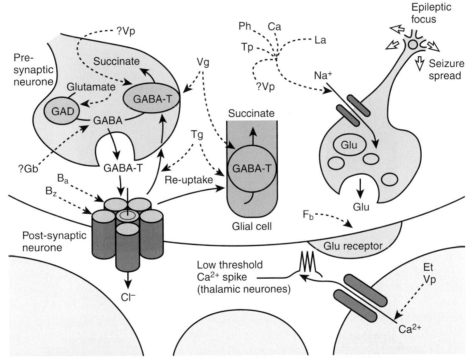

Fig. 17-19. Mechanism of action of some of the anticonvulsants. Ba, barbiturates; Bz, benzodiazepine; Ca, carbamazepine; Et, ethosuximide; Fb, felbamate; Gb, gabapentin; La, lamotrigine; Ph, phenytoin; Tg, tiagabine; Tp, topiramate; Vg, vigabatrin; Vp, valproate.

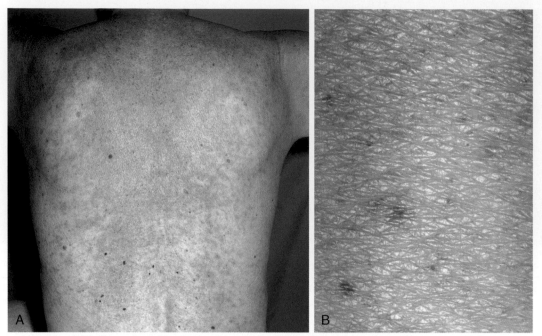

Fig. 17-20. Skin rash resulting from carbamazepine therapy. **A,** Patient's back. **B,** Close-up view of skin.

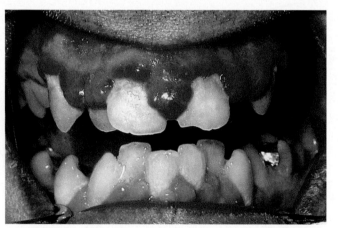

Fig. 17-21. Gum hypertrophy secondary to phenytoin therapy.

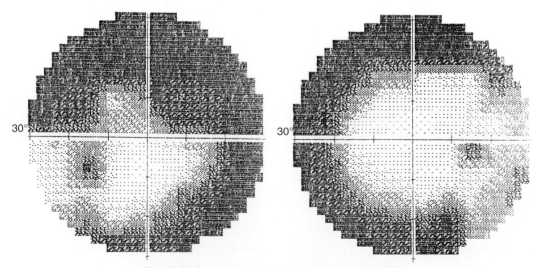

Fig. 17-22. Binasal visual field defects caused by vigabatrin.

FIGURE CREDITS

Chapter 1 Acknowledgements

Fig. 1.03 Dr B R Muller, Principle Biochemist, Charing Cross Hospital, London, UK

Fig. 1.09 Professor Hugh Markus, Department of Neurosciences, St. George's Hospital, London, UK

Fig. 1.43 Dr S Sato, Chief, EEG Laboratory, National Institute of Neurological Disorders and Stroke, Bethesda, Maryland, USA

Fig. 1.66a,b, 1.67 Dr Jean Jacobs, Emeritus Senior Lecturer in Neuropathology, The National Hospital, Queen Square, London, UK

Chapter 2 Acknowledgements

Fig. 2.3, 2.4 Professor Nigel Leigh, Department of Neurosciences, King's College Hospital, London, UK

Fig. 2.14, 2.17 The Late Professor P K Thomas, Emeritus Professor of Neurology, The Royal Free Hospital, London, UK

Fig. 2.15A, 2.18 Dr M Reilly, Consultant Neurologist, The National Hospital, Queen Square, London, UK

Fig. 2.7, 2.15B Dr R Guiloff, Consultant Neurologist, Charing Cross and Chelsea and Westminster Hospitals, London, UK

Fig. 2.21, 2.34, 2.39, 2.41, 2.42 Dr J Jacobs, Emeritus Senior Lecturer in Neuropathology, The National Hospital, Queen Square, London, UK

Fig. 2.27 Dr LF Hass

Fig. 2.28, 2.29, 2.30, 2.31 The Late Dr B Gibberd, Emeritus Consultant Neurologist, Chelsea and Westminster Hospital, London, UK

Fig. 2.32, 2.33 Professor A S Cohen, Chief of Medicine, Boston University School of Medicine, Boston, MA, USA

Fig. 2.40 Dr B R Muller, Principal Biochemist, Charing Cross Hospital, London, UK

Fig. 2.49 Dr W Schady, Senior Lecturer, Neurology, Manchester Royal Infirmary, UK

Fig. 2.52 Dr F Roncaroli, Senior Lecturer in Neuropathology, Charing Cross Hospital, London, UK

Fig. 2.67, 2.75, 2.87 Dr N Khalil, Consultant Neurophysiologist, Charing Cross Hospital, London, UK

Fig. 2.68, 2.71 Mr D Peterson, Consultant Neurosurgeon, Charing Cross Hospital, London, UK

Fig. 2.76 Dr M Donaghy, Reader in Clinical Neurology, The Radcliffe Infirmary, Oxford, UK

Chapter 3 Acknowledgements

Figs. 3.11, 3.12, 3.13, 3.14, 3.26, 3.32, 3.33, 3.35, 3.44, 3.45, 3.46, 3.75, 3.76, 3.81, are reproduced from the *Handbook of Muscle Disease 1996,* Edited by Russell JM Lane, by permission of Marcel Dekker Inc.

Figures 3.26, 3.29, 3.40, 3.51, 3.56, 3.62, 3.66, 3.67, 3.69, 3.70, 3.71, 3.73, 3.86, 3.87 are provided courtesy of Dr Federico Roncaroli, Charing Cross Hospital, Imperial College, London, UK.

Fig. 3.24, 3.51, 3.86 provided courtesy of Professor Sewry, Imperial College, London

Fig. 3.15 provided courtesy of Dr Federico Roncaroli, Charing Cross Hospital, Imperial College, London, UK.

Fig. 3.21 provided courtesy of the late Dr Louise Anderson, University of Newcastle upon Tyne, UK

Fig. 3.23 provided courtesy of Professor Francesco Muntoni, Consultant Paediatric Neurologist, Hammersmith Hospital, Imperial College, London.

Fig. 3.40 provided courtesy of Dr Federico Roncaroli, Charing Cross Hospital, Imperial College, London, UK.

Fig. 3.41 provided courtesy of Professor Haluk Topaloglu, Hacettepe Children's Hospital, Ankara, Turkey

Fig. 3.61 provided courtesy of Dr Wojtek Ralowicz, Consultant Neurologist, Charing Cross Hospital, Imperial College London

Fig. 3.78 provided courtesy of Professor Caroline Sewry, Imperial College, London

Fig. 3.79 provided courtesy of Dr Jill Moss, Imperial College, London

Fig. 3.87 provided courtesy of Professor Caroline Sewry, Imperial College, London

Fig. 3.88 provided courtesy of Dr Emilio Panagua, Madrid)

Fig. 3.90 provided courtesy of Dr. Winnie Wong, University of Hong Kong).

Chapter 4 Acknowledgements

Fig. 4.11 Dr H Bokura, Department of Neurology, Shimane University School of Medicine, 89-1, Enya, Izumo, Shimane 693-8501, Japan

Fig. 4.29 Professor Jean-Claude Baron, Department of Clinical Neurosciences, Addenbrooke's Hospital, Cambridge, UK

Fig. 4.34 Dr Michael J Mullen, Consultant Cardiologist, Royal Brompton Hospital, London, UK

Fig. 4.44 Mary Ellis, Senior Vascular Technician, Department of Vascular Surgery, Charing Cross Hospital, London, UK

Fig. 4.45 Professor Hugh Markus, Clinical Neurosciences Department, St George's Hospital, London, UK

Fig. 4.51 Leclerc X and Pruvo J-P, Recent advances in magnetic resonance angiography of carotid and vertebral arteries. Current Opinion in Neurology 2000; 13: 75-82, by permission of the publishers

Fig. 4.55 Heiss W-D, Grond M, Thiel A, et al. Permanent cortical damage detected by flumazenil positron emission tography in acute stroke. Stroke 1998; 29: 454-461, by permission of the publishers

Chapter 5 Acknowledgements

Fig. 5.6 Tanaka A, Ueno Y, Nakayama Y et al. Small chronic hemorrhages and ischemic lesions in association with spontaneous intracerebral hematomas. Stroke 1999; 30: 1637-1642, by kind permission

Fig. 5.9 Dr G Budzilovich, NYU Medical Center, New York, USA

Fig. 5.20 Lee C C, Ward H A, Sharbrough F W et al. Assessment of functional MR imaging in neurosurgical planning. American Journal of Neuroradiology 1999; 20: 1511-1519, by kind permission

Fig. 5.46 Dr B R Muller, Department of Clinical Chemistry, Charing Cross Hospital, London, UK

Fig. 5.53 Mr P Richards, Consultant Neurosurgeon, The Radcliffe Infirmary, Oxford, UK

Fig. 5.54 Kahara V J, Seppanen S K, Ryymin P S et al. MR angiography and three-dimensional time-of-flight and targeted maximum-intensity-projection reconstructions in the follow-up of intracranial aneurysms embolized with Guglielmi detachable coils. American Journal of Neuroradiology 1999; 20: 1470-1475, by kind permission

Fig. 5.55 Dr Irwin Feigin, NYU Medical Center, New York, USA

Chapter 6 Acknowledgements

Fig. 6.6, 6.11, 6.15 Dr Komatani, Department of Radiology, School of Medicine, Japan

Fig. 6.7 Dr James Lowe, Department of Histopathology, Queen's Medical Centre, University of Nottingham, UK

Fig. 6.12 Dr D M A Mann, Senior Lecturer in Neuropathology, Department of Pathological Sciences, University of Manchester, UK

Chapter 7 Acknowledgements

Fig. 7.4, 7.5, 7.6 Dr W R G Gibb, Previously Senior Lecturer in Neurology, Institute of Psychiatry, Denmark Hill, London, UK

Fig. 7.7, 7.14, 7.15 Dr D B Calne, Previously Division of Neurology, Faculty of Medicine, University of British Columbia, Vancouver, Canada

Fig. 7.8, 7.19 Dr P Piccini, Senior Lecturer in Neurology, The Hammersmith Hospital, London, UK

Fig. 7.23, 7.34, 7.40, 7.54, 7.61 Ellison D, et al. Neuropathology. A reference text of CNS pathology, 2004. Mosby, by kind permission

Fig. 7.27 Dr K C Wilhelmson, Fronto-temporal dementia. Archives of Neurology 2004; 61: 398-406, by kind permission

Fig. 7.28 Dr Jon Stoessel, Neurodegenerative Disorders Centre, University of British Columbia, Vancouver, Canada

Fig. 7.33 Dr G U Sawle, Previously Clinical Lecturer, MRC Cyclotron Unit, Hammersmith Hospital, London, UK. First published in Brain 1991; 114: 541-556

Fig. 7.35 Professor Sid Gilman, Department of Neurology, The University of Michigan, Ann Arbor, USA

Fig. 7.42 Dr I Chinchon, Neuropathologist, Hospital Universitario, Virgen Del Rocio, Sevilla, Spain

Fig. 7.64 Dr J C Mazziotta, Professor of Neurology and Radiological Sciences, Department of Neurology, Reed Neurological Research Centre, UCLA School of Medicine, Los Angeles, USA

Chapter 8 Acknowledgements

Fig. 8.11 Dr B Badie, Associate Professor, Department of Neurological Surgery, University of Wisconsin Hospital, Madison, USA

Fig. 8.12 (by kind) Chang S-C, Lai P-H, Chen W-L, et al. Diffusion-weighted MRI features of brain abscess and cystic or necrotic brain tumors. Comparison with conventional MRI. Journal of Clinical Imaging, 2002; 26: 227-236

Fig. 8.22 (by kind) Geijer B et al. Neuroradiology 2002; 44: 568-573

Fig. 8.87, 8.88 Mr D J Spalton, Consultant Ophthalmic Surgeon, St Thomas' Hospital, London, UK. First published in Spalton D J, Hitchings R A, Hunter P A. Atlas of Clinical Ophthalmology. Mosby 1984, by kind permission

Fig. 8.107 Vincent A, Buckley C, Schott M J, et al. Potassium channel antibody-associated encephalopathy: a potentially immunotherapy-responsive form of limbic encephalitis. Brain 2004; 127: 701-712, by kind permission

Fig. 8.110 Rees J H, Hain S F, Johnson M R, et al. The role of [18F] fluoro-2-deoxyglucose-PET scanning in the diagnosis of para neoplastic neurological disorders. Brain 2001; 124: 2223-2231, by kind permission

Chapter 9 Acknowledgements

Fig. 9.21, 9.27 Dr Fred Epstein, Chief of Paediatric Neurosurgery, NYU Medical Center, New York, USA

Fig. 9.37 Dr Keith Wood, Consultant Haematologist, Leicester Royal Infirmary, Leicester, UK

Chapter 10 Acknowledgements

Fig. 10.12 Mr Martin Rice-Edwards, Emeritus Consultant Neurosurgeon, Charing Cross Hospital, London, UK

Fig. 10.50 Dr J K Wood, Consultant Haematologist, The Leicester Royal Infirmary, Leicester, UK

Fig. 10.58, 10.59 Dr T E Feinberg, Neuro Behaviour Center, Beth Israel Medical Center, New York, USA

Chapter 11 Acknowledgements

Fig. 11.3 From Doyle E, Vote B J, Casswell A G. British Journal of Ophthalmology 2004; 88: 301-302, by permission from BMJ Publishing Group Ltd

Fig. 11.5 From Afridi S, Matharu M S, Lee L et al. Brain 2005; 128; 932-939, by permission of Oxford University Press

Fig. 11.8a and c From Lance J W, Zagami A S. Ophthalmoplegic Migraine: A Recurrent Demyelinating Neuropathy? Cephalalgia 2001; 21: 84-89, by permission from Wiley-Blackwell, Oxford

Fig. 11.10 From Madjikhanani N, Sanchez Del Rio M, Wu O et al. Proceedings of the National Academy of Sciences 2001; 98: 4687-4692, by permission

Fig. 11.11 From Buzzi M G, Dimitriadou V, Theoharides TC et al. Brain Research 1992; 583: 137-139, by permission from Elsevier

Fig. 11.19 From Higgins J N P, Cousins C, Owler B K et al. Journal of Neurology, Neurosurgery and Psychiatry, 2003; 74: 1662-1666, by permission from BMJ Publications

Fig. 11.30 Courtesy of Dr Peter Evans, Consultant Anaesthetist, Charing Cross Hospital, London, UK

Fig. 11.36 Copyright Dr Charles Gomersall 2007. Reproduced with permission from ICU Web www.aic.cuhk.edu.hk/web8

Fig. 11.38 Copyright Dr Charles Gomersall 2007. Reproduced with permission from ICU Web www.aic.cuhk.edu.hk/web8

Fig. 11.50 From Smith C M. The Neuropathology of Head Injury. Advances in Clinical Neuroscience and Rehabilitation 2005; 5: 22-24, by permission from Neuroco Ltd

Chapter 12 Acknowledgements

Fig. 12.23a Dr R Shakir, Consultant Neurologist, Charing Cross Hospital, London, UK

Fig. 12.46a Dr G Budzilovich, Consultant Pathologist, NYU Medical Center, New York, USA

Fig. 12.47 The late Dr Marius Valsamis

Fig. 12.73, 12.74 Dr N F Lawton, Consultant Neurologist, Southampton General Hospital, Southampton, UK

Chapter 13 Acknowledgements

Fig. 13.7, 13.8 Professor Lassmann, Brain Research Institute, University of Vienna, Austria. First published in Annals of Neurology 2000; 47: 707-717

Fig. 13.9 Dr Grahame Kidd, Department of Neurosciences, Lerner Research Institute, Cleveland, USA. First published in Annals of Neurology 2000; 48: 893-901

Fig. 13.10, 13.11 Dr D Gay, Department of Microbiology and Pathology, Colchester General Hospital, Colchester, UK. First published in Brain 1991; 114: 557-572

Fig. 13.13 Dr N Khalil, Consultant Neurophysiologist, Charing Cross Hospital, London, UK

Fig. 13.14 The late Professor W I McDonald, modified from fig. 1 in Nature 1980; 286: 154-155

Fig. 13.29 Dr J Dick, Consultant Neurologist, Manchester Royal Infirmary, Manchester, UK

Fig. 13.42, 13.48, 13.50 Dr David Ellison, Consultant Neuropathologist, Newcastle General Hospital, UK. First published in Neuropathology by Ellison D, Love S, Chimelli L, et al. Mosby 2004

Chapter 14 Acknowledgements

Fig. 14.37, 14.38 Professor P L A Bill, Professor of Neurology, Wentworth Hospital, University of Natal, Durban, South Africa

Fig. 14.47, 14.60 Dr David Ellison, Consultant Neuropathologist, Newcastle General Hospital, UK. First published in Neuropathology by Ellison D, Love S, Chimelli L, et al. Mosby 2004

Chapter 15 Acknowledgements

Fig. 15.3 Dr David Ellison, Consultant Neuropathologist, Newcastle General Hospital, UK. First published in Neuropathology by Ellison D, Love S, Chimelli L et al. Mosby 2004

Fig. 15.11, 15.12, 15.36, 15.38 Mr D J Spalton, Consultant Ophthalmologist, St Thomas's Hospital, London, UK. First published in Spalton D J, Hitchins R A, Hunter P A. Atlas of Clinical Opththalmology, London. Gowers Medical Publishing, 1984

Fig. 15.68 The Late Dr S Meadows

Chapter 16 Acknowledgements

Fig. 16.27 Dr Margaret Burke, Mount Vernon Hospital, Northwood, Middlesex, UK

Chapter 17   Acknowledgements

Fig. 17.7   Dr T Van Oertzen, Consultant Neurologist/Epileptologist, St George's Hospital, London, UK. First published in The Journal of Neurology, Neurosurgery and Psychiatry 2002; 73: 643-647, by permission from BMJ publications

Fig. 17.9, 17.11   Images from The National Society for Epilepsy MRI Unit, UK

Fig. 17.17   Dr Alexander Hammers. First published in Brain 2003; 26: 1300-1318, by permission of Oxford University Press

Fig. 17.18   Dr P Piccini. First published in The Journal of Neurology, Neurosurgery and Psychiatry 2004, 75: 669-676, by permission from BMJ publications

Fig. 17.19   From Oxford Textbook of Medicine, Fourth Edition, edited by Warrell D A, Cox T M, Firth J D and Benj Jr. E J, 2003